Role of Genetics in Pulmonary Diseases

Role of Genetics in Pulmonary Diseases

Edited by Summer Goodwin

hayle medical

New York

Hayle Medical,
750 Third Avenue, 9th Floor,
New York, NY 10017, USA

Visit us on the World Wide Web at:
www.haylemedical.com

ISBN: 9978-1-63241-616-2

The publisher's policy is to use permanent paper from mills that operate a sustainable forestry policy. Furthermore, the publisher ensures that the text paper and cover boards used have met acceptable environmental accreditation standards.

Printed in China.

Cataloging-in-Publication Data

Role of genetics in pulmonary diseases / edited by Summer Goodwin.
p. cm.
Includes bibliographical references and index.
ISBN 978-1-63241-616-2
1. Lungs--Diseases--Genetic aspects. 2. Lungs--Diseases. 3. Genetic disorders.
4. Medical genetics. I. Goodwin, Summer.
RC756 .R65 2019
616.24--dc23

Table of Contents

Preface

The pulmonary circulation is the part of the circulatory system, which transports deoxygenated blood away from the right ventricle of the heart to the lungs, and then returns the oxygenated blood to the left ventricle and atrium of the heart. The vessels involved in pulmonary circulation are pulmonary veins and pulmonary arteries. Pulmonary circulation can be affected by a number of conditions, chief among which are pulmonary hypertension, pulmonary embolus, vascular resistance, cardiac shunt and pulmonary shunt. Any disease that damages the lungs and affects their function may be called a chronic lung disease. It encompasses a number of clinical conditions which include idiopathic pulmonary fibrosis, chronic obstructive pulmonary disease, cystic fibrosis, emphysema, etc. Studies have shown a strong association of certain gene variants with impaired lung function. This book includes some of the vital pieces of work being conducted across the world, on various topics related to pulmonary diseases. It provides significant information of this discipline to help develop a good understanding of the role of genetics in the incidence of these disorders. Coherent flow of topics, student-friendly language and extensive use of examples make this book an invaluable source of knowledge.

The information contained in this book is the result of intensive hard work done by researchers in this field. All due efforts have been made to make this book serve as a complete guiding source for students and researchers. The topics in this book have been comprehensively explained to help readers understand the growing trends in the field.

I would like to thank the entire group of writers who made sincere efforts in this book and my family who supported me in my efforts of working on this book. I take this opportunity to thank all those who have been a guiding force throughout my life.

Editor

1

The Mucoid Switch in *Pseudomonas aeruginosa* Represses Quorum Sensing Systems and Leads to Complex Changes to Stationary Phase Virulence Factor Regulation

Ben Ryall[1], Marta Carrara[1], James E. A. Zlosnik[1¤b], Volker Behrends[1,2], Xiaoyun Lee[1¤a], Zhen Wong[1], Kathryn E. Lougheed[1], Huw D. Williams[1]*

1 Department of Life Sciences, Faculty of Natural Sciences, Imperial College London, Sir Alexander Fleming Building, London, United Kingdom, **2** Department of Surgery and Cancer, Faculty of Medicine, Imperial College London, Sir Alexander Fleming Building, London, United Kingdom

Abstract

The opportunistic pathogen *Pseudomonas aeruginosa* chronically infects the airways of Cystic Fibrosis (CF) patients during which it adapts and undergoes clonal expansion within the lung. It commonly acquires inactivating mutations of the anti-sigma factor MucA leading to a mucoid phenotype, caused by excessive production of the extracellular polysaccharide alginate that is associated with a decline in lung function. Alginate production is believed to be the key benefit of *mucA* mutations to the bacterium in the CF lung. A phenotypic and gene expression characterisation of the stationary phase physiology of *mucA22* mutants demonstrated complex and subtle changes in virulence factor production, including cyanide and pyocyanin, that results in their down-regulation upon entry into stationary phase but, (and in contrast to wildtype strains) continued production in prolonged stationary phase. These findings may have consequences for chronic infection if mucoid *P. aeruginosa* were to continue to make virulence factors under non-growing conditions during infection. These changes resulted in part from a severe down-regulation of both AHL-and AQ (PQS)-dependent quorum sensing systems. *In trans* expression of the cAMP-dependent transcription factor Vfr restored both quorum sensing defects and virulence factor production in early stationary phase. Our findings have implications for understanding the evolution of *P. aeruginosa* during CF lung infection and it demonstrates that *mucA22* mutation provides a second mechanism, in addition to the commonly occurring *lasR* mutations, of down-regulating quorum sensing during chronic infection this may provide a selection pressure for the mucoid switch in the CF lung.

Editor: Martin Pavelka, University of Rochester, United States of America

Funding: BBSRC PhD studentship. The funders had no role in study design, data collection and analysis, decision to publish, or preparation of the manuscript.

Competing Interests: The authors have declared that no competing interests exist.

* E-mail: h.d.williams@imperial.ac.uk

¤a Current address: Departement de Microbiologie Fondamentale, Universite de Lausanne, Lausanne, Switzerland
¤b Current address: Centre for Understanding and Preventing Infection in Children and Department of Pediatrics/Faculty of Medicine, University of British Columbia, Vancouver, British Columbia, Canada

Introduction

Pseudomonas aeruginosa forms intractable, chronic infections in around 80% of Cystic Fibrosis (CF) sufferers and is associated with decreased lung function and an increased risk of respiratory failure and death [1,2]. It's success as a CF lung pathogen is aided by the expression of a range of virulence factors including the potent toxin hydrogen cyanide, which is regulated by quorum sensing and expressed maximally under low oxygen tension, a condition that *P. aeruginosa* is believed to experience in the thickened mucus of the CF lung [3,4]. *P. aeruginosa* cyanide production is the mediating factor in the paralytic killing of *Caenorhabditis elegans* [5], is toxic to *Drosophila melanogaster* [6] and cyanide has been detected in burn wound infections caused by *P. aeruginosa* [7]. The potential clinical significance of cyanide in CF lung infections was recently demonstrated by the detection of cyanide in sputum from cystic fibrosis patients infected with *P. aeruginosa* and its presence is associated with a decline in lung function [8,9]. However, the clinical significance of cyanogenesis and its consequences for the host remain unclear [10,11]. Cyanide is volatile and its usefulness as a surrogate marker for the diagnosis of *P. aeruginosa* and *Bcc* infection in children who cannot expectorate sputum is currently being investigated [12,13]. Cyanide has the potential to inhibit aerobic and anaerobic respiration [16]. *P. aeruginosa* avoids the toxic effects of cyanide in part by synthesising a respiratory chain terminated by a cyanide insensitive terminal oxidase [14,15] and by the action of detoxification mechanisms [16,17].

A major event in the course of chronic *P. aeruginosa* lung infection is a switch of infecting strains to an alginate over-producing, mucoid phenotype that is often associated with a poor prognosis for the patient [2,18]. Understanding the consequences of the switch to alginate overproduction is important to an understanding of how *P. aeruginosa* is able to achieve such persistent and problematic CF infections. The mucoid switch most commonly results from loss of regulation of the alternate sigma factor AlgU via mutation in the anti-sigma factor *mucA* [2,19]. The *P. aeruginosa* MucA protein along with MucB sequesters AlgU to the cytoplasmic membrane. Loss of function mutations of *mucA* result in AlgU being constitutively free to interact with core RNA polymerase and direct transcription from its target genes, which include the alginate biosynthetic genes located in the *algD* operon as well as AlgU's own operon [20,21], leading to alginate over production and elevated levels of AlgU. One of the most common mutations in *mucA* in CF clinical isolates is the *mucA22* mutation, which results in the truncation of MucA [20,21].

It is believed that alginate overproduction *per se* provides a major benefit to *P. aeruginosa* of the mucoid switch in the CF lung, due to it providing the bacterium with protection from the host immune response by inhibiting phagocytosis, protecting it against the oxidative burst and providing an immunomodulatory role [22,23]. However, AlgU regulates genes in addition to the alginate biosynthetic genes, including other transcriptional regulators, such as *algR* and the heat shock sigma factor *rpoH* [24,25]. Previous studies have shown an increase in type III secretion systems, a decrease in flagellum production and the decrease in C4-HSL-dependent quorum sensing in biofilms are associated with *mucA* mutation [26–28]. Recently it was shown that the *mucA22* mutation also affects the osmotic stress sensitivity of *P. aeruginosa* but only in stationary phase, suggesting that *mucA22*, in addition to affecting alginate production during growth, affects cellular physiology in non-growing cells, a factor that could be significant during chronic infections [29,30].

Given the evidence for the presence of cyanide in the CF lung together with its stationary phase synthesis and the chronic nature of *P. aeruginosa* CF lung infection, our aim was to investigate the effect of the switch to mucoidy on cyanide production by *P. aeruginosa*. We show here that *mucA* mutation causes a more complex and subtle change in cyanide and pyocyanin production than previously recognised, resulting in down-regulation upon entry into early stationary phase and, in contrast to wildtype strains, continued production in prolonged stationary phase. We further show that *mucA* mutation is associated with a profound down regulation of the three major quorum sensing systems of *P. aeruginosa*. We argue that these findings have significant implications in terms of chronic CF lung infection.

Materials and Methods

Bacterial strains and growth conditions

The bacterial strains used are listed in Table S1. Overnight starter cultures were prepared by inoculating several colonies into 5 ml LB broth in a 25 ml sterile universal bottle at 37°C with shaking at 200 rpm. For all assays and RNA extractions strains were grown by inoculating 1 ml of overnight culture into 50 ml LB broth in 250 ml conical flasks incubated in an orbital shaker at 200 rpm and 37°C.

Construction of *mucA22* mutants

Unmarked *mucA22* mutants (loss of a single base) were made in two *P. aeruginosa* wild type backgrounds: PAO1 and PAO381 by gene replacement of the wildtype allele as described previously [29], with the presence of the correct mutation checked by sequencing of PCR amplicons of the putative *mucA22* mutants. Non-mucoid suppressor strains were isolated from *mucA22* strains by growing on LBA plates for several days at 37°C, after which time non-mucoid outgrowths appeared from the edge of the mucoid colony. Suppressor strains are denoted by adding an S to the end of the name of the *mucA22* mutant they were isolated from.

Cyanide, pyocyanin and elastase assays

Cyanide measurement was performed using a cyanide ion-selective micro-electrode (Lazar Research Laboratories, L.A., CA, USA) as described in [31] and elastase was assayed using the elastin-congo red method of Ohman et al [32]. Pyocyanin was assayed as described by Essar et al [33]. Briefly, the culture supernatant was extracted into chloroform, which was then acidified with 0.2M HCl and the pyocyanin-containing acidic, aqueous layer was removed and it's absorbance determining at 520 nm. The A520 reading was then normalised by dividing by the final OD600 reading of the culture.

Quorum sensing signal molecule bioluminescent assay

lux-reporter strains were used to assay the levels of quorum sensing signal molecules in culture supernatants. Plasmid pSB401 in *E. coli* S17.1 was used for assaying 2-oxo-C12-HSL, plasmid pSB536 in *E. coli* S17.1 was used for assaying C4-HSL and PAO1Δ*pqsA*:*pqsA*::*CTXlux* [34,35] was used for assaying PQS. Luminescence and OD was measured in a FLUOstar Omega plate Reader (BMG Labtech). The luminescence output for each well was blank corrected and normalised to OD. Concentrations of 2-oxo-C12HSL and C4HSL were calculated with reference to an AHL standard curve. PQS levels were calculated relative to PAO1 8 hour supernatant levels.

qRT-PCR

RNA was extracted using RNeasy Protect Bacteria Mini Kit (Qiagen) using enzymatic lysis and proteinase K digestion with on column DNAase treatment. qRT-PCR was carried out using Rotor-Gene SYBR Green PCR Kit (Qiagen) in a Rotor-Gene 3000 quantitative PCR machine (Corbett). Expression of the target genes was normalised to the expression of 16S RNA.

Results

mucA22 mutants and isolation and use of spontaneous suppressor strains

Isogenic *mucA22* mutants were constructed in PAO1 and PAO381 backgrounds and spontaneous mucoid suppressor strains were isolated from each of the *mucA22* mutants as described in Materials and Methods. We used these as control strains in this study as we wanted to know whether suppression of mucoidy affected key phenotypes associated with *mucA* mutation, particularly as suppressors are likely to accumulate in the CF lung [36]. We did not complement or repair the *mucA22* mutations as a control, because the high frequency of spontaneous mucoid to non-mucoid conversion in our hands made it difficult to be confident that a change to non-mucoidy did not result from the acquisition of a secondary mutation. By gene sequencing we confirmed that the suppressor strains, for which data is reported here, did not have a *mucA22* reverting mutation and neither did they have mutations in *algU*, *algR*, *algD2*, or *lasR*.

P. aeruginosa mucA22 strains are deficient in cyanide, pyocyanin and elastase production in early stationary phase

As an initial test cyanide levels were measured in 13 independently isolated *mucA22* strains 2 hours after entry of the cultures into stationary phase. Each of the *mucA22* strains had markedly reduced culture cyanide levels compared to their isogenic wildtype strain equating to an approximate 75% reduction in peak cyanide levels (comparing mean cyanide concentration for each *mucA22* strain to their respective wild type, t-test, all p values<0.001; Fig. S1A). All spontaneous non-mucoid suppressor strains isolated from *mucA22* strains showed a return to wildtype cyanide production. PAO579, a mucoid PAO381 derivative that has made the switch to mucoidy by an *algU/mucA22* independent mechanism [37], produces ~3 times the cyanide levels of the PAO381 *mucA22* strains (data not shown), strongly suggesting that the phenotype observed is a consequence of *mucA22* mutation rather than alginate over production *per se*. At 2 h into stationary phase the *mucA22* strains produced significantly less pyocyanin than their wild type parents (t-test p<0.001 for each pair; Fig. S1B). In contrast, the suppressor strains showed wild type pyocyanin production. In stationary phase *mucA22* mutants were also defective in elastase production (p<0.01 for each pair) and this phenotype was partially reversed in suppressor strain (Fig. S1C).

P. aeruginosa mucA22 strains maintain cyanide and pyocyanin production in late stationary phase

Investigating the kinetics of cyanide production throughout growth indicated marked differences between wildtype and *mucA22* mutants (Fig. 1A; Fig. S2). For the wild type strain PAO1, cyanide concentrations in culture media increased rapidly at the onset of stationary phase and reached a maximum of ~300 μM after 8–9 hours in culture, followed by a steady decrease in levels until cyanide was no longer detectable after 20 hours. In contrast, the *mucA22* mutant (M04) had the expected lower peak-level of ~100 μM cyanide, but these levels were maintained into late stationary phase. The suppressor strains behave similarly to PAO1 and a similar pattern of cyanide production was found in *mucA22* mutants isolated in PAO381 background (Fig. S2). Culture pH was similar for all strains throughout growth, indicating that cyanide gas formation, was not responsible for the differential levels of solution cyanide. We conclude that the wildtype strains switch off cyanide production a few hours into stationary phase and any remaining cyanide is lost from the culture, presumably by blowing off or being metabolised [15]. The kinetics of pyocyanin production was affected in a similar way in *mucA22* mutants, with a decrease relative to wildtype and suppressor in early stationary phase followed by continued production leading to 3 –fold higher levels than the wildtype and suppressor strain in late stationary phase cultures (Fig. 1B). Turning to elastase activity, levels were negligible in mid-log phase but throughout stationary phase the *mucA22* strains were deficient in elastase production compared to their parental strain (p<0.01 for each pair) (Fig. 1C), this being reversed in most of the suppressor strains. These findings indicate that *mucA22* mutation is associated with a global alteration of virulence factor regulation in stationary phase, although, the regulation of elastase production appears to differ from that of cyanide and pyocyanin.

The *mucA22* mutation alters the expression of cyanide, pyocyanin and elastase biosynthetic genes

qRT-PCR was used to determine whether the phenotypic changes observed in *mucA22* mutants resulted from changes in gene expression. PAO1 and the suppressor strain M04S (Fig. 2A) showed similar *hcnA* expression levels to each other, with highest levels at 2 hours (mid-log phase) and 6 hours (early stationary phase) and decreased levels in late stationary phase (24 hours). It is interesting that significant *hcnA* expression is observed in the mid-log phase cultures at a time when no cyanide was detectable in the culture medium (Fig. 1), indicating that *hcnA* expression is induced in exponential phase well ahead of cyanide production in stationary phase. Expression in the *mucA22* mutant M04 was significantly lower at 2 and 6 hours and markedly increased at 24 hours. Overall, the pattern of *hcnA* expression is consistent with the cyanide production data presented in Fig. 1 (and Figs. S1 and S2) suggesting that the low-level cyanide production in early stationary phase followed by continued production in later stationary phase seen in *mucA22* strains results from differences in the expression of the cyanide synthase genes. *hcnA* transcripts were still evident in PAO1 at 24 hours even though cyanide levels in culture supernatant had dropped to zero (Fig. 2), suggesting that either post-transcriptional regulation is affecting cyanide production or it is being lost from culture as fast as it is being made.

The expression of *phzM* and *phzS* genes was very low in mid-log phase cultures, although lowest in *mucA22* strains (Fig. 2B and C), but was expressed at similar levels in early stationary phase cultures, suggesting that deceased pyocyanin production in *mucA22* strains may be a consequence of a delay in induction of pyocyanin gene expression (but this is not as marked as with the *hcnA* gene) or it may not be wholly explained by changes in gene expression. However, the *mucA22* strain M04 showed significantly increased expression of *phzM* and *phzS* compared to the wild type and suppressor strains at 24 hours, indicating that increased pyocyanin levels in late stationary phase cultures of mucoid strains correlated with increased pyocyanin gene expression.

lasB expression was detected only at very low levels in exponential phase cultures (2 h), but there was significantly increased *lasB* expression in all strains at 6 h and a significant difference between the wild type and *mucA22* strain (M04). At 24 h, all strains showed similar *lasB* expression.

The qRT-PCR gene expression data are broadly consistent with the phenotypic data and in particular show markedly increased levels of the *hcnA* and *phz* genes that are consistent with maintenance of increased cyanide and pyocyanin levels in late stationary phase.

The *mucA22* mutation results in suppression of quorum sensing signal molecule production throughout growth

As cyanide, pyocyanin and elastase are quorum sensing-(QS)-regulated [38], we tested whether *mucA22* mutation led to a defect in the two N-acyl homoserine lactone (AHL)-dependent QS systems of *P. aeruginosa*; the *lasRI* and *rhlRI* systems that synthesise 3-oxo-C12-HSL and C4–HSL respectively [38]. The *mucA22* mutant M04 was greatly impaired in the production of both these AHL molecules (Fig. 3A and B; as were other independently isolated *mucA22* mutants of PAO1 and PAO381, Fig. S3). Wild type levels of both AHLs were observed in the non-mucoid suppressor strain.

The third quorum sensing system in *P. aeruginosa* is the 2-alkyl-4-quinolone (AQ or PQS)-dependent quorum sensing system (mediated by PQS; 2-heptyl-3-hydroxy-4-quinolone and HHQ; 2-heptyl-4-quinolone) and we found that the *mucA22* mutant M04 was also impaired in production of PQS (Fig. 3C). This was most apparent in early to mid-stationary phase (8 hours, t-test, p<0.05), whereas in late stationary phase (24 hours), the differences between wildtype and *mucA22* and the suppressor strain are less marked but still significant (t-test, p<0.05). These data are consistent with a quorum sensing defect being responsible for the changes in cyanide, pyocyanin and elastase production in early stationary phase cultures of mucoid strains.

We used qRT-PCR to determine the expression of *lasR*, *lasI* (2-oxo-C12-HSL system), *rhlR*, *rhlI* (C4-HSL system) and the *pqsA*, *pqsH* and *pqsR* genes (PQS system) (Fig. 4). In early stationary phase (6 h), M04 had a significant reduction in expression of AHL and PQS quorum sensing genes compared to the wild-type (Fig. 4), which suggested that reduced AHL and PQS levels in early

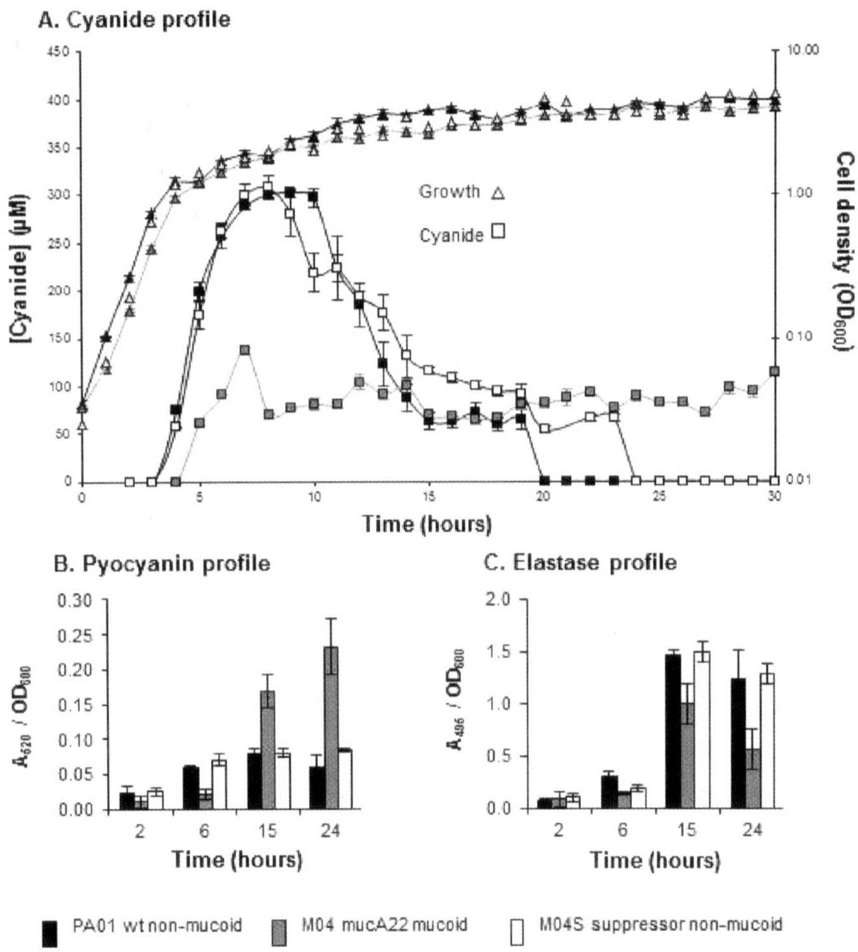

Figure 1. ***mucA22*, mucoid strains show differential regulation of virulence factor production throughout grow. A**, Change in cyanide concentration in liquid culture supernatant (primary y axis, square markers) throughout growth (secondary y axis, triangle markers) for PAO1 (wild type, non-mucoid) (black); M04 (*mucA22*, mucoid) (dark grey); and M04S (non-mucoid suppressor isolated from M04) (light grey). **B** and **C** respectively, pyocyanin and elastase levels in culture supernatant normalised to OD_{600} of culture at 2 hours (mid-exponential phase), 6 hours (early stationary phase),15 hours (mid stationary phase) and 24 hours (late stationary phase). Values are means of 3 independent replicates with SE error bars. Culture conditions and cyanide, pyocyanin and elastase assays were as described in Figure 1.

stationary phase (Fig. 3) result from gene expression changes. However, quorum-sensing gene expression levels in the suppressor strain M04S was similar to M04 and did not reflect the levels of AHL and PQS molecules detected (Fig. 3); the reason for this is unclear. The correlation between the levels of quorum sensing gene expression and the AHL and PQS levels is less clear at 24 hours (Fig. 4).

We also tested whether adding back C4-HSL or 3-oxo-C12-HSL was able to recover the early stationary phase cyanide-production phenotype of *mucA22* strains. However, supplementing the culture medium with 100 μM C4-HSL or 3-oxo-C12 HSL did not recover early stationary phase (6–8 h) cyanide production in *mucA22* mutants (data not shown). However, as *rhlR* and *lasR* expression is repressed in *mucA22* strains (Fig. 4), it is likely that the levels of the RhlR and LasR proteins are too low to respond effectively to the added AHLs. We also considered the possibility that our *mucA22* mutants had acquired a *lasR* mutation, but PCR amplification and sequencing of the *lasR* gene from mutants showed none to be present.

These experiments demonstrate that the switch to mucoidy has a profound effect on the multiple quorum sensing systems of *P. aeruginosa*.

mucA22 mutation does not act through disruption of the *rsmY/rsmZ* regulatory network

Next we explored further how a defect in *mucA* could lead to a loss of quorum sensing and affect cyanide production. We reasoned that a defect in *mucA*, leading to increased expression of *algU* might act through disruption of *rsmY* and *rsmZ* regulatory systems, which through sequestration of the negative regulator of quorum sensing RsmA activate quorum sensing and cyanide production [39–43] and that this might occur through competition with an unidentified sigma factor that is a proposed component of the HptB -mediated region of this regulatory pathway [44]. To test this we introduced *rsmY*-and *rsmZ-lacZ* fusions into wild type (PAO1), *mucA22* mutant (M04) and suppressor strain (M04S) and measured β-galactosidase activity of reporter strains through growth into stationary phase. No significant differences in *rsmY*- and *rsmZ-lacZ* fusion expression were observed between wild type and *mucA22* strains at any stage during growth, indicating that expression *rsmY* and *rsmZ* is not compromised by *mucA22* mutation (Fig. S4).

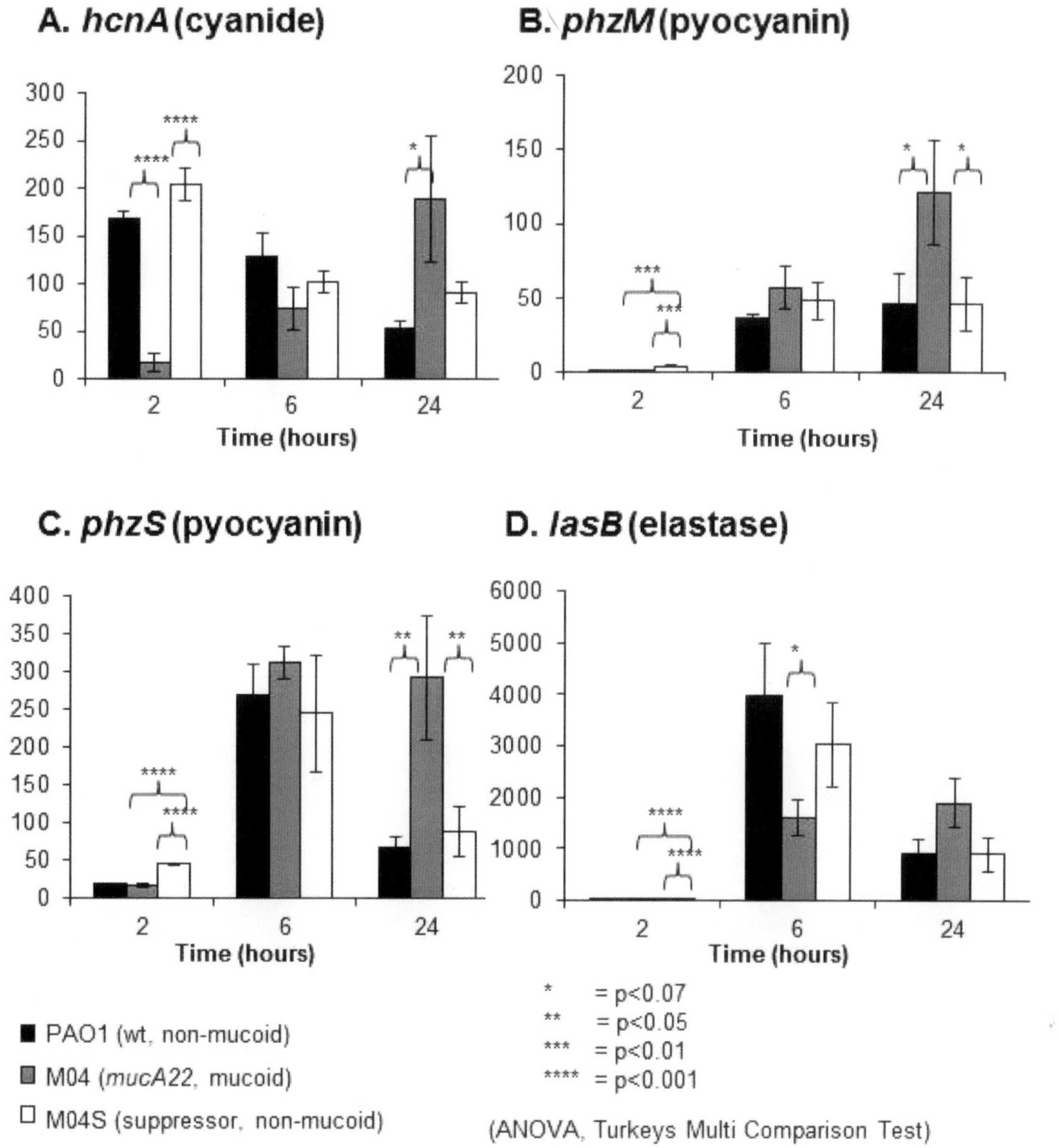

Figure 2. *mucA* mutation alters the expression of cyanide, pyocyanin and elastase genes. Expression profiles of *hcnA* (A), *phzM* (B), *phzS* (C) and *lasB*, (D) for PAO1 (wild type, non-mucoid) (black); M04 (*mucA22*, mucoid) (dark grey); and M04S (non-mucoid suppressor isolated from M04) (light grey). Values are averages of 3 biological replicates and the value for each replicate was the average of duplicate qRT-PCR technical replicates. Error bars are ±SEM. Data were analysed by ANOVA and post-hoc by Tukey's Multiple Comparison Test.

Plasmid expression of the cAMP-dependent transcription factor Vfr restores the quorum sensing defect and early stationary phase cyanide production in the *mucA22* mutant

AlgU activates the expression of a number of genes, including the gene encoding the AlgR response regulator and together they activate the transcription of the alginate biosynthetic genes [45,46]. The cAMP-dependent Vfr signalling system has been shown to be defective in *mucA* mutants at the level of *vfr* expression via a mechanism involves AlgU and AlgR [47]. Given that plasmid encoded Vfr restores cAMP-dependent Vfr signalling in a *mucA22* mutant [47], we investigated whether introduction of pPa-*vfr* into our isogenic strains resulted in the restoration of cyanide production. It is clear that cyanide production in early stationary phase is restored to wildtype levels in the *mucA22* mutant by pPa-*vfr* (Fig. 5A), suggesting that loss of Vfr contributes to the reduced peak cyanide production in *mucA22* mutants. The presence of pPa-*vfr* in wildtype and suppressor strains leads to them maintaining the production of cyanide into late stationary phase (24 h) in a way similar to M04, rather than the complete loss of cyanide production associated with the wildtype in the absence of pPa-*vfr* (Fig. 5B, Fig. 1). Furthermore, we found that plasmid borne expression of Vfr was able to restore 3-oxo-C12-HSL and C4-HSL and PQS levels to wildtype in 6 h stationary phase cultures of M04 (Fig. 5C–E).

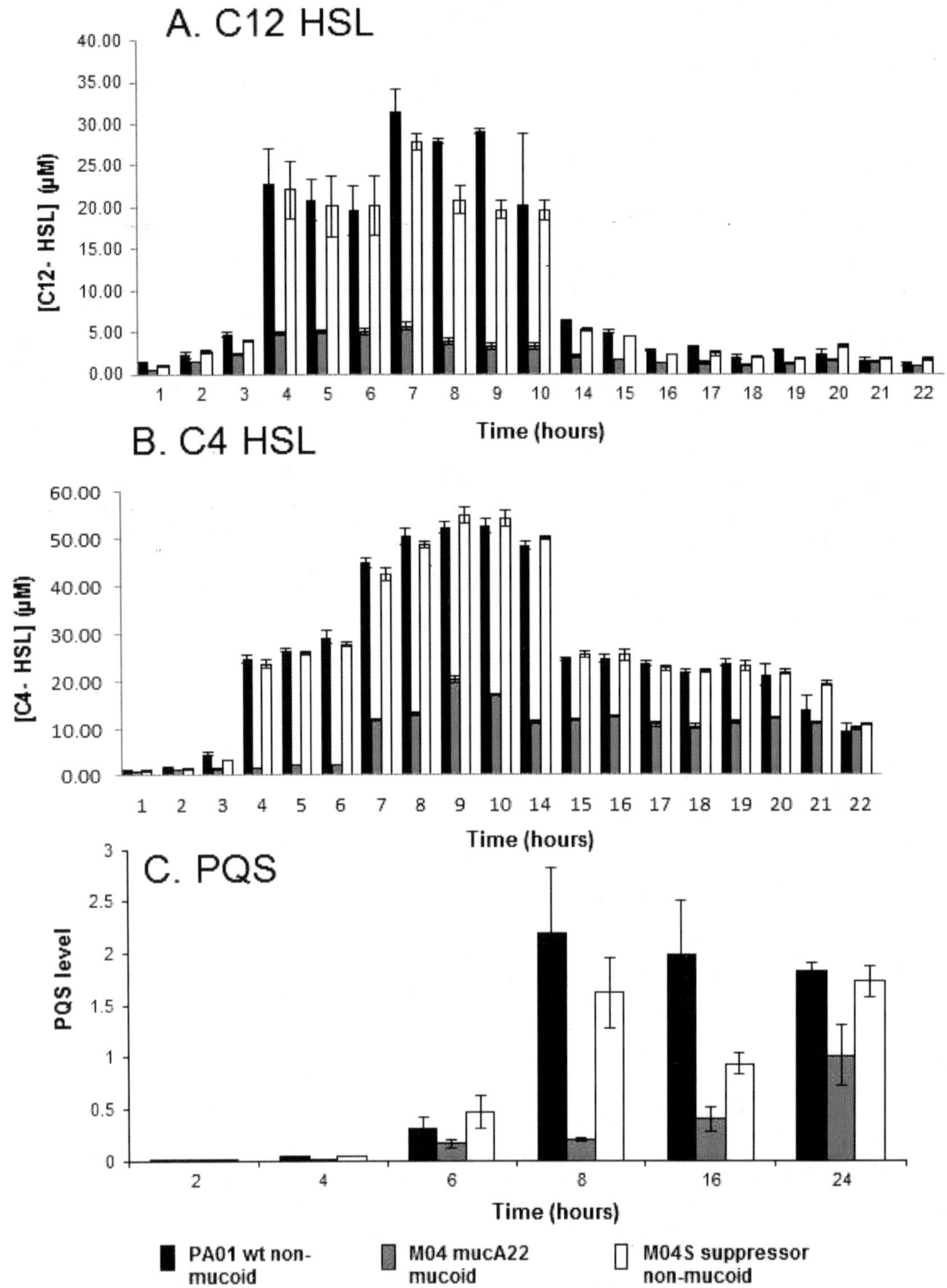

Figure 3. *mucA* mutation leads to suppression of quorum sensing signal molecule production throughout growth. Activities of the LasIR (A) RhlIR (B) and PQS (C) systems was compared in PAO1 (wild type, non-mucoid) (black), M04 (*mucA22*, mucoid) (dark grey) and M04S (non-mucoid suppressor isolated from MucA04) (light grey) using bioluminescent reporter strains to assay 3-oxo-C_{12} (lasIR) C_4-HSL (RhlIR) and PQS signal molecule levels in supernatant. Bioluminescence was measured using a luminometer. Culture conditions were as described in Figure 1. Values are means of 3 independent replicates and error bars are ±SEM.

Discussion

The *mucA22* mutation is the predominant mutation leading to mucoidy in *P. aeruginosa* during chronic CF lung infections. In this present work we report that the switch to a mucoid phenotype via a *mucA22* mutation has a profound effect on stationary phase physiology. An important finding is that a persistent low-level production of cyanide and pyocyanin occurs in mucoid strains in

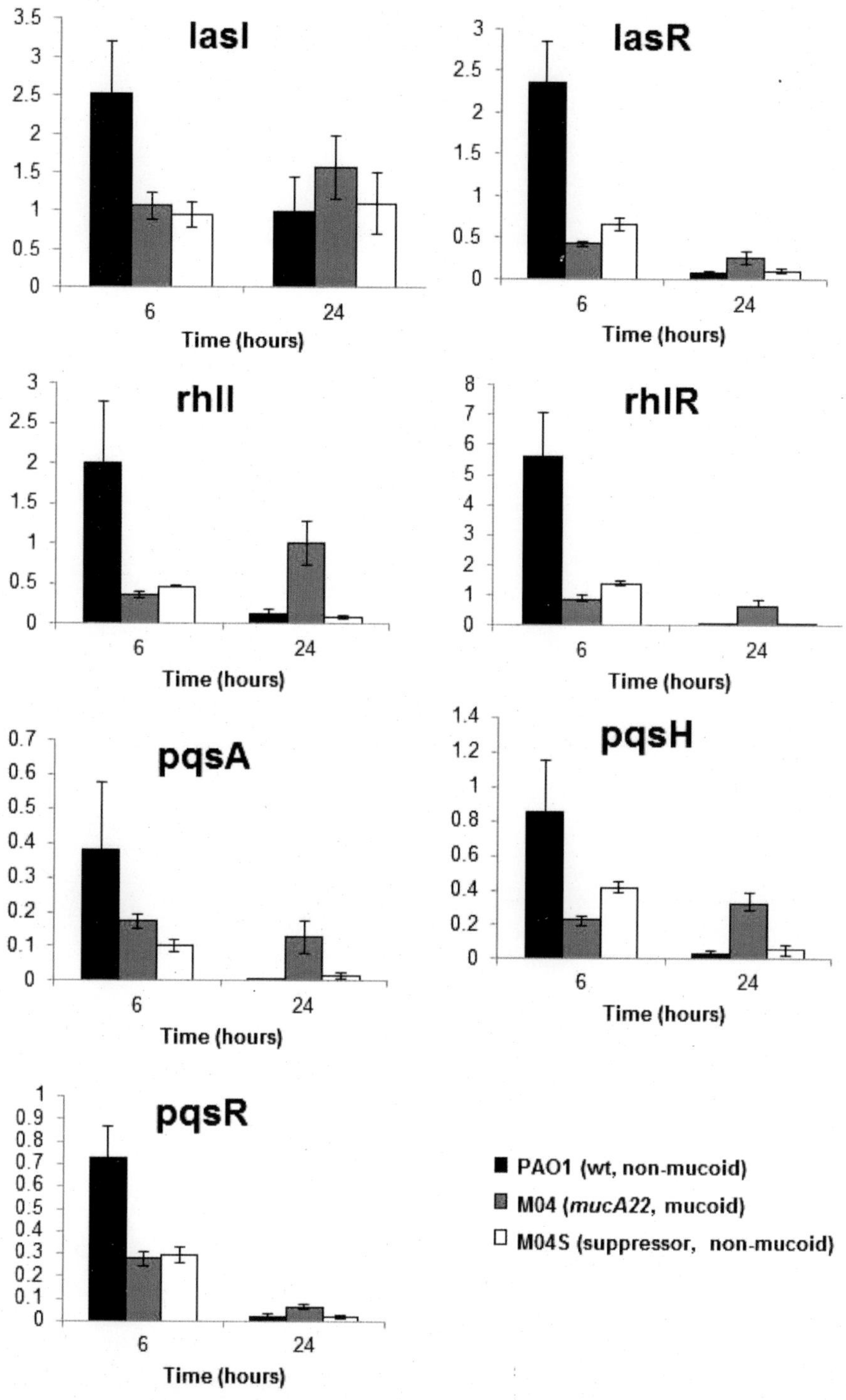

Figure 4. *mucA* mutation leads to suppression of quorum sensing gene expression. qRT-PCR expression profiles of quorum sensing regulatory genes for: PAO1 (wild type, non-mucoid) (black); M04 (*mucA22*, mucoid) (dark grey); and M04S (non-mucoid suppressor isolated from MucA04) (light grey). Values are averages of 3 biological replicates and the value for each replicate was the average of duplicate qRT-PCR technical replicates Error bars are ±SE and data were analysed by ANOVA and post-hoc by Tukey's Multiple Comparison Test.

late stationary phase compared to non-mucoid strains. We used spontaneous non-mucoid revertants of mucoid strains in this study due to the problematic nature of complementing or repairing *mucA22* mutations in the context of the unstable nature of the mucoid phenotype. The mucoid phenotype is frequently reported as unstable and non-mucoid variants emerge through suppressor mutations in culture and in the CF lung and where both phenotypes can coexist [36,48–51]. Suppressor mutations in the *algU* gene have been described [51], but we did not find *algU* mutations in any of the suppressor stains used in this study and neither did they have identifiable mutations in known regulars of mucoidy including; *mucA*, *algD*, *algR*, and *lasR*.

Cody et al (2009) have reported the regulation of *hcnABC* genes by the AlgZ-AlgR two component regulatory systems and

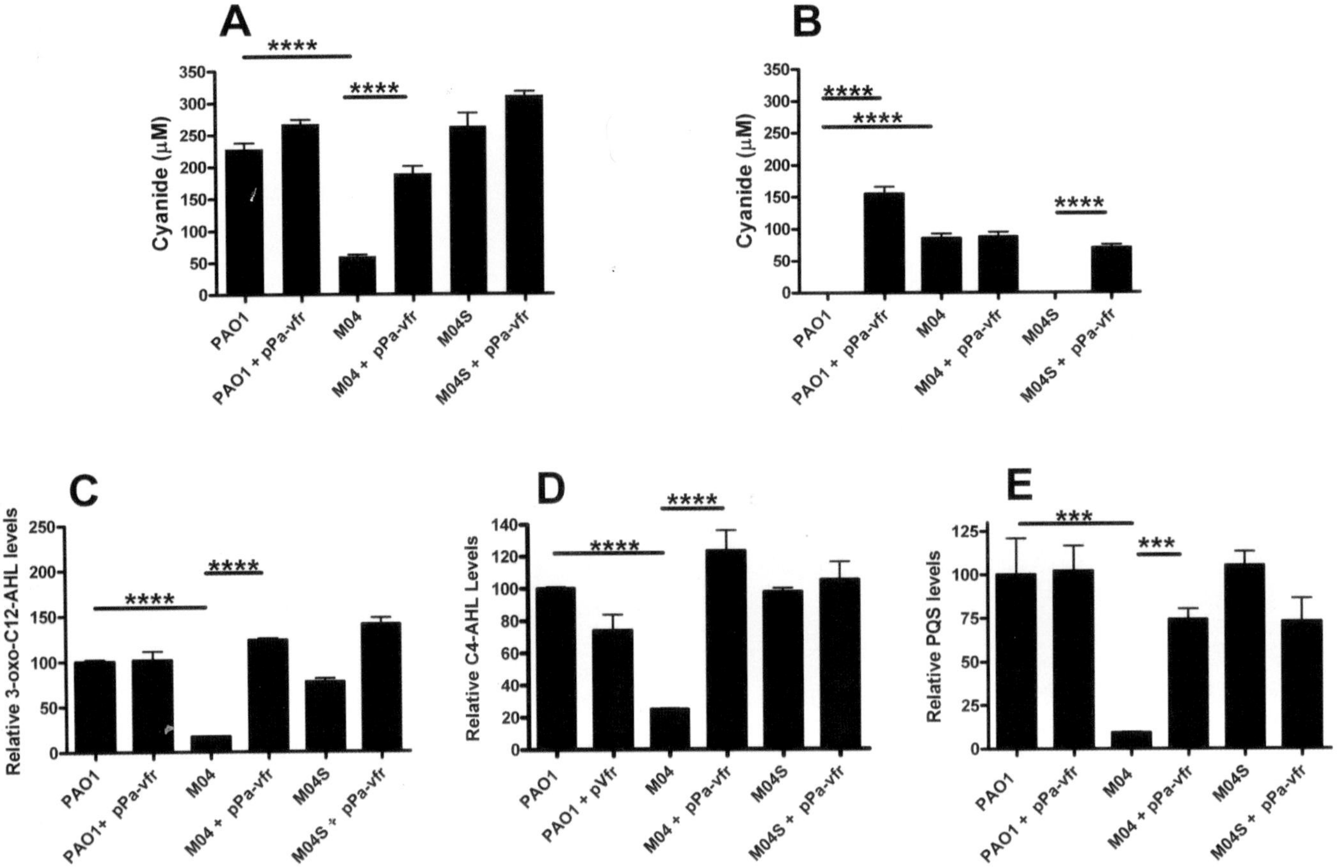

Figure 5. Plasmid expression of the cAMP-dependent transcription factor Vfr restores the early stationary phase cyanide production and the quorum sensing defect in the *mucA22* mutant. Cyanide concentration and QS molecule levels were measured in culture supernatants of wildtype (PAO1), *muc22* mutant (M04) and its suppressor strain (M04S) with or without the plasmid pPa-vfr. Cyanide levels after (A) 6 hours growth (early stationary phase) and (B) 24 hours growth (late stationary phase). (C) Relative 3-oxo-C12 AHL levels; (D) relative C4-AHL levels; (E) relative PQS levels after 8 hours growth (early stationary phase). Values are relative to the PAO1 8 hour value. All experiments are averages of three independent replicates error bars are ±SEM and data were analysed by ANOVA and post-hoc by Tukey's Multiple Comparison Test. **** $p < 0.001$; *** $p < 0.01$.

demonstrated the presence of HCN in cultures after 36 hours of growth [52]. This contrasts with our findings, which were highly reproducible in our hands. The only time we have seen cyanide in late stationary phase was using sealed flasks that prevent loss of cyanide gas by blowing off [15].Previously, mucoid CF isolates have been reported to be deficient in motility (due to inhibition of flagella production), pyocyanin production, elastase and total protease production, and decreased exotoxin A and exoenzyme S production as well as having reduced expression of type III secretion systems and type IV pili [26,53–56]. Here we demonstrate that *mucA22* mutation and the consequent increased availability of the sigma factor AlgU leads to a more complex and subtle change in the stationary phase regulation of virulence factor production than previously recognised (Figs. 1, 2 and S1). We show that *mucA22* mutation results in repression of AHL- and AQ-dependent quorum sensing systems (Figs. 3 and 4) leading to decreased production of the virulence factors cyanide, pyocyanin and elastase in early stationary phase, but also changes the regulation of cyanide and pyocyanin in late stationary phase leading to their continued production in non-growing cultures which is in stark contrast to non-mucoid strains (Fig. 1). qRT-PCR data indicates that *mucA22* mutation leads to changes in the regulation of expression of the HCN synthase genes (*hcnABC*), the *phz* genes involved in pyocyanin synthesis and the elastase encoding *lasB* gene (Fig. 2). The effects of *mucA* mutation on stationary phase properties that we observe fit with the recent finding that MucA modulates osmotic stress tolerance in stationary phase, but not exponential phase, cultures of *P. aeruginosa* [29].

Previous publications provide contradictory findings regarding cyanide production in mucoid and non-mucoid strains. Carterson et al found that mucoid strains produced seven times **more** cyanide than non-mucoid strains [57]. This is in contrast with a study [58] that found a **decrease** in expression of the *hcnABC* genes in mucoid *P. aeruginosa*, and a recent survey of hydrogen cyanide (HCN) released into the gas phase by 96 genotyped *P. aeruginosa* strains that found reduced cyanide accumulation by mucoid strains [59]. The apparent incongruous nature of these reports is explained by our data. While Carterson *et al* [57] measured cyanide given off from plate grown cultures (most cells of which will have reached stationary phase), Rau *et al* [58] performed a transcriptomic study on mid-exponential phase cultures. Our data shows that in exponential phase cultures the *hcnA* gene is expressed in non-mucoid strains (in advance of cyanide being detectable in the growth medium), but there is a 10-fold lower level of expression in *mucA22* mucoid strains, which is consistent with data of Rau *et al* [58]. This differential gene expression is maintained into early stationary phase when cyanide levels peak at a 2.5-fold lower level in *mucA* strains (Fig. 1 and 2). There is complete loss of cyanide production in non-mucoid strains in late stationary phase (Fig. 1), whereas mucoid strains maintain cyanide production, which explains, we suggest, the high levels of cyanide trapped from the plate grown cultures by Carterson *et al* [57]. Indeed when we assayed cyanide in our strains by the same plate assay method we obtained a similar result to Carterson *et al* (2004) (data not shown). In an earlier study, Firoved and Deretic [25] reported an increase in expression of *lasB*, *hcnA* and *hcnC* in a *mucA* strain, grown to mid-exponential phase, compared to its non-mucoid parent, but cyanide levels were not measured. These data are different to both our findings and those of Rau et al [58], and are not easily explained other than by possible growth condition and strain differences.

Elastase peak levels were also reduced in *mucA22* mutants, but *lasB* showed different regulation in late stationary phase to cyanide and pyocyanin, indicating operation of a different regulatory mechanism.

As cyanide, pyocyanin and elastase are all positively regulated by quorum sensing we tested whether the change in their regulation in a *mucA22* mutant might be through an effect on quorum sensing. We found that while *mucA22* strains showed induction of LasR/3-oxo-C12-HSL, RhlR/C4-HSL and AQ-dependent quorum sensing systems their levels were reduced to approximately 17%, 35%, and 10% respectively of wild type levels at the time of peak production in early stationary phase (Fig. 3), which can explain the decreased cyanide, pyocyanin and *lasB* expression in early stationary phase in *mucA* strains. In late stationary phase (22 to 24 hours) *mucA* strains have comparable or lower levels of QS molecules compared to wild type and suppressor strains, and so the maintenance of cyanide and pyocyanin production at these time points must be dependent on other regulatory factors. Morici et al have previously demonstrated a link between the AlgR response regulator (a positive regulator of *hcnABC*) and the RhlR/C4-HSL quorum sensing system [28]. They showed by both transcriptomic and gene fusion studies that AlgR partly suppressed the RhlR/C4-HSL quorum sensing system, but in a biofilm specific manner; it did not affect planktonic cultures. Rau et al [58] reported an effect of *mucA* mutation on the RhlR/C4-AHL quorum sensing system, showing decreased *rhlR* and *rhlI* expression at a single time point in mid-exponential phase cultures and also decreased C4-HSL production when cultures reached an OD_{600} of 1.0. Our study has confirmed and extended these findings through the growth cycle from early exponential phase to late stationary phase and to effects on the *lasR* and PQS quorum sensing systems.

We next addressed how the *mucA22* mutation could lead to such marked effects on quorum sensing? We found no evidence for a role for the regulatory small RNAs *rsmY* and *rsmZ* in this regulation, but we did find data supporting a role for Vfr, the cAMP-dependent positive regulator of the Las quorum sensing system (Fig. 5). Vfr has recently been shown to be down regulated in *mucA* strains via an AlgR dependant mechanism [47] and we found that plasmid expression of Vfr restored the quorum sensing defect in *mucA22* mutants and consequently restored cyanide production. So while at this stage a complete mechanism to explain our findings is not deducible, a testable model building on these findings is shown in Fig. 6.

The switch to a mucoid phenotype is one of the most frequently encountered and clinically significant changes undergone by *P. aeruginosa* and occurs during chronic infection of the cystic fibrosis lung. It occurs in most CF lung infections and is concurrent with a decrease in the clinical condition of the patient [2,18]. Evidence indicates that alginate provides *P. aeruginosa* with protection from the host immune response by inhibiting phagocytosis, protecting against the oxidative burst and by providing an immunomodulatory role and so provides a selective advantage in the lung [60,61]. However the pleiotropic effects of *mucA22* mutation on quorum sensing and virulence factor regulation may also provide a powerful selection pressure for the mucoid switch. Genetic analysis of *P. aeruginosa* isolates from the airways of multiple CF patients has revealed that one of the most common targets of mutation in CF isolates is the *lasR* gene [62], suggesting a strong selection for the loss of *lasR* function and subsequent down-regulation of quorum sensing pathways in the CF airways. Our data indicates that the switch to mucoidy provides a second route for down regulation of quorum sensing pathways, which could provide a selection pressure for the switch to mucoidy during CF lung infections. Whether these findings are of significance *in vivo* requires further study in appropriate model systems and of clinical strains.

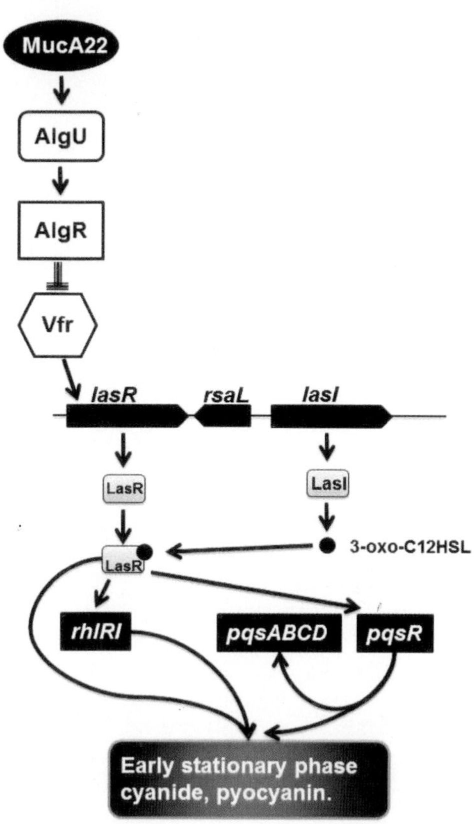

Figure 6. Model to explain early stationary phase down regulation of cyanide, pyocyanin and elastase production by mucA22 mutation of *P. aeruginosa*. This figure is an adaptation and extension of Figure 7 from [47]. Solid arrows indicate positive regulation and T-bar negative regulation. *MucA22* mutation results in release of AlgU, which is then free to associate with core RNA polymerase and direct expression from its target genes, which include the gene for the transcriptional regulator AlgR. AlgR is a repressor of the cAMP-dependent transcriptional regulator, VfR, which is a positive regulator of the LasRI quorum sensing system. AlgR inhibition Vfr transcription will result in down regulation of the LasRI quorum sensing system, which since it is the dominant QS system will act to down regulate both the RhlRI and AQ (PQS) QS systems, resulting in suppression of the entire QS network and decreased expression of virulence factors in early stationary phase.

If this mechanism was reproduced in vivo during CF lung infection it would lead to continued production and cyanide and pyocyanin in non-growing populations of *P. aeruginosa*, which could be significant as these compounds can damage lung tissue and provide a source of nutrients for growth and survival. While cyanide is only synthesised aerobically HCN made by P. aeruginosa in oxic regions of the lung that diffuse into anoxic areas would potentially inhibit anaerobic respiration in the absence of protective mechanism against HCN [16,63].

Supporting Information

Figure S1 *mucA22*, mucoid strains are deficient in cyanide, pyocyanin and elastase production in early stationary phase. Cyanide (**A**), Pyocyanin (**B**) and Elastase (**C**) in supernatant of liquid cultures of non-mucoid wild type (black), mucoid *mucA22* (dark grey) and non-mucoid suppressor (light grey) strains at 2 hours post stationary phase initiation. Cultures were incubated in 50 ml LB in 250 ml conical flasks in orbital shaker at 200 rpm and 37°C and grown until 2 hour post stationary phase initiation (6 hours in all cases); growth was followed by determining OD_{600} every hour. Cyanide concentrations were measured with an ion selective micro electrode. Pyocyanin levels were determined by chloroform/HCl extraction followed by absorbance measurement 520 nm. Elastase levels were determined by assaying enzymatic breakdown of Elastin-Congo red then measurement of liberated Congo red in a spectrophotometer at A_{495}. Values are means of 3 independent replicates and error bars are ±SEM.

Figure S2 Growth and Cyanide production for PA0381 and PAO578 (*mucA22*). Optical density on primary y axis, (solid markers) cyanide concentration on secondary y axis, (empty markers) for (A) PAO381 (wild type, non-mucoid) (black); and PAO578 (*mucA22*, mucoid derivative of PAO381) (dark grey).

Figure S3 *mucA* mutation leads to suppression of quorum sensing signal molecule production in independently isolated *mucA22* mutants isolated in PAO1 and PAO381 backgrounds. Activities of the C4-AHL (A) and 3-oxo-C12-AHL (B) was compared in wild type, non-mucoid strains (WT), *mucA22* (MUCOID) and suppressor strains after 2 hours (mid-log) and 6 hours (early stationary phase) of growth in LB medium. Values are means of 3 independent replicates and error bars are ±SEM.

Figure S4 *mucA22* mutation does not act through disruption of the *rsmY*/*rsmZ* regulatory network. The wildtype strain PAO1, the *mucA22* mutant M04 and its suppressor strain M04S carrying the *rsmY-lacZ* or *rsmZ-lacZ* gene fusions [44] were grown in LB and growth followed (A) and samples assayed for β-galactosidase (B), the values plotted being ±SEM (n = 3 biological replicates).

Table S1 Bacterial strains and plasmids.

Acknowledgments

We thank Alain Filloux, John Govan, Paul Williams and Matthew Wolfgang for kindly providing strains and plasmids.

Author Contributions

Conceived and designed the experiments: BR JEAZ HDW. Performed the experiments: BR MC JEAZ VB XL ZW KEL. Analyzed the data: BR MC JEAZ VB XL ZW KEL HDW. Wrote the paper: BR HDW.

References

1. Schaedel C, de Monestrol I, Hjelte L, Johannesson M, Kornfalt R, et al. (2002) Predictors of deterioration of lung function in cystic fibrosis. Pediatr Pulmonol 33: 483–491.
2. Govan JR, Deretic V (1996) Microbial pathogenesis in cystic fibrosis: mucoid *Pseudomonas aeruginosa* and *Burkholderia cepacia*. Microbiol Rev 60: 539–574.
3. Castric PA (1983) Hydrogen cyanide production by Pseudomonas aeruginosa at reduced oxygen levels. Can J Microbiol 29: 1344–1349.
4. Worlitzsch D, Tarran R, Ulrich M, Schwab U, Cekici A, et al. (2002) Effects of reduced mucus oxygen concentration in airway *Pseudomonas* infections of cystic fibrosis patients. J Clin Invest 109: 317–325.
5. Gallagher LA, Manoil C (2001) *Pseudomonas aeruginosa* PAO1 kills *Caenorhabditis elegans* by cyanide poisoning. J Bacteriol 183: 6207–6214.
6. Broderick KE, Chan A, Balasubramanian M, Feala J, Reed SL, et al. (2008) Cyanide produced by human isolates of *Pseudomonas aeruginosa* contributes to lethality in *Drosophila melanogaster*. J Infect Dis 197: 457–464.
7. Goldfarb WB, Margraf H (1967) Cyanide production by *Pseudomonas aeruginosa*. Ann Surg 165: 104–110.
8. Ryall B, Davies JC, Wilson R, Shoemark A, Williams HD (2008) *Pseudomonas aeruginosa*, cyanide accumulation and lung function in CF and non-CF bronchiectasis patients. Eur Respir J 32: 740–747.
9. Sanderson K, Wescombe L, Kirov SM, Champion A, Reid DW (2008) Bacterial cyanogenesis occurs in the cystic fibrosis lung. Eur Respir J 32: 329–333.
10. Anderson RD, Roddam LF, Bettiol S, Sanderson K, Reid DW (2010) Biosignificance of bacterial cyanogenesis in the CF lung. J Cyst Fibros 9: 158–164.
11. Lenney W, Gilchrist FJ (2011) *Pseudomonas aeruginosa* and cyanide production. Eur Respir J 37: 482–483.
12. Enderby B, Smith D, Carroll W, Lenney W (2009) Hydrogen cyanide as a biomarker for *Pseudomonas aeruginosa* in the breath of children with cystic fibrosis. Pediatr Pulmonol 44: 142–147.
13. Stutz MD, Gangell CL, Berry LJ, Garratt LW, Sheil B, et al. (2011) Cyanide in bronchoalveolar lavage is not diagnostic for *Pseudomonas aeruginosa* in children with cystic fibrosis. Eur Respir J 37: 553–558.
14. Cunningham L, Pitt M, Williams HD (1997) The *cioAB* genes from *Pseudomonas aeruginosa* code for a novel cyanide-insensitive terminal oxidase related to the cytochrome *bd* quinol oxidases. Molecular Microbiology 24: 579–591.
15. Zlosnik JE, Tavankar GR, Bundy JG, Mossialos D, O'Toole R, et al. (2006) Investigation of the physiological relationship between the cyanide-insensitive oxidase and cyanide production in *Pseudomonas aeruginosa*. Microbiology 152: 1407–1415.
16. Williams HD, Zlosnik JEA, Ryall B (2007) Oxygen, cyanide and energy generation in the cystic fibrosis pathogen *Pseudomonas aeruginosa*. Advances in Microbial Physiology, Vol 52 52: 1–71.
17. Cipollone R, Ascenzi P, Tomao P, Imperi F, Visca P (2008) Enzymatic detoxification of cyanide: clues from *Pseudomonas aeruginosa* Rhodanese. J Mol Microbiol Biotechnol 15: 199–211.
18. Lyczak JB, Cannon CL, Pier GB (2002) Lung infections associated with cystic fibrosis. Clin Microbiol Rev 15: 194–222.
19. Martin DW, Schurr MJ, Mudd MH, Govan JRW, Holloway BW, et al. (1993) Mechanism of conversion to mucoidy in *Pseudomonas-aeruginosa* infecting cystic fibrosis patients. Proceedings of the National Academy of Sciences of the United States of America 90: 8377–8381.
20. Rowen DW, Deretic V (2000) Membrane-to-cytosol redistribution of ECF sigma factor AlgU and conversion to mucoidy in *Pseudomonas aeruginosa* isolates from cystic fibrosis patients. Mol Microbiol 36: 314–327.
21. Martin DW, Schurr MJ, Mudd MH, Govan JR, Holloway BW, et al. (1993) Mechanism of conversion to mucoidy in *Pseudomonas aeruginosa* infecting cystic fibrosis patients. Proc Natl Acad Sci U S A 90: 8377–8381.
22. Mathee K, Ciofu O, Sternberg C, Lindum PW, Campbell JIA, et al. (1999) Mucoid conversion of *Pseudomonas aeruginosa* by hydrogen peroxide: a mechanism for virulence activation in the cystic fibrosis lung. Microbiology-Sgm 145: 1349–1357.
23. Pedersen SS, Moller H, Espersen F, Sorensen CH, Jensen T, et al. (1992) Mucosal immunity to *Pseudomonas aeruginosa* alginate in cystic fibrosis. APMIS 100: 326–334.
24. Firoved AM, Boucher JC, Deretic V (2002) Global genomic analysis of AlgU (sigma(E)-dependent promoters (sigmulon) in *Pseudomonas aeruginosa* and implications for inflammatory processes in cystic fibrosis. J Bacteriol 184: 1057–1064.
25. Firoved AM, Deretic V (2003) Microarray analysis of global gene expression in mucoid *Pseudomonas aeruginosa*. J Bacteriol 185: 1071–1081.

26. Wu WH, Badrane H, Arora S, Baker HV, Jin SG (2004) MucA-mediated coordination of type III secretion and alginate synthesis in *Pseudomonas aeruginosa*. Journal of Bacteriology 186: 7575–7585.
27. Tart AH, Blanks MJ, Wozniak DJ (2006) The AlgT-dependent transcriptional regulator AmrZ (AlgZ) inhibits flagellum biosynthesis in mucoid, nonmotile *Pseudomonas aeruginosa* cystic fibrosis isolates. J Bacteriol 188: 6483–6489.
28. Morici LA, Carterson AJ, Wagner VE, Frisk A, Schurr JR, et al. (2007) *Pseudomonas aeruginosa* AlgR represses the Rhl quorum-sensing system in a biofilm-specific manner. J Bacteriol 189: 7752–7764.
29. Behrends V, Ryall B, Wang X, Bundy JG, Williams HD (2010) Metabolic profiling of *Pseudomonas aeruginosa* demonstrates that the anti-sigma factor MucA modulates osmotic stress tolerance. Mol Biosyst 6: 562–569.
30. Williams HD, Behrends V, Bundy JG, Ryall B, Zlosnik JE (2010) Hypertonic saline therapy in cystic fibrosis: do population shifts caused by the osmotic sensitivity of infecting bacteria explain the effectiveness of this treatment? Front Microbiol 1: 120.
31. Zlosnik JE, Williams HD (2004) Methods for assaying cyanide in bacterial culture supernatant. Lett Appl Microbiol 38: 360–365.
32. Ohman DE, Cryz SJ, Iglewski BH (1980) Isolation and characterization of *Pseudomonas aeruginosa* PAO mutant that produces altered elastase. J Bacteriol 142: 836–842.
33. Essar DW, Eberly L, Hadero A, Crawford IP (1990) Identification and characterization of genes for a second anthranilate synthase in *Pseudomonas aeruginosa*: interchangeability of the two anthranilate synthases and evolutionary implications. J Bacteriol 172: 884–900.
34. Winson MK, Swift S, Fish L, Throup JP, Jorgensen F, et al. (1998) Construction and analysis of *luxCDABE*-based plasmid sensors for investigating N-acyl homoserine lactone-mediated quorum sensing. FEMS Microbiol Lett 163: 185–192.
35. Fletcher MP, Diggle SP, Crusz SA, Chhabra SR, Camara M, et al. (2007) A dual biosensor for 2-alkyl-4-quinolone quorum-sensing signal molecules. Environ Microbiol 9: 2683–2693.
36. Hauser AR, Jain M, Bar-Meir M, McColley SA (2011) Clinical significance of microbial infection and adaptation in cystic fibrosis. Clin Microbiol Rev 24: 29–70.
37. Boucher JC, Schurr MJ, Deretic V (2000) Dual regulation of mucoidy in *Pseudomonas aeruginosa* and sigma factor antagonism. Mol Microbiol 36: 341–351.
38. Williams P, Camara M (2009) Quorum sensing and environmental adaptation in *Pseudomonas aeruginosa*: a tale of regulatory networks and multifunctional signal molecules. Curr Opin Microbiol 12: 182–191.
39. Pessi G, Haas D (2000) Transcriptional control of the hydrogen cyanide biosynthetic genes *hcnABC* by the anaerobic regulator ANR and the quorum-sensing regulators LasR and RhlR in *Pseudomonas aeruginosa*. J Bacteriol 182: 6940–6949.
40. Heurlier K, Williams F, Heeb S, Dormond C, Pessi G, et al. (2004) Positive control of swarming, rhamnolipid synthesis, and lipase production by the posttranscriptional RsmA/RsmZ system in *Pseudomonas aeruginosa* PAO1. J Bacteriol 186: 2936–2945.
41. Burrowes E, Baysse C, Adams C, O'Gara F (2006) Influence of the regulatory protein RsmA on cellular functions in *Pseudomonas aeruginosa* PAO1, as revealed by transcriptome analysis. Microbiology 152: 405–418.
42. Kay E, Humair B, Denervaud V, Riedel K, Spahr S, et al. (2006) Two GacA-dependent small RNAs modulate the quorum-sensing response in *Pseudomonas aeruginosa*. J Bacteriol 188: 6026–6033.
43. Brencic A, McFarland KA, McManus HR, Castang S, Mogno I, et al. (2009) The GacS/GacA signal transduction system of *Pseudomonas aeruginosa* acts exclusively through its control over the transcription of the RsmY and RsmZ regulatory small RNAs. Mol Microbiol 73: 434–445.
44. Bordi C, Lamy MC, Ventre I, Termine E, Hachani A, et al. (2010) Regulatory RNAs and the HptB/RetS signalling pathways fine-tune *Pseudomonas aeruginosa* pathogenesis. Mol Microbiol 76: 1427–1443.
45. Martin DW, Schurr MJ, Yu H, Deretic V (1994) Analysis of promoters controlled by the putative sigma factor AlgU regulating conversion to mucoidy in *Pseudomonas aeruginosa*: relationship to sigma E and stress response. J Bacteriol 176: 6688–6696.
46. Mohr CD, Leveau JH, Krieg DP, Hibler NS, Deretic V (1992) AlgR-binding sites within the *algD* promoter make up a set of inverted repeats separated by a large intervening segment of DNA. J Bacteriol 174: 6624–6633.
47. Jones AK, Fulcher NB, Balzer GJ, Urbanowski ML, Pritchett CL, et al. (2010) Activation of the *Pseudomonas aeruginosa* AlgU regulon through *mucA* mutation inhibits cyclic AMP/Vfr signaling. J Bacteriol 192: 5709–5717.
48. Schurr MJ, Martin DW, Mudd MH, Deretic V (1994) Gene cluster controlling conversion to alginate-overproducing phenotype in *Pseudomonas aeruginosa*: functional analysis in a heterologous host and role in the instability of mucoidy. J Bacteriol 176: 3375–3382.
49. Ohman DE, Goldberg JB, Flynn JL (1990) Molecular analysis of the genetic switch activating alginate production In: Silver S, Chakrabarty AM, Iglewski B, Kaplan S, editors. *Pseudomonas*: biotransformations, pathogenesis, and evolving biotechnology. Washington D.C.: American Society for Microbiology.
50. Govan JRW (1988) Alginate biosynthesis and other unusual characterisatics associated with the pathogenesis of *Pseudomonas aeruginosa* in cystic fibrosis. In: Griffiths E, Donachie W, Stephen J, editors. Bacterial infections od respiratory and gastrointestinal mucosae. Oxford: IRL Press.
51. Sautter R, Ramos D, Schneper L, Ciofu O, Wassermann T, et al. (2012) A complex multilevel attack on Pseudomonas aeruginosa algT/U expression and algT/U activity results in the loss of alginate production. Gene 498: 242–253.
52. Cody WL, Pritchett CL, Jones AK, Carterson AJ, Jackson D, et al. (2009) *Pseudomonas aeruginosa* AlgR controls cyanide production in an AlgZ-dependent manner. J Bacteriol 191: 2993–3002.
53. Elston HR, Hoffman KC (1967) Increasing incidence of encapsulated Pseudomonas aeruginosa strains. Am J Clin Pathol 48: 519–523.
54. Garrett ES, Perlegas D, Wozniak DJ (1999) Negative control of flagellum synthesis in *Pseudomonas aeruginosa* is modulated by the alternative sigma factor AlgT (AlgU). J Bacteriol 181: 7401–7404.
55. Mohr CD, Rust L, Albus AM, Iglewski BH, Deretic V (1990) Expression patterns of genes encoding elastase and controlling mucoidy: co-ordinate regulation of two virulence factors in *Pseudomonas aeruginosa* isolates from cystic fibrosis. Mol Microbiol 4: 2103–2110.
56. Woods DE, Sokol PA, Bryan LE, Storey DG, Mattingly SJ, et al. (1991) In vivo regulation of virulence in *Pseudomonas aeruginosa* associated with genetic rearrangement. J Infect Dis 163: 143–149.
57. Carterson AJ, Morici LA, Jackson DW, Frisk A, Lizewski SE, et al. (2004) The transcriptional regulator AlgR controls cyanide production in *Pseudomonas aeruginosa*. J Bacteriol 186: 6837–6844.
58. Rau MH, Hansen SK, Johansen HK, Thomsen LE, Workman CT, et al. (2010) Early adaptive developments of *Pseudomonas aeruginosa* after the transition from life in the environment to persistent colonization in the airways of human cystic fibrosis hosts. Environ Microbiol 12: 1643–1658.
59. Gilchrist FJ, Alcock A, Belcher J, Brady M, Jones A, et al. (2011) Variation in hydrogen cyanide production between different strains of *Pseudomonas aeruginosa*. Eur Respir J 38: 409–414.
60. Pedersen SS (1992) Lung infection with alginate-producing, mucoid *Pseudomonas aeruginosa* in cystic fibrosis. APMIS Suppl 28: 1–79.
61. Simpson JA, Smith SE, Dean RT (1989) Scavenging by alginate of free radicals released by macrophages. Free Radic Biol Med 6: 347–353.
62. Smith EE, Buckley DG, Wu Z, Saenphimmachak C, Hoffman LR, et al. (2006) Genetic adaptation by *Pseudomonas aeruginosa* to the airways of cystic fibrosis patients. Proc Natl Acad Sci U S A 103: 8487–8492.
63. Filiatrault MJ, Tombline G, Wagner VE, Van Alst N, Rumbaugh K, et al. (2013) *Pseudomonas aeruginosa* PA1006, which plays a role in molybdenum homeostasis, is required for nitrate utilization, biofilm formation, and virulence. PLoS One 8: e55594.

2

Candidate Markers Associated with the Probability of Future Pulmonary Exacerbations in Cystic Fibrosis Patients

Gabriella Wojewodka[1], Juan B. De Sanctis[2], Joanie Bernier[3], Julie Bérubé[4], Heather G. Ahlgren[5], Jim Gruber[3], Jennifer Landry[3], Larry C. Lands[6], Dao Nguyen[5], Simon Rousseau[5], Andrea Benedetti[5,7], Elias Matouk[3], Danuta Radzioch[1,5]*

1 Department of Human Genetics, McGill University, Montreal, Quebec, Canada, **2** Institute of Immunology, Central University of Venezuela, Caracas, Venezuela, **3** Adult Cystic Fibrosis Clinic, Montreal Chest Institute, McGill University Health Center, Montreal, Quebec, Canada, **4** McGill University Health Center Research Institute, Montreal, Quebec, Canada, **5** Department of Medicine, McGill University, Montreal, Quebec, Canada, **6** Division of Pediatric Respiratory Medicine, Montreal Children's Hospital, McGill University Health Center Research Institute, Montreal, Quebec, Canada, **7** Department of Epidemiology, Biostatistics and Occupational Health, Montreal Chest Institute, McGill University Health Center, Montreal, Quebec, Canada

Abstract

Introduction: Pulmonary exacerbations (PEs) cause significant morbidity and can severely impact disease progression in cystic fibrosis (CF) lung disease, especially in patients who suffer from recurrent PEs. The assessments able to predict a future PE or a recurrent PE are limited. We hypothesized that combining clinical, molecular and patient reported data could identify patients who are at risk of PE.

Methods: We prospectively followed a cohort of 53 adult CF patients for 24 months. Baseline values for spirometry, clinical status using the Matouk Disease Score, quality of life (QOL), inflammatory markers (C-reactive protein (CRP), interleukins (IL)-1β, -6, -8, -10, macrophage inflammatory protein (MIP)-1β, tumor necrosis factor (TNF) and vascular endothelial growth factor (VEGF)), polyunsaturated fatty acids and lipid peroxidation in blood plasma were collected for all patients during periods of stable disease, and patients were monitored for PE requiring PO/IV antibiotic treatment. Additionally, we closely followed 13 patients during PEs collecting longitudinal data on changes in markers from baseline values. We assessed whether any markers were predictors of future PE at baseline and after antibiotic treatment.

Results: Out of 53 patients, 37 experienced PEs during our study period. At baseline, we found that low lung function, clinical scoring and QOL values were associated with increased risk of PE events. PEs were associated with increased inflammatory markers at Day 1, and these biomarkers improved with treatment. The imbalance in arachidonic acid and docosahexaenoic acid levels improved with treatment which coincided with reductions in lipid peroxidation. High levels of inflammatory markers CRP and IL-8 were associated with an early re-exacerbation.

Conclusion: Our results demonstrate that worse clinical and QOL assessments during stable disease are potential markers associated with a higher risk of future PEs, while higher levels of inflammatory markers at the end of antibiotic treatment may be associated with early re-exacerbation.

Editor: Erich Gulbins, University of Duisburg-Essen, Germany

Funding: GW received funding from the Frederick Banting and Charles Best Canada Graduate Scholarships Doctoral Award from the Canadian Institutes of Health Research. JBdS received funding from FONACIT (G2005000389). DR received funding from Ministère du Développement Économique, de l'Innovation et de l'Exportation (MDEIE/MESRST), MSBi Valorisation and Cystic Fibrosis Canada. The funders had no role in study design, data collection and analysis, decision to publish, or preparation of the manuscript.

Competing Interests: The authors have declared that no competing interests exist.

* E-mail: danuta.radzioch@mcgill.ca

Introduction

Cystic fibrosis (CF) patients often suffer acute exacerbations of their pulmonary symptoms, necessitating more aggressive treatment. Pulmonary exacerbations (PEs) are major events contributing to the morbidity and progression of CF lung disease. The recovery from PEs is largely based on the reversal of symptoms and improvement in lung function. However, pre-PE lung function levels are not recovered in 15% to 25% of CF patients[1,2]. Even when pulmonary function tests return to normal values, experiencing a PE contributes to long-term decline in lung disease with similar impacts on survival as would a 12% reduction in lung function[3,4]. Higher frequencies of PEs were associated with greater rates of decline in forced expiratory volume in one second percent predicted ($FEV_1\%$), especially having more than two PEs per year could increase the need for transplant and the risk of death[5]. The survival model characterized by Liou et al. also predicted that the impact on 5-year mortality of four PE events in a single year was as detrimental as *Bulkholderia cepacia* infection or a 48% reduction in FEV_1%[3]. Given the substantial morbidity and mortality associated with PEs, there is an urgent need to identify patients at risk of PE, particularly recurrent PEs. Improving the clinicians' ability to stratify patients based on their risk to develop PEs will allow for more effective prevention (eg. treatment of CF related diabetes or allergic bronchopulmonary aspergillosis) and early intervention to prevent irreversible lung damage. Although standards of care that include inhaled antibiotics, azithromycin, recombinant human deoxyribonuclease and hypertonic saline contribute in reducing the frequency of exacerbations, there is currently no effective and reproducible diagnostic marker for the identification of early stages of PE. The standard criteria used to monitor PEs are mainly focused on lung function indicators such as FEV_1% which are mostly reflective of disease severity and not necessarily disease activity[6]. Patient reported symptoms are important complements to physician-documented clinical signs in the diagnosis of PE. In fact, newly developed diaries are being validated for the purpose of early intervention to quickly reduce the development of a full and vigorous inflammatory response and to shorten and reduce the severity of PE with the hope of preventing the development of irreversible lung damage[7].

The events that trigger PEs are still poorly understood and may include respiratory viral infections[8,9] and air pollution[10]. Bacterial pathogens already present in the patients' lungs may be causing PEs by adapting their virulence or colonizing new areas of the lung[11]. Retrospective studies have found risk factors for developing PEs which include the female sex, nutritional status, CF co-morbidities such as CF related diabetes, pancreatic insufficiency, and lung microbiology (eg. *Aspergillus fumigatus, Bulkholderia cepacia*)[2,3,5,12,13]. Due to the nature of data available to perform retrospective analyses, these risk factors are based on clinical information which help to identify a population of CF patients more likely to have PEs. However on an individual basis, it remains difficult to assess which patients will experience a PE.

There have been few prospective studies looking at factors associated with risk of PEs which included molecular markers as predictors. A study by Sequeiros et al. found that the time to the next PE was shorter in patients with allergic bronchopulmonary aspergillosis and CF related diabetes. The authors also described that high C-reactive protein (CRP) and low FEV_1 values at the end of antibiotic PE treatment were associated with shorter times until the next PE. They did not find any other molecular markers of significance[14]. Gray et al. demonstrated that serum calprotectin levels at the end of PE treatment rather than CRP were linked to the time until next PE[15]. These two studies show the potential of inflammatory markers in predicting risk of future PE.

For this study, we asked two questions: 1) In a period of stable disease, who is more likely to have a PE in the future? and 2) After PE treatment, who is at risk of an early re-exacerbation? We hypothesized that combining clinical and patient reported data with inflammatory markers and fatty acids may result in a better evaluation of patient disease activity. More specifically, we describe that worse disease-specific patient reported quality of life (QOL) and clinical assessments during stable disease indicated risk of PE, while higher levels of inflammation at the end of PE treatment were associated with early re-exacerbation.

Materials and Methods

Study design

Primary study: Markers at stable disease associated with risk of future PE. CF patients from the Adult Cystic Fibrosis Clinic at the Montreal Chest Institute (Montreal, Qc, Canada) were approached during their regular clinic visit to participate in the study. Fifty-three patients were enrolled in our prospective cohort study and were followed for a 12 month period from enrollment. The study duration was 24 months in total. Baseline data was recorded during a period of stable disease defined by the absence of any PE requiring intravenous (IV) or oral antibiotic therapy in the preceding month. One patient was excluded from the study after baseline data was collected due to lung transplantation, thus we had 52 patients in our patient group. Inhaled antibiotics (tobramycin or aztreonam) were prescribed as maintenance therapy to 39 patients enrolled in the study (75% of the cohort: 32 patients that had PE and 7 that had no PE). A PE was defined as any change in patients' symptoms (increased cough, sputum production and breathlessness, and decreases in lung function, weight, appetite and energy) requiring additional oral or IV antibiotic therapy [5]. The decision to treat was at the physicians' discretion and was not influenced by this study. All patients were treated with β-lactams and/or fluoroquinolones in addition to tobramycin. Some received additional antibiotics such as doxycycline, clindamycin or trimethoprim. Nine patients were given corticosteroids during their first PE of the study based on previous response and/or severe bronchospasm.

Secondary study: Markers at the end of PE treatment associated with early re-exacerbation. Among patients that experienced PE ($n = 37$), we collected serial longitudinal clinical data and blood samples throughout the PEs of 13 randomly selected patients. Data and samples were collected at Day 1 (within 24 hours prior to PE treatment, $n = 13$), and on follow-up assessments on Days 7 ($n = 12$), 14 ($n = 11$), 21 ($n = 9$) and 42 ($n = 8$). Four patients received treatment for 14 days and nine for 21 days. Patient compliance limited the sampling of all patients for Days 7, 14 and 21 time points. By Day 42, four patients had already re-exacerbated and were not included in this follow-up time point.

Volunteers serving as healthy controls (HC) were recruited from the McGill University Health Centre. CF patients and healthy controls gave written consent to participate in the study which was approved by the Institutional Review Board of the McGill University Health Centre.

Clinical data and clinical scoring

At enrollment, patients' information on age, sex, weight and body mass index (BMI) was recorded. At baseline ($n = 52$) and at all defined time points during PEs ($n = 8$–13), the patients' weight, BMI, complete blood cell counts and clinical information for the Matouk Disease Score were assessed. The Matouk Disease Score (Matouk Modified N. Huang Disease Score), previously described and validated[16,17], was used to quantify disease activity of CF patients. Briefly, the total score comprises of four subscores: Clinical (weight, weight change, dyspnoea, cough, sputum, physical exam, respiratory rate/breathing pattern/cardiac frequency, bacterial culture, appetite and general condition), Pulmonary Function (PFT: forced vital capacity percent predicted (FVC%), FEV_1% predicted, FEV_1/FVC, forced expiratory flow $(FEF)_{25-75\%}$ predicted, $FEF_{50\%}$ predicted, RV/TLC), Chest Radiography (CXR) score (based on the Bradsfield method for radiography scoring, comprised of scores for air trapping, linear markings, nodular cystic lesions, parenchymal lesions, general impression) and Complications score (number of previous PEs, pneumothorax, hemoptysis, respiratory failure, cardiac enlargement, pulmonary surgery). Healthier patients have higher scores for Clinical, PFT and CXR categories and lower values for the Complications score. To calculate the total score: Total score = Clinical+PFT+CXR−Complications. A full description of the scoring method can be found in File S1.

Measures of lung function

At baseline (n = 52) and at all defined time points during PEs (n = 8–13), lung function was assessed by spirometry, and included FEV_1% and FVC%. Spirometry was performed according to the American Thoracic Society standards[18,19].

Patient reported quality of life (QOL)

The QOL evaluation was recorded at baseline (n = 52) and at defined time points during PE (n = 8–13) by a self-administered questionnaire using the CF Questionnaire-Revised (CFQ-R) which comprised of 50 items associated with 3 symptom scales (Weight, Respiratory Function and Digestion) and 9 QOL domains (Physical, Vitality, Emotional, Eating Disturbances, Treatment Burden, Health Perceptions, Body Image, Social Functioning and Role/School Functioning) [20]. Higher scores reflect healthier disease status. The total score is the sum of scores for all items in the questionnaire.

Plasma inflammatory biomarker analysis

At baseline (n = 52) and each defined time points during PEs (n = 8–13), blood samples were collected in ethylenediaminetetra-acetic acid (EDTA) coated tubes and spun at 3000 rpm for 10 min at 4°C for plasma isolation. Plasma CRP levels were quantified in the hospital's clinical laboratory using ELISA. Cytokines were measured in plasma with the MILLIPLEX® Map multiplex assay kit (Millipore, Mississauga, ON, Canada) and the MAGPIX® multiplex system (Millipore) according to the manufacturer's instructions. The data was assessed for interleukin (IL)-1β, IL-6, IL-8, IL-10, macrophage inflammatory protein 1β (MIP-1β, also known as CCL4), tumor necrosis factor (TNF) and vascular endothelial growth factor (VEGF) using the MILLIPLEX® Analyst software, version 4.2 (Millipore). The concentrations of cytokines are expressed as pg/ml.

Plasma polyunsaturated fatty acid and lipid peroxidation analysis

After plasma isolation as described above, 100 µl of plasma was added to 900 µl 2:1 chloroform/methanol solution with added 1 mM of butylated hydroxyanisole (BHA) to prevent oxidation of the fatty acids. Samples were stored in −80°C until analysis. Lipids were isolated using the method described by Folch[21]. The polyunsaturated fatty acids (PUFA) in this fraction were esterified as described by Schlenk and Gellerman[22] and the esters were identified by gas chromatography/mass spectrometry (Hewlett Packard 5880A, WCOT capillary column (Supelco-10, 35 m×0.5 mm, 1 µm thick)) using commercial standards (Sigma-Aldrich, Oakville, ON, Canada)[23]. In addition, the total protein content of the aqueous phase was analysed using the bicinchoninic assay (Pierce Biotechnology, Rockford, IL, USA). The concentrations of arachidonic acid (AA) and docosahexaenoic acid (DHA) are expressed as nmol/µg of protein. The AA/DHA ratio represents the amount of AA to DHA in each patient. The AA/DHA ratio represents the amount of AA to DHA in each sample. Lipid peroxidation was assessed by indirectly measuring malondialdehyde (MDA) using the thiobarbituric acid reactive species (TBARS) assay[23] and is expressed as nmol of TBARS/mg of protein.

Statistical analysis

The Cox proportional hazards and Kaplan-Meier models were used for survival analysis with time to first PE used as the outcome. For the Cox proportional hazards models, models were adjusted for age and sex. For the Kaplan-Meier method, continuous covariates were dichotomized at the median, and a log rank test was conducted (Figure 1). For comparisons of two groups, the Student's t-test or the Mann-Whitney test and Chi-square were used. For changes from baseline during PE, statistical analysis was performed using the percentage change with the one sample t-test or Wilcoxon signed-rank test (Figures 2 and 3, Table S1). The percentage change was calculated as: $(\text{Value}_{\text{PE time point}} - \text{Value}_{\text{baseline}})/\text{Value}_{\text{baseline}} \times 100$.

The ANOVA test with Bonferroni post-tests were used to evaluate differences between the PUFA levels at all PE time points (Figure 4) and Pearson correlations were estimated for this data. Significance was set at $p<0.05$. See File S1 for additional description.

Results

Patient demographics, baseline clinical and biomarker characteristics

We prospectively followed our adult CF cohort for a total of 24 months, and 37 out of 52 patients experienced at least one PE during the follow-up period. The patient demographics and baseline values of the cohort are described in Tables 1 and 2. At baseline, CF patients that experienced at least one PE ("PE group") had lower lung function, weight, BMI and Matouk Disease Score compared to the patients who did not have a PE ("no PE group") (Table 1). The baseline levels of white blood cells and blood neutrophils, although still within the normal range, were higher in the "PE group", suggesting higher levels of systemic inflammation even during a stable disease state. These patients also had lower QOL assessments for total score, Weight, Physical, Emotion, Health Perceptions, Body Image and Role items (Table 1). IL-6 and IL-10 levels were higher in the "PE group" compared to the "no PE group" (Table 2). Consistent with previously reported data from our group and other investigators[24–26] there was a lipid imbalance in PUFA with high AA levels and low DHA levels CF patients compared to HC. Overall the AA/DHA ratio was higher in CF patients than in HC. However, there were no differences in fatty acids between the "no PE group" and "PE group" during stable disease. Overall, these characteristics suggest that the "PE group" has more severe and active disease, and a lower QOL at baseline, compared the "no PE group".

Worse clinical disease severity and activity, and QOL are associated with PE events

Using the Cox proportional hazards model adjusting for age and sex, we tested the association between our markers and the risk of PE (Table 3). Better lung function (FEV_1% and FVC%) and higher Clinical, PFT, CXR subscores and total Matouk Disease Score were associated with a lower risk of PE. A lower Complications subscore was associated with lower risk of PE. The Matouk Disease Score incorporates patients' symptoms as well as physician-recorded clinical parameters and other complications adding to disease activity beyond spirometric evaluations. Thus a high degree of disease severity as measured by lung spirometry was associated with high risk of PE as was high disease

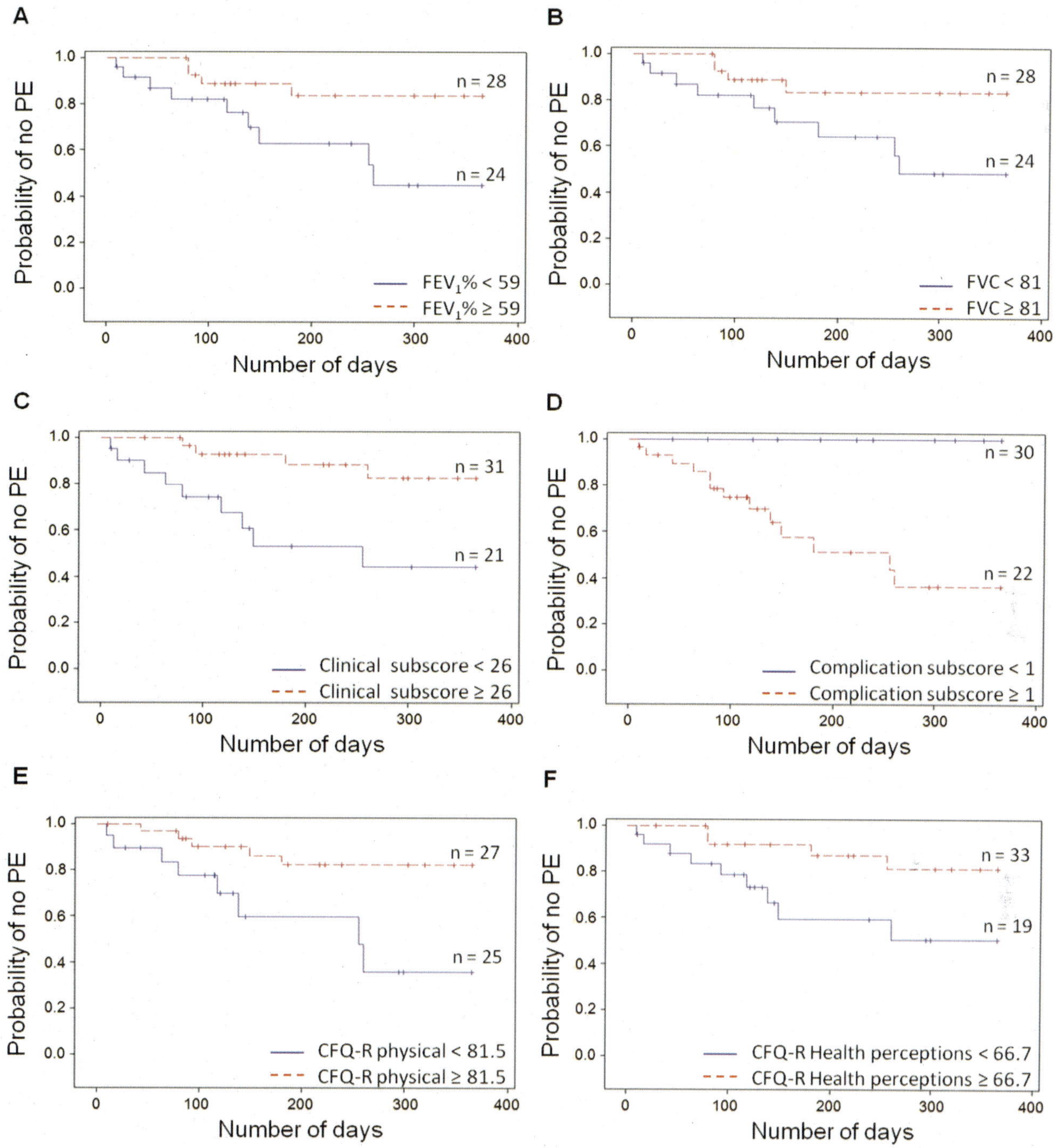

Figure 1. Probability of having a PE is associated with low clinical and QOL assessments. Using the Kaplan-Meier survival analysis, we evaluated whether the markers were associated with the risk of a PE. Continuous covariates were dichotomized at the median. The parameters illustrated here were all influencing the probability of having a PE. Lower risks of PE were associated with A) higher FEV1% predicted ($p = 0.020$), B) higher FVC% predicted ($p = 0.032$), C) higher Clinical subscore of the Matouk Disease Score ($p = 0.004$), D) lower Complications subscore of the Matouk Disease Score ($p = 0.000$), E) higher assessments of QOL physical ($p = 0.030$) and F) higher health perceptions ($p = 0.006$) domains.

activity assessed by the Matouk Disease Score. The analysis also showed that low CFQ-R symptom scores (Weight and Respiratory) and low QOL domains (Physical, Vitality, Health Perceptions and Role) indicated higher risk of PE. No inflammatory markers or PUFA were found to be associated with risk of PE using the Cox proportional hazard model.

To illustrate these relationships, we used the Kaplan-Meier survival model, with patients dichotomized based on median values (Figure 1). We obtained similar results to the Cox proportional hazards model. Lower lung function (FEV_1%, Figure 1A and FVC%, Figure 1B), worse subscores of the Matouk Disease Score (low Clinical subscore, Figure 1C and high Complications subscore Figure 1D, data not shown for other

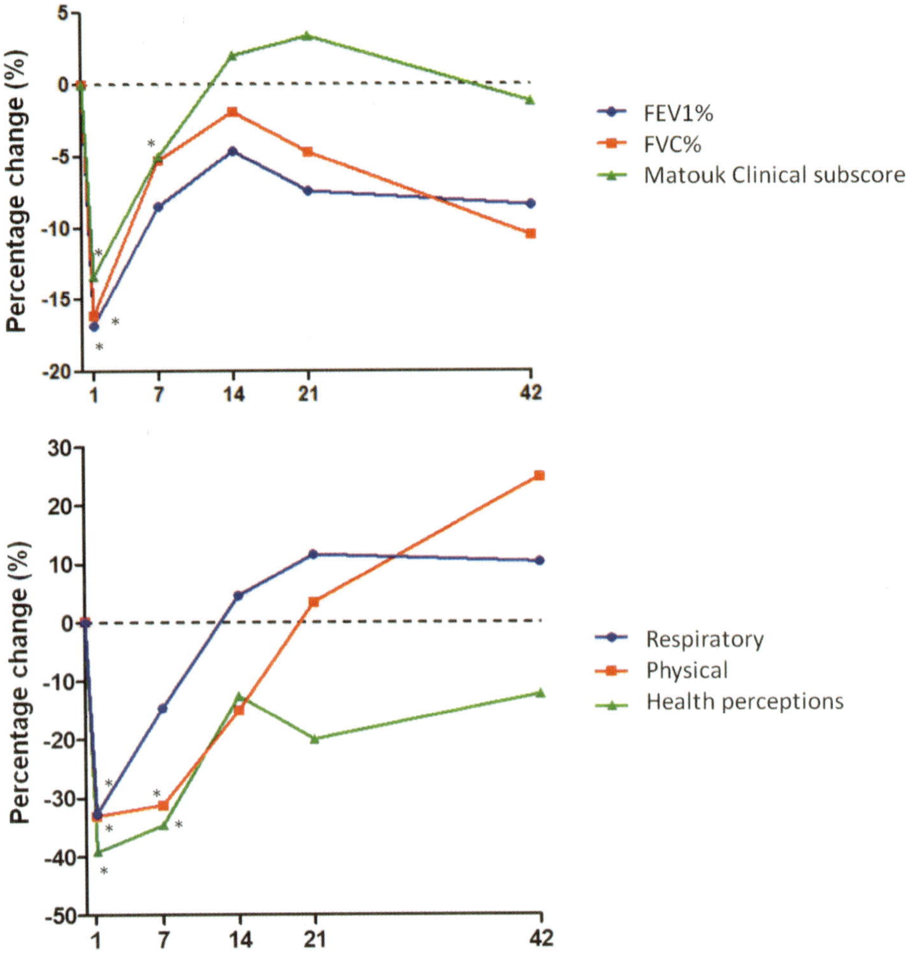

Figure 2. Percentage change of clinical and QOL parameters throughout PEs in CF. A) FEV1% (*blue, circles*) and FVC% (*red, squares*) were significantly reduced from baseline values at Day 1 of PE (FEV1% p = 0.001; FVC% p = 0.010). Both parameters subsequently improved with treatment however, FVC% significantly declined at Day 42 (p = 0.028). The Clinical subscore of the Matouk Disease score (*green, triangles*) was significantly decreased from baseline values on Day 1 (p = 0.000) and Day 7 (p = 0.045). See Table S1 for the results of other Matouk Disease subscores. B) QOL items also decreased with PE onset, Day 1, such as Respiratory (*blue, circles*, p = 0.002), Physical (*red, squares*, p = 0.025) and Health Perceptions domains (*green, triangles*, p = 0.000). The Physical and Health Perceptions domains remained decreased at Day 7 (p = 0.025 and p = 0.001, respectively). Other QOL domains which decreased at Day 1 include: Vitality, Health Perceptions, Social and Role (Table S1). The dotted horizontal line indicates a 0% change or no change from baseline values. * indicates a significant difference from baseline. Day 1, n = 13; Day 7, n = 12, Day 14, n = 11; Day 21, n = 9; Day 42, n = 8. Full table of results can be found in Table S1.

subscores) and low scores for the CFQ-R QOL domains Physical and Health Perceptions were also related to a higher risk of a future PE (Figures 1E and 1F, respectively). No baseline inflammatory markers or PUFA were associated with increased risk of PE events, although there was a trend with higher CRP levels (median 5.3 mg/L, p = 0.0537, data not illustrated).

Changes in clinical parameters and QOL during PE

We performed a second study with 13 patients to evaluate whether any of our markers at the end of PE treatment would be predictive of an early re-exacerbation. We first calculated the percentage change at each time point for each patient compared to their baseline values obtained during a period of stable disease (Figure 2 and full data set is presented in Table S1). As expected, lung function was most reduced at Day 1 of a PE (−16.8% FEV_1% and −16.1% FVC% compared to baseline), and steadily improved over the course of PE treatment lasting either 14 or 21 days (Figure 2A). FEV_1% and FVC% approached pre-PE baseline values at Day 14. However, both values decreased again by Day 21 and 42 where FVC% values were 10.5% lower than baseline values (p = 0.028)(Figure 2A). At the onset of PE (Day 1), all components of the Matouk Disease Score worsened compared to baseline (Clinical subscore illustrated in Figure 2A). The Clinical subscore steadily improved with PE treatment where it was 3.4% above baseline on Day 21. The CXR subscore did not decrease at PE onset, however showed a trend toward improvement on Day 21, attesting to the limited sensitivity of the Bradsfield radiologic scoring to capture small CXR changes (Table S1). The QOL evaluation revealed that patients recognized a decline of their health on Day 1 with improvements on Days 7, 14, 21 and 42 (Respiratory, Physical and Health Perceptions illustrated in Figure 2B).

Changes in inflammatory markers during PE

In previous studies, inflammatory markers such as CRP, IL-1β, IL-6, IL-8 and VEGF were found to increase with PE onset and to respond to antibiotic treatment for PEs [14,15,27–32]. We calculated the percentage change for the concentrations of

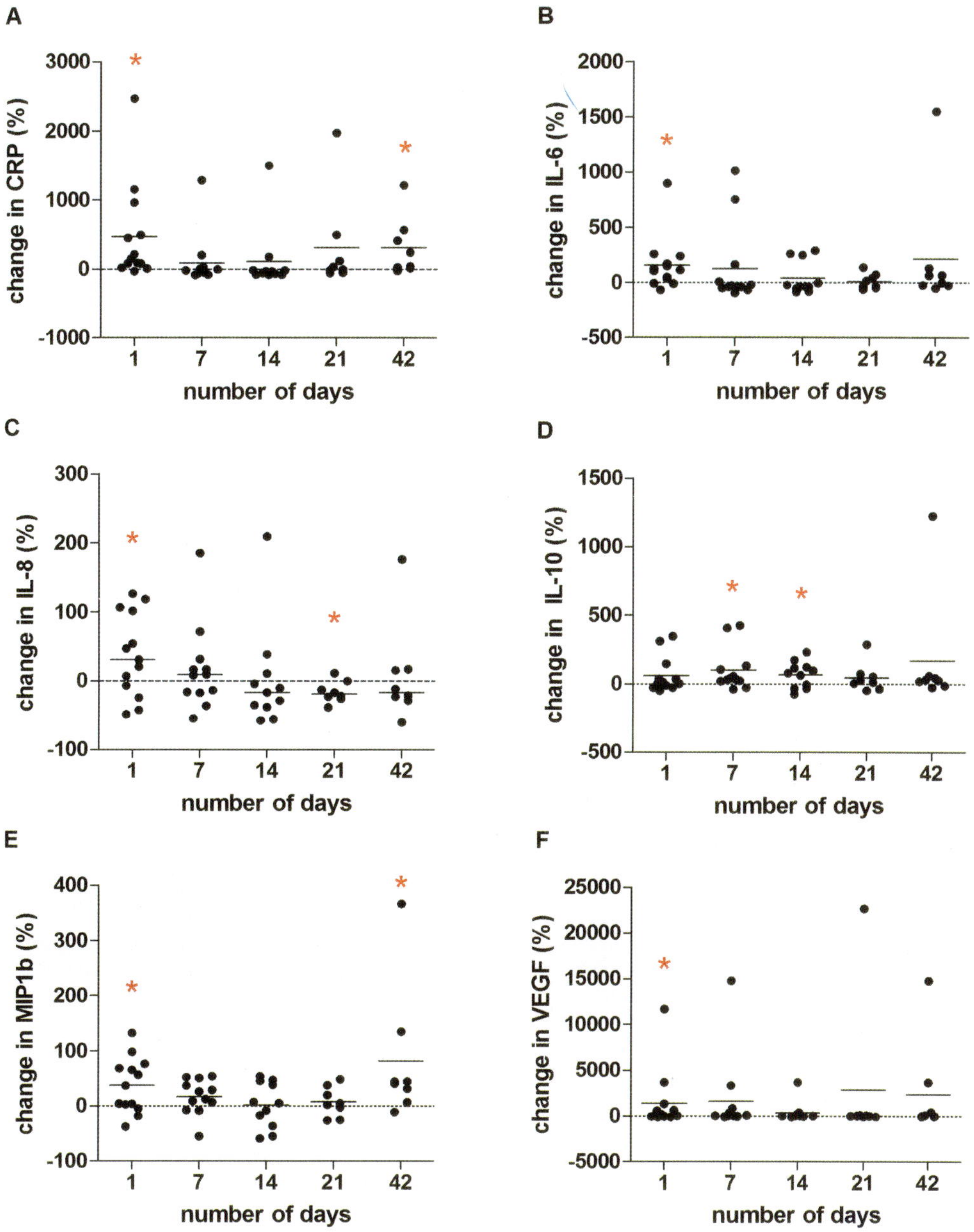

Figure 3. Percentage change in inflammatory markers throughout PEs in CF. Inflammatory markers were measured in blood plasma from CF patients throughout PE. The percentage change was calculated at each time point and compared to a 0% change which indicates no change from baseline (represented by dotted horizontal line). A) CRP levels were significantly increased from baseline values on Day 1 of PE ($p = 0.001$) and Day 42 ($p = 0.039$). B) IL-6 levels were significantly higher on Day 1 of PE ($p = 0.006$). C) IL-8 concentrations were significantly higher on Day 1 ($p = 0.047$) and significantly lower than baseline values after treatment on Day 21 ($p = 0.022$). D) IL-10 levels rose significantly on Days 7 ($p = 0.021$) and Day 14 ($p = 0.046$). E) MIP-1β increased from baseline on Days 1 ($p = 0.020$) and Day 42 ($p = 0.023$). F) VEGF levels were significantly higher on Day 1 of PE ($p = 0.043$). Solid horizontal lines are set at the mean * indicates a significant difference from 0% change from baseline. Day 1, n = 13; Day 7, n = 12, Day 14, n = 11; Day 21, n = 9; Day 42, n = 8. Full data set is found in Table S2.

inflammatory markers at each time point, in comparison to baseline values for each patient. In general, we also found PE onset induced an inflammatory response which returned to baseline values toward the end of treatment (Days 14 and 21). Once off aggressive treatment for PE, inflammatory markers tended to increase again in some patients at Day 42. More specifically, we found the elevated CRP levels from baseline values on Day 1 decreased during treatment and significantly worsened once again post-treatment by Day 42 (Figure 3A). Similarly, IL-6, IL-8, MIP-1β and VEGF also increased on Day 1 and improved over the course of treatment (Figure 3B, C, E, F, respectively). IL-10 increased on Days 7 and 14 from baseline values, suggesting that anti-inflammatory mechanisms were activated (Figure 3D). Interestingly, MIP-1β levels significantly increased again post-treatment on Day 42 (Figure 3F). All other inflammatory markers tended to increase at Day 42, although with a large variation between patients. IL-1β and TNF were not significantly changed throughout PE (Table S2).

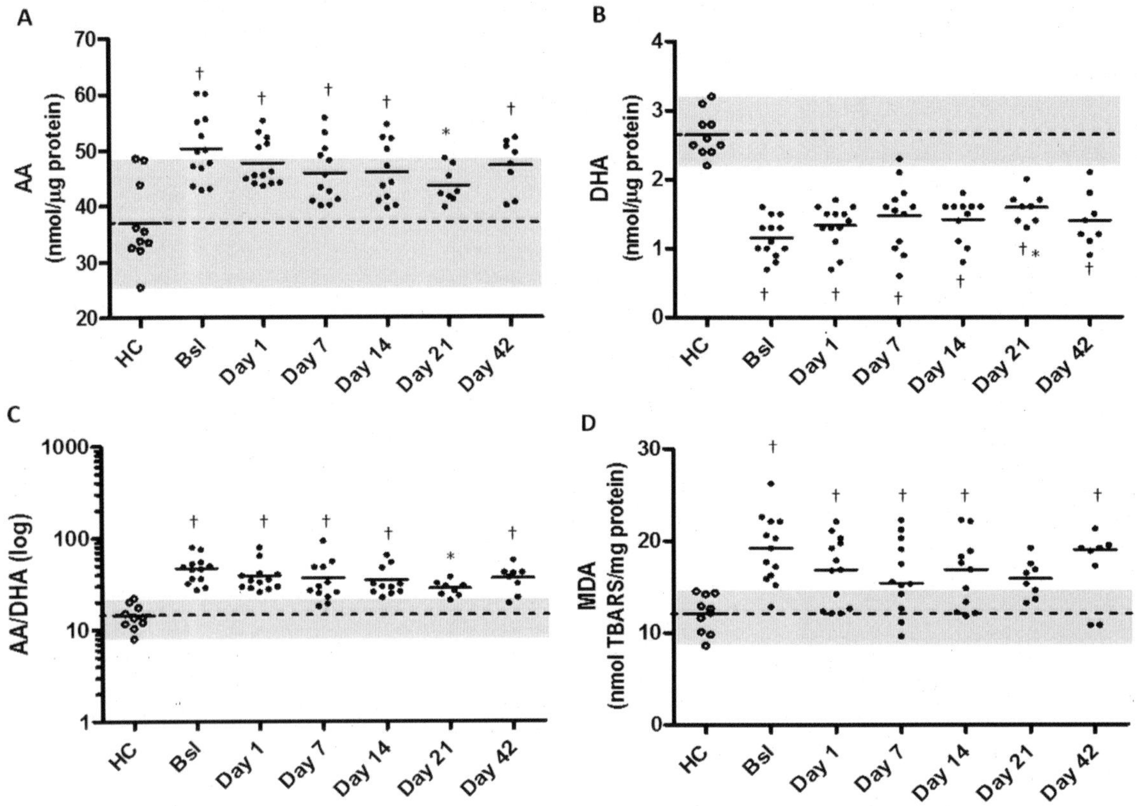

Figure 4. The levels of PUFA and peroxidation improve with treatment for PE in CF. PUFA concentrations were measured in blood plasma of healthy controls (HC, *white circles*) and CF patients (*black circles*) at stable disease (Bsl), at PE onset (Day 1), throughout PE treatment (Days 7, 14 and 21) and post treatment (Day 42). A) AA levels decreased during PE treatment and were significantly different from Bsl values at Day 21 ($p<0.05$). All PE time points including Bsl were significantly different from HC, except on Day 21 where there was no longer a difference with HC. B) DHA levels improved with PE treatment and were significantly increased from Bsl values at Day 21 ($p<0.05$). All PE time points including Bsl were significantly different from HC. C) Overall, the AA/DHA ratio was significantly decreased from Bsl values on Day 21 ($p<0.05$). All PE time points including Bsl were significantly different from HC, except on Day 21 where there was no difference with HC. D) MDA levels improved with treatment however no statistical difference was detected from Bsl. All PE time points including Bsl were significantly different from HC, except on Day 21 where there was no difference with HC. Solid lines indicate the means of the groups. Dotted lines indicate the HC mean and grey shadowing illustrates the min-max range for HC values. * represents significant difference from Bsl group using the Bonferroni post-test after ANOVA. † indicates significant difference from HC group using the Bonferroni post-test after ANOVA. Significance set as $p<0.05$. HC $n=10$, CF $n=8$–13.

Improvements in PUFA levels and lipid peroxidation during PE

A hallmark of CF disease is the imbalance in PUFAs with high levels of AA and low levels of DHA[24-26,33,34]. AA is pro-inflammatory and its metabolites include prostaglandins and eicosanoids which are also increased in CF[35,36]. DHA is anti-inflammatory and its metabolites include resolvins and protectins. This imbalance in PUFAs may contribute to the inflammatory status observed in CF[37,38]. In fact, our previous studies in a CF mouse model showed improvements in AA and DHA after treatment with fenretinide, a semi-synthetic retinoid, which were concurrent with reductions in inflammatory markers and better clearance of lung infections[25,39].

Unexpectedly, we found improvements in the PUFA imbalance compared to baseline on Day 21 for both AA (Figure 4A) and DHA (Figure 4B). At this time point, AA levels dropped to normal values, the AA/DHA ratio improved (Figure 4C), and both were no longer significantly different from HC concentrations. It is important to note that these improvements were not permanent as AA levels and AA/DHA ratios increased by Day 42. Lipid peroxidation decreased with treatment for PE and, MDA levels were no longer different from HC at Day 21(Figure 4D). We found a significant positive correlation between MDA and AA in plasma at the end of treatment ($r=0.6917$, $p=0.013$) and an inverse correlation between MDA and DHA, however this trend did not reach significance ($r=-0.3392$, $p=0.290$).

Potential promising markers of early re-exacerbation

To determine whether any of our markers assessed on the last day of treatment (either Day 14, $n=4$, or Day 21, $n=8$) could indicate an early re-exacerbation, the patient cohort was divided based on whether their next PE was under or over 42.5 days from the last day of treatment, which was the median number of days for the group (Table 4). "Early PE" refers to the patient group which had their next PE less than 42.5 days after the last day of treatment, while the group which developed no subsequent PE or a second PE more than 42.5 days after the last day of treatment was called "Late PE". One patient was excluded from the analysis since information on their next PE was not available, thus 12 patients were included. The "Early PE" group had a trend towards lower lung spirometry values, total Matouk Disease Score and QOL total score at end of treatment compared to the "Late PE" group, but this did not result in a statistical significance. More importantly, we found increased levels of inflammatory markers in

Table 1. Patient demographics and baseline values of studied parameters.

		Total CF patient group	Non-exacerbating (no PE)	Exacerbating (PE)	p-value no PE vs. PE
Demographics	**Number of patients**	52	15	37	
	Sex (F/M)	24/28	5/10	19/18	0.358
	Age	32.8 (1.8)	36.1 (3.4)	31.5 (2.3)	0.112
	Age range	18–64	18–59	18–64	
	Weight (kg)	60.8 (2.1)	**64.9 (2.8)**	**59.1 (2.6)**	**0.031***
	BMI (kg/m^2) (NR: 18.5–24.9)	21.9 (0.6)	**23.4 (0.7)**	**21.3 (0.7)**	**0.009***
Clinical assessments	**FEV1% predicted (%)**	63.0 (3.8)	**78.5 (5.0)**	**56.8 (4.6)**	**0.009***
	FVC% predicted (%)	79.8 (3.7)	**95.1 (5.2)**	**73.6 (4.4)**	**0.008***
	White blood cells (10^9/L) (NR: 4.8–10.8)	9.4 (0.4)	**8.1 (0.6)**	**10.0 (0.4)**	**0.018***
	Neutrophils (10^9/L) (NR: 1.6–7.7)	6.7 (0.3)	**5.6 (0.5)**	**7.1 (0.4)**	**0.033***
	Eosinophils (10^9/L) (NR: 0.0–0.5)	0.2 (0.02)	0.2 (0.07)	0.2 (0.01)	0.562
	Platelets (10^9/L) (NR: 140–440)	284.6 (8.4)	**244.0 (14.6)**	**301.6 (9.0)**	**0.001***
Matouk Disease Score	**Clinical** (0–50 points)	36.3 (0.6)	**39.3 (1.0)**	**35.1 (0.7)**	**0.002***
	PFT (0–25 points)	16.6 (0.9)	**19.9 (1.1)**	**15.2 (1.0)**	**0.018***
	CXR (0–25 points)	16.5 (0.4)	**18.2 (0.9)**	**15.8 (0.4)**	**0.008***
	Complication (0–37 points)	2.6 (0.5)	**0.3 (0.2)**	**3.5 (0.7)**	**0.000***
	Total	66.9 (2.0)	**77.3 (2.3)**	**62.6 (2.4)**	**0.001***
Quality of life	**Weight**	64.1 (5.2)	**84.5 (5.5)**	**55.9 (6.5)**	**0.016***
	Respiratory	68.3 (2.3)	74.8 (4.5)	65.6 (2.6)	0.072
	Digestion	78.0 (2.5)	84.5 (4.0)	75.4 (3.1)	0.064
	Physical	71.8 (3.4)	**83.3 (3.8)**	**67.2 (4.4)**	**0.041***
	Vitality	64.4 (2.2)	67.8 (4.4)	63.1 (2.6)	0.341
	Emotion	81.7 (2.2)	**90.7 (2.6)**	**78.0 (2.7)**	**0.008***
	Eating	90.3 (2.3)	91.1 (4.8)	89.9 (2.7)	0.537
	Treatment burden	66.2 (3.4)	74.8 (6.7)	62.8 (3.9)	0.113
	Health Perceptions	69.5 (2.8)	**80.8 (4.0)**	**54.9 (3.3)**	**0.009***
	Body Image	73.5 (3.5)	**88.9 (3.1)**	**67.3 (4.3)**	**0.004***
	Social	74.6 (2.5)	81.5 (4.4)	71.8 (2.9)	0.074
	Role	82.8 (2.8)	**91.7 (3.0)**	**79.2 (3.6)**	**0.044***
	Total (0–1200 points)	885.2 (21.8)	**994.2 (28.9)**	**841.0 (25.1)**	**0.001***

Data represented as mean (SEM). * p-value designates significant statistical difference between non-exacerbating (no PE) and exacerbating patients (PE) using Student's t-test or Mann-Whitney t-test when values were not normally distributed. NR indicates normal range for cell counts. BMI normal range from Health Canada (http://www.hc-sc.gc.ca).

"Early PE" patients with significantly higher CRP and IL-8, indicating that these markers may contribute to assessing which patients could rapidly re-exacerbate.

Discussion

The importance of PEs in CF disease progression is well established however the triggers of these events are still being understood which limits the means for prevention. Retrospective studies have identified patient groups at risk of PEs such as those with liver disease, CF related diabetes, low FEV_1 values [5,12]. However, the difficulty remains in determining on an individual basis which patient has a high risk of a future PE.

Our prospective study is unique for two main reasons: 1) the large panel of data that were collected at stable disease and 2) the extensive sampling throughout PEs. With these results, we assessed markers predicting future PE in two distinct cases: from stable disease and at the last day of treatment for PE.

Assessing risk from stable disease

Patients who developed PEs had worse baseline disease severity (based on lung spirometry and BMI), greater baseline disease activity (based on the Matouk Disease Score) and worse self-reported QOL at stable disease. Interestingly, this was associated with higher inflammatory markers (Tables 1 and 2). Using survival models, the clinical (lung spirometry and Matouk Disease score) and QOL assessments were predictive of future PE with better scores associated with lower risk of PE (Figure 1 and Table 3). The inflammatory markers we assessed were not associated with future PE when measured at stable disease. Noteworthy, there was a trend with low CRP associated with low risk of PE, which merits further investigation with a larger cohort of patients. Monitoring changes in these markers may lead to an early recognition of PEs which would allow for earlier intervention. This, in turn, would reduce the impact of heightened and prolonged inflammation on lung tissue.

Table 2. Baseline values of inflammatory markers and fatty acids.

	Healthy controls (HC) n = 3–11	Total CF patients group (CF) n = 52	Non-exacerbating CF patients (no PE) n = 15	Exacerbating CF patients (PE) n = 37
CRP (mg/L)	2.0 (1.1)	7.4 (1.0)	6.04 (1.7)	8.0 (1.2)
IL-1β (pg/ml)	3.8 (2.7)	0.9 (0.1)	0.79 (0.2)	0.9 (0.1)
IL-6 (pg/ml)	2.7 (1.1)	5.2 (1.2)	2.93 (0.6)	**6.0 (1.6)**†
IL-8 (pg/ml)	3.6 (0.9)	5.0 (0.5)	4.08 (0.6)	5.8 (0.6)
IL-10 (pg/ml)	2.1 (0.9)	**29.1 (3.2)***	19.04 (2.6)	**38.8 (7.2)**†
MIP-1β (pg/ml)	31.8 (6.9)	24.3 (1.6)	24.83 (3.2)	24.2 (1.9)
TNF (pg/ml)	5.3 (0.5)	**3.8 (0.3)***	3.45 (0.5)	3.9 (0.4)
VEGF (pg/ml)	129.5 (46.7)	95.7 (16.5)	82.45 (17.3)	101.0 (22.2)
AA (nmol/μg of protein)	37.0 (2.4)	**49.5 (0.8)***	48.45 (1.5)	49.9 (1.0)
DHA (nmol/mg of protein)	2.7 (0.1)	**1.2 (0.1)***	1.30 (0.1)	1.2 (0.1)
AA/DHA ratio	14.4 (1.4)	**48.8 (4.6)***	40.92 (3.8)	51.8 (6.1)

Data represented as mean (SEM). * p-value represents statistically significant difference between HC and CF groups. † represents statistically significant difference between "no PE" and "PE" groups. Significance was set at $p<0.05$.

Presently, there are no known methods which could prevent the occurrence of PEs. Current treatments for CF have shown impacts on reducing the number of PEs, such as routine inhaled antibiotic therapy for infected patients, human recombinant deoxyribonuclease and inhaled hypertonic saline [40]. Some CF centers advocate the routine use of IV antibiotics for two weeks every three months, rather than in only response to PE symptoms. They report improved survival rates using this protocol, however its impact on the rate of PEs is unclear [41,42]. Elborn et al. reported no significant effect of elective IV antibiotics every three months (four/year) in a randomized control trial compared to treating patients because of PEs. Patients in the control group were prescribed IV antibiotics three times per year while 40% of the elective treatments were in response to PEs. Thus it is unclear whether elective IV antibiotics had a significant impact on reducing the rate of PE [43,44]. However, the number of PEs in each group were not directly compared, thus based on the reports currently available, it is difficult to conclude whether the rate of PEs can be reduced by preventative aggressive antibiotics. These treatments were assigned at specific times (every three months) which may come too early to prevent PEs. Rather patients may benefit from obtaining IV antibiotics as soon as a change is detected in their clinical status or QOL assessments. Previous studies have shown that CF patients who recorded their lung spirometry using a daily diary had lower rates of lung function decline than those who did not [45]. A new study by Lechtzin et al. looking at twice weekly electronic symptom recording by CF patients may help determine the usefulness of a more frequent symptom and lung function monitoring for early recognition of PEs[7].

Table 3. Markers influencing time to first PE during stable disease.

Marker		Hazard ratio[1]	95% hazard ratio confidence limits	p-value
Clinical assessment	FEV1% predicted	0.97	0.94–0.99	0.006
	FVC% predicted	0.97	0.95–0.99	0.010
Matouk Disease Score	Clinical	0.74	0.63–0.86	0.000
	PFT	0.88	0.80–0.98	0.015
	CXR	0.71	0.50–0.94	0.017
	Complication	1.33	1.17–1.51	0.000
	Total	0.92	0.88–0.96	0.000
Quality of life	Weight	0.97	0.95–0.99	0.006
	Respiratory	0.96	0.92–0.99	0.024
	Physical	0.96	0.93–0.99	0.003
	Vitality	0.96	0.93–1.00	0.043
	Health perceptions	0.95	0.92–0.99	0.005
	Role	0.96	0.94–0.99	0.020
	Total	0.99	0.99–1.00	0.004

[1]HR<1 is associated with lower risk of future PE.

Table 4. Markers associated with early re-exacerbation at the end of PE treatment.

	Early PE (n = 6)	Late PE (n = 6)	p- value
Days until next PE mean (min – max)	17.3 (1–29)	142.5 (56–365)	N/A
FEV1% predicted (%)	38.5 (7.2)	50.0 (8.5)	0.328
FVC% predicted (%)	56.5 (9.9)	64.0 (10.0)	0.606
Matouk Total score	46.5 (6.2)	56.8 (3.7)	0.180
QOL Total score	752.0 (86.7)	765.5 (62.8)	0.902
CRP (mg/L)	42.5 (26.1)	5.2 (2.7)	**0.045***
IL-6 (pg/ml)	4.9 (1.6)	2.6 (0.6)	0.199
IL-8 (pg/ml)	3.9 (0.4)	2.7 (0.3)	**0.034***
IL-10 (pg/ml)	24.4 (2.5)	77.0 (37.8)	0.195

Data presented as mean (SEM) unless specified. * indicates significant difference between the groups using Student's t-test or Mann-Whitney test if values were not normally distributed.

Prediction from end of treatment

Each PE significantly decreases lung function in CF patients, even more with PEs in rapid succession [4]. In our study, we found that higher inflammation at the end of treatment may be a better indication of early re-exacerbation rather than clinical or patient QOL assessments (Table 4). The few prospective studies looking at predictors of future PEs used measurements at the end of PE treatment. CRP was previously shown to be correlated to the number of days until the next PE [14], a finding not universally reported[15]. Regardless of the discrepancies, these studies showed the usefulness of inflammatory markers such as CRP and calprotectin in assessing risk of future PE [14,15]. Sequeiros et al. also showed that early re-exacerbation was correlated with more symptoms after 14 days of treatment such as cough, sputum production, breathlessness and fatigue [14].

We found that FEV_1% values tended to be lower in patients that quickly re-exacerbated, and due to our small patient group, we cannot disregard this as a marker of recurring PE. Thus, inflammatory markers such as CRP and IL-8, in conjunction with patient reported symptoms, clinical evaluations and spirometry, could be additional indicators of a recurring PE. And, although symptoms and clinical picture (lung function and Matouk Disease score) have returned to baseline at the end of treatment, patients may still be experiencing some level of unresolved inflammation indicating the PE has not been cleared completely. There has been evidence that extending the course of antibiotics may only offer a small improvement in symptoms but not lung function or inflammation[46]. In these cases, perhaps a change in antibiotics and/or the use of anti-inflammatory agents to aid in the resolution of inflammation would benefit the patient and prevent early re-exacerbation. However, based on our study, we cannot determine whether the unresolved inflammation itself triggers a new PE or whether it is a response to other underlying active processes such as a poorly controlled infection. We did not look at causes of PEs such as viral infections which have been reported to impact recovery from PE[9].

Kinetics of inflammation and PUFA throughout PE

We found in general inflammatory markers increased at PE onset such as CRP, IL-6, IL-8, MIP-1β and VEGF compared to values at stable disease periods, and responded to treatment as soon as Day 7 (Figure 3). This corroborates previous findings regarding resolution of inflammation with antibiotic treatment[14,27,32,47]. MIP-1β, a chemoattractant for monocytes, has rarely been assessed in CF and, to our knowledge, this is the first time reported to respond to treatment in the context of PEs in CF.

Our study design allowed us to monitor whether improvements during PE treatment are maintained after treatment was completed. Five patients out of 13 were not available for Day 42 assessments due to a re-exacerbation (n = 4) or other complications (n = 1, same patient that was excluded from the second study on markers associated with early re-exacerbation). Even with this small number of patients, we were able to observe decreases in FVC% values and increases in CRP and MIP-1β at Day 42 compared to baseline values. Due to the small sample size and large variation at this time point, we could not conclude whether these changes are indicative of future exacerbations and further studies are necessary. However, it is important to recognize that improvements at the end of treatment, a time point assessed in many PE studies, may not be representative of the patient's disease status on the long term.

Few studies have assessed the changes in PUFAs at PE onset and throughout treatment[48,49]. Similar to our results regarding lipid peroxidation, McGrath and colleagues demonstrated a decrease MDA in CF patients after antibiotic treatment for PE[50]. The improvements in PUFA during PE occur during treatment but worsen at Day 42, when patients are no longer treated for PE. Thus the improvements in the AA/DHA ratio may be due to the effects of the treatment itself in reducing lipid peroxidation, also observed in this study. Antibiotics have been shown to protect lung epithelial cells from oxidative damage[51]. Tobramycin in particular was found to act as a potent reactive oxygen species scavenger[52]. In general, PUFAs are very susceptible to peroxidation due to their high content of double bonds compared to other types of fatty acids causing DHA to be more affected than AA[53]. The increase in anti-inflammatory DHA may contribute to the resolution of inflammation. Additionally, the reduction in lipid peroxidation may itself be a factor. Oxidized fatty acids such as DHA were found to act on Toll-Like Receptor 4 much like its ligand lipopolysaccharide activating downstream NF-κB signalling[54]. It is important to note that changes in PUFA were not permanent and routine treatments for disease maintenance do not normalize PUFA levels since CF patients at stable disease still have defects in AA and DHA levels (Figure 4 and Table 2). Currently, no antibiotic or steroid therapy for CF has proven to be successful in correcting

PUFA abnormalities, which could improve disease status of patients.

Limitations

Our study has several limitations that are important to consider. Among the 52 patients included in our analysis, we had longitudinal clinical and molecular marker measurements in only 13 patients during their PEs. Due to the extensive testing and the availability of the clinical coordinator, this was the volume of patients we could handle for the study period. However, due to the large panel of markers we assessed and the prospective nature of the study design, this study remains an important exploratory analysis generating many hypotheses about predictive markers of PE.

The median time to next PE was somewhat low suggesting that our patient group had high disease activity. Parkins et al. described that 13% of their patient cohort re-exacerbated in 45 days. They used this time point as a definition of non-response to treatment which may be another way to describe the six patients with early re-exacerbations since they had higher levels of inflammation[1]. Our Day 42 time point was also affected when it overlapped with new PEs. Noteworthy, our definition of PE was more inclusive than the other definitions used[5,14,27] as it included any event needing additional IV or oral therapy thereby including mild and severe types of exacerbations.

Conclusions

This study demonstrates that monitoring changes in clinical and patient reported assessments during stable disease may help in determining which patients are at risk for PEs. Our longitudinal analysis of inflammation throughout PEs suggests that, at the end of antibiotic treatment for PE, inflammatory markers could contribute to monitoring patients at risk of early recurring PE. The imbalance in PUFA levels improve after treatment for PE possibly due to a decrease in lipid peroxidation. Regarding early re-exacerbation, our analysis reveals that CRP and IL-8 in particular can be important in assessing patients at risk of early recurring PEs, which needs to be confirmed in a larger study. The data presented here offer more insight into potential markers of PEs which, in conjunction with clinical data, may improve earlier recognition of PEs in CF.

Supporting Information

File S1 Additional explanation of methods including a full description of the scoring method and points allocated for the Matouk Disease Score, and additional information regarding the statistical methods used.

Table S1 Percentage change of clinical parameters throughout exacerbations in CF. Includes percentage change, standard errors and statistical evaluation of clinical parameters, Matouk Disease Score and QOL assessments throughout PE time points.

Table S2 Percentage change of inflammatory markers during PE. Includes percentage change, standard errors and statistical evaluation of inflammatory markers throughout PE time points.

Acknowledgments

We would like to thank all the personnel at the Adult Cystic Fibrosis Clinic at the Montreal Chest Institute, all the patients and healthy volunteers participating in this study.

Author Contributions

Conceived and designed the experiments: GW HGA JG JL LCL DN SR EM DR. Performed the experiments: GW JBS. Analyzed the data: GW AB. Contributed reagents/materials/analysis tools: JBS SR DR. Wrote the paper: GW DR. Clinical assessments of patients: J. Bernier EM. Administration of quality of life questionnaire: J. Bernier. Blood sample processing: J. Bérubé.

References

1. Parkins MD, Rendall JC, Elborn JS (2012) Incidence and risk factors for pulmonary exacerbation treatment failures in patients with cystic fibrosis chronically infected with Pseudomonas aeruginosa. Chest 141: 485–493.
2. Sanders DB, Bittner RC, Rosenfeld M, Hoffman LR, Redding GJ, et al. (2010) Failure to recover to baseline pulmonary function after cystic fibrosis pulmonary exacerbation. Am J Respir Crit Care Med 182: 627–632.
3. Liou TG, Adler FR, Fitzsimmons SC, Cahill BC, Hibbs JR, et al. (2001) Predictive 5-year survivorship model of cystic fibrosis. Am J Epidemiol 153: 345–352.
4. Waters V, Stanojevic S, Atenafu EG, Lu A, Yau Y, et al. (2012) Effect of pulmonary exacerbations on long-term lung function decline in cystic fibrosis. Eur Respir J 40: 61–66.
5. de Boer K, Vandemheen KL, Tullis E, Doucette S, Fergusson D, et al. (2011) Exacerbation frequency and clinical outcomes in adult patients with cystic fibrosis. Thorax 66: 680–685.
6. Hakimi Shoki A, Mayer-Hamblett N, Wilcox PG, Sin DD, Quon BS (2013) Systematic Review of Blood Biomarkers in Cystic Fibrosis Pulmonary Exacerbations. Chest epub Jul 18.
7. Lechtzin N, West N, Allgood S, Wilhelm E, Khan U, et al. (2013) Rationale and design of a randomized trial of home electronic symptom and lung function monitoring to detect cystic fibrosis pulmonary exacerbations: The early intervention in cystic fibrosis exacerbation (eICE) trial. Contemp Clin Trials 36: 460–469.
8. Hoek RA, Paats MS, Pas SD, Bakker M, Hoogsteden HC, et al. (2013) Incidence of viral respiratory pathogens causing exacerbations in adult cystic fibrosis patients. Scand J Infect Dis 45: 65–69.
9. Etherington C, Naseer R, Conway SP, Whitaker P, Denton M, et al. (2013) The role of respiratory viruses in adult patients with cystic fibrosis receiving intravenous antibiotics for a pulmonary exacerbation. J Cyst Fibros epub Jul 23.
10. Farhat SC, Almeida MB, Silva-Filho LV, Farhat J, Rodrigues JC, et al. (2013) Ozone is associated with an increased risk of respiratory exacerbations in patients with cystic fibrosis. Chest 144: 1186–1192.
11. Fodor AA, Klem ER, Gilpin DF, Elborn JS, Boucher RC, et al. (2012) The adult cystic fibrosis airway microbiota is stable over time and infection type, and highly resilient to antibiotic treatment of exacerbations. PLoS One 7: e45001.
12. Sawicki GS, Ayyagari R, Zhang J, Signorovitch JE, Fan L, et al. (2013) A pulmonary exacerbation risk score among cystic fibrosis patients not receiving recommended care. Pediatr Pulmonol 48: 954–961.
13. Sutton S, Rosenbluth D, Raghavan D, Zheng J, Jain R (2013) Effects of puberty on cystic fibrosis related pulmonary exacerbations in women versus men. Pediatr Pulmonol epub Mar 4.
14. Sequeiros IM, Jarad N (2012) Factors associated with a shorter time until the next pulmonary exacerbation in adult patients with cystic fibrosis. Chron Respir Dis 9: 9–16.
15. Gray RD, Imrie M, Boyd AC, Porteous D, Innes JA, et al. (2010) Sputum and serum calprotectin are useful biomarkers during CF exacerbation. J Cyst Fibros 9: 193–198.
16. Matouk E, Ghezzo RH, Gruber J, Hidvegi R, Gray-Donald K (1997) Internal consistency reliability and predictive validity of a modified N. Huang clinical scoring system in adult cystic fibrosis patients. Eur Respir J 10: 2004–2013.
17. Matouk E, Ghezzo RH, Gruber J, Hidvegi R, Gray-Donald K (1999) Construct and longitudinal validity of a modified Huang clinical scoring system in adult cystic fibrosis patients. Eur Respir J 13: 552–559.
18. Society AT (1987) Standardization of Spirometry, a Statement of the American Thoracic Society. Am Rev Respir Dis 136: 1285–1298.
19. Knudson RJ, Lebowitz MD, Holberg CJ, Burrows B (1983) Changes in the normal maximal expiratory flow-volume curve with growth and aging. Am Rev Respir Dis 127: 725–734.

20. Quittner AL, Sweeny S, Watrous M, Munzenberger P, Bearss K, et al. (2000) Translation and linguistic validation of a disease-specific quality of life measure for cystic fibrosis. J Pediatr Psychol 25: 403–414.
21. Folch J, Lees M, Sloane Stanely GH (1957) A simple method for the isolation and purification of total lipides from animal tissues. J Biol Chem 226: 497–509.
22. Schlenk H, Gellerman J (1960) Esterification of fatty acids with diazomethane on a small scale. Anal Chem 32: 1412–1414.
23. Oborna I, Wojewodka G, De Sanctis JB, Fingerova H, Svobodova M, et al. (2010) Increased lipid peroxidation and abnormal fatty acid profiles in seminal and blood plasma of normozoospermic males from infertile couples. Hum Reprod 25: 308–316.
24. Freedman SD, Blanco PG, Zaman MM, Shea JC, Ollero M, et al. (2004) Association of cystic fibrosis with abnormalities in fatty acid metabolism. N Engl J Med 350: 560–569.
25. Guilbault C, Wojewodka G, Saeed Z, Hajduch M, Matouk E, et al. (2009) Cystic Fibrosis Fatty Acid Imbalance is Linked to Ceramide Deficiency and Corrected by Fenretinide. Am J Respir Cell Mol Biol 41: 100–106.
26. Gilljam H, Strandvik B, Ellin A, Wiman LG (1986) Increased mole fraction of arachidonic acid in bronchial phospholipids in patients with cystic fibrosis. Scand J Clin Lab Invest 46: 511–518.
27. Horsley AR, Davies JC, Gray RD, Macleod KA, Donovan J, et al. (2013) Changes in physiological, functional and structural markers of cystic fibrosis lung disease with treatment of a pulmonary exacerbation. Thorax 68: 532–539.
28. Downey DG, Brockbank S, Martin SL, Ennis M, Elborn JS (2007) The effect of treatment of cystic fibrosis pulmonary exacerbations on airways and systemic inflammation. Pediatr Pulmonol 42: 729–735.
29. Nixon LS, Yung B, Bell SC, Elborn JS, Shale DJ (1998) Circulating immunoreactive interleukin-6 in cystic fibrosis. Am J Respir Crit Care Med 157: 1764–1769.
30. Liou TG, Adler FR, Keogh RH, Li Y, Jensen JL, et al. (2012) Sputum biomarkers and the prediction of clinical outcomes in patients with cystic fibrosis. PLoS One 7: e42748.
31. Chiron R, Grumbach YY, Quynh NV, Verriere V, Urbach V (2008) Lipoxin A(4) and interleukin-8 levels in cystic fibrosis sputum after antibiotherapy. J Cyst Fibros 7: 463–468.
32. Colombo C, Costantini D, Rocchi A, Cariani L, Garlaschi ML, et al. (2005) Cytokine levels in sputum of cystic fibrosis patients before and after antibiotic therapy. Pediatr Pulmonol 40: 15–21.
33. Lloyd-Still JD, Powers CA, Hoffman DR, Boyd-Trull K, Lester LA, et al. (2006) Bioavailability and safety of a high dose of docosahexaenoic acid triacylglycerol of algal origin in cystic fibrosis patients: a randomized, controlled study. Nutrition 22: 36–46.
34. Strandvik B, Bronnegard M, Gilljam H, Carlstedt-Duke J (1988) Relation between defective regulation of arachidonic acid release and symptoms in cystic fibrosis. ScandJGastroenterolSuppl 143: 1–4.
35. Konstan MW, Walenga RW, Hilliard KA, Hilliard JB (1993) Leukotriene B4 markedly elevated in the epithelial lining fluid of patients with cystic fibrosis. AmRevRespirDis 148: 896–901.
36. Lucidi V, Ciabattoni G, Bella S, Barnes PJ, Montuschi P (2008) Exhaled 8-isoprostane and prostaglandin E(2) in patients with stable and unstable cystic fibrosis. Free RadicBiolMed 45: 913–919.
37. Lawrence RH, Sorrell TC (1994) Eicosapentaenoic acid modulates neutrophil leukotriene B4 receptor expression in cystic fibrosis. Clin Exp Immunol 98: 12–16.
38. Weldon SM, Mullen AC, Loscher CE, Hurley LA, Roche HM (2007) Docosahexaenoic acid induces an anti-inflammatory profile in lipopolysaccharide-stimulated human THP-1 macrophages more effectively than eicosapentaenoic acid. J Nutr Biochem 18: 250–258.
39. Guilbault C, De Sanctis JB, Wojewodka G, Saeed Z, Lachance C, et al. (2008) Fenretinide corrects newly found ceramide deficiency in cystic fibrosis. AmJRespirCell MolBiol 38: 47–56.
40. Flume PA, O'Sullivan BP, Robinson KA, Goss CH, Mogayzel PJ Jr., et al. (2007) Cystic fibrosis pulmonary guidelines: chronic medications for maintenance of lung health. AmJRespirCrit Care Med 176: 957–969.
41. Szaff M, Hoiby N, Flensborg EW (1983) Frequent antibiotic therapy improves survival of cystic fibrosis patients with chronic Pseudomonas aeruginosa infection. Acta Paediatr Scand 72: 651–657.
42. Nir M, Lanng S, Johansen HK, Koch C (1996) Long-term survival and nutritional data in patients with cystic fibrosis treated in a Danish centre. Thorax 51: 1023–1027.
43. Elborn JS, Prescott RJ, Stack BH, Goodchild MC, Bates J, et al. (2000) Elective versus symptomatic antibiotic treatment in cystic fibrosis patients with chronic Pseudomonas infection of the lungs. Thorax 55: 355–358.
44. Breen L, Aswani N (2012) Elective versus symptomatic intravenous antibiotic therapy for cystic fibrosis. Cochrane Database Syst Rev 7: CD002767.
45. Finkelstein SM, Wielinski CL, Kujawa SJ, Loewenson R, Warwick WJ (1992) The impact of home monitoring and daily diary recording on patient status in cystic fibrosis. Pediatr Pulmonol 12: 3–10.
46. Sequeiros IM, Jarad NA (2012) Extending the course of intravenous antibiotics in adult patients with cystic fibrosis with acute pulmonary exacerbations. Chron Respir Dis 9: 213–220.
47. McColley SA, Stellmach V, Boas SR, Jain M, Crawford SE (2000) Serum vascular endothelial growth factor is elevated in cystic fibrosis and decreases with treatment of acute pulmonary exacerbation. Am J Respir Crit Care Med 161: 1877–1880.
48. Durieu I, Abbas-Chorfa F, Drai J, Iwaz J, Steghens JP, et al. (2007) Plasma fatty acids and lipid hydroperoxides increase after antibiotic therapy in cystic fibrosis. Eur Respir J 29: 958–964.
49. Durieu I, Vericel E, Guichardant D, Roth H, Steghens JP, et al. (2007) Fatty acids platelets and oxidative markers following intravenous n-3 fatty acids administration in cystic fibrosis: An open pilot observational study. J Cyst Fibros 6: 320–326.
50. McGrath LT, Mallon P, Dowey L, Silke B, McClean E, et al. (1999) Oxidative stress during acute respiratory exacerbations in cystic fibrosis. Thorax 54: 518–523.
51. Cantin A, Woods DE (1993) Protection by antibiotics against myeloperoxidase-dependent cytotoxicity to lung epithelial cells in vitro. J Clin Invest 91: 38–45.
52. Gziut M, MacGregor HJ, Nevell TG, Mason T, Laight D, et al. (2013) Anti-inflammatory effects of tobramycin and a copper-tobramycin complex with superoxide dismutase-like activity. Br J Pharmacol 168: 1165–1181.
53. Halliwell B, Chirico S (1993) Lipid peroxidation: its mechanism, measurement, and significance. Am J Clin Nutr 57: 715S–724S.
54. Mutoh A, Ueda S (2013) Peroxidized unsaturated fatty acids stimulate Toll-like receptor 4 signaling in endothelial cells. Life Sci 92: 984–992.

3

Insulin-Like Growth Factor 1 (IGF-1) Enhances the Protein Expression of CFTR

Ha Won Lee[1], Jie Cheng[1], Olga Kovbasnjuk[2], Mark Donowitz[1], William B. Guggino[1]*

1 Department of Physiology, Johns Hopkins University, School of Medicine, Baltimore, Maryland, United States of America, **2** Department of Medicine, Johns Hopkins University, School of Medicine, Baltimore, Maryland, United States of America

Abstract

Low levels of insulin-like growth factor 1 (IGF-1) have been observed in the serum of cystic fibrosis (CF) patients. However, the effects of low serum IGF-1 on the cystic fibrosis transmembrane conductance regulator (CFTR), whose defective function is the primary cause of cystic fibrosis, have not been studied. Here, we show in human cells that IGF-1 increases the steady-state levels of mature wildtype CFTR in a CFTR-associated ligand (CAL)- and TC10-dependent manner; moreover, IGF-1 increases CFTR-mediated chloride transport. Using an acceptor photobleaching fluorescence resonance energy transfer (FRET) assay, we have confirmed the binding of CAL and CFTR in the Golgi. We also show that CAL overexpression inhibits forskolin-induced increases in the cell-surface expression of CFTR. We found that IGF-1 activates TC10, and active TC10 alters the functional association between CAL and CFTR. Furthermore, IGF-1 and active TC10 can reverse the CAL-mediated reduction in the cell-surface expression of CFTR. IGF-1 does not increase the expression of ΔF508 CFTR, whose processing is arrested in the ER. This finding is consistent with our observation that IGF-1 alters the functional interaction of CAL and CFTR in the Golgi. However, when ΔF508 CFTR is rescued with low temperature or the corrector VRT-325 and proceeds to the Golgi, IGF-1 can increase the expression of the rescued ΔF508 CFTR. Our data support a model indicating that CAL-CFTR binding in the Golgi inhibits CFTR trafficking to the cell surface, leading CFTR to the degradation pathway instead. IGF-1-activated TC10 changes the interaction of CFTR and CAL, allowing CFTR to progress to the plasma membrane. These findings offer a potential strategy using a combinational treatment of IGF-1 and correctors to increase the post-Golgi expression of CFTR in cystic fibrosis patients bearing the ΔF508 mutation.

Editor: Effie C. Tsilibary, National Center for Scientific Research Demokritos, Greece

Funding: This work was supported by the Cystic Fibrosis Foundation GUGGINO5X0, Korea Science and Engineering Foundation (KOSEF), and the National Institutes of Health (NHLBI PO1 HL51811 to WBG, NIDDK PO1 DK072084 to WBG, MD, OK; and RO1 DK 58928 to OK). The funders had no role in study design, data collection and analysis, decision to publish, or preparation of the manuscript.

Competing Interests: The authors declare that there are no completing interests.

* E-mail: wguggino@jhmi.edu

Introduction

Cystic fibrosis is a genetic disease caused by mutations in CFTR [1]. CFTR's primary function is to move chloride ions across the plasma membrane of epithelial cells; this is a key function in the normal operation of several organs, including the airways, the intestinal tract, the pancreas, the epididymis, and the sweat duct (see [2] for a review). Dysfunctional chloride transport of mutant CFTRs leads to pathologically low levels of fluid, accompanied by altered composition in the airways, pancreatic duct, and intestinal tract, and it causes symptoms such as bacterial airway infections, chronic inflammation, growth retardation, male infertility, and obstruction of pancreatic ducts and the gastrointestinal tract. Failure to absorb fluid in the sweat ducts leads to high sweat chloride in patients, a symptom that has been used as a defining factor prior to the identification of the CF gene [3].

Because CFTR is localized at the cell surface to transport chloride ions, CFTR mutations resulting in improper localization (e.g., the most common mutation, ΔF508 CFTR) are particularly severe [4,5]. Therefore, the processes involved in the trafficking of both wildtype and ΔF508 CFTR have been studied extensively (see [6] for a review). It is now well known that CFTR trafficking to the cell surface is regulated by PDZ proteins (the Golgi reassembly stacking protein [GRASP], CFTR-associated ligand [CAL], Na^+/H^+ exchanger regulatory factor [NHERF1/2], and CFTR-associated protein 70 [CAP70]), which bind to CFTR [7–10]. These proteins assemble CFTR into protein complexes in the ER, Golgi, or plasma membrane in polarized epithelial cells [8,10] and ultimately regulate CFTR localization at the apical membrane by allowing CFTR to reach the plasma membrane, sequestering it within the cell, or targeting it for degradation (see [11] for review). For example, GRASP is localized to the Golgi [12]. When ER stress occurs, GRASP is phosphorylated and then binds to CFTR, leading to CFTR trafficking from the ER to the cell surface through a unique trafficking pathway [9]. CAL regulates the total and cell-surface expression of CFTR, either by enhancing the lysosomal degradation of CFTR [7] or allowing it to traffic to the plasma membrane, depending on which secondary proteins are bound to CAL [13]. At the plasma membrane, NHERF and CAP70 stabilize CFTR and allow CFTR to form an efficient functional complex [8,14,15].

As previously mentioned, CAL and its associated binding proteins regulate the lysosomal degradation and surface expression of CFTR [13,16]. CAL is an adaptor protein that has multiple protein-interacting domains, including a PDZ domain that binds CFTR and two coiled-coil domains that are responsible for its

Golgi localization. Syntaxin 6 (STX6), a soluble N-ethylmaleimide-sensitive factor-activating protein receptor protein (SNARE) protein, and TC10, a small GTPase of the Rho family, are known to bind to CAL in the region of the coiled-coil domains [17,18].

STX6 is involved in intracellular vesicle trafficking [16,18,19]. Binding of STX6 to CAL reduces CFTR protein expression by increasing the transport of CFTR to the lysosome and thus promoting the lysosomal degradation of CFTR. Therefore, when bound to STX6, CAL is a negative regulator of both the total and cell surface expression of CFTR. In contrast, TC10 is a positive regulator of CFTR surface expression: By binding to CAL, it promotes the trafficking of CFTR to the plasma membrane and increases the total and cell-surface expression of CFTR [13]. Although the interaction of CFTR with CAL, TC10, and STX6 has been studied, how these pathways are regulated is not known. Information on how this regulation occurs certainly has implications for our understanding of both wildtype CFTR and the mutant ΔF508 CFTR.

Given that active TC10 promotes the trafficking of CFTR to the cell surface [13], the question to be asked is how TC10 is activated to increase the surface expression of CFTR.? IGF-1 and insulin activate TC10 through a GTP exchange factor in neurons and adipocytes [20,21]. IGF-1 activates TC10 in neurons for neuronal growth, and insulin increases GLUT4 vesicle translocation in adipocytes for glucose uptake by activating TC10 [21–23]. Thus, it is likely that IGF-1 and/or insulin is(are) the upstream activator(s) of TC10 that ultimately regulate(s) CFTR protein expression. CF patients as well as CF pig models have low IGF-1 levels in their serum [24–27], an observation that also has implications for the pathophysiology of CF. Therefore, in this report, we tested whether IGF-1 alters CFTR expression. Dominant-negative TC10 was used to determine whether TC10 activation is required for any of the IGF-1-induced changes in CFTR protein expression. Our results showed that TC10, activated via IGF-1, does indeed alter the functional interaction between CFTR and CAL, ultimately increasing CFTR surface expression. We also suggest that IGF-1 may have therapeutic value in patients bearing the ΔF508 CFTR mutation.

Materials and Methods

Reagents and Antibodies

IGF-1, forskolin, and brefeldin A were obtained from Sigma. cDNAs encoding EYFP-tagged wildtype or mutant CFTR were subcloned with the pEYFP-C1 plasmid (Clontech), and cDNA encoding ECFP-tagged CAL was subcloned with the pECFP-C1 plasmid (Clontech), in the same manner that GFP was tagged to CFTR and CAL in previous studies [7,28]. Anti-CFTR antibodies were obtained from the University of North Carolina (217) and Upstate (M3A7). Anti-GFP antibody (ab290) and anti-Na,K-ATPase antibody (464.6) were purchased from Abcam, anti-HA antibody (12CA5) from Roche, and anti-HA antibody conjugated with HRP from Sigma. Anti-GM130 antibody (35/GM130) was obtained from BD Bioscience and Alexa-647 goat anti-mouse IgG from Invitrogen.

Cell Culture and Transfection

HeLa cells were cultured in Dulbecco's modified Eagle's medium (DMEM, Invitrogen) supplemented with 10% fetal bovine serum (FBS, Invitrogen) and penicillin/streptomycin (Invitrogen) in a humidified 37°C CO_2 incubator. CFBE41o- cells (a cell line from bronchial epithelial cells of a cystic fibrosis patient [29,30], kindly provided by Dr. Gruenert) were cultured in minimum essential medium Eagle (MEM, Invitrogen) with 10% FBS and penicillin/streptomycin, and CFBE-WTCFTR cells (CFBE41o- cells stably transfected with wildtype CFTR [30], kindly provided by Dr. Gruenert) were cultured in MEM with 10% FBS, penicillin/streptomycin and 300 µg/ml hygromycin B. For serum starvation, HeLa cells were cultured in DMEM with 0.5% FBS, and CFBE and CFBE-WTCFTR cells were cultured in MEM without FBS. Cells were transiently transfected with Lipofectamine 2000 reagent (Invitrogen) according to the manufacturer's instruction and incubated for 24–48 hours.

Coimmunoprecipitation and Western Blotting

Cells were washed twice with cold Dulbecco's phosphate buffered saline (DPBS, Invitrogen), and then resuspended in lysis buffer (150 mM Tris, 50 mM NaCl, 1% Nonidet P-40, pH 7.4) with protease inhibitor cocktail (Roche). After 20 minutes on ice, the lysates were cleared by centrifugation at 15,000 g for 20 minutes. Pellets were discarded, and supernatants were used for further experiments. Protein G-Sepharose (GE Healthcare) was mixed with cleared lysates and primary antibodies and incubated on a rotary shaker at 4°C overnight. The beads were washed three times with lysis buffer and incubated in Laemmli buffer at 95°C for 5 minutes or at 42°C for 20 minutes. Total cleared lysates were denatured in Laemmli buffer at 42°C for 20 minutes. The protein concentration of each sample was measured with a BCA protein assay kit (Thermo Scientific), and equal amounts of total proteins were loaded on HCl-Tris gels.

Proteins were separated by SDS-PAGE and transferred to PVDF membranes (BioRad). After the transfer, the membranes were blocked with 5% nonfat milk in Tris-buffered saline with 0.05% Tween 20 (TBST) for 1 hour. The membranes were incubated with primary antibodies in 5% milk in TBST at 4°C overnight. The membranes were washed four times with TBST and incubated with Clean-Blot IP Detection Reagent (Thermo Scientific) or appropriate horseradish peroxidase-conjugated secondary antibodies (GE Healthcare).

Cell-surface Biotinylation

After cells were washed four times with cold DPBS containing 1 mM Ca^{2+} and 1 mM Mg^{2+}, they were incubated with 0.5 mg/ml sulfo-NHS-SS-biotin (Thermo Scientific) in DPBS with Ca^{2+} and Mg^{2+} at 4°C for 30 minutes. Free sulfo-NHS-SS-biotin was then quenched by washing with cold 192 mM glycine in DPBS four times. Cells were lysed with lysis buffer, and the lysates were centrifuged at 15,000 g at 4°C for 20 minutes. The supernatants were incubated with NeutrAvidin UltraLink Resin (Thermo Scientific) at 4°C for 5 hours or overnight. The beads were washed twice with lysis buffer, and proteins were eluted with Laemmli buffer at 42°C for 20 minutes. Biotinylated protein samples were analyzed by western blotting as described above.

TC10 Activity Assays

HA-tagged TC10 [13] was transfected into cells. The transfected cells were serum-starved, and after 24 hours, the cells were treated with 0.1 µg/ml IGF-1 for another 24 hours. After a wash with cold DPBS, the cells were scraped in magnesium-containing lysis buffer (Millipore), and the cell lysates were incubated with GST-PAK-1 PBD-conjugated agarose beads (Millipore) for 1 hour and washed with the lysis buffer three times [31,32]. Laemmli buffer was added to the beads and boiled for 5 minutes.

Fluorescence Microscope and Acceptor Photobleaching Fluorescence Resonance Energy Transfer (FRET)

A Zeiss LSM 510 laser scanning system and 40x oil-immersion lens were used. Cells were seeded onto cover glasses or a glass-bottom dish. The following steps were done at room temperature: After a wash with cold DPBS, cells were fixed with 4% paraformaldehyde for 10 minutes. For immunostaining, after the fixation, cells were permeabilized with DPBS containing 0.1% Triton X-100 for 20 minutes and blocked with 1% bovine albumin serum or 5% goat serum (both from Sigma) for 1 hour. After blocking, the cells were incubated with primary antibodies and then with secondary antibodies conjugated to Alexa 647. Cells were mounted using ProLong Gold with DAPI (Invitrogen).

CFP was excited by a 458-nm Argon/2 laser, and the emission was detected with a 465–510 filter; YFP was excited by a 514-nm Argon/2 laser, and the emission was detected with a 520–555 filter. Alexa 647 was excited by a 633-nm HeNe633 and detected with a 646–700 filter. The 16-bit look-up table originally provided with ImageJ was applied to CFP images taken for FRET.

CFP/YFP pairs were used for acceptor photobleaching FRET. Images for CFP and YFP were collected before and after photobleaching with the 514-nm Argon/2 laser at the maximum intensity. From the images, the signal intensity of CFP was measured with ImageJ image software (NIH), and FRET efficiency was calculated using the following formula: $\mathit{FRET\ efficiency}\ (\%) = \left(1 - \frac{I_{Pre}}{I_{Post}}\right) \times 100$, where I_{Pre} and I_{Post} correspond to the CFP signal intensity (background signal was subtracted) before and after photobleaching, respectively.

For quantification of the colocalization, Pearson's correlation coefficients were calculated with an ImageJ plugin, Colocalization Test (Wright Cell Image Facility, Canada).

Short-circuit Current Measurements

Short-circuit current (I_{SC}) measurements were performed in a six-channel Easy-Mount chamber system (Physiologic Instruments, San Diego, CA) that accepts Snapwell filters (Corning Costar, Acton, MA; 3407). I_{SC} was measured with a VCCMC6 multichannel voltage-current clamp amplifier (Physiologic Instruments) in the voltage-clamp mode. Data were acquired on an 1.71-GHz PC running Windows XP (Microsoft, Redmond, WA) and equipped with DI-720 (DATAQ Instruments, Akron, OH), with Acquire and Analyze version 2.3.159 (Physiologic Instruments) software. Cells were cultured to confluence on Snapwell filters before measurement. The cell monolayers were bathed on both sides with solution containing 115 mM NaCl, 25 mM sodium gluconate, 5 mM potassium gluconate, 1.2 mM $MgCl_2$, 1.2 mM $CaCl_2$, 10 mM D-glucose and 10 mM HEPES (pH 7.4 with NaOH). The mucosal side was replaced with a low Cl^- solution containing 139 mM sodium gluconate, 1.2 mM NaCl, 5 mM potassium gluconate, 1.2 mM $MgCl_2$, 1.2 mM $CaCl_2$, 10 mM D-glucose, and 10 mM HEPES (pH 7.4 with NaOH). The solution was constantly circulated, maintained at 37°C, and bubbled gently with air. Amiloride (20 μM) was added to the mucosal solution, and after stabilization, forskolin (10 μM) was added to the serosal chamber, followed by the CFTR channel inhibitor CFTRinh-172 (5 μM).

Statistical Analysis

All quantitative results are given as averages ± standard error (SE). Statistical significance was determined using Student's *t*-test. Values of $p<0.05$ were considered significant.

Results

CAL Binds to CFTR at the Golgi

To find out how CAL regulates CFTR trafficking, we investigated the interaction between CAL and CFTR by using an acceptor photobleaching FRET assay. For the assay, expression vectors of CFP-tagged CAL and YFP-tagged CFTR were constructed. As a first step, the binding of CAL-CFP and YFP-CFTR was confirmed by coimmunoprecipitation in HeLa cells (Fig. 1A). Next, CAL-CFP was transiently transfected into HeLa cells with YFP-CFTR or with YFP-ΔTRL CFTR, which does not bind CAL, and their FRET efficiency was then measured. The FRET results (Fig. 1B-E) confirmed the binding of YFP-CFTR and CAL-CFP, showing that the FRET efficiency of CAL-CFP and YFP-wildtype CFTR was significantly higher than that of the negative controls (CAL-CFP alone or with YFP-ΔTRL CFTR). These results demonstrate that CAL binds CFTR, but not ΔTRL CFTR, *in vivo* and that the detected FRET is specific for the binding of CAL to CFTR.

The cell compartment in which CAL binds CFTR was determined by immunostaining for GM130, a Golgi marker. CAL-CFP and YFP-CFTR were colocalized with GM130 (Fig. 1F). Their colocalization within the Golgi and their binding suggest that CAL-CFP binds to YFP-CFTR in the Golgi. To support this result, we examined the FRET between CAL-CFP and YFP-CFTR after treatment with brefeldin A (BFA), a chemical that disrupts Golgi structure. Following treatment of cells with 10 μg/ml BFA at 37°C for 30 minutes, CAL-CFP was expressed throughout the cells, and the FRET between CAL-CFP and YFP-CFTR was reduced markedly (Fig. 2C,E). Thus, the *in vivo* binding of CAL-CFP and YFP-CFTR appears to depend upon the Golgi being intact, again suggesting that the Golgi apparatus is required for the binding of CAL-CFP and YFP-CFTR.

In order to examine more closely the trafficking of CAL and CFTR after forskolin treatment, we cotransfected 1.5 μg of YFP-CFTR and 0.5 μg of CAL-CFP expression plasmids into HeLa cells. After a 24-hour incubation, we treated the cells with 100 μM forskolin at 37°C for 30 minutes and immunostained the cells with an anti-GM130 antibody. We then used a plugin of ImageJ to calculate Pearson's correlation coefficients to determine the quantitative colocalization of GM130 with CAL-CFP and YFP-CFTR. Interestingly, forskolin did not change the Pearson's correlation coefficient between GM130 and CAL-CFP but reduced the coefficient between GM130 and YFP-CFTR (Fig. 3). Thus, following forskolin treatment, less CFTR was localized to the Golgi. Surprisingly, forskolin did not change the localization of CAL (Fig. 3), suggesting that the binding of CAL to CFTR occurs in the Golgi as shown above, but CAL does not move with CFTR out of the Golgi.

To verify that CFTR and CAL were not moving together to the plasma membrane in response to forskolin treatment, we examined the interaction between CFTR and CAL by the acceptor photobleaching FRET assay, utilizing the experimental conditions described above. More CFTR was present at the cell surface after forskolin treatment (Fig. 2D, Fig. 3, and CFTR-only sample results of Fig. 4), whereas CAL-CFP was still located in the cytosol (Fig. 2D and Fig. 3). Moreover, the treatment of forskolin reduced the FRET of CAL-CFP and YFP-CFTR (Fig. 2D, E), suggesting that forskolin reduces the association of CAL-CFP with YFP-CFTR and enhances CFTR movement to the cell surface, while CAL remains in the Golgi.

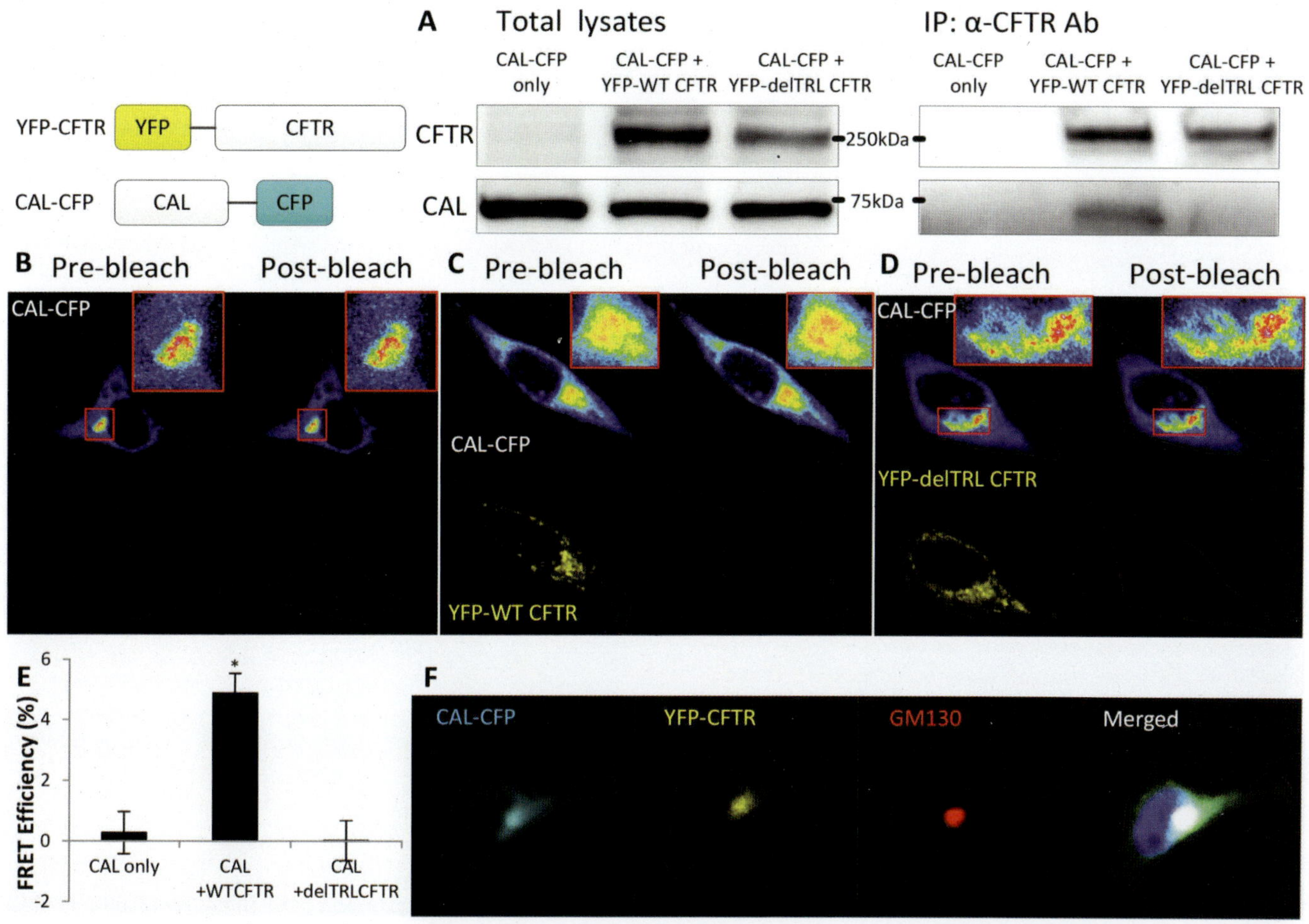

Figure 1. CAL-CFP binds YFP-CFTR in vivo, and CAL and CFTR are colocalized in the Golgi in HeLa cells. The N terminus of CFTR was tagged with YFP, and CFP was tagged to the C terminus of CAL was tagged with CFP. In HeLa cells, CAL-CFP was transiently expressed alone (A,B), with YFP-wildtype CFTR (A,C), or with YFP-delTRL CFTR (A,D). (A) Left panel: CAL-CFP, YFP-wildtype CFTR, and YFP-delTRL CFTR from total lysates were immunoblotted with anti-GFP antibody. Right panel: The cell lysates were immunoprecipitated with anti-CFTR antibody. (B-D) The left columns are the images before photobleaching with a 514-nm laser, and the right columns are the images after photobleaching. CFP and YFP are pseudocolored with a 16-bit lookup table (provided with ImageJ) and yellow, respectively. E shows the statistical analysis of the FRET efficiency obtained from the images. Results are means ±SE. (n = 11–13) *$p<0.001$. (F) YFP-CFTR and CAL-CFP were colocalized with GM130. HeLa cells that had been transfected with YFP-CFTR and CAL-CFP were immunostained with anti-GM130 antibody. The right-most panel shows the merged image of CAL-CFP, YFP-CFTR, GM130, and DAPI. (B–D, F). Cell outlines are drawn with gray lines.

Overexpression of CAL Inhibits the Forskolin-induced Promotion of CFTR Trafficking to the Cell Surface

To study the effect of CAL on the cell-surface expression of CFTR, we varied the doses of the CAL-CFP *versus* YFP-CFTR cDNA cotransfected into HeLa cells. We also performed a cell-surface biotinylation assay to measure the forskolin-induced changes in the cell-surface expression of CFTR. Fig. 4 shows that when YFP-CFTR was expressed alone, the 30-minute treatment with forskolin enhanced the CFTR expression at the cell surface, as previously shown [33,34]. When the ratio of the transfected amount of CAL-CFP cDNA to YFP-CFTR cDNA was 1:3, the same ratio we used in both the FRET assay and cell imaging studies, forskolin still increased the cell-surface expression of CFTR. However, when we transfected three times more CAL-CFP than YFP-CFTR cDNA (3:1), forskolin no longer increased the surface expression of CFTR (Fig. 4). In all cases, forskolin did not change the total expression of CFTR (Fig. 4). Therefore, changes in CAL expression levels regulate CFTR's progress to the cell surface.

Active TC10 Alters CAL-CFTR Binding and Increases the Steady-state Levels of CFTR at the Cell Surface, Even with Highly Overexpressed CAL

Previously, we showed that the constitutively active form of TC10 increases the surface expression of CFTR by binding to CAL [13]. We were curious to see whether active TC10 would also alter the CAL-CFTR interaction. The FRET assay showed that a constitutively active TC10 mutant, Q75L TC10, which remains in the GTP-bound form, does indeed reduce the FRET between CAL-CFP and YFP-CFTR. Importantly, the dominant-negative mutant T31N TC10, which remains in the GDP form, did not affect the FRET (Fig. 5A). These results indicate that active TC10 does indeed alter the binding of CFTR and CAL.

To test this possibility further, we cotransfected 1.5 μg of CAL-CFP cDNA with 1.5 μg of YFP-CFTR cDNA. This ratio inhibited the effects of forskolin on CFTR surface expression (Fig. 5B), as in Fig. 4. However, when the same amounts of CAL-CFP and YFP-CFTR cDNAs were cotransfected along with the active form of TC10 (Q75L TC10), forskolin was able to increase the surface

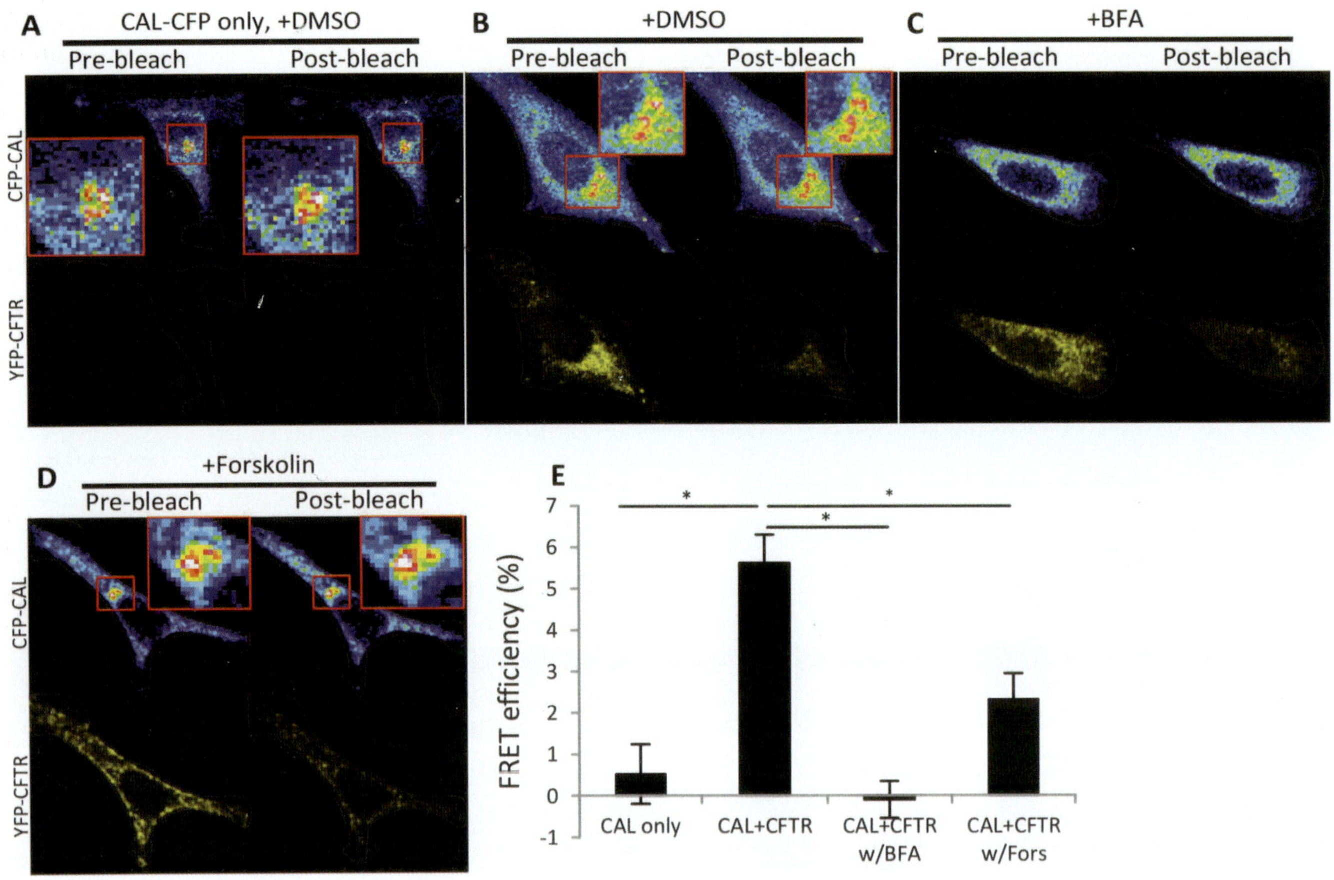

Figure 2. Disrupting the Golgi structure with brefeldin A and increasing the cell-surface expression of CFTR with forskolin diminish the FRET of CAL and CFTR. HeLa cells were transfected with CAL-CFP (0.5 µg) only (A) or with CAL-CFP (0.5 µg) and YFP-CFTR (1.5 µg) (B–D). DMSO (A, B), 10 µg/ml brefeldin A (BFA) (C), or 100 µM forskolin (D) was added at 37°C for 30 minutes. Images before (left columns) and after (right columns) photobleaching with a 514-nm laser are shown. CFP and YFP are pseudocolored with a 16-bit lookup table and yellow, respectively. Cell outlines are drawn with gray lines. (E) is the statistical analysis of the FRET efficiency of CAL and CFTR. The FRET efficiency of CAL and CFTR was reduced when BFA or forskolin was added. Results are means ±SE. (n = 44–68) *p<0.001.

expression of CFTR. Note that co-transfection of the dominant-negative form of TC10, T31N TC10, did not counter the effects of CAL overexpression, and in that case, forskolin did not increase CFTR surface expression (Fig. 5B). These data suggest that active TC10 enhances CFTR expression at the cell surface, even when CAL is overexpressed.

IGF-1 increases the Steady State Levels of CFTR via TC10 and CAL

To determine whether the effects of TC10 are physiological, we utilized IGF-1, which is known to activate TC10 in neurons [21]. HeLa cells were transfected with YFP or YFP-CFTR, and after a 24-hour serum starvation, 0.1 µg/ml IGF-1 was applied for an additional 24 hours. IGF-1 increased the protein expression of YFP-CFTR but not of YFP alone (Fig. 6A); moreover, IGF-1 increased the CFTR expression level at the cell surface in HeLa cells (Fig. 6B). Because the two vector constructs share the same CMV promoter in the same backbone vector, the effects of IGF-1 on YFP-CFTR must be the result of post-transcriptional regulation. Furthermore, our results support the specificity of IGF-1′s effects on CFTR, in that IGF-1 treatment of HeLa cells did not change the protein expression of an endogenous plasma membrane protein, Na,K-ATPase (Fig. 6A).

To determine whether this regulation occurs in bronchial epithelial cells from cystic fibrosis patients (CFBE41o-, referred to as CFBE), we treated CFBE-WTCFTR cells (CFBE cells stably transfected with CFTR) with IGF-1. The effect was identical to that observed in the HeLa cells; IGF-1 increased the protein expression of CFTR but not of Na,K-ATPase (Fig. 6A). These data demonstrate that the effects of IGF-1 are not general, but specific for CFTR, and perhaps other proteins that share the same IGF-1-specific trafficking pathway.

To assess the function of CFTR in CFBE-WTCFTR cells, we measured CFTR-mediated Cl^- transport activity in IGF-1-treated cells. CFBE-WTCFTR cells grown on permeable supports were serum-starved for 24 hours, then treated with 0.1 µg/ml IGF-1 for 24 hours. High-resistance epithelial layers of CFBE-WTCFTR cells (whose average resistance was >1,200 Ω•cm^2 for both control and IGF-1-treated cells) were mounted in Ussing chambers to measure the short-circuit current (I_{SC}). As shown in Fig. 6C and D, the forskolin-activated I_{SC} in IGF-1 treated cells was significantly higher than the control cells. I_{SC} was completely inhibited by the CFTR inhibitor CFTRinh-172, showing that the currents were indeed CFTR-dependent.

To determine whether IGF-1 activates TC10 in CFBE and HeLa cells, we used a peptide (PAK-1 PBD) that binds selectively to activated TC10 [31,32]. Treatment with IGF-1 increased the

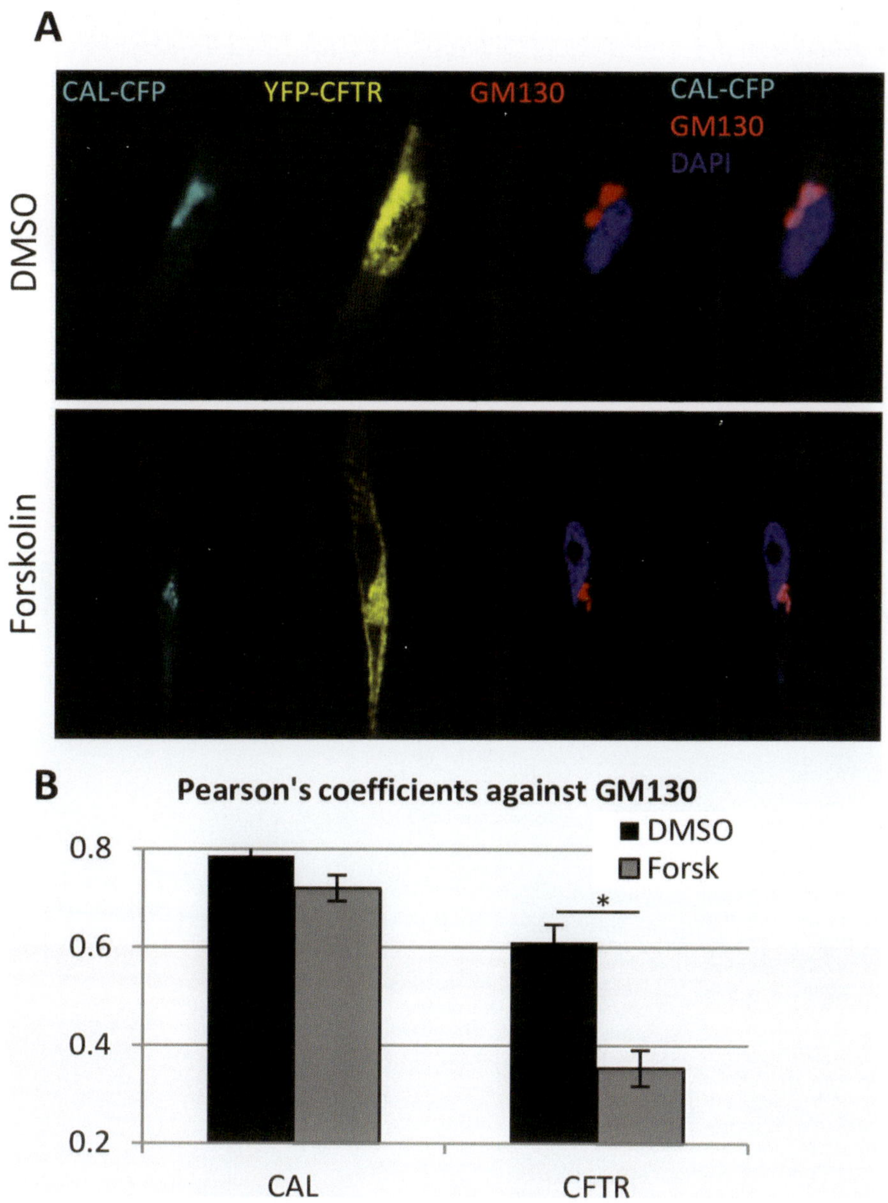

Figure 3. Forskolin treatment relocates CFTR, but not CAL, out of the Golgi in HeLa cells. HeLa cells were transfected with CAL-CFP (0.5 μg) and YFP-CFTR (1.5 μg). GM130 was immunostained with anti-GM130 antibody, followed by secondary antibody conjugated with Alexa-647. DMSO (A, upper panel) or 100 μM forskolin (A, lower panel) was added at 37°C for 30 minutes. (B) The graph shows Pearson's correlation coefficients of GM130 and CAL or of GM130 and CFTR. The coefficients were calculated using an ImageJ plugin, the Colocalization Test. Pearson's correlation coefficients of GM130 and CAL-CFP were not altered in the presence of forskolin, but those of GM130 and YFP-CFTR were reduced by forskolin treatment. Results are means ±SE. (n = 6–9) *$p < 0.01$.

level of activated TC10 in HeLa cells and in CFBE cells transfected with HA-tagged TC10 (Fig. 7A). When T31N TC10 was coexpressed with CFTR to suppress the endogenous activity of TC10, the IGF-1-induced increase of YFP-CFTR expression was abolished (Fig. 7B). Thus, activation of TC10 is required for IGF-1 to increase CFTR expression.

Given our observation that active TC10 reduced the FRET of CAL and CFTR, we reasoned that a similar mechanism might be involved in the IGF-1-mediated regulation of the steady-state levels of CFTR. Indeed, CAL-CFTR FRET was also reduced by IGF-1 (Fig. 7C). Therefore, we surmised that if IGF-1 increases the expression of CFTR by suppressing CAL, overexpression of CAL would reduce the effects of IGF-1. As expected, overexpression of CAL reduced the increase in CFTR expression induced by IGF-1 in HeLa cells (Fig. 7D). The effect of CAL overexpression could be reversed by the co-overexpression of TC10. In this case, IGF-1 still increased the steady-state levels of CFTR even when CAL was overexpressed (Fig. 7D). This result demonstrates that TC10, activated by IGF-1, can increase the steady-state levels of CFTR in a dominant fashion over CAL.

As shown in HeLa cells and also in CFBE-WTCFTR cells, IGF-1 increased CFTR protein expression via TC10 (Fig. 6A, Fig. 7B). This increase by IGF-1 was inhibited by CAL overexpression. However, CAL's inhibition of IGF-1 was overcome by co-overexpression of TC10, again showing the dominance of TC10 in this process (Fig. 7E).

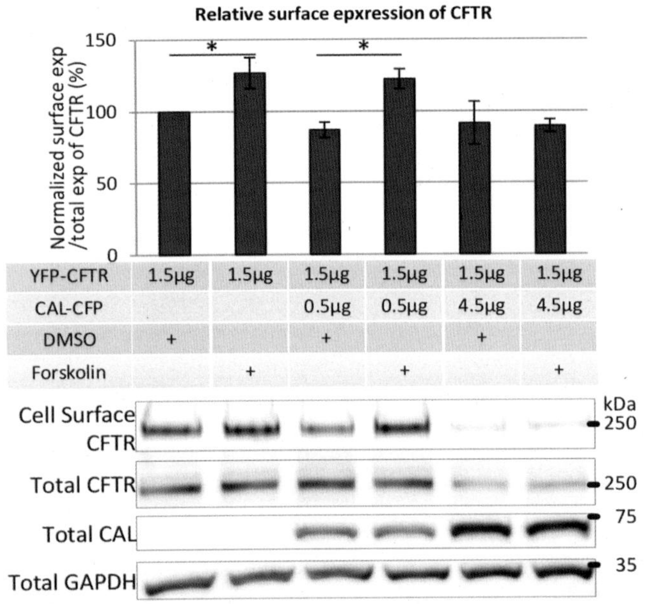

Figure 4. Forskolin fails to increase the cell-surface expression of CFTR with highly overexpressed CAL. HeLa cells were transfected with YFP-CFTR and CAL-CFP as indicated in the table. At 48 hours after transfection, cells were treated with DMSO or 100 μM forskolin at 37°C for 30 minutes. CFTR at the cell surface was then biotinylated. Cell surface-biotinylated CFTR, total CFTR, and total CAL were immunoblotted with anti-GFP antibody, and GAPDH was immunoblotted with anti-GAPDH antibody. The graph shows the ratio of the cell surface-biontinylated CFTR expression level to the total CFTR expression level, normalized by the ratio of the YFP-CFTR-alone samples with the DMSO treatment (%). When CAL was not overexpressed or 0.5 μg of CAL was transfected, forskolin increased the cell-surface expression of CFTR. However, when 4.5 μg of CAL was transfected, forskolin did not increase the cell-surface expression of CFTR. The total expression of CFTR was not altered by the forskolin treatment in all cases. Results are means ±SE. (n = 4) *p<0.05.

IGF-1 Increases the Expression of Rescued ΔF508 CFTR, but not ΔF508 CFTR

ΔF508 CFTR is misfolded and resides primarily in the ER [4]. Most of the misfolded ΔF508 CFTR is degraded by ER-associated degradation and does not proceed to the Golgi. However, incubating cells at the low temperature [35] or treating with correctors [36–39] allows ΔF508 CFTR to proceed to the Golgi and the cell surface. Because ΔF508 CFTR is only core-glycosylated in the ER, it is detected by western blotting as a lower molecular weight B band, which resides primarily in ER; rescued ΔF508 CFTR, in contrast, is detected as a B band and a higher molecular weight C band, which is the Golgi-processed glycoform. We therefore transfected HeLa cells and CFBE cells with YFP-tagged ΔF508 CFTR and then rescued ΔF508 by incubating the cells at 27°C for 2 days [35] (Fig. 8). ΔF508 CFTR in CFBE cells was also rescued by incubating the cells with a corrector, VRT-325, at 37°C for 2 days [36] (Fig. 8B). IGF-1 did not increase the expression of ΔF508 CFTR; however, it did increase the expression of the C band of rescued ΔF508 CFTR as well as the B band of rescued ΔF508 CFTR (Fig. 8).

Discussion

The question of how CAL regulates the trafficking of CFTR to the lysosome for degradation and, at the same time, to the cell surface remains unanswered. Where CAL molecules bind would be important information for understanding how CAL regulates CFTR. Our data have confirmed that CFTR and CAL are colocalized to the Golgi. We have also developed an acceptor photobleaching FRET assay to assess the binding of CAL and CFTR in the Golgi. Initially, we obtained FRET between CFTR labeled on the N-terminus with YFP and CAL labeled on the C-terminus with CFP and confirmed that the FRET assay showed the *in vivo* binding of CAL and CFTR. We then observed that when the normal structure of the Golgi was chemically disrupted, FRET was reduced, implying that the binding of CAL and CFTR was also disrupted and that the Golgi is required for their binding. When a decreased amount of CFTR was found in the Golgi after treatment with forskolin, which promotes the movement of CFTR from the Golgi to the cell surface, FRET between CAL and CFTR

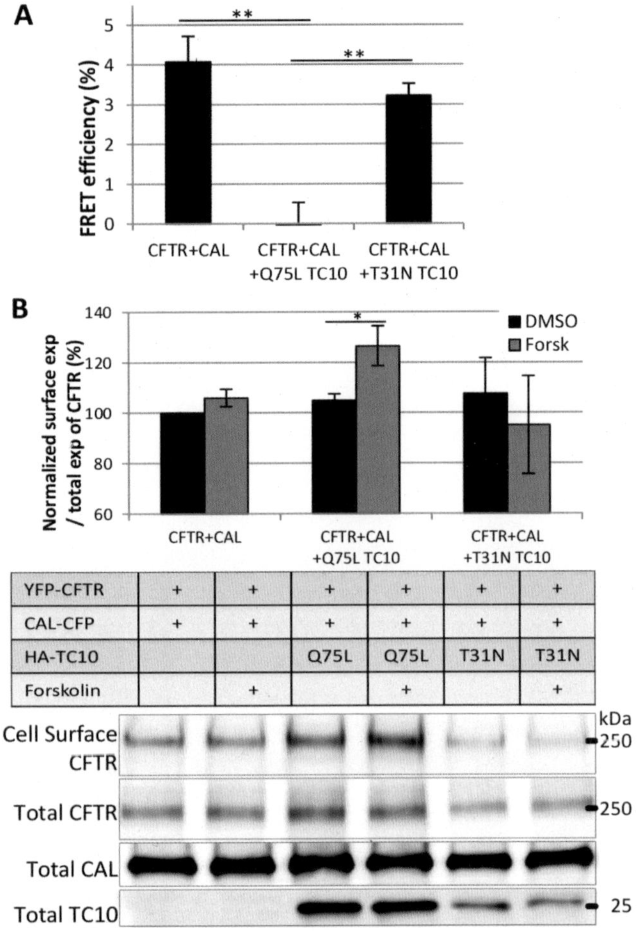

Figure 5. Active TC10 enhances CFTR expression at the cell surface, and this effect is impeded by highly overexpressed CAL HeLa cells were transfected with 1.5 μg of YFP-CFTR plus 0.5 μg (A) or 1.5 μg (B) of CAL-CFP expression vector without HA-TC10, with HA-Q75L TC10, or with HA-T31N TC10, as indicated. (A) The FRET efficiency of CAL and CFTR was reduced by a constitutively active mutant of TC10 (Q75L TC10) but not by a dominant-negative mutant, T31N TC10. (B) HeLa cells were treated with DMSO or 100 μM forskolin at 37°C for 30 minutes as described in the table. CFTR at the cell surface was biotinylated. The graph shows the ratio of cell surface-biontinylated CFTR to total CFTR, normalized by the ratio of the samples with YFP-CFTR and CAL-CFP treated with DMSO (%). Results are means ±SE. (In A, n = 7–13; B, n = 4) *p<0.05 and **p<0.005.

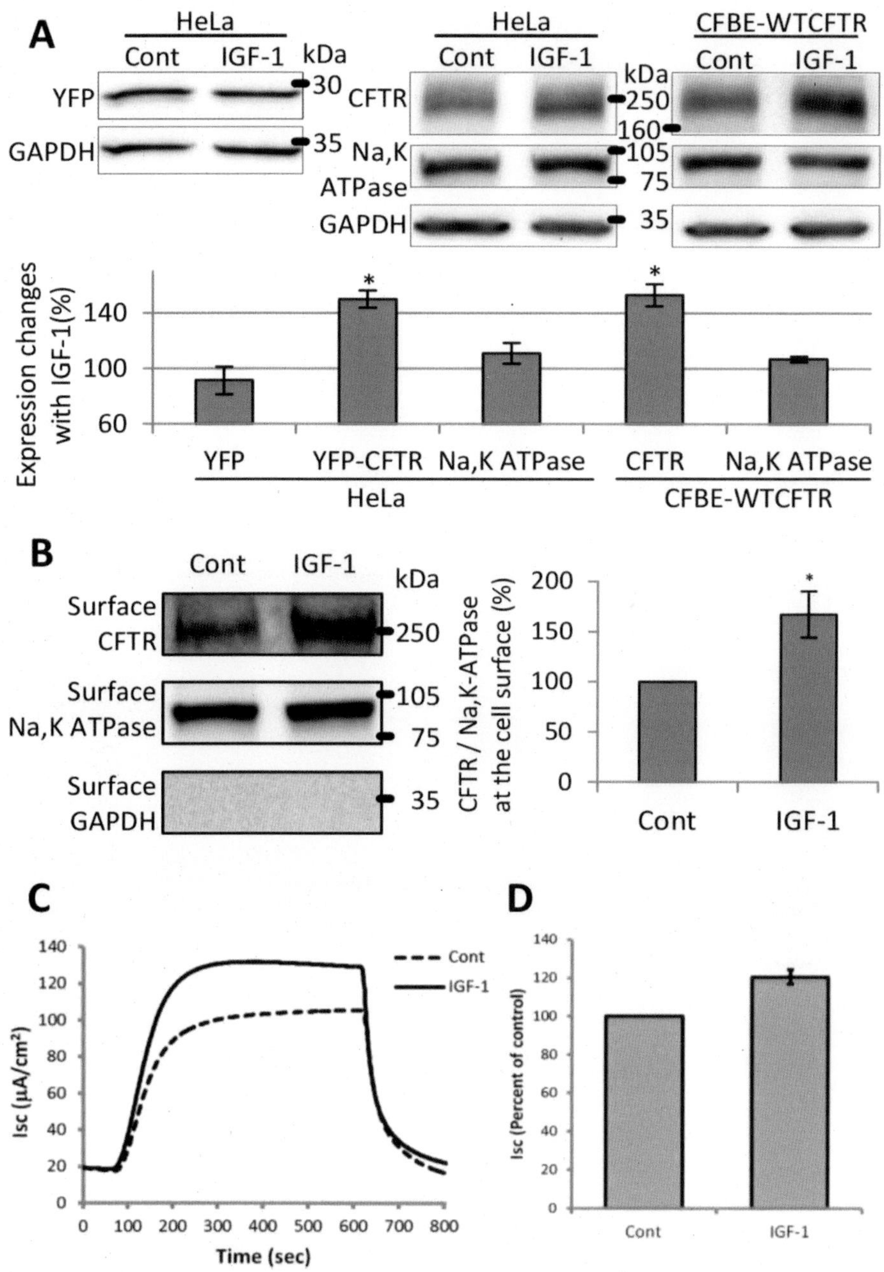

Figure 6. IGF-1 increases the protein expression level of CFTR and increases CFTR-mediated chloride transport in bronchial epithelial cells. (A) IGF-1 specifically increases the expression level of CFTR. HeLa cells were transfected with YFP or YFP-CFTR and incubated for one day, or confluent CFBE-WTCFTR cells were used. The graph in the right lower panel shows the expression of YFP, YFP-CFTR, CFTR, or Na,K-ATPase normalized by the GAPDH expression and normalized again by the corresponding control samples (%). (B) CFTR expression at the cell surface was increased by IGF-1 in HeLa cells. Proteins at the cell surface were cell surface-biotinylated. The graph in the right panel shows the expression of YFP-CFTR at the cell surface normalized by the Na,K-ATPase expression at the cell surface and normalized again by the corresponding control samples (%). (A,B) Cells were starved for 24 hours and then treated with 0.1 μg/ml IGF-1 for the next 24 hours. Results are means ±SE. (n = 3) (C) CFBE-WTCFTR cells grown on permeable supports were starved for 24 hours, then treated with 0.1 μg/ml IGF-1 for 24 hours. Cells were then mounted on the Ussing chamber setup, where short-circuit currents were measured as described in Materials and Methods. In the graph, 10 μM forskolin was added at the first arrow, and 5 μM CFTRinh-172 was added at the second arrow. (D) Ratio of I_{SC} between cells treated with 0.1 μg/ml IGF-1 (IGF-1) and untreated cells (Cont). Error bars represent SE. (n = 5). *p<0.05 and **p<0.005.

was also reduced. This finding supports the hypothesis that CAL binds CFTR and regulates the trafficking of CFTR at the Golgi.

Active TC10 has been shown to enhance CFTR expression [13], and we have found that it promotes the trafficking of CFTR to the cell surface, even in the presence of highly overexpressed CAL, suggesting that the role of TC10 is dominant over CAL. One possible mechanism to explain these findings is that active TC10 disrupts the binding of CAL to CFTR by proceeding with CFTR to the plasma membrane and leaving CAL behind in the Golgi. Alternatively, TC10 could alter the conformation of the CFTR-CAL complex, thereby increasing the distance between the fluorescent tags on the N-terminus of CFTR and on CAL that

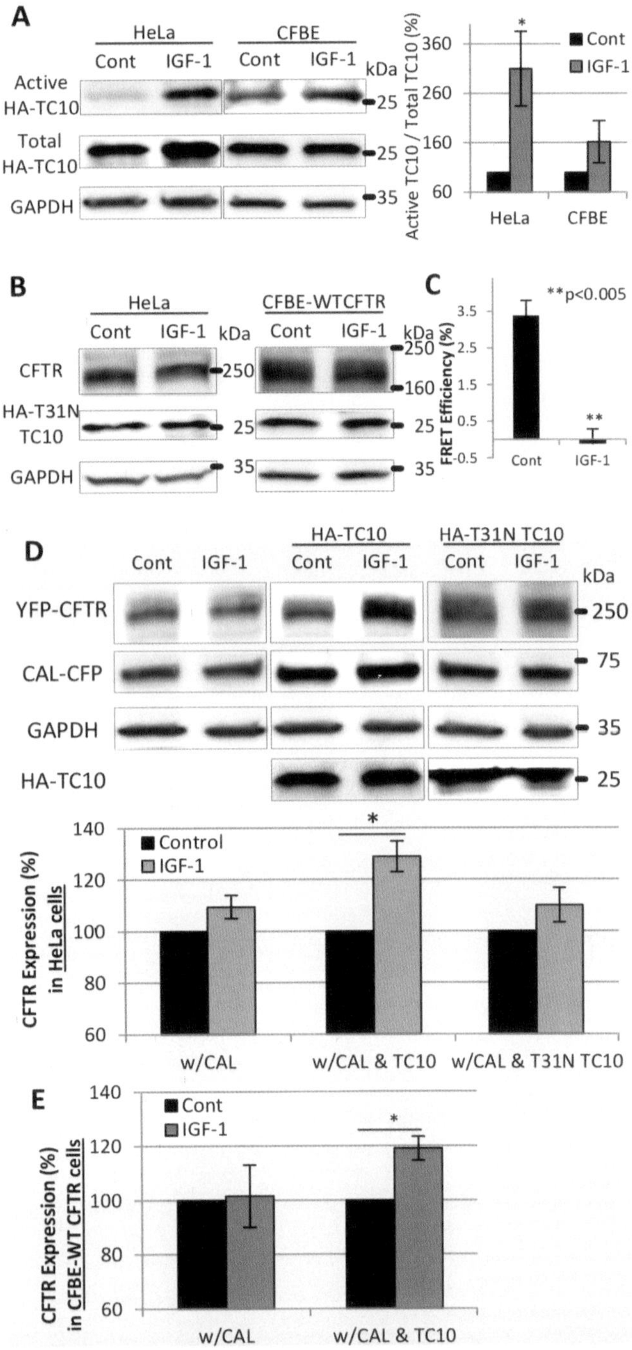

Figure 7. TC10 and CAL are involved in the IGF-1-mediated increase in CFTR expression level. (A) IGF-1 activates TC10. After HeLa cells or CFBE cells were transfected with HA-TC10, active TC10 was pulled down from the cell lysates with GST-PAK1 PBD peptide-conjugated beads. Total TC10 and GAPDH are from total cell lysates. The graph shows the amount of active TC10 normalized by the amount of total TC10 expression (%). (B) Dominant-negative TC10 (T31N TC10) inhibited the effects of IGF-1, increasing the CFTR expression. HeLa cells were cotransfected with YFP-CFTR and HA-T31N TC10, or CFBE-WTCFTR cells were transfected with HA-T31N TC10. Shown are representative images. (C) The FRET efficiency of CAL and CFTR was reduced by IGF-1. HeLa cells transfected with CAL and CFTR were starved for 4 hours and treated with 0.1 μg/ml IGF-1 for 30 minutes. (D,E) The CAL overexpression inhibited effects of IGF-1 increasing the CFTR expression, but the cotransfection with wildtype TC10 recovered the effects of IGF-1 on the CFTR expression in HeLa cells (D) and CFBE-WT CFTR cells (E). HeLa cells were transfected with YFP-CFTR and CAL-CFP without or with TC10 or T31N TC10. CFBE-WT CFTR cells were transfected with CAL-CFP without or with TC10. The CFTR expression level was normalized by the GAPDH expression level and normalized again by the corresponding control samples (%). (A,B,D,E) Cells were starved for 24 hours, and then 0.1 μg/ml IGF-1 was added for the next 24 hours. (A,C–E) Results are means ±SE. (n = 3) *p<0.05 and **p<0.005.

bind to the C-terminus of CFTR. This alteration in conformation would also reduce the FRET of CAL and CFTR by active TC10, while CAL still binds CFTR. Indeed, our lab has shown in a previous report by coimmunoprecipitation that CAL and CFTR remain associated following active TC10 overexpression [13]. TC10 is known to bind to the N-terminal coiled-coil domain of CAL and not to the PDZ domain where CFTR binds [17]; thus, it is not surprising that CAL can still bind CFTR in the presence of TC10. TC10, by inducing conformational changes, might move the whole CAL-CFTR complex away from the Golgi toward the plasma membrane, since our previous report showed that active TC10 relocates CAL toward the plasma membrane in COS7 cells [13]. At or near the plasma membrane, CFTR would competitively bind to NHERF, which has a higher affinity for the PDZ domain of CFTR than does CAL [40], and thereby enhance the CFTR expression at the plasma membrane by stabilizing CFTR [41].

TC10 has two known mechanisms for regulating membrane trafficking: It recruits excocyst complex proteins (e.g., Exo70, Sec6, and Sec8) to GLUT4 vesicles in adipocytes and to plasmalemmal precursor vesicles in neurons [21–23]. These complexes are involved in the exocytosis of membrane vesicles. Secondly, TC10 uses PI3K-dependent signaling by increasing phosphatidylinositol 3-phosphate (PI3P) [42–44]. The increased PI3P level induces exocytosis of membrane vesicles and raises the intriguing possibility that when present together in cells, GLUT4 and CFTR may traffic together to the plasma membrane in the same TC10 activated pathway. The current study proposes a novel, third mechanism for TC10 regulation whereby active TC10 alters the binding of a cargo molecule, CFTR, to an adaptor protein, CAL, and thereby enhances the trafficking of the cargo (i.e., CFTR) to the plasma membrane.

TC10 is located downstream of the IGF-1 receptor cascade [21–23]. We show here that IGF-1 activates TC10 and increases CFTR expression in CFBE and HeLa cells, but does not increase CFTR expression in the presence of the dominant-negative TC10. Furthermore, we have shown that IGF-1 increases CFTR expression by activating TC10. As we saw in the case of constitutively active TC10, IGF-1 alters the CFTR-CAL interaction and enhances CFTR expression.

In bronchial epithelial cells, adequate expression of the CFTR protein is required to prevent bacterial infection, which is the most common CF symptom [45,46]. The reports that bronchial epithelial cells express the IGF-1 receptor [47] and react to IGF-1 [48,49] suggest that these cells may have IGF-1 signaling. Our results also indicate that that IGF-1 selectively increases CFTR protein expression and CFTR-mediated chloride transport in a cell line model, CFBE cells (the bronchial epithelial cell line from cystic fibrosis patients). Therefore, our results raise the possibility that IGF-1 treatment could increase CFTR expression in vivo.

Serum IGF-1 levels vary physiologically and pathologically in individuals in response to aging, caloric uptake, injury, and other conditions, and they regulate IGF-1 signaling, causing mitogenic effects such as cell proliferation, tissue regeneration, and body growth [50–53]. According to our present results, changes in the level of IGF-1 would be expected to alter CFTR protein expression. CAL also binds other plasma membrane proteins

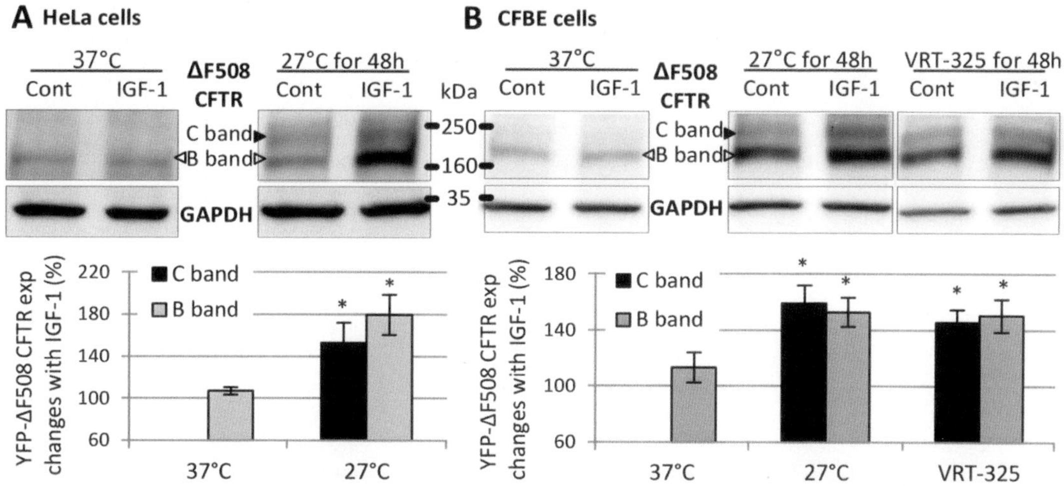

Figure 8. IGF-1 increases the expression level of rescued ΔF508 CFTR but not unrescued ΔF508 CFTR. HeLa cells (A) and CFBE cells (B) were transfected with YFP-ΔF508 CFTR, and after 1 day, plates of both cell lines were incubated at 37°C or at 27°C for 2 days; additional plates of CFBE cells were incubated with 5 μM VRT-325 at 37°C for 2 days. At the same time, 1 day after the transfection, these cells were serum-starved, and on next day, 0.1 μg/ml IGF-1 was added for 1 day. The expression level of ΔF508 CFTR in the cell lysates was assessed by western blotting. When unrescued (incubated at 37°C), ΔF508 CFTR showed one band (the B band), but when rescued (incubated at 27°C or with VRT-325 at 37°C), it showed two bands (B and C). IGF-1 did not increase the expression level of unrescued ΔF508 CFTR but did increase the expression level of rescued ΔF508 CFTR. The ΔF508 CFTR expression level was normalized by the GAPDH expression level, and the ΔF508 CFTR expression change as a result of IGF-1 treatment was then calculated by normalizing again with the non-treated control samples (%). Results are means ±SE. (n = 6 for HeLa at 27°C and CFBE at 37°C, n = 3 for all the others) *$p<0.05$.

such as the β1-adrenergic receptor, ClC-3B, somatostatin receptor subtype 5, and cadherin 23, and enhances their lysosomal degradation [54–57]. If TC10 also regulates the CAL-dependent degradation of these proteins, IGF-1 could also post-translationally regulate the expression levels of these plasma membrane proteins. IGF-1 levels are low in the serum of CF patients and the CF pig model [26,27]; therefore, IGF-1 has been studied and used in a clinical trial to reverse growth retardation in CF patients [25,58].

ΔF508 CFTR, the most common CF mutation, is degraded by ER-associated degradation and does not reach the Golgi or plasma membrane [59]. Our results show that IGF-1 does not change the expression level of ΔF508 CFTR, consistent with our proposal that IGF-1 alters the binding of CAL to CFTR at the Golgi, since almost all of ΔF508 CFTR is sequestered in the ER and does not proceed to the Golgi [60]. However, IGF-1 does increase the expression of rescued ΔF508 CFTR, because when ΔF508 CFTR is rescued by correctors or low temperature, it moves out of the ER to the Golgi and the cell surface [35,38,61]. Interestingly, IGF-1 does not increase the intensity of un-rescued ΔF508 CFTR band B, whose N-glycosylation is initiated in the ER but not finalized in the Golgi; however, it does increase its intensity when ΔF508 CFTR is corrected by low temperature or VRT-325. These data suggest that the rescued immature B band of ΔF508 CFTR may in some instances exit the ER through an unconventional trafficking pathway, perhaps enhanced by TC10 acting through IGF-1, and reach the plasma membrane in an immature form [62]. However, more work is needed to establish this effect conclusively. Correctors have been developed and are currently in clinical trials [37,38]. Thus, it is possible that an additive treatment combining IGF-1 with a corrector would be more effective for cystic fibrosis than a corrector alone.

Acknowledgments

We thank Dr. B. Cha for assistance with setting up the FRET assay and Dr. Deborah McClellan for editorial assistance.

Author Contributions

Conceived and designed the experiments: HWL OK MD WG. Performed the experiments: HWL JC. Analyzed the data: HWL WBG. Contributed reagents/materials/analysis tools: OK. Wrote the paper: HWL WBG.

References

1. Riordan JR, Rommens JM, Kerem B, Alon N, Rozmahel R, et al. (1989) Identification of the cystic fibrosis gene: cloning and characterization of complementary DNA. Science 245: 1066–1073.
2. Rowe SM, Miller S, Sorscher EJ (2005) Cystic Fibrosis. New England Journal of Medicine 352: 1992–2001.
3. Gibson LE, Cooke RE (1959) A test for concentration of electrolytes in sweat in cystic fibrosis of the pancreas utilizing pilocarpine by iontophoresis. Pediatrics 23: 545–549.
4. Cheng SH, Gregory RJ, Marshall J, Paul S, Souza DW, et al. (1990) Defective intracellular transport and processing of CFTR is the molecular basis of most cystic fibrosis. Cell 63: 827–834.
5. Kerem BS, Buchanan JA, Durie P, Corey ML, Levison H, et al. (1989) DNA marker haplotype association with pancreatic sufficiency in cystic fibrosis. Am J Hum Genet 44: 827–834.
6. Bertrand CA, Frizzell RA (2003) The role of regulated CFTR trafficking in epithelial secretion. Am J Physiol Cell Physiol 285: C1–18.
7. Cheng J, Moyer BD, Milewski M, Loffing J, Ikeda M, et al. (2002) A Golgi-associated PDZ Domain Protein Modulates Cystic Fibrosis Transmembrane Regulator Plasma Membrane Expression. Journal of Biological Chemistry 277: 3520–3529.
8. Wang S, Yue H, Derin RB, Guggino WB, Li M (2000) Accessory Protein Facilitated CFTR-CFTR Interaction, a Molecular Mechanism to Potentiate the Chloride Channel Activity. Cell 103: 169–179.
9. Gee Heon Y, Noh Shin H, Tang Bor L, Kim Kyung H, Lee Min G (2011) Rescue of ΔF508-CFTR Trafficking via a GRASP-Dependent Unconventional Secretion Pathway. Cell 146: 746–760.
10. Sun F, Hug MJ, Lewarchik CM, Yun CHC, Bradbury NA, et al. (2000) E3KARP Mediates the Association of Ezrin and Protein Kinase A with the

Cystic Fibrosis Transmembrane Conductance Regulator in Airway Cells. Journal of Biological Chemistry 275: 29539–29546.

11. Guggino WB, Stanton BA (2006) New insights into cystic fibrosis: molecular switches that regulate CFTR. Nat Rev Mol Cell Biol 7: 426–436.
12. Shorter J, Watson R, Giannakou ME, Clarke M, Warren G, et al. (1999) GRASP55, a second mammalian GRASP protein involved in the stacking of Golgi cisternae in a cell-free system. EMBO J 18: 4949–4960.
13. Cheng J, Wang H, Guggino WB (2005) Regulation of cystic fibrosis transmembrane regulator trafficking and protein expression by a Rho family small GTPase TC10. J Biol Chem 280: 3731–3739.
14. Moyer BD, Duhaime M, Shaw C, Denton J, Reynolds D, et al. (2000) The PDZ-interacting Domain of Cystic Fibrosis Transmembrane Conductance Regulator Is Required for Functional Expression in the Apical Plasma Membrane. Journal of Biological Chemistry 275: 27069–27074.
15. Bezprozvanny I, Maximov A (2001) PDZ domains: More than just a glue. Proceedings of the National Academy of Sciences 98: 787–789.
16. Cheng J, Cebotaru V, Cebotaru L, Guggino WB (2010) Syntaxin 6 and CAL Mediate the Degradation of the Cystic Fibrosis Transmembrane Conductance Regulator. Mol Biol Cell 21: 1178–1187.
17. Neudauer CL, Joberty G, Macara IG (2001) PIST: A Novel PDZ/Coiled-Coil Domain Binding Partner for the Rho-Family GTPase TC10. Biochemical and Biophysical Research Communications 280: 541–547.
18. Charest A, Lane K, McMahon K, Housman DE (2001) Association of a Novel PDZ Domain-containing Peripheral Golgi Protein with the Q-SNARE (Q-solubleN-Ethylmaleimide-sensitive Fusion Protein (NSF) Attachment Protein Receptor) Protein Syntaxin 6. Journal of Biological Chemistry 276: 29456–29465.
19. Kuliawat R, Kalinina E, Bock J, Fricker L, McGraw TE, et al. (2004) Syntaxin-6 SNARE Involvement in Secretory and Endocytic Pathways of Cultured Pancreatic {beta}-Cells. Mol Biol Cell 15: 1690–1701.
20. Chiang SH, Baumann CA, Kanzaki M, Thurmond DC, Watson RT, et al. (2001) Insulin-stimulated GLUT4 translocation requires the CAP-dependent activation of TC10. Nature 410: 944–948.
21. Dupraz S, Grassi D, Bernis ME, Sosa L, Bisbal M, et al. (2009) The TC10-Exo70 complex is essential for membrane expansion and axonal specification in developing neurons. J Neurosci 29: 13292–13301.
22. Inoue M, Chang L, Hwang J, Chiang SH, Saltiel AR (2003) The exocyst complex is required for targeting of Glut4 to the plasma membrane by insulin. Nature 422: 629–633.
23. Inoue M, Chiang SH, Chang L, Chen XW, Saltiel AR (2006) Compartmentalization of the Exocyst Complex in Lipid Rafts Controls Glut4 Vesicle Tethering. Molecular Biology of the Cell 17: 2303–2311.
24. Taylor AM, Bush A, Thomson A, Oades PJ, Marchant JL, et al. (1997) Relation between insulin-like growth factor-I, body mass index, and clinical status in cystic fibrosis. Archives of Disease in Childhood 76: 304–309.
25. Taylor AM, Thomson A, Bruce-Morgan C, Ahmed ML, Watts A, et al. (1999) The relationship between insulin, IGF-I and weight gain in cystic fibrosis. Clinical Endocrinology 51: 659–665.
26. Hardin DS, Ferkol T, Ahn C, Dreimane D, Dyson M, et al. (2005) A retrospective study of growth hormone use in adolescents with cystic fibrosis. Clinical Endocrinology 62: 560–566.
27. Rogan MP, Reznikov LR, Pezzulo AA, Gansemer ND, Samuel M, et al. (2010) Pigs and humans with cystic fibrosis have reduced insulin-like growth factor 1 (IGF1) levels at birth. Proceedings of the National Academy of Sciences 107: 20571–20575.
28. Moyer BD, Loffing J, Schwiebert EM, Loffing-Cueni D, Halpin PA, et al. (1998) Membrane Trafficking of the Cystic Fibrosis Gene Product, Cystic Fibrosis Transmembrane Conductance Regulator, Tagged with Green Fluorescent Protein in Madin-Darby Canine Kidney Cells. Journal of Biological Chemistry 273: 21759–21768.
29. Bruscia E, Sangiuolo F, Sinibaldi P, Goncz KK, Novelli G, et al. (2002) Isolation of CF cell lines corrected at DeltaF508-CFTR locus by SFHR-mediated targeting. Gene Ther 9: 683–685.
30. Illek B, Maurisse R, Wahler L, Kunzelmann K, Fischer H, et al. (2008) Cl transport in complemented CF bronchial epithelial cells correlates with CFTR mRNA expression levels. Cell Physiol Biochem 22: 57–68.
31. Taylor SJ, Shalloway D (1996) Cell cycle-dependent activation of Ras. Current Biology 6: 1621–1627.
32. Benard V, Bohl BP, Bokoch GM (1999) Characterization of Rac and Cdc42 Activation in Chemoattractant-stimulated Human Neutrophils Using a Novel Assay for Active GTPases. Journal of Biological Chemistry 274: 13198–13204.
33. Bradbury N, Jilling T, Berta G, Sorscher E, Bridges R, et al. (1992) Regulation of plasma membrane recycling by CFTR. Science 256: 530–532.
34. Denning GM, Ostedgaard LS, Cheng SH, Smith AE, Welsh MJ (1992) Localization of cystic fibrosis transmembrane conductance regulator in chloride secretory epithelia. J Clin Invest 89: 339–349.
35. Denning GM, Anderson MP, Amara JF, Marshall J, Smith AE, et al. (1992) Processing of mutant cystic fibrosis transmembrane conductance regulator is temperature-sensitive. Nature 358: 761–764.
36. Yu GJ, Yoo CL, Yang B, Lodewyk MW, Meng L, et al. (2008) Potent s-cis-Locked Bithiazole Correctors of ΔF508 Cystic Fibrosis Transmembrane Conductance Regulator Cellular Processing for Cystic Fibrosis Therapy. Journal of Medicinal Chemistry 51: 6044–6054.
37. Van Goor F, Hadida S, Grootenhuis PD, Burton B, Stack J, et al. (2009) VX-809, a CFTR corrector, increases the cell surface density of functional F508del-CFTR in pre-clinical models of cystic fibrosis. Pediatric Pulmonology 44: 154–155.
38. Van Goor F, Hadida S, Grootenhuis PDJ, Burton B, Stack JH, et al. (2011) Correction of the F508del-CFTR protein processing defect in vitro by the investigational drug VX-809. Proceedings of the National Academy of Sciences 108: 18843–18848.
39. Pedemonte N, Lukacs GL, Du K, Caci E, Zegarra-Moran O, et al. (2005) Small-molecule correctors of defective Î"F508-CFTR cellular processing identified by high-throughput screening. The Journal of Clinical Investigation 115: 2564–2571.
40. Cushing PR, Fellows A, Villone D, Boisguérin P, Madden DR (2008) The Relative Binding Affinities of PDZ Partners for CFTR: A Biochemical Basis for Efficient Endocytic Recycling. Biochemistry 47: 10084–10098.
41. Moyer BD, Denton J, Karlson KH, Reynolds D, Wang S, et al. (1999) A PDZ-interacting domain in CFTR is an apical membrane polarization signal. The Journal of Clinical Investigation 104: 1353–1361.
42. Maffucci T, Brancaccio A, Piccolo E, Stein RC, Falasca M (2003) Insulin induces phosphatidylinositol-3-phosphate formation through TC10 activation. EMBO J 22: 4178–4189.
43. Lodhi IJ, Bridges D, Chiang SH, Zhang Y, Cheng A, et al. (2008) Insulin Stimulates Phosphatidylinositol 3-Phosphate Production via the Activation of Rab5. Molecular Biology of the Cell 19: 2718–2728.
44. Kelly KL, Ruderman NB (1993) Insulin-stimulated phosphatidylinositol 3-kinase. Association with a 185-kDa tyrosine-phosphorylated protein (IRS-1) and localization in a low density membrane vesicle. Journal of Biological Chemistry 268: 4391–4398.
45. Guggino WB (1999) Cystic Fibrosis and the Salt Controversy. Cell 96: 607–610.
46. Vij N, Mazur S, Zeitlin PL (2009) CFTR Is a Negative Regulator of NFκB Mediated Innate Immune Response. PLoS ONE 4: e4664.
47. Kim WY, Jin Q, Oh SH, Kim ES, Yang YJ, et al. (2009) Elevated Epithelial Insulin-like Growth Factor Expression Is a Risk Factor for Lung Cancer Development. Cancer Research 69: 7439–7448.
48. Siegfried JM, Kasprzyk PG, Treston AM, Mulshine JL, Quinn KA, et al. (1992) A mitogenic peptide amide encoded within the E peptide domain of the insulin-like growth factor IB prohormone. Proceedings of the National Academy of Sciences 89: 8107–8111.
49. Shoji S, Ertl RF, Linder J, Koizumi SI, Duckworth WC, et al. (1990) Bronchial Epithelial Cells Respond to Insulin and Insulin-like Growth Factor-I as a Chemoattractant. Am J Respir Cell Mol Biol 2: 553–557.
50. Thissen JP, Ketelslegers JM, Underwood LE (1994) Nutritional Regulation of the Insulin-Like Growth Factors. Endocrine Reviews 15: 80–101.
51. Corpas E, Harman SM, Blackman MR (1993) Human Growth Hormone and Human Aging. Endocrine Reviews 14: 20–39.
52. Florini JR, Ewton DZ, Coolican SA (1996) Growth Hormone and the Insulin-Like Growth Factor System in Myogenesis. Endocrine Reviews 17: 481–517.
53. Le Roith D, Bondy C, Yakar S, Liu JL, Butler A (2001) The Somatomedin Hypothesis: 2001. Endocrine Reviews 22: 53–74.
54. He J, Bellini M, Xu J, Castleberry AM, Hall RA (2004) Interaction with Cystic Fibrosis Transmembrane Conductance Regulator-associated Ligand (CAL) Inhibits β1-Adrenergic Receptor Surface Expression. Journal of Biological Chemistry 279: 50190–50196.
55. Gentzsch M, Cui L, Mengos A, Chang XB, Chen JH, et al. (2003) The PDZ-binding Chloride Channel ClC-3B Localizes to the Golgi and Associates with Cystic Fibrosis Transmembrane Conductance Regulator-interacting PDZ Proteins. Journal of Biological Chemistry 278: 6440–6449.
56. Wente W, Stroh T, Beaudet A, Richter D, Kreienkamp Jr H (2005) Interactions with PDZ Domain Proteins PIST/GOPC and PDZK1 Regulate Intracellular Sorting of the Somatostatin Receptor Subtype 5. Journal of Biological Chemistry 280: 32419–32425.
57. Xu Z, Oshima K, Heller S (2010) PIST regulates the intracellular trafficking and plasma membrane expression of Cadherin 23. BMC Cell Biology 11: 80.
58. Bucuvalas JC, Chernausek SD, Alfaro MP, Krug SK, Ritschel W, et al. (2001) Effect of Insulinlike Growth Factor-1 Treatment in Children With Cystic Fibrosis. Journal of Pediatric Gastroenterology and Nutrition 33: 576–581.
59. Jensen TJ, Loo MA, Pind S, Williams DB, Goldberg AL, et al. (1995) Multiple proteolytic systems, including the proteasome, contribute to CFTR processing. Cell 83: 129–135.
60. McKone EF, Emerson SS, Edwards KL, Aitken ML (2003) Effect of genotype on phenotype and mortality in cystic fibrosis: a retrospective cohort study. The Lancet 361: 1671–1676.
61. Loo TW, Bartlett MC, Clarke DM (2005) Rescue of ΔF508 and Other Misprocessed CFTR Mutants by a Novel Quinazoline Compound. Molecular Pharmaceutics 2: 407–413.
62. Luo Y, McDonald K, Hanrahan JW (2009) Trafficking of immature DeltaF508-CFTR to the plasma membrane and its detection by biotinylation. Biochem J 419: 211–219.

4

Cystic Fibrosis Transmembrane Conductance Regulator (CFTR) Allelic Variants Relate to Shifts in Faecal Microbiota of Cystic Fibrosis Patients

Serena Schippa[1]☙, Valerio Iebba[1*]☙, Floriana Santangelo[1], Antonella Gagliardi[1], Riccardo Valerio De Biase[2], Antonella Stamato[2], Serenella Bertasi[2], Marco Lucarelli[3], Maria Pia Conte[1¶], Serena Quattrucci[2¶]

1 Public Health and Infectious Diseases Department, Microbiology Unit, 'Sapienza' University of Rome, Rome, Italy, **2** Regional Cystic Fibrosis Centre, Paediatrics and Infant Neuropsychiatry Department, 'Sapienza' University of Rome, Rome, Italy, **3** Department of Haematology and Cellular Biotechnologies, Sapienza University of Rome, Rome, Italy

Abstract

Introduction: In this study we investigated the effects of the Cystic Fibrosis Transmembrane conductance Regulator (*CFTR*) gene variants on the composition of faecal microbiota, in patients affected by Cystic Fibrosis (CF). *CFTR* mutations (F508del is the most common) lead to a decreased secretion of chloride/water, and to mucus sticky secretions, in pancreas, respiratory and gastrointestinal tracts. Intestinal manifestations are underestimated in CF, leading to ileum meconium at birth, or small bowel bacterial overgrowth in adult age.

Methods: Thirty-six CF patients, fasting and under no-antibiotic treatment, were *CFTR* genotyped on both alleles. Faecal samples were subjected to molecular microbial profiling through Temporal Temperature Gradient Electrophoresis and species-specific PCR. Ecological parameters and multivariate algorithms were employed to find out if *CFTR* variants could be related to the microbiota structure.

Results: Patients were classified by two different criteria: 1) presence/absence of F508del mutation; 2) disease severity in heterozygous and homozygous F508del patients. We found that homozygous-F508del and severe CF patients exhibited an enhanced dysbiotic faecal microbiota composition, even within the CF cohort itself, with higher biodiversity and evenness. We also found, by species-specific PCR, that potentially harmful species (*Escherichia coli* and *Eubacterium biforme*) were abundant in homozygous-F508del and severe CF patients, while beneficial species (*Faecalibacterium prausnitzii*, *Bifidobacterium spp.*, and *Eubacterium limosum*) were reduced.

Conclusions: This is the first report that establishes a link among *CFTR* variants and shifts in faecal microbiota, opening the way to studies that perceive CF as a 'systemic disease', linking the lung and the gut in a joined axis.

Editor: Neeraj Vij, Johns Hopkins School of Medicine, United States of America

Funding: This study was funded by Cystic Fibrosis Lazio Regional Center, Italy, and MIUR Italian Minister for Research. The funders had no role in study design, data collection and analysis, decision to publish, or preparation of the manuscript.

Competing Interests: The authors have declared that no competing interests exist.

* E-mail: valerio.iebba@uniroma1.it

☙ These authors contributed equally to this work.

¶ These authors also contributed equally to this work.

Introduction

Cystic fibrosis (CF; OMIM 219700) is an autosomal recessive disorder affecting the exocrine glands of the respiratory, digestive and reproductive systems. The clinical manifestations of CF in affected individuals vary widely, with both age at diagnosis and lethality ranging from the first year of life to the third (and later) decade [1]. In CF, the chronic infection of respiratory tract leads to progressive respiratory deficiency [2]. Mutations in the cystic fibrosis transmembrane conductance regulator (*CFTR*) gene lead to the accumulation of mucus on epithelial surfaces mainly in pancreas, respiratory and gastrointestinal tracts [3,4]. The *CFTR* gene (OMIM 602421) functions as a chloride channel that regulates ions and water transport across epithelial cell membranes. Around 1500 mutations and 300 polymorphisms in the *CFTR* gene are known (Cystic Fibrosis Mutation Database; http://www.genet.sickkids.on.ca/cftr/), usually grouped in five classes representative of all the possible alterations in the maturation process and/or transfer of the CFTR protein [1,5]. In this five-class system, mutations belonging to classes I, II, and III are predicted to have severe functional consequences on CFTR function via different molecular mechanisms. Mutations belonging to classes IV and V, on the other hand, are expected to confer some residual function to CFTR channel, and thus to give milder symptoms. Based on the residual functionality of the protein, mutations are classified as mild or severe, even if a direct

Table 1. Patients' genetics and demographics.

Patient	Sex	Age (years)	CFTR allele, ♂	CFTR allele, ♀	Criterion I[a]	Criterion II (1 = severe, 0 = mild)[b]	Pancreatic status[d]	FEV1%	BMI
1	M	17	F508del	M1V	2	(1)	1	65	17.91
2	F	23	F508del	Y569D	2	(1)	0	97	18.66
3 (s1)[c]	F	20	P1013L	F508del	2	(0)	0	87	18.67
4	M	11	F508del	L997F (without R117L)	2	0	0	110	21.33
5 (s1)[c]	M	11	P1013L	F508del	2	(0)	0	100	23.14
6	M	8	R553X	F508del	2	1	0	80	15.87
7	M	3	F508del	unknown	2	(0)	0	nd	nd
8	F	33	F508del	F508del	1	1	1	73	18.61
9	M	10	F508del	L1077P	2	1	0	94	19.79
10	M	9	F508del	G542X	2	1	1	100	16.00
11	F	9	4167delCTAAGCC	L1065P	3	nd	1	76	14.57
12	F	14	R117C (without $(TG)_{12}T_5$)	F508del	2	0	0	94	18.44
13	F	11	F508del	991del5	2	1	1	109	17.80
14	M	42	$(TG)_{12}T_5$	F508del	2	0	0	106	23.78
15 (s2)[c]	M	9	F508del	F508del	1	1	1	82	15.45
16	M	10	F508del	R347P	2	(0)	0	89	15.91
17 (s2)[c]	F	6	F508del	F508del	1	1	1	110	15.20
18 (s3)[c]	M	39	2789+5G>A	N1303K	3	nd	0	105	19.33
19 (s3)[c]	F	41	2789+5G>A	N1303K	3	nd	0	80	19.47
20	F	26	N1303K	W1282X	3	nd	1	90	19.57
21	M	7	*CFTR*dele2,3 (21 kb)	N1303K	3	nd	1	107	12.85
22	F	9	F508del	L997F (without R117L)	2	0	0	113	25.21
23	M	7	P5L	W1282X	3	nd	0	89	22.31
24	M	9	2789+5G>A	F508del	2	(1)	1	97	15.60
25	F	2	F508del	F508del	1	1	1	nd	nd
26	F	32	N1303K	N1303K	3	nd	1	107	21.22
27	M	14	L1065R	T338I	3	nd	0	116	21.50
28	M	12	711+3A>G	S549R(A>C)	3	nd	0	97	20.00
29	M	13	unknown	R117H (without $(TG)_{12}T_5$)	3	nd	0	104	19.36
30	M	14	F508del	G542X	2	1	1	84	21.87
31	F	13	F508del	F508del	1	1	1	85	18.00
32	F	41	2789+5G>A	N1303K	3	nd	1	84	21.08
33	F	21	L1065P	F508del	2	(0)	0	62	18.29
34	F	50	D1152H	F508del	2	(0)	0	63	23.74
35	M	29	F508del	2790-2A>G	2	(1)	0	92	24.46
36	F	45	unknown	W1282X	3	nd	0	69	23.42

[a](Hm = 1; Ht = 2; N = 3).
[b]when the value is indicated in parenthesis tentative data are available.
[c]s1, s2 a s3 denote a sibling relationship for these three couples of patients.
[d]1 = pancreas insufficiency, 0 = pancreas sufficiency.

correlation among *CFTR* genotype and severity of clinical manifestations is known only for the pancreatic status, not for the lung status [4]. In the gastrointestinal (GI) tract, the loss of the CFTR function results in a dehydrated state of the lumen that is believed to contribute to the insolubility of secreted mucus and glycoproteins. The GI tract represents an additional site where the CF pathology is early manifested, with severe consequences [4,6]. In CF patients many factors predispose to the onset of the small bowel bacterial overgrowth (SBBO) condition, characterized by a high bacterial load in the small intestine [7]. Such a condition could lead to impairment of quality of life at an early stage and also later in the lifespan of an individual. Among the many factors influencing the microbiota composition, the genetic background could act a specific role, as already assessed in other studies [8,9]. Under this hypothesis, the present study aimed to find out a correlation between faecal microbiota composition and the *CFTR* gene mutations in a cohort of CF patients. To this end, the presence of a control cohort was not necessary, because we aimed to depict the variability in microbiota composition mainly driven by different *CFTR* alleles, related to different clinical forms of CF disease. To this purpose, we selected a cohort of 36 CF patients and classified them by means of two different criteria: 1) presence/absence of F508del mutation; 2) disease severity in heterozygous and homozygous F508del patients. Dominant microbiota of faecal samples was characterized by Temporal Temperature Gradient Gel Electrophoresis (TTGE), a semi-quantitative technique useful for comparative purposes, and by species-specific PCR of cultivable bacterial species usually found in faeces. The results obtained were correlated to the two CF patients classifications, through statistical analysis, in order to find out if mutations in the *CFTR* gene could be related to the microbiota population structure. We also described shifts in faecal microbiota composition driven by *CFTR* genetic background in terms of ecological structure.

Materials and Methods

Ethics Statement

Faecal samples were obtained from hospitalized patients and external controls within the 'Cystic Fibrosis Centre' of the Department of Paediatrics at Hospital 'Policlinico Umberto I' of Rome. Ethics approval for this study was granted by the Ethics Committees of the 'Sapienza' University and 'Policlinico Umberto I' Hospital, Italy. Written informed consent was obtained from parents of all subjects enrolled in this study who were under 18 years of age, while the written informed consent was given autonomously by subjects over (or equal to) 18 years. In any case, written informed consent was obtained upon instructions on ethics, aims, and methodologies employed in the study.

Patients and Classification Criteria

Thirty-six CF patients referred to the 'Regional Cystic Fibrosis Centre' of the Department of Paediatrics at Hospital 'Policlinico Umberto I' of Rome, were enrolled after written informed consent (Table 1). The study protocol was approved by the Committee on Ethical Practice of the 'Policlinico Umberto I' hospital. All patients enrolled did not received antibiotics during 2 month prior to the beginning of the study: this was a rigorous selection criterion, due to the difficulties in not providing antibiotics to CF patients, who usually undergo such a therapy. All patients underwent the same antibiotic treatment (200 mg of ciprofloxacin every 12 hours), suspended 2 months before faecal sampling. All patients enrolled did not suffer from ileum meconium in early stage of life. Furthermore, all patients were fasting one day prior the faecal sampling. All these criteria were chosen to homogenise and reduce the internal variability of microbiota response, in order to have a 'common background' to investigate the role of CFTR genetics on microbiota composition itself. The diagnostic work up of CF was according to international protocols.

Genetic, Biochemical and Clinical Characterization of CF Patients

For all patients a mutational analysis was performed. A first-level genetic investigation was achieved by an ABI PRISM 3100 Avant genetic analyser (Applied Biosystems), through the multiplex DNA test 'PCR/OLA/SCS' (Brinson et al., 1997; Grossman et al., 1994), encompassing the 32 most frequent mutations of the CFTR gene. All patients who had not been characterized by PCR/OLA/SCS were subjected to a second-level genetic investigation, by an ABI PRISM 3130 xl genetic analyser (Applied Biosystems), with direct sequencing of the CFTR gene [10]. The effect of CFTR mutations found and, whenever possible, the functional class, were deduced from literature data [1]. In order to classify the patients we used as criteria of severity: 1) patients characterized by the presence of severe mutations (if known, of class I, II, III) in homozygous or compound heterozygous state and pancreas insufficiency (severe, annotated as 1 in Table 1); 2) patients characterized by the presence of mild mutations (if known, of class IV and V) in homozygous or compound heterozygous state and pancreatic sufficiency (mild, annotated as 0 in Table 1). The mutations found within this case series may be classified as follows. Class I, II or III: G542X, W1282X, F508del, N1303K, L1065P, L1077P, Y569D, S549R(A>C). Class IV or V: R117H, 2789+5G>A, TG12T5, R347P, D1152H, R117C. For the growth evaluation, for patients from birth to 20 years, the weight and height percentiles, the IBW (weigh for height index), and the Body Mass Index (BMI) were assessed, as valid criteria to give assessment of patients nutritional status for all patients age [11]. The assessment of body weight is easy to perform and very useful because the weight gain may be compromised in patients with CF. The height is generally less frequently compromised than the body weight, so its deficit is indicative of a serious and persistent malnutrition. Lung function was assessed by the quantity of air exhaled in one second during a forced breath (FEV1), expressed as a percentage of the theoretical value [12]. As a tool for assessing spirometry was used the Sensor Medics Vmax229. The sweat test was performed with the method of Gibson and Cooke pilocarpine iontophoresis [13], by using Macroduct Collection System and Chloride Meter Jenway System for lecture. The test is considered positive for Cl concentrations above 60 mmol/L, considered negative with values below 40 mmol/L (30 mmol/L for infants). The sweat test with values ranging between 40–60 mmol/L (30–60 mmol/L for infants) were considered borderline. The faecal elastase assay, ELISA stool test Schebo Pancreatic Elastase 1, was used to evaluate the pancreatic exocrine function. Faecal elastase values were considered normal in the range 200–500 mg/g of faeces, borderline between 100–200 mg/g, pathological if less than 100 mg/g of faeces.

Faecal DNA Extraction

Faecal samples were taken from fasting CF patients in a sterile environment placed into the 'Policlinico Umberto I' hospital, directly collected in a 500 mL sterile bottle with large neck, transferred to a 50 mL sterile tube, and immediately frozen at −80°C. Total DNA was extracted within 1 hour from sampling by QIAmp Stool Mini Kit (QIAGEN, Hilden, Germany) following manufacturer's instructions. Starting faecal amount was set at 500 mg, picked up from different chunks within the sample itself, in order to minimize the sampling error. Upon extraction, total DNA concentration was quantified by a NanoDrop spectrophotometer (Thermo Fisher Scientific, Wilmington, Delaware, U.S.A.) at 260 nm, along with the 260/280 ratio, and integrity checked through 1% agarose gel electrophoresis containing EtBr 0.5 μg/ml. We obtained similar DNA concentrations after kit extraction from all CF patients, as assessed by Mann-Whitney U test ($P = 0.348$).

PCR Amplification of Bacterial Gene Coding for 16S rRNA

Universal primers GCclamp-U968 (5′-CGC CCG GGG CGC GCC CCG GGC GGG GCG GGG GCA CGG GGG GAA CGC GAA GAA CCT TAC-3′) and L1401 (5′-GCG TGT GTA CAA GAC CC-3′) were used to amplify the V6–V8 region of bacterial gene coding for 16S rRNA [14]. PCR was performed with Taq DNA-polymerase (Hot Star Taq Plus, QIAGEN). PCR reaction (25 μL) contained 1× buffer per PCR, 2.5 mM $MgCl_2$, 200 μM for each dNTP, 0.5 μM of GCclamp-U968 and L1401 primers, 1.25 U of Taq polymerase and 100 ng of total DNA. The samples were amplified under the following conditions: 95°C for

5 min, cycles at 94°C for 45″, 53°C for 45″, 72°C for one min and 10″, and a final step of 72°C for 30 min. This final elongation step was employed to minimize artefactual 'double bands', which could lead to an overestimation of the actual bacterial diversity. To rule out unspecific products a 'touchdown PCR' was performed with a starting annealing temperature of 58°C and decreasing it by 0.5°C each cycle to reach 53°C, followed by 30 cycles at 53°C. In order to minimize the PCR bias, three 'touchdown PCR' reactions were performed for each sample and subsequently pooled. To minimize hetero-duplex formation and single-stranded DNA (ssDNA) contamination during PCR amplification, that might cause sequence heterogeneity in a single TTGE band, 5 additional cycles of 'reconditioning PCR' were performed, taking 1/10 of the previous pooled PCR volume as template in a new reaction. In order to minimize the PCR bias, three 'reconditioning PCR' reaction were done for each sample and subsequently pooled for TTGE experiments. Successful reaction and DNA concentration was quantified by spectrophotometer measurements at 260 nm and DNA integrity checked through 1% agarose gel electrophoresis containing EtBr 0.5 μg/ml. 500 ng of DNA of PCR product from each sample was used to perform the subsequent TTGE experiments.

TTGE Analysis of Amplified 16S rRNA V6-V8 Region

The DCode Universal Mutation Detection System was used for sequence-specific separation of PCR products. Electrophoresis was performed through a 1 mm thick, 16×16 cm 8% polyacrylamide gel, 7 M urea, 1.25×TAE (Tris-Acetic acid-EDTA, ethylenediaminetetraacetic acid), and, respectively, 40 μL and 400 μL of TEMED (Tetramethylethylenediamine) and 10% ammonium persulfate, using 7 litres of 1.25×TAE as the electrophoresis buffer. Electrophoresis was run at 69 V for 18 hours with an initial temperature of 66°C and a ramp rate of 0.2°C/h. For better resolution, a pre-run of 20 V for 15 minutes were held at the beginning of electrophoresis. Each well was loaded with 500 ng of amplified DNA plus a 2X gel loading dye (0.05% bromophenol blue, 0.05% xylene cyanol, and 70% glycerol). Gels were stained in the dark by immersion for 30 minutes in a solution of 6 μg/ml of EtBr in TAE 1X, de-stained in fresh TAE buffer 1.25X for 30 minutes, and photographed with DigiDoc-It system (UVP, Cambridge, UK). In order to minimize the inter-run variance, TGGE runs were conducted in triplicate.

Species-specific PCR of Bacterial 16S rRNA

We choose to detect, by species-specific PCR, a panel of bacterial species particularly present in human faeces as reported by different authors [15,16]. 16S rRNA gene-targeted primers were utilized to detect them (Table 2). The PCR experiments were performed as previously described [17], with some modifications. Briefly, the PCR was done in triplicate, the starting amount of DNA was 100 ng, and the total number of cycles was 25. The three PCR amplifications for each sample were subsequently pooled, concentrated with Speed Vac (Savant, Holbrook, NY, USA) to reach a final volume approximately equal to 1/3 of the original. The unified PCR reactions were titrated using two different methods: firstly, twenty-five microliters of each concentrated PCR were loaded on a 1% agarose gel containing EtBr 0.5 μg/ml, run for 1 hour at 80 V, photographed with DigiDoc-It system (UVP, Cambridge, UK), and analysed for densitometry with Phoretix 1D software (TotalLab, Newcastle upon Tyne, United Kingdom); secondly, measure of DNA concentration was performed with NanoDrop spectrophotometer (Thermo Fisher Scientific, Wilmington, Delaware, U.S.A.) at 260 nm, using one microliter of unified PCR. DNA titration values obtained from both methods were expressed as nanograms of DNA amount per microliter of PCR. A correction for number of 16S rRNA operons within each bacterial species was done, in order to ensure a suitable inter-species data normalization and interpretation. Mann-Whitney U test was employed to assess differences in relative abundances of bacterial species. A *P* value equal or less to 0.05 was considered statistically significant.

Statistical Methods

Multivariate analysis. Two supervised classification methods, Partial Least Square Discriminant Analysis (PLS-DA) and Orthogonal Projection on Latent Structure Discriminant Analysis (OPLS-DA), were performed on a presence/absence matrix of TTGE bands, derived from the overall 36 TTGE profiles. These multivariate statistical analyses were employed to test the grouping behaviour of the TTGE profiles from CF patients, accordingly to two particular classification criteria: i) F508del homozygous/heterozygous/absence, ii) disease severity upon the non-F508del allele. Three-dimensional score plots were generated on a presence/absence TTGE matrix data by means of PLS-DA/OPLS-DA algorithms implemented in Simca-P+ software (Umetrics, Umeå, Sweden), taking into account two principal components and one orthogonal component. The number of useful components was determined by five-fold cross-validation. Data were automatically mean-centred and unit-variance (UV) scaled by the statistical software. These analyses correlated a number of X variables (TTGE bands) to a set of Y variables (CF patients' category), obtaining the covariance between X and Y. PLS-DA/OPLS-DA approaches created a predictive model, validated through Fisher's test, useful to classify CF patients according to their faecal microbiota composition, as assessed through TTGE and species-specific PCR. A *P* value less than or equal to 0.05 was considered statistically significant. *Clustered Image Mapping (CIM).* A resuming heatmap figure, to figure out the putative *CFTR* action in shaping faecal bacterial community, was obtained by the on-line software 'CIMminer' (http://discover.nci.nih.gov/cimminer) based on a scaled and centred dataset of TTGE bands and their OPLS-DA coefficient loadings. Weight coefficients were computed by PLS-DA/OPLS-DA algorithm with Simca-P+ software (Umetrics) for each TTGE band (87 X-variables) on each CF patients' classification group. X and Y variables were 2D clustered, based on Euclidean distance dissimilarity matrix and agglomeration method of Ward.

Ecological Features

Five ecological parameters were computed for each faecal TTGE profile, taking into account the number of bands, their relative position, and their volume (in pixels): Simpson biodiversity (*Hsi*), Simpson evenness (*Esi*), carrying capacity (*Rr*), Gini coefficient of concentration (*C*), and normalized area under Pareto-Lorenz curves (*PL*0.5). Simpson biodiversity index (*Hsi*), reflecting the number and relative abundances of the bacterial species within a sample, was calculated for each TTGE lane by the equation $H_{si} = 1 - \sum_{i=1}^{S} p_i^2$, where $p_i = n_i/N$, n_i = volume (in pixels) of ith TTGE band, N = sum of total TTGE bands pixel volumes, and S = number of TTGE bands. Simpson evenness index (*Esi*), reflecting the distribution of species density within a sample, was calculated by the formula $E_{si} = (1 - \sum_{i=1}^{S} p_i^2) \Big/ (1 - 1/S)$, where symbols were the same as above.

The range-weighted richness (*Rr*), reflecting the carrying capacity of the faecal habitat and richness of microbial commu-

Table 2. Group- and species-specific primers based on 16S rRNA sequences.

Target bacteria	Primer	Sequence (5′ to 3′)	Product size (bp)
Bacteroides fragilis group	g-Bfra-F	ATAGCCTTTCGAAAGRAAGAT	501
	g-Bfra-R	CCAGTATCAACTGCAATTTTA	
Prevotella group	g-Prevo-F	CACRGTAAACGATGGATGCC	529
	g-Prevo-R	GGTCGGGTTGCAGACC	
Bifidobacterium group	g-Bifid-F	CTCCTGGAAACGGGTGG	563
	g-Bifid-R	GGTGTTCTTCCCGATATCTACA	
Clostridium coccoides group	g-Ccoc-F	AAATGACGGTACCTGACTAA	441
	g-Ccoc-R	CTTTGAGTTTCATTCTTGCGAA	
Bifidobacterium adolescentis	BIA-1	GGAAAGATTCTATCGGTATGG	244
	BIA-2	CTCCCAGTCAAAAGCGGTT	
Bifidobacterium longum	BIL-1	GTTCCCGACGGTCGTAGAG	153
	BIL-2	GTGAGTTCCCGGCATAATCC	
Eubacterium biforme	EBI-1	GCTAAGGCCATGAACATGGA	463
	EBI-2	GCCGTCCTCTTCTGTTCTC	
Eubacterium limosum	ELI-1	GGCTTGCTGGACAAATACTG	274
	ELI-2	CTAGGCTCGTCAGAAGGATG	
Fusobacterium prausnitzii	FPR-1	AGATGGCCTCGCGTCCGA	199
	FPR-2	CCGAAGACCTTCTTCCTCC	
Peptostreptococcus productus	PSP-1	AACTCCGGTGGTATCAGATG	268
	PSP-2	GGGGCTTCTGAGTCAGGTA	
Lactobacillus acidophilus	LAA-1	CATCCAGTGCAAACCTAAGAG	286
	LAA-2	GATCCGCTTGCCTTCGCA	
Escherichia coli	ECO-1	GACCTCGGTTTAGTTCACAGA	585
	ECO-2	CACACGCTGACGCTGACCA	
Bacteroides thetaiotaomicron	BT-1	GGCAGCATTTCAGTTTGCTTG	423
	BT-2	GGTACATACAAAATTCCACACGT	
Bacteroides vulgatus	BV-1	GCATCATGAGTCCGCATGTTC	287
	BV-2	TCCATACCCGACTTTATTCCTT	
Bacteroides distasonis	BD-1	GTCGGACTAATACCGCATGAA	273
	BD-2	TTACGATCCATAGAACCTTCAT	
Clostridium clostridiiforme	CC-1	CCGCATGGCAGTGTGTGAAA	255
	CC-2	CTGCTGATAGAGCTTTACATA	

nity, was computed by the equation $Rr = S^2 * Tg$, where S is the total number of TTGE bands in a profile and Tg the temperature gradient comprised between the first and the last band of the same pattern [18]. Rr index was subsequently normalized (Rr_{norm}) to the value of 400, the maximum Rr value achievable for a faecal bacterial habitat, as found in this study and in literature [18]. Gini coefficient of concentration (C), reflecting the inequality of the bacterial population structure was computed by the formula $C = \frac{S}{S-1}\left\{\left(\frac{2}{S^2\bar{n}}\right) * \sum_{i=1}^{S}\left[\left(i^{th} - \frac{S+1}{2}\right)n_i\right]\right\}$, where the portion within curly braces is the Gini coefficient (G), S is the number of TTGE bands, $\bar{n} = \sum_{i=1}^{S} n_i \Big/ S$, n_i is the volume (in pixels) of ith TTGE band, and i^{th} is the number of ith band ($i^{th} = 1,2,\ldots S$) found in a TTGE profile. Surface area between the diagonal and the Pareto-Lorenz curve ($PL0.5$), that measures the structure of the community in terms of its evenness, or the dominance of particular bacterial species, was calculated for each TTGE profile in two step. Firstly, Pareto-Lorenz curve was graphed putting on x-axis the cumulative normalized number of TTGE bands and on y-axis their cumulative normalized volume-intensities (in pixels). Secondly, aforementioned surface area was computed using the macro 'area under curve' employed in SigmaPlot 9.0 (SigmaStat), and subsequently normalized to 0.5 value (the surface area under the diagonal itself): values so obtained are comparable to the Fo functional organization parameter previously proposed [18]. The Mann-Whitney U test was used to assess putative differences among the ecological parameters, and a P value less than or equal to 0.05 was considered significant.

Results

Patients and CFTR Genotyping

A cohort of 36 CF patients was enrolled and underwent to *CFTR* genotyping, as described in Materials and Methods. Both maternal and paternal *CFTR* alleles were sequenced (Table 1), and prevalence of each allele in the entire CF cohort was assessed

(Figure S1). The enrolled 36 CF patients had an overall of 26 different *CFTR* alleles, with a major prevalence of the mutation F508del (24/36, 66.7%), and, at a lesser extent, N1303K (6/36, 16.7%), 2789+5G>A (5/36, 13.9%) and W1282X (3/36, 8.3%), accordingly with literature (Table 1) [1,5]. The other mutations were found in our case series to an allele frequency below 5.6%. Some of them are characteristic of certain ethnic groups, such as W1282X in the original Jews of Central Europe, 3659delC in Sweden and, to come to the Italian reality, T338I in Sardinia, 2183AA>G and R1162X in Northern Italy [1,5]. In order to assess the influence of *CFTR* genotype on faecal microbiota, the unique cohort of patients was divided by two specific classification criteria. Following the first criterion, all the 36 CF patients were divided in three classes: Hom-F508del (homozygous F508del) (n = 5), Het-F508del (heterozygous F508del) (n = 19), and Non-F508del (absence of F508del) (n = 12). Following the second criterion, only patients with homozygosis (n = 5) or heterozygosis (n = 19) for F508del mutation were taken into account. For this second criterion, a combination of the two *CFTR* alleles plus a clinical evaluation (Forced expiratory volume - FEV1%, exocrine pancreas function, and Body mass index - BMI) were taken into account, and a final score of 'mild' (n = 10) and 'severe' (n = 14) was given to each patient (Table 1). The first criterion encompassed all 36 CF patients, whilst the second one comprehended 24 CF patients harbouring at least one F508del allele.

F508del Mutation Drives a Different Faecal Microbiota Composition

Our cohort consisted of 26 *CFTR* genotypes (Table 1, Figure S1), allowing the examination of putative relationships existing among *CFTR* alleles and faecal bacterial community composition. Due to the high prevalence of F508del mutation (Figure S1), we choose to divide patients in 3 classes: homozygous-F508del (n = 5), heterozygous-F508del (n = 19) or non-F508del mutation (n = 12). Their TTGE profiles of faecal microbiota were regressed against this first criterion by means of PLS-DA algorithm, to assess if F508del mutation could affect the faecal microbiota structure in a particular way. We reported representative mean TTGE profiles for each of the three classes, along with a heatmap based on Euclidean distance generated by means of the online tool CIMminer (Figure 1, panel A). In this latter, the red areas correspond to the TTGE bands with higher importance in dividing the three classes, showing how the different genetic background, due to the homozygous-F508del, heterozygous-F508del and non-F508del, arise different faecal microbiota compositions in CF patients. A score plot obtained by the PLS-DA analysis was also depicted (Figure 1, panel B), showing a significant separation among the three classes of CF patients (Total error = 0%, Fisher's $P = 3.1*10^{-14}$).

Faecal Microbiota Composition is Shaped by CF Disease Severity

CFTR gene mutations are commonly divided in 5 classes, upon their phenotypic/clinical severity [1,5]. In order to assess if the faecal microbiota structure would be affected by CF disease severity, we choose all the CF patients harbouring at least one F508del mutation. Once established that F508del drives a different faecal microbiota composition (see above), we focused our attention on homozygous-F508del (n = 5) and heterozigous-F508del (n = 19) patients, dividing them into two distinct classes: mild (n = 10) and severe (n = 14). Their TTGE profiles of faecal microbiota were regressed against this second criterion by means of OPLS-DA algorithm: this criterion was chosen because F508del mutation was found in 24/36 (66.7%) of CF patients, thus allowing a common background to investigate the role of the other *CFTR* allele on faecal microbiota composition. We reported representative mean TTGE profiles for each of the two classes, along with a heatmap based on Euclidean distance generated by means of the online tool CIMminer (Figure 2, panel A). In the heatmap, red areas correspond to the TTGE bands with higher importance in dividing the severe and mild classes, showing how the different genetic background, due to the other non-F508del allele, could shape a different faecal microbiota compositions in CF patients. A score plot obtained by the OPLS-DA analysis was also drawn (Figure 2, panel B), showing a significant separation among the two classes of CF patients (Total error = 0%, Fisher's $P = 1.2*10^{-6}$). Thus, CFTR mutations, driving a mild or severe clinical phenotype in CF patients, could also drive, in some measure, the faecal microbiota composition.

Ecological Parameters Describe the Faecal Microbiota Structure in CF Patients

To determine which aspects of community composition were most related to CFTR mutation, specific ecological parameters were computed for each TTGE profile: Simpson biodiversity (*Hsi*), Simpson equipartition index (*Esi*), normalized carrying capacity (Rr_{norm}), Gini coefficient of inequality (*C*), and normalized Pareto-Lorenz curves (*PL*0.5). Even if the TTGE is considered a semi-quantitative technique, it can describe bacteria that constitute up to 1% of the total bacterial community [19,20]: thus, due to this resolution power, it can properly describe changes in bacterial community structure. Taking into account all CF patients, without any classification, we found linear correlations among the ecological parameters: *Esi* and *Hsi* ($R^2 = 0.925$), *C* and *PL*0.5 ($R^2 = 0.926$) were linearly and positive correlated, whilst *Esi* and *C*, *Hsi* and *C* were linearly correlated with a negative slope (Figure 3). Rr_{norm} parameter showed no correlation with *Esi*, *Hsi*, *C*, or *PL*0.5 (results not shown). Mann-Whitney U test was used to calculate putative ecological differences among faecal microbiota of homozygous-F508del, heterozygous-F508del and non-F508del groups (criterion I). The same test was used to quantify differences in ecological parameters among severe and mild CF patients (criterion II). In Table 3 are the results. Homozygous F508del mutation led the faecal microbiota to higher evenness (*Esi*) ($P = 0.027$) and higher biodiversity (*Hsi*), compared to heterozygous-F508del and non-F508del. Severe CF patients showed a faecal microbiota with lesser inequality of the bacterial population structure (*C*) and lesser dominance of particular bacterial species (*PL*0.5), compared to the mild one ($P = 0.024$). At a microbial community level, these results could explain why F508del mutation led to a different faecal microbiota composition, as well as the CF disease severity did.

Particular Bacterial Species are Related to the CF Disease Phenotype

Once established that F508del mutation and CF disease severity drive a particular faecal microbiota composition, showing different values of ecological parameters, we shifted our attention from the microbiota to some of its constituting bacterial species. Species-specific PCR assays were performed to achieve a presence/absence and a relative quantification of some cultivable bacterial species usually found in faeces, as reported in literature [15,16]. After an accurate correction for the intra-species number of 16S rDNA operons, a matrix of relative quantification based on 1% agarose gel densitometry was built, combined with species-specific

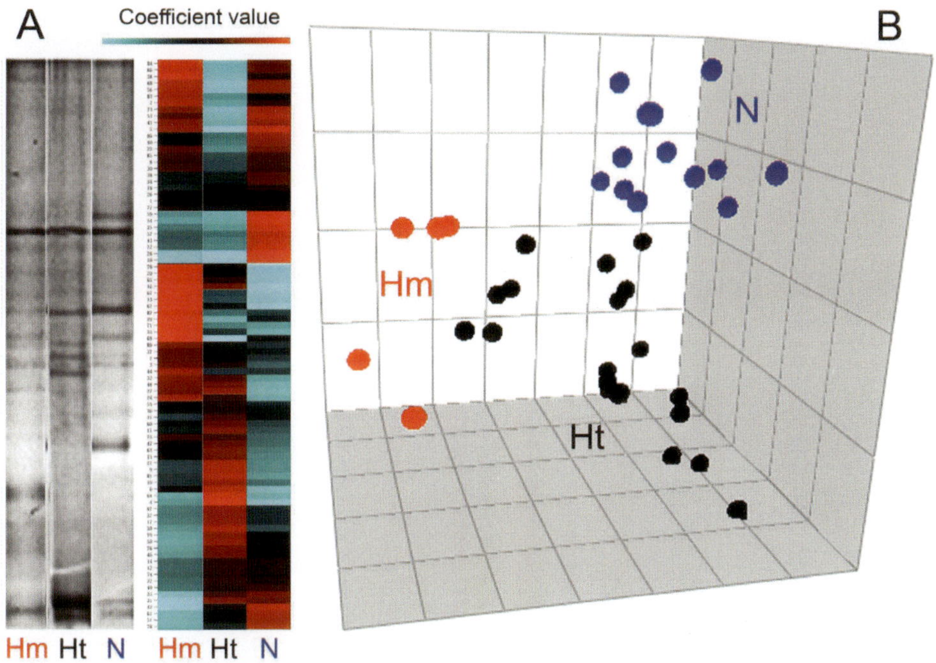

Figure 1. PLS-DA analysis of TTGE profiles, according to F508del mutation. Panel A) On the left are reported representative TTGE profiles from homozygous-F508del (Hm), heterozygous-F508del (Ht) and non-F508del (N) patients. Simca-P+ software was used to compute weight coefficients for each TTGE band (87 *x* variables) on the three different sub-groups of CF patients (3 *y* variables, Hm-Ht-N), with a scaled and centred data set. These coefficients were useful to interpret the influence of the x variables on the y ones. A clustered image heatmap was generated with CIMminer online software (panel A, right). As depicted in the color-coded legend, the higher that the coefficient value is, the higher the weight (red), while the lower that the value is, the lower the weight (turquoise). Panel B) Faecal TTGE profiles of all 36 CF patients were analysed by PLS-DA, and the resulting 3D score plot model gave a significant separation between the three sub-groups: homozygous-F508del (Hm, red circles); heterozygous-F508del (Ht, black circles), and non-F508del (N, blue circles).

prevalence data, and processed with Mann-Whitney U test to assess putative differences in bacterial relative abundances. Among sixteen bacterial species or groups examined (Table 2), only five were found to be differentially distributed, in terms of relative abundance, in faecal samples of CF patients divided by the two classification criteria: *Escherichia coli*, *Faecalibacterium prausnitzii*, *Bifidobacterium* group, *Eubacterium limosum*, *Eubacterium biforme*. We found higher levels of *E. coli* and *E. biforme* in homozygous-F508del patients, and, at the same time, higher levels of *F. prausnitzii*, *Bifidobacterium*, and *E. limosum* in non-F508del patients (Figure 4). Taking into account the criterion II, we found that severe CF patients harboured more *E. coli* and *E. biforme* than mild one, which, in turn, had higher levels of *F. prausnitzii*, *Bifidobacterium*, and *E. limosum* in their faecal samples (Figure 5).

Discussion

Recently, the intricate molecular mechanisms underpinning the host-microbe cross-talk has begun to emerge. Gut microbiota, the biggest bacterial community in our body, exerts many beneficial effects on our health, acting like an 'organ' with peculiar characteristics in its composition and function [21]. Many features can shape the gut microbiota structure: sex [22], diet [23], birth delivery [24], feeding mode [25], and disease status [26]. Up to date, only two studies focused on the role of human genetics as a modifier agent of gut microbiota composition: the first, in Inflammatory Bowel Diseases (IBD) [9], and the second, in Familiar Mediterranean Fever (FMF) [8]. Like FMF, Cystic fibrosis is a good candidate to assess how the genetic background could shape the gut microbiota, due to its monogenic nature (unlike IBD, where 99 loci are known to play a role [27]). During development, intestine is the first district in which high levels of CFTR mRNA are expressed, and are constitutively maintained during all the lifetime [28]. The intestine usually presents high protein or mucous loads, together with low flow rates, and CFTR defects lead to abnormalities in: gastrointestinal tissue morphology, electrolytes secretion, mucus secretion, protein concentration, and protein folding [28]. For this reason, a loss of function of CFTR protein can lead to intestinal obstruction (called ileum meconium) as the earliest clinical phenotype of CF, and to intestinal complications in paediatric/adult age as a secondary site of CF manifestations (after the lung) [28]. Recently, it was found how a diminished pH in airway epithelia from $CFTR^{-/-}$ pigs impaired bacterial killing [29], and it could be speculated a similar event also in the gastrointestinal tract, where a particular microbiota could arise [30].

Our study hypothesis was that *CFTR* genetic background could act as a selective force, able to drive a different gut microbiota, as well as the faecal one, in CF patients. Gut microbiota encompasses mucosa-associated and luminal microbiota, while faeces mainly harbor the luminal part of the gut microbiota. Therefore, we showed here how *CFTR* gene variants were related to shifts in faecal microbiota profiles of CF patients. Particularly, we found that the most common *CFTR* mutation, F508del, found in 66.7% of our patients, led to a peculiar composition of faecal microbiota, especially in the homozygous state (Fig. 1), in which *E. coli* and *E. biforme* species prevailed (Fig. 4). The potential effect that differences in sample size could have on data interpretation, e.g. in the case of the five homozygous F508del patients, was considered and taken into account in the multivariate statistical

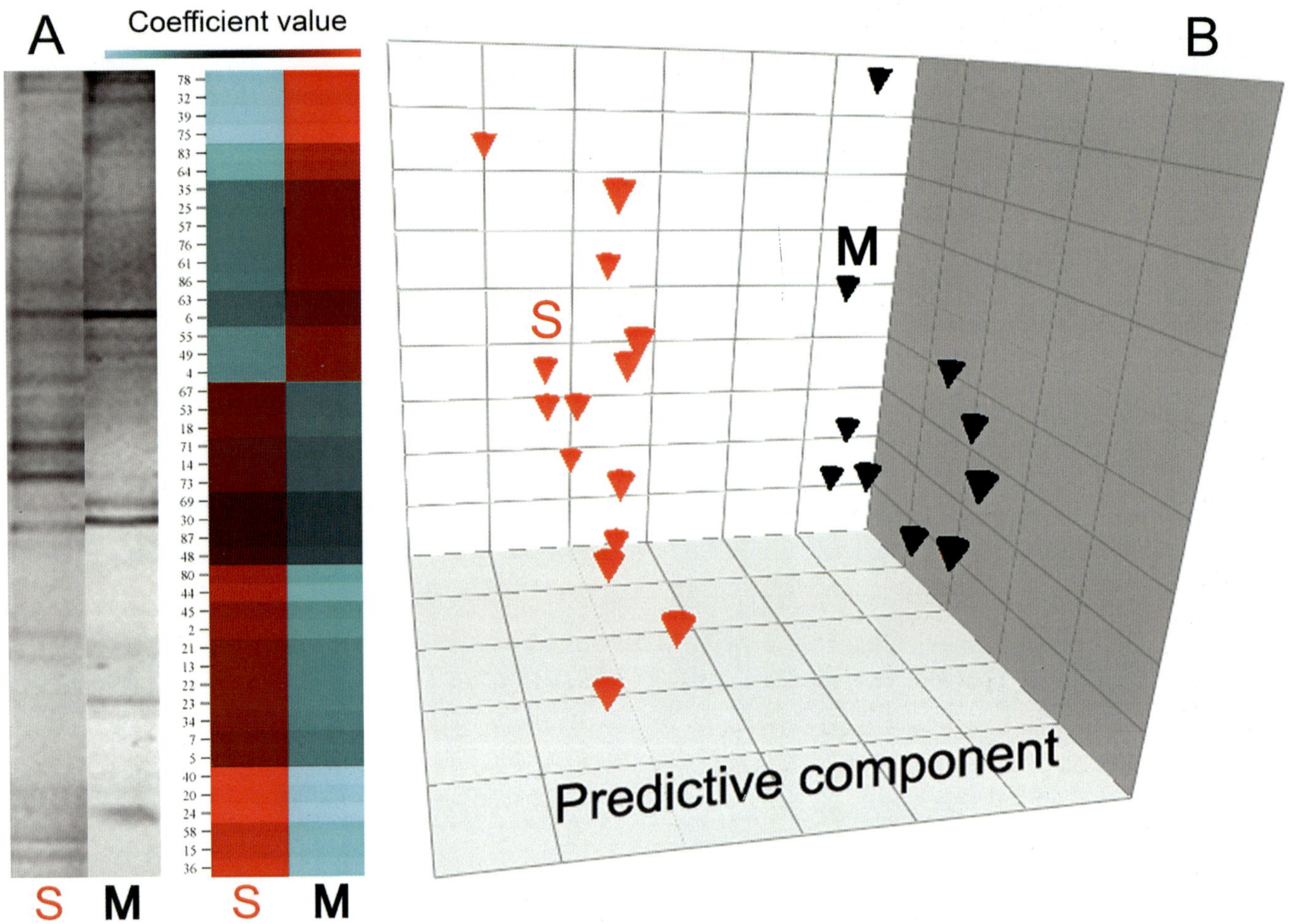

Figure 2. OPLS-DA analysis of TTGE profiles, according to disease severity. Panel A) On the left are reported representative TTGE profiles from severe and mild CF patients. Simca-P+ software was used to compute weight coefficients for each TTGE band (87 *x* variables) on the two subgroups of CF patients (2 *y* variables) harbouring at least one F508del mutation in one allele: severe (S) and mild (M), with a scaled a centred data set. A clustered image heatmap was generated with CIMminer online software (panel A, right). As depicted in the color-coded legend, the higher that the coefficient value is, the higher the weight (red), while the lower that the value is, the lower the weight (turquoise). Panel B) Faecal TTGE profiles of all 24 CF patients harbouring at least one F508del allele were analysed by OPLS-DA, and the resulting 3D score plot model gave a significant separation among the two sub-groups: severe (S, black diamonds) and mild (M, red diamonds).

analysis by intra-variance correction. Such results are to be considered indicative for future studies addressed to investigate the role of homozygous F508del state in human subjects more deeply. F508del mutation arose around 11000 years ago, spreading out during the Neolithic human expansion, due to a putative selective advantage of heterozygous F508del state [31]. Following literature data, F508del mutation belongs to the second class of *CFTR* mutations, in which loss of function of the resulting CFTR protein heavily impairs chloride secretion, leading to a higher thickness and viscosity of the mucus layer [1,5]. It could be arguable that such a peculiar intestinal habitat, along with an inflamed mucosal state, could enhance the adhesion capability of particular bacterial species, such as *E. coli* and *E. biforme*, leading to higher counts in their populations, as already established for *E. coli* strains in Inflammatory Bowel Diseases [32]. Indeed, we found these two bacterial species to be prevalent also in faecal samples from severe CF patients, not from mild (Fig. 5). The mean percentages of *E. coli* and *E. biforme* in faecal samples are usually 1.21% [33] and 1.00% [34], respectively. Thus, the expected *E. coli*/*E. biforme* ratio of the mean relative abundances in a faecal sample from healthy subjects should be around 1.2. Actually, in a parallel on-going study, we found that *E. coli*/*E. biforme* mean ratio within our cohort of healthy subjects was 1.6, and this ratio grew up to 50.4 in an age- and sex-matched CF cohort (unpublished data, not shown here). Notably, *E. coli* differs from *E. biforme* not only for the cell wall properties (the former is Gram-negative, the latter is Gram-positive), but also for antibiotic susceptibility [35].

E. coli was found to be highly prevalent in homozygous-F508del and severe CF patients, which also harboured a different faecal microbiota (Fig. 1 and 2). The high prevalence of *E. coli* found could be due to its enhanced fitness in the CF intestinal habitat as already observed in Celiac disease [36] and IBD [32,37]. We could hypothesize that high levels of *E. coli* in homozygous F508del and severe CF patients would be related to a 'pathobiont' sub-population. Since there is an increasing evidence of intestinal inflammation in CF [38], this habitat could be at the origin of a positive selection for inflammation-adapted *E. coli* 'pathobionts', as well as it happens in other disorders. In IBD patients with underlying genetic mutations, inflammation is targeted to specific members of the microbiota and not to infectious pathogens [39]. Moreover, other authors found that *Escherichia* genus, as well as *Clostridium* and *Enterococcus*, that reside in all people, are usually

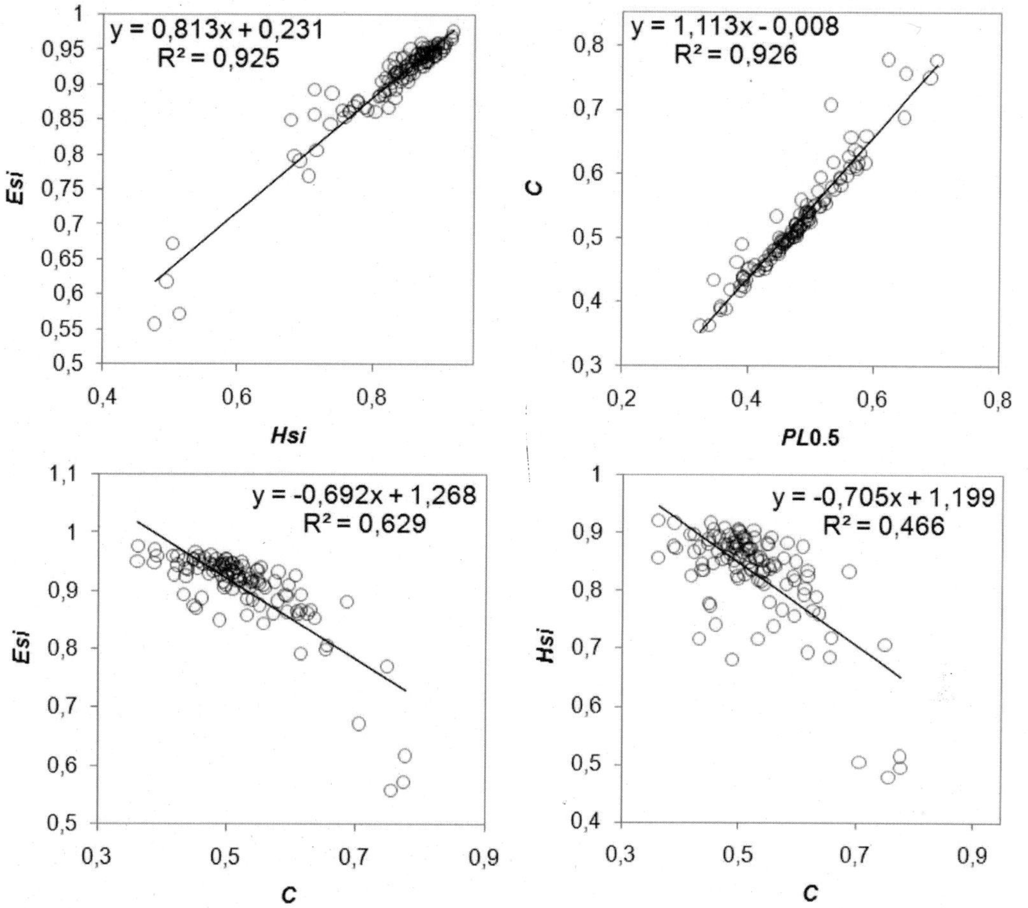

Figure 3. Correlations among ecological features. Faecal TTGE profiles were used to compute five ecological parameters: Simpson biodiversity (*Hsi*), Simpson equiripartition index (*Esi*), normalized carrying capacity (Rr_{norm}), Gini coefficient of inequality (*C*), and normalized Pareto-Lorenz curves (*PL0.5*). Each panel reports the linear equation y = mx+q and the R^2 value, to assess a positive or negative correlation and the goodness of linear fit. Rr_{norm} gave no correlation with any of the other ecological parameters (correlation not shown).

targeted by T cell response in an inflamed intestinal habitat, leading to the 'pathobiont' hypothesis [40,41]. *E. biforme* resulted to be significantly present in homozygous-F508del (Fig. 4) and severe CF patients (Fig. 5). This bacterial species was isolated from human faeces, rumen, sewage and soil, but it was occasionally isolated from wounds, abscesses and periodontitis, thus it may be considered an opportunistic pathogen [34,42]. At the same time, both in homozygous-F508del and severe CF patients, we also found a marked reduction in beneficial bacterial species, as stated in literature, such as *Faecalibacterium prausnitzii* [43], *Bifidobacterium spp.*, and *Eubacterium limosum* [44] (Fig. 4 and 5). Interestingly, it is conceivable that *E. biforme* doesn't belong to the same genus of *E. limosum*, because the former belongs to Erysipelotrichi class, while the latter belongs to Clostridia class, both within the Firmicutes phylum. Thus, a within-the-genus different bacterial habit should be taken unambiguously, albeit *E. biforme* and *E. limosum* apparently have the same 'genus' designation. From the aforementioned results, one could realize that *CFTR* genetic back-

Table 3. Ecological parameters.

Parameter	Homozygous F508del	Heterozygous F508del	Non-F508del	*P* value[a]	Severe	Mild	*P* value
Hsi	0.863±0.008	0.820±0.011	0.829±0.016	**0.048** (Hm-Ht)	0.840±0.009	0.813±0.019	0.398
Esi	0.933±0.005	0.897±0.010	0.905±0.012	**0.027** (Hm-Ht)	0.917±0.007	0.888±0.017	0.112
Rr_{norm}	0.503±0.071	0.370±0.028	0.407±0.040	**0.019** (Hm-Ht)	0.398±0.038	0.398±0.039	0.936
C	0.492±0.015	0.525±0.011	0.538±0.013	0.142 (Hm-N)	0.502±0.013	0.539±0.014	**0.024**
PL0.5	0.456±0.015	0.478±0.011	0.489±0.010	0.179 (Hm-N)	0.460±0.012	0.493±0.013	**0.024**

[a]Hm, homozygous F508del; Ht, heterozygous F508del; N, non-F508del. The lowest *P* value was reported for all comparisons (within round brackets is reported the corresponding match). In bold are the significant *P* values.

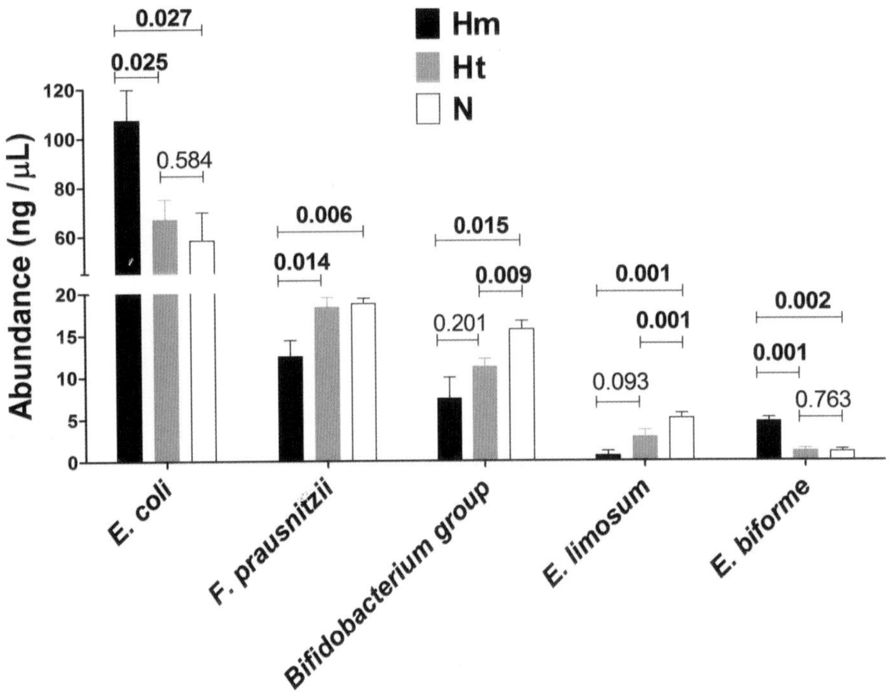

Figure 4. Species-specific PCR, according to F508del mutation. Species-specific PCR were performed on 16 bacterial species or groups, and a Mann-Whitney U test was employed to assess putative differences in their relative abundances (expressed as ng/μL) among homozygous-F508del (Hm, black bars), heterozygous-F508del (Ht, grey bars) and non-F508del (N, white bars) patients. In figure were reported the five bacterial species (or groups) with significant *P* values (in bold) among sub-groups.

ground in homozygous-F508del and severe patients led to an enhanced dysbiosis, with the prevalence of *E. coli* and *E. biforme* species, even within the CF cohort itself. Indeed, we found that biodiversity (*Hsi*), evenness (*Esi*), and carrying capacity (Rr_{norm})

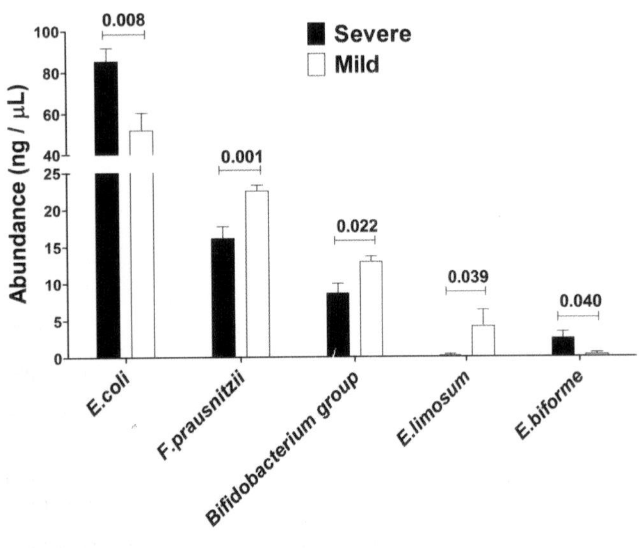

Figure 5. Species-specific PCR, according to disease severity. Species-specific PCR were performed on 16 bacterial species or groups, and a Mann-Whitney U test was employed to assess putative differences in their relative abundances (expressed as ng/μL) among severe (black bars) and mild (white bars) CF patients. In figure were reported the five bacterial species (or groups) with significant *P* values (in bold) among sub-groups.

were significantly higher in homozygous-F508del patients, while inequality (C) and community dominance (*PL0.5*) were lower in severe CF patients (Table 3). These results are in agreement with the hypothesis of an enhanced SBBO in the gut of CF patients [7], eventually leading to a major load of bacterial counts and by-products that could stimulate an exaggerated mucosal response in the gut. Owing to faeces that mainly represent the luminal bacteria, in order to properly assess an *in situ* dysbiotic event, further experiments should be done on intestinal biopsies from CF patients, similarly to what has recently been done on samples from transplanted lungs [45]. Such a requirement could be difficult to be achieved, because CF patients usually don't undergo gastro-duodenoscopy or endoscopy in their clinical follow-up, and, most importantly, intestinal symptoms are commonly underestimated [2,6,28]. It is noteworthy that our cohort was not under antibiotic treatment for two months before faecal sampling, nor the patients underwent a probiotic usage: thus, the role of the *CFTR* gene on shaping the faecal microbiota was not influenced by such treatments. Previously, it was demonstrated a relation among *CFTR* gene mutations and modifications induced in the airway microbiota in 51 CF patients [46], thus, the common genetic background could establish a link among the two main body districts in which CFTR mRNA is expressed: the lung and the gut [28]. Recent studies evidenced an emerging view of an intimate cross-talk [47] existing among the lung and the gut, especially in CF [48]. Thus, CF disease could be perceived as a 'systemic disease', in which pulmonary and intestinal habitats are inter-connected in a 'lung-gut axis' by immunological system, common genetic background (like *CFTR*), and, ultimately, some bacterial or viral species, or they by-products [47]. Clinical studies should be pointed towards a holistic view of the comorbidities existing within a disease: such an effort should also ameliorate the CF treatment regimens. The present study was only on an observational basis: further experiments with mice, or pigs, carrying mutated *CFTR* variants, would shed light on the actual microbiota-modulating properties of *CFTR* gene. This kind of study would improve the knowledge on the refined interactions existing among host and microbiota, important step to set up new therapy strategies aimed at restoring and maintaining an healthy intestinal microbiota in CF patients, and to ameliorate their clinical conditions.

Supporting Information

Figure S1 CFTR alleles prevalence. All *CFTR* mutations found in this study are reported in descending order of prevalence. On *x*-axis is shown the percentage of patients (n = 36, black bars), or the percentage of *CFTR* alleles (n = 72, white bars), harbouring almost one copy of the mutation depicted on *y*-axis.

Author Contributions

Conceived and designed the experiments: VI SS. Performed the experiments: VI FS AG. Analyzed the data: VI. Contributed reagents/materials/analysis tools: RDB AS SB ML MPC SQ. Wrote the paper: VI SS.

References

1. Castellani C, Cuppens H, Macek M Jr, Cassiman JJ, Kerem E, et al. (2008) Consensus on the use and interpretation of cystic fibrosis mutation analysis in clinical practice. J Cyst Fibros 7: 179–196.
2. Davis PB, Drumm M, Konstan MW (1996) Cystic fibrosis. Am J Respir Crit Care Med 154: 1229–1256.
3. Boucher RC (2002) An overview of the pathogenesis of cystic fibrosis lung disease. Adv Drug Deliv Rev 54: 1359–1371.
4. Ahmed N, Corey M, Forstner G, Zielenski J, Tsui LC, et al. (2003) Molecular consequences of cystic fibrosis transmembrane regulator (CFTR) gene mutations in the exocrine pancreas. Gut 52: 1159–1164.
5. Rowntree RK, Harris A (2003) The phenotypic consequences of CFTR mutations. Ann Hum Genet 67: 471–485.
6. Casaccia G, Trucchi A, Nahom A, Aite L, Lucidi V, et al. (2003) The impact of cystic fibrosis on neonatal intestinal obstruction: the need for prenatal/neonatal screening. Pediatr Surg Int 19: 75–78.
7. Fridge JL, Conrad C, Gerson L, Castillo RO, Cox K (2007) Risk factors for small bowel bacterial overgrowth in cystic fibrosis. J Pediatr Gastroenterol Nutr 44: 212–218.
8. Khachatryan ZA, Ktsoyan ZA, Manukyan GP, Kelly D, Ghazaryan KA, et al. (2008) Predominant role of host genetics in controlling the composition of gut microbiota. PloS one 3: e3064.
9. Frank DN, Robertson CE, Hamm CM, Kpadeh Z, Zhang T, et al. (2011) Disease phenotype and genotype are associated with shifts in intestinal-associated microbiota in inflammatory bowel diseases. Inflamm Bowel Dis 17: 179–184.
10. Lucarelli M, Narzi L, Piergentili R, Ferraguti G, Grandoni F, et al. (2006) A 96-well formatted method for exon and exon/intron boundary full sequencing of the CFTR gene. Anal Biochem 353: 226–235.
11. Borowitz D, Baker RD, Stallings V (2002) Consensus report on nutrition for pediatric patients with cystic fibrosis. J Pediatr Gastroenterol Nutr 35: 246–259.
12. Lewiston N, Moss R, Hindi R, Rubinstein S, Sullivan M (1987) Interobserver variance in clinical scoring for cystic fibrosis. Chest 91: 878–882.
13. Gibson LE, Cooke RE (1959) A test for concentration of electrolytes in sweat in cystic fibrosis of the pancreas utilizing pilocarpine by iontophoresis. Pediatrics 23: 545–549.
14. Nubel U, Engelen B, Felske A, Snaidr J, Wieshuber A, et al. (1996) Sequence heterogeneities of genes encoding 16S rRNAs in *Paenibacillus polymyxa* detected by temperature gradient gel electrophoresis. J Bacteriol 178: 5636–5643.
15. Wang RF, Cao WW, Cerniglia CE (1996) PCR detection and quantitation of predominant anaerobic bacteria in human and animal fecal samples. Appl Environ Microbiol 62: 1242–1247.
16. Matsuki T, Watanabe K, Fujimoto J, Miyamoto Y, Takada T, et al. (2002) Development of 16S rRNA-gene-targeted group-specific primers for the detection and identification of predominant bacteria in human feces. Appl Environ Microbiol 68: 5445–5451.
17. Conte MP, Schippa S, Zamboni I, Penta M, Chiarini F, et al. (2006) Gut-associated bacterial microbiota in paediatric patients with inflammatory bowel disease. Gut 55: 1760–1767.
18. Marzorati M, Wittebolle L, Boon N, Daffonchio D, Verstraete W (2008) How to get more out of molecular fingerprints: practical tools for microbial ecology. Environ Microbiol 10: 1571–1581.
19. Zoetendal EG, Akkermans AD, De Vos WM (1998) Temperature gradient gel electrophoresis analysis of 16S rRNA from human fecal samples reveals stable and host-specific communities of active bacteria. Appl Environ Microbiol 64: 3854–3859.
20. Zoetendal EG, Cheng B, Koike S, Mackie RI (2004) Molecular microbial ecology of the gastrointestinal tract: from phylogeny to function. Curr Issues Intest Microbiol 5: 31–47.
21. Ley RE, Peterson DA, Gordon JI (2006) Ecological and evolutionary forces shaping microbial diversity in the human intestine. Cell 124: 837–848.
22. Li M, Wang B, Zhang M, Rantalainen M, Wang S, et al. (2008) Symbiotic gut microbes modulate human metabolic phenotypes. Proc Natl Acad Sci U S A 105: 2117–2122.
23. De Filippo C, Cavalieri D, Di Paola M, Ramazzotti M, Poullet JB, et al. (2010) Impact of diet in shaping gut microbiota revealed by a comparative study in children from Europe and rural Africa. Proc Natl Acad Sci U S A 107: 14691–14696.
24. Biasucci G, Rubini M, Riboni S, Morelli L, Bessi E, et al. (2010) Mode of delivery affects the bacterial community in the newborn gut. Early Hum Dev 86 Suppl 1: 13–15.
25. Adlerberth I (2008) Factors influencing the establishment of the intestinal microbiota in infancy. Nestle Nutr Workshop Ser Pediatr Program 62: 13–29; discussion 29–33.
26. Iebba V, Aloi M, Civitelli F, Cucchiara S (2011) Gut microbiota and pediatric disease. Dig Dis 29: 531–539.
27. Lees CW, Barrett JC, Parkes M, Satsangi J (2011) New IBD genetics: common pathways with other diseases. Gut 60: 1739–1753.
28. Tizzano EF, Buchwald M (1995) CFTR expression and organ damage in cystic fibrosis. Ann Intern Med 123: 305–308.
29. Pezzulo AA, Tang XX, Hoegger MJ, Alaiwa MH, Ramachandran S, et al. (2012) Reduced airway surface pH impairs bacterial killing in the porcine cystic fibrosis lung. Nature 487: 109–113.
30. Duytschaever G, Huys G, Bekaert M, Boulanger L, De Boeck K, et al. (2011) Cross-sectional and longitudinal comparisons of the predominant fecal microbiota compositions of a group of pediatric patients with cystic fibrosis and their healthy siblings. Appl Environ Microbiol 77: 8015–8024.
31. Wiuf C (2001) Do delta F508 heterozygotes have a selective advantage? Genet Res 78: 41–47.
32. Iebba V, Conte MP, Lepanto MS, Di Nardo G, Santangelo F, et al. (2012) Microevolution in *fimH* gene of mucosa-associated *Escherichia coli* strains isolated from pediatric patients with inflammatory bowel disease. Infect Immun 80: 1408–1417.
33. Moore WE, Moore LH (1995) Intestinal floras of populations that have a high risk of colon cancer. Appl Environ Microbiol 61: 3202–3207.
34. Schwiertz A, Le Blay G, Blaut M (2000) Quantification of different *Eubacterium* spp. in human fecal samples with species-specific 16S rRNA-targeted oligonucleotide probes. Appl Environ Microbiol 66: 375–382.
35. Le Blay G, Lacroix C, Zihler A, Fliss I (2007) In vitro inhibition activity of nisin A, nisin Z, pediocin PA-1 and antibiotics against common intestinal bacteria. Lett Appl Microbiol 45: 252–257.
36. Schippa S, Iebba V, Barbato M, Di Nardo G, Totino V, et al. (2010) A distinctive 'microbial signature' in celiac pediatric patients. BMC Microbiol 10: 175.
37. Schippa S, Iebba V, Totino V, Santangelo F, Lepanto M, et al. (2012) A potential role of *Escherichia coli* pathobionts in the pathogenesis of pediatric inflammatory bowel disease. Can J Microbiol 58: 426–432.
38. Lee JM, Leach ST, Katz T, Day AS, Jaffe A, et al. (2012) Update of faecal markers of inflammation in children with cystic fibrosis. Mediators Inflamm 2012: 948367.
39. Packey CD, Sartor RB (2009) Commensal bacteria, traditional and opportunistic pathogens, dysbiosis and bacterial killing in inflammatory bowel diseases. Curr Opin Infect Dis 22: 292–301.
40. Chow J, Mazmanian SK (2010) A pathobiont of the microbiota balances host colonization and intestinal inflammation. Cell Host Microbe 7: 265–276.
41. Chow J, Lee SM, Shen Y, Khosravi A, Mazmanian SK (2010) Host-bacterial symbiosis in health and disease. Advances in immunology 107: 243–274.
42. Harper-Owen R, Dymock D, Booth V, Weightman AJ, Wade WG (1999) Detection of unculturable bacteria in periodontal health and disease by PCR. J Clin Microbiol 37: 1469–1473.
43. Sokol H, Pigneur B, Watterlot L, Lakhdari O, Bermudez-Humaran LG, et al. (2008) *Faecalibacterium prausnitzii* is an anti-inflammatory commensal bacterium identified by gut microbiota analysis of Crohn disease patients. Proc Natl Acad Sci U S A 105: 16731–16736.
44. Roh H, Ko HJ, Kim D, Choi DG, Park S, et al. (2011) Complete genome sequence of a carbon monoxide-utilizing acetogen, *Eubacterium limosum* KIST612. J Bacteriol 193: 307–308.

45. Goddard AF, Staudinger BJ, Dowd SE, Joshi-Datar A, Wolcott RD, et al. (2012) Direct sampling of cystic fibrosis lungs indicates that DNA-based analyses of upper-airway specimens can misrepresent lung microbiota. Proc Natl Acad Sci U S A 109: 13769–13774.
46. Cox MJ, Allgaier M, Taylor B, Baek MS, Huang YJ, et al. (2010) Airway microbiota and pathogen abundance in age-stratified cystic fibrosis patients. PloS one 5: e11044.
47. Keely S, Talley NJ, Hansbro PM (2012) Pulmonary-intestinal cross-talk in mucosal inflammatory disease. Mucosal Immunol 5: 7–18.
48. Rogers GB, Carroll MP, Hoffman LR, Walker AW, Fine DA, et al. (2010) Comparing the microbiota of the cystic fibrosis lung and human gut. Gut Microbes 1: 85–93.

5

Loss of Social Behaviours in Populations of *Pseudomonas aeruginosa* Infecting Lungs of Patients with Cystic Fibrosis

Natalie Jiricny[1], Søren Molin[2], Kevin Foster[1], Stephen P. Diggle[3], Pauline D. Scanlan[1], Melanie Ghoul[1], Helle Krogh Johansen[4], Lorenzo A. Santorelli[1], Roman Popat[5], Stuart A. West[1], Ashleigh S. Griffin[1]*

1 Department of Zoology, Oxford University, Oxford, United Kingdom, **2** Department of Systems Biology, Technical University of Denmark, Lyngby, Denmark, **3** School of Life Sciences, Centre for Biomolecular Sciences, University Park, University of Nottingham, Nottingham, United Kingdom, **4** Institute for International Health, Immunology and Microbiology, University of Copenhagen, Copenhagen, Denmark, **5** Centre for Immunity, Infection and Evolution, University of Edinburgh Ashworth Labs, King's Buildings, West Mains Road, Edinburgh, United Kingdom

Abstract

Pseudomonas aeruginosa, is an opportunistic, bacterial pathogen causing persistent and frequently fatal infections of the lung in patients with cystic fibrosis. Isolates from chronic infections differ from laboratory and environmental strains in a range of traits and this is widely interpreted as the result of adaptation to the lung environment. Typically, chronic strains carry mutations in global regulation factors that could effect reduced expression of social traits, raising the possibility that competitive dynamics between cooperative and selfish, cheating strains could also drive changes in *P. aeruginosa* infections. We compared the expression of cooperative traits - biofilm formation, secretion of exo-products and quorum sensing (QS) - in *P. aeruginosa* isolates that were estimated to have spent different lengths of time in the lung based on clinical information. All three exo-products involved in nutrient acquisition were produced in significantly smaller quantities with increased duration of infection, and patterns across four QS signal molecules were consistent with accumulation over time of mutations in *lasR*, which are known to disrupt the ability of cells to respond to QS signal. Pyocyanin production, and the proportion of cells in biofilm relative to motile, free-living cells in liquid culture, did not change. Overall, our results confirm that the loss of social behaviour is a consistent trend with time spent in the lung and suggest that social dynamics are potentially relevant to understanding the behaviour of *P. aeruginosa* in lung infections.

Editor: Gunnar F. Kaufmann, The Scripps Research Institute and Sorrento Therapeutics, Inc., United States of America

Funding: Work was funded by BBSRC studentship to NJ; ERC to SAW; Royal Society and L'Oreal/UNESCO Fellowship for Women in Science to ASG; NERC grant to SAW and SPD Grant Ref: NE/J007064/. The funders had no role in study design, data collection and analysis, decision to publish, or preparation of the manuscript.

Competing Interests: The authors would like to declare here that this work was supported in part by a commercial funder - L'Oreal - through a Fellowship for Women in Science to Ashleigh Griffin in 2008. This does not alter the authors' adherence to all the PLOS ONE policies on sharing data and materials.

* E-mail: ashleigh.griffin@zoo.ox.ac.uk

Introduction

Research at the interface of microbiology and evolutionary biology has revealed that populations of bacterial cells are complex communities of individuals that communicate, compete and cooperate with one another [1,2]. Many basic functions of bacterial cells involve interaction with neighbouring cells through the release of extra-cellular products. Biofilm formation, for example, involves the production of exo-polysaccharides, nutrient acquisition involves the release of degrading enzymes and iron chelators, and cell-to-cell communication involves the release of quorum sensing (QS) signal molecules. Exo-products are often costly to produce, and laboratory experiments show that cells which cheat by avoiding these costs, can outcompete cooperative neighbours, resulting in reduced survival and viability of the population as a whole [3,4,5]. The competitive dynamics of cooperators and cheats have been the subject of detailed study in the lab, but little is known about these dynamics in natural populations. In particular, very little is known about social behaviours during pathogenic infections, despite the fact that many virulence factors involve the release of exo-products and are, therefore, potentially subject to exploitation [6,7].

The bacterium, *Pseudomonas aeruginosa*, has emerged as a model experimental system for studying social behaviour using strains that either cheat or cooperate to perform a number of important functions. *P. aeruginosa* is also widely studied as an opportunistic pathogen of plants, animals and humans and in particular, as a pathogen causing persistent and frequently fatal lung infections in patients with cystic fibrosis (CF) [8]. There is, however, a lack of studies combining these two fields of research to understand how social evolution influences the behaviour of *P. aeruginosa* as a pathogen [6,9,10].

There is evidence to suggest that a number of traits that have been shown to be cooperative and exploitable in laboratory cultures, may not be expressed, or have reduced expression in strains isolated from the sputa of CF patients with long-term *P. aeruginosa* infections: biofilm formation [11], the siderophore pyoverdin [12], exo-polysaccharide [13,14], pyocins [15]; pyocyanin [16], and quorum sensing signal molecules [17,18,19]. The evidence is inconsistent, however other studies show that the ability to form biofilms is maintained in chronic isolates [20] and that exo-polysaccharide production is increased in chronic infections [21]. Furthermore, sequence analysis shows that mutations found to accumulate in lung isolates are primarily involved in regulation, making it difficult to assess what phenotypic characteristics are beneficial in the lung environment [18,22,23,24].

The loss of cooperative traits has been shown to confer a competitive advantage over cooperative, wildtype strains in the lab under certain conditions, raising the possibility that the same competitive dynamics are favouring invasion of non-cooperative cheats in the lung [3,5,6,25]. These observations are currently understood, however, to result exclusively from adaptation to the lung environment following colonisation from outside the lung [22,23,24,26]. One difficulty in distinguishing possible explanations arises from the lack of studies that (1) explicitly characterise how putatively social traits change with the duration of time spent in the lung, (2) assess whether there is a general trend across putatively social traits, and (3) determine to what extent this trend is replicated across patients.

In this paper, we report the results of a series of assays designed to provide a general picture of how traits demonstrated to be cooperative in the lab [3,4,5,27] are expressed in strains isolated from different stages of infection. Our sample included isolates from the sputa samples of sixteen patients and eleven isolates from outside the lung (naïve). By treating patients as independent data points, we avoid the common problem of pseudoreplication that results from treating sputa samples or isolates from the same patient as independent data points. As it is not possible without frequent and comprehensive sampling regime to determine the exact length of time a particular genotype has spent in the lung, we estimated this from the clinically defined duration of infection. The strains used in our study were either naïve strains isolated from outside the lung or from three different clinically defined stages of CF lung infection: acute - isolates that have caused a single, acute infection in a child with CF; chronic (<6 months) - isolates that have caused a single, chronic infection for less than six months in an adult with CF; and chronic (>6 months) isolates that have caused chronic infection of more than six month duration in adults with CF (Table S1 in File S1). We assayed three categories of traits shown to be cooperative and exploitable in the lab: (1) the production of extra-cellular products involved in nutrient uptake – protease, elastase and the iron-chelating siderophore, pyoverdin; (2) biofilm formation – a composite trait involving many genes and (3) communication through the production of QS cell-to-cell signalling molecules.

Materials and Methods

Origin of isolates

Our collection of *P. aeruginosa* isolates comprised of 11 harvested from outside the lung, either from the environment or different PA01 strains [28] originally isolated from a burn wound [29,30], six lung isolates from children with CF, four lung isolates from adult CF patients with chronic infections (<6 months duration) and six lung isolates identified as either the transmissible DK-1 or DK-2 strains [22] (Table S1 in File S1) from adult CF patients with chronic infections of >6 months duration (Table S1 in File S1). All clinical isolates were from sputum samples obtained by endolaryngeal suction if the patients are not sputum producers or by sputum cough [31]. Patients were randomly selected from the Copenhagen CF Centre at Rigshospitalet and all have been previously described elsewhere [32,33,34].The sample size for all statistical analyses was 27.

To minimise potential for adaptation to the lab environment following isolation from source, all isolates were stored at −80C until required.

Classification of isolates

We categorised 40 *P. aeruginosa* isolates according to whether they were isolated from the lung and the duration of infection: naïve (external), acute, chronic (<6 months) or chronic (>6 months) for a number of traits (Table S1 in File S1). Where multiple isolates per category were obtained from the same lung, their trait profiles were averaged before analysis to avoid pseudoreplication [35].

Measuring pyoverdin production

We prepared isolate cultures from freezer stock in 200 μL volumes of King's B medium (20 g Proteose peptone N°3, 10 mL Glycerol, 1.5 g $K_2HPO_4.3H_2O$, and 1.5 g $MgSO_4.7H_2O$ per litre) in a 96-well microtitre plate incubated at 37°C, 200 rpm for 24 h. After 24 h we transferred 1 μL of each culture to a 200 μL volume of iron-limited CAA (5 g Casamino acids, 1.18 g $K_2HPO_4.3H_2O$, 0.25 g $MgSO_4.7H_2O$, per litre with 100 μg mL^{-1} human apo-transferrin (Sigma) and 20 mM sodium bicarbonate [36,37] in a 96-well microtitre plate. The apo-transferrin in the CAA binds iron, triggering siderophore production in iron-starved bacteria. We incubated the cultures statically at 37°C for 24 h and then measured their cell density at an absorbance of 600 nm (A_{600}) [36,38], and pyoverdin production in relative fluorescence units (RFU), at an excitation wavelength of 400 nm and an emission wavelength of 460 nm [38] using a fluorimeter (SpectraMax M2, Molecular Devices, UK). We replicated each assay seven times per culture, and calculated the mean pyoverdin production per cell by RFU/A_{600}. We determined siderotypes using multiplex PCR to identify each isolate's ferripyoverdin receptor profile, as described by Bodilis *et al.* [39] (Figure S1 in File S1).

Measuring pyocyanin production

We assayed for pyocyanin production based on the method described by Essar *et al.* [40]. We cultured isolates from freezer stock in 10 mL King's B (KB) media (KB medium: 20 g Proteose peptone N°3, 10 mL Glycerol, 1.5 g $K_2HPO_4.3H_2O$, and 1.5 g $MgSO_4.7H_2O$ per litre) in glass 25-mL vials and incubated these for 24 h at 37°C, 180 rpm. We then vortexed and dispensed 100 μL of each culture into 1 mL cuvettes containing 900 μL dH_2O to measured A_{600} and then sub-cultured all isolates into 10 mL fresh KB in 100 mL conical flasks to maximise pyocyanin production, with final cell densities standardised to an A_{600} value of 1, using 10 mL of sterile KB as the control. Cultures were then incubated at 37°C, 180 rpm for 18 h before measuring A_{600} as above; 10 mL of each culture was transferred into 15 mL Falcon tubes and centrifuged at 1,470 *g* for 15 min. We then filter-sterilised (0.2 μm pore size) the supernatant and aliquoted 5 mL into a second set of Falcon tubes to which was added 3 mL chloroform before being vortexed for 5 sec and centrifuged at 1,120 *g* for 10 min. We transferred 2 mL of the bottom extraction layer of chloroform into a new 15 mL Falcon and added 2 mL 0.2 M HCl to each for re-extraction. After vortexing for 5 sec, we centrifuged these extraction layers at 1,120 *g* for 1 min, transferred 1 mL of each top layer to a 1.5 mL Eppendorf before centrifuging at 15,490 *g* for 1 min and removed 900 μL of the top layer of each Eppendorf to a cuvette to read the A_{520} of the pyocyanin in acidic solution, using the control as the blank. We then quantified pyocyanin production per culture as μg.mL^{-1} as (A_{520}/

TRAIT	ANOVA/ Non-parametric test	Ordered Heterogeneity test (with Bonferroni critical P-values)	Tests with Merged Groups	Trend
Exo-products				
Pyoverdin	$F_{(1,3)}$ =18.415, **P=1.391^{e-05}** (P<0.0125)	P<0.0125		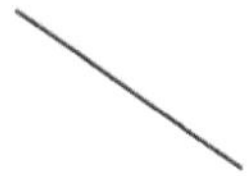
Pyocyanin	(ln transformed) $F_{(1,3)}$ =4.9232, P=0.01217, n.s.	n.s.		
Protease	Kruskal-Wallis chi-squared = 12.8516, df=3, **P=0.004969** (P<0.0125)	P<0.0125		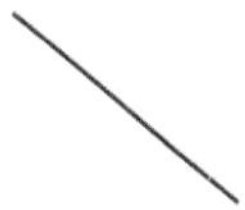
Elastase	(exp transformed) $F_{(1,3)}$ =6.955, **P=0.002935** (P<0.0125)	P<0.0125		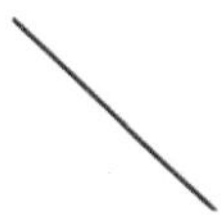
Biofilm formation				
Proportion of cells in Biofilm	(ln transformed) $F_{(1,3)}$ =1.3672, P= 0.2885, n.s.	n.s.	1-3 merged vs 4 t = 1.693, P= 0.1386 n.s.	
Communication				
3-oxo-C_{12}-HSL (LC/MS)	(ln (x+1) transformed) Kruskal-Wallis χ-squared = 10.3996, df=3, P=0.01546, n.s.	P<0.0125		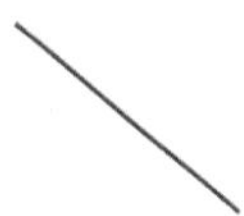
PQS (LC/MS)	$F_{(1,3)}$=4.4192, P=0.01912, n.s.	n.s.	1-3 merged vs 4 t = 4.386, **P=0.0005509** (P<0.0125)	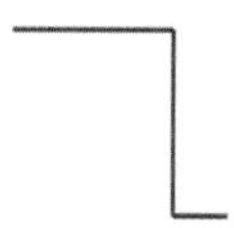
C_4-HSL (LC/MS)	$F_{(1,3)}$= 4.0669, P=0.0252, n.s.	n.s.	Groups could not be merged	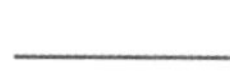
C_7-HHQ (LC/MS)	(sqrt transformed) $F_{(1,3)}$=10.996, **P=0.0003640** (P<0.0125)	n.s.	Groups 1-3 merged vs 4; t = -5.0885, **P=0.0002145** (P<0.0125)	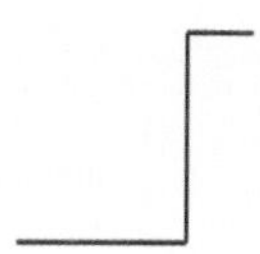

Figure 1. A table summarising statistical analyses and trends in expression over time across all traits.

A_{600})17.072 [41] then multiplied the result by 0.66, as only $^2/_3$ of the chloroform extraction layer was sampled [40,41].

Measuring total protease activity

We dispensed 250 µL Azocasein solution (2% Azocasein: Sigma, 2 mM $CaCl_2$, 40 mM tris-HCl, pH 7.8) into 2 mL Eppendorfs and added 150 µL filter-sterilised supernatant and the control supernatant (as described in the pyocyanin protocol) to each. We vortexed the Azocasein-treated supernatants for 5 sec before incubating them statically at 37°C for 45 min before stopping the reaction by precipitating out the undigested substrate in 1.2 mL trichloroacetic acid (10%) for 15 min and centrifuging at 15,490 *g* for 10 min. We then added 900 µL of each supernatant to 750 µL 1 M NaOH (1 M) in fresh Eppendorfs, vortexed for 5 sec then transferred 100 µL of each acid-treated supernatant into a cuvette containing 900 µL dH_2O and read A_{440} of each using the control as the blank. We calculated the protease activity of each isolates A_{440}/A_{600} of pre-filtered culture [42,43].

Measuring elastase activity

Methods for measuring elastase production was based on Ohman et al. (1980) [44]. We dispensed 900 µL Elastin Congo-Red (ECR) buffer (0.0275 g ECR:Sigma, 1 mM $CaCl_2$, 100 mM Tris, pH 7.5) into 2 mL Eppendorf tubes and added 100 µL of filter-sterilised supernatant and the control supernatant (as described in the pyocyanin protocol) to each. We then incubated ECR-treated supernatants at 37°C with shaking for 4 h before spinning-down the ECR granules (13,000 rpm for 1 min), transferring 100 µL supernatant off the top of each Eppendorf into 900 µL dH_2O in a cuvette and reading A_{495} of each, using the control as the blank.

Extraction of quorum sensing molecules

QS molecules extraction methods based on Ortori et al [45,46]. Isolates were cultured from freezer stock in 10 mL Luria Broth (LB, Sigma) media in glass 25-mL vials and incubated these for 24 h at 37°C, 180rpm, with 10 mL of sterile LB as the control. Cultures were then vortexed and 100 µL dispensed into 1 mL cuvettes containing 900 µL dH_2O for measuring cell density at A_{600}. We then transferred the 9.9 mL of each culture and the control into 15 mL Falcon tubes and centrifuged these at 1,470 *g* for 15 min before filter-sterilising (0.2 µm pore size) the supernatants and aliquoting 9 mL of each into a second set of Falcon tubes. We extracted QS molecules from the supernatants by adding 9.5 mL of acidified ethyl acetate (100 µl glacial acetic acid, 1 L ethyl acetate), vortexing these mixtures for 30 s and then centrifuging them for 10 min at 1,470 *g* to separate the organic and aqueous phases. We then removed 7 mL of the organic phase of each treated supernatant and dried them using a centrifugal evaporator (Jouan, RC10 22) for 2 h at 50°C. We reconstituted the dried samples in 1 mL methanol and aliquoted 500 µl of each into two 1.5 mL Eppendorfs. Samples were stored at −20°C.

Quantifying proportion of the cell population in biofilm

We quantified the proportion of cells growing as a biofilm in a microtitre plate using a BacTiter-Glo assay (BacTiter-Glo™ Microbial Cell Viability Assay kit, Promega). Cultures were inoculated from freezer stock and grown overnight, in 3 mL Luria Broth (LB) at 37°C, 200 rpm. We normalised the cultures to 0.05 A_{600} in 3 mL fresh LB, incubated them for 2 h to reach exponential phase, then diluted them to 0.0025 A_{600} in 10 mL 1% Bacto Tryptone media (TB: 10 g Bacto™ Tryptone (Becton, Dickinson & Co, Franklin Lakes, NJ, USA) in 1 L distilled H_2O (dH_2O)). We aliquoted eight 150 µL volumes of each culture into a flat-bottomed 96-well microtitre plate (plate A), filling one column with sterile TB as a negative control. Plates were sealed in

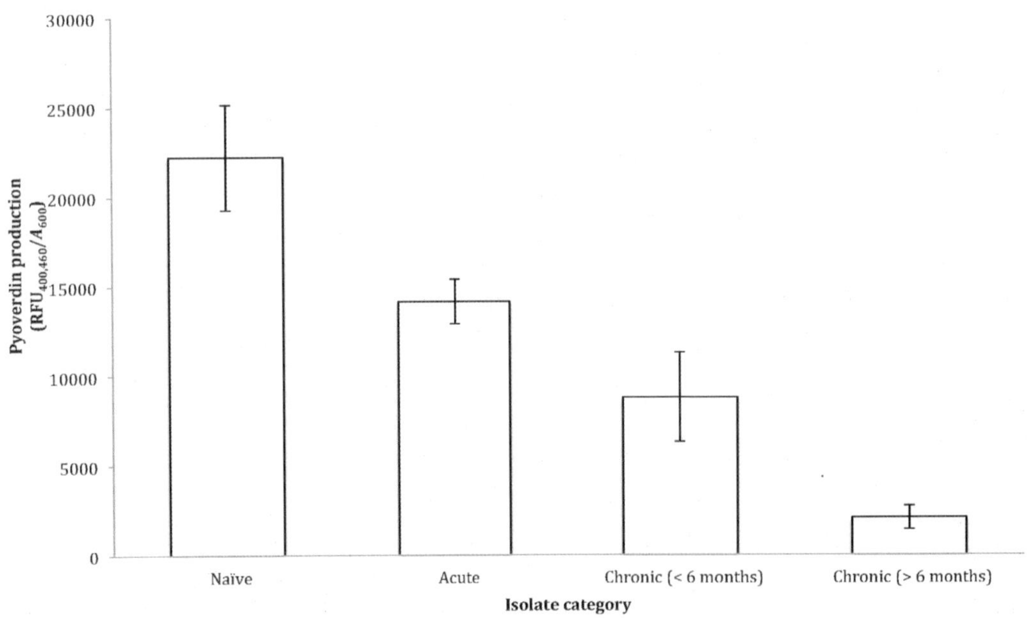

Figure 2. The estimated pyoverdin production per cell of the four *P. aeruginosa* isolate categories. Pyoverdin production calculated as $RFU_{400,460}/A_{600}$. Data shown as untransformed averages of five replicates per isolate per category ±SE.

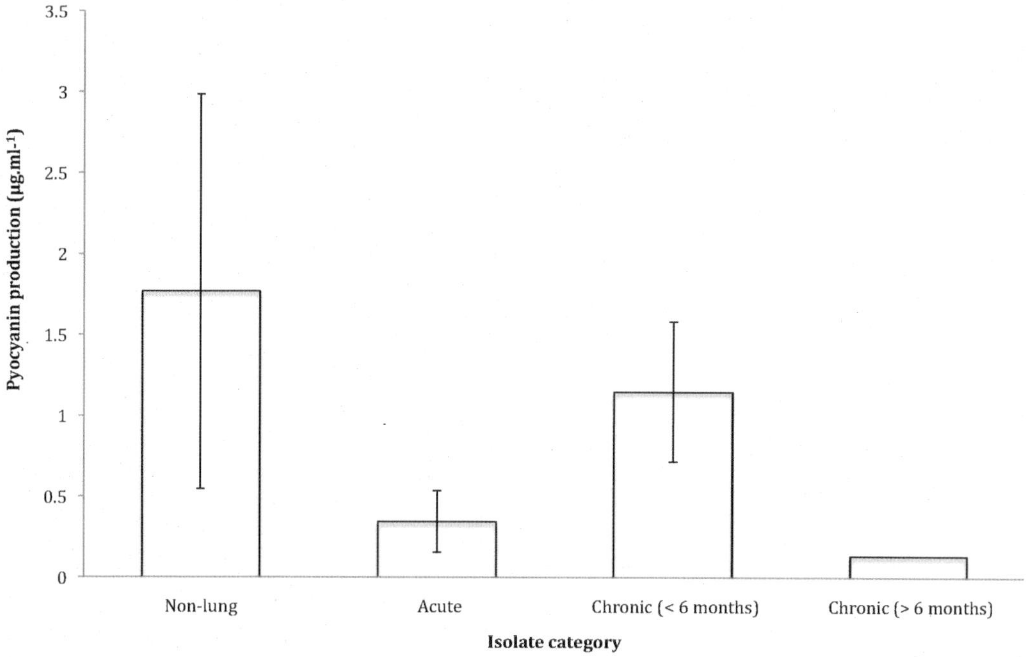

Figure 3. Pyocyanin production of the four *P. aeruginosa* isolate categories. Data shown as untransformed averages of five replicates per isolate per category ±SE.

an airtight container and incubated at room temperature (RT) for 24 h. BacTiter-Glo (BTG) substrate and buffer was thawed and mixed before being left for a further 1 h 30 min to allow time for trace amounts of ATP in the reagent to burn-off – maximising the assay's sensitivity. After 24 h incubation we removed 40 μL of supernatant from each well of plate A and diluted these 1:2.5 in a 96-well plate containing 60 μL dH_2O (plate B). We then transferred 66 μL of the plate B dilutions to a black 96-well microtitre plate (plate C), and added 33 μL of BTG. We then washed plate A three times in distilled water (dH_2O) to remove the remaining supernatants, dried the plate on paper towels and loaded each well with 50 μL equilibrated BTG, quickly followed by 100 μL Phosphate Buffered Saline (PBS: dH_2O). We then placed plate A on a 750 rpm shaking platform for 5 min and then transferred 100 μL of each well of plate A to a black 96-well plate (plate D). We then read the luminescence per well of plates D and E immediately (t_1) in counts per minute (CPM) on a Top-Count.NXT™ Microplate Scintillation & Luminescence counter. A second CPM reading was taken of both plates 2–4 h later (t_2). The two CPM readings were used to calculate the total luminescence emitted by the supernatant and biofilm populations of each culture, and these totals were used to back-calculate signal strength of each population at time 0 when the BTG was first added to each well ($[CPM]_0$). $[CPM]_0$ was calculated as:

$$\left(\frac{(CPM_1 - CPM_2)}{In(CPM_1/CPM_2)}\right) * e(kt_1)$$

where $k = \ln(CPM_1/CPM_2)/(t_2\text{-}t_1)$.

We then corrected the $[CPM]_0$ values for dilution factors and calculated the proportion of cells in a microtitre culture existing in biofilm as: biofilm $[CPM]_0$/(biofilm $[CPM]_0$ + planktonic$[CPM]_0$), using the average for the 8 replicates of each isolate for further analysis.

Quantification of QS signal molecules by liquid chromatography/mass spectrometry (LC/MS)

We prepared reconstituted organic extracts for isolates as described above. After sonicating for 5 min followed by centrifuging at 9,500 *g* for 10 min, we transferred extracted supernatant (described above) of each into a glass insert within a high performance liquid chromatography (HPLC) vial and sealed these with screw caps. For the liquid chromatography (LC) analysis of QS molecules *N*-(3-oxo-dodecanoyl)-L-homoserine lactone (3-oxo-C_{12}-HSL), *N*-butanoyl-L-homoserine lactone (C_4-HSL), 2-heptyl-4(1*H*)-quinolone (C_7-HHQ), and 2-heptyl-3-hydroxy-4(1*H*)-quinolone (PQS), we used a mobile phase run through a pre-primed and equilibrated HPLC Agilent instrument, series 1200, with an Ascentis Express C18 column (150×2.1 mm internal diameter, 2.7 μm particle size). We then cleaned the Agilent HPLC system and recalibrated it into the positive ion mode to run full mass spectrometry (MS) scans on the samples for the same QS molecule range. We then used the Bruker DataAnalysis programme version 3.3 to interpret the LC/MS data. The programme matched LC retention times and MS peak spectra to the 10 μM QS standards injected at intervals throughout both assay methods to produce an LC/MS profile for each isolate.

Statistical analyses

We tested for significant differences with time spent in the lung (as estimated by source of isolate) using a one-way ANOVA analysis. We normalised residuals prior to analyses: data from biofilm and pyocyanin assys were transformed by natural log ($\ln(x)$), and data from the elastase and the C_7-HHQ assays by exponential ($\exp(x)$) and square root ($\text{sqrt}(x)$) respectively. We performed Kruskal-Wallis tests for non-parametric data sets to test for significant differences in production of protease and 3-oxo-C_{12}-HSL. We log-transformed 3-oxo-C_{12}-HSL data by ($\ln(x+1)$) to normalise residuals. Ordered heterogeneity (OH) tests were used to test for the occurrence of a trend in the production levels of each

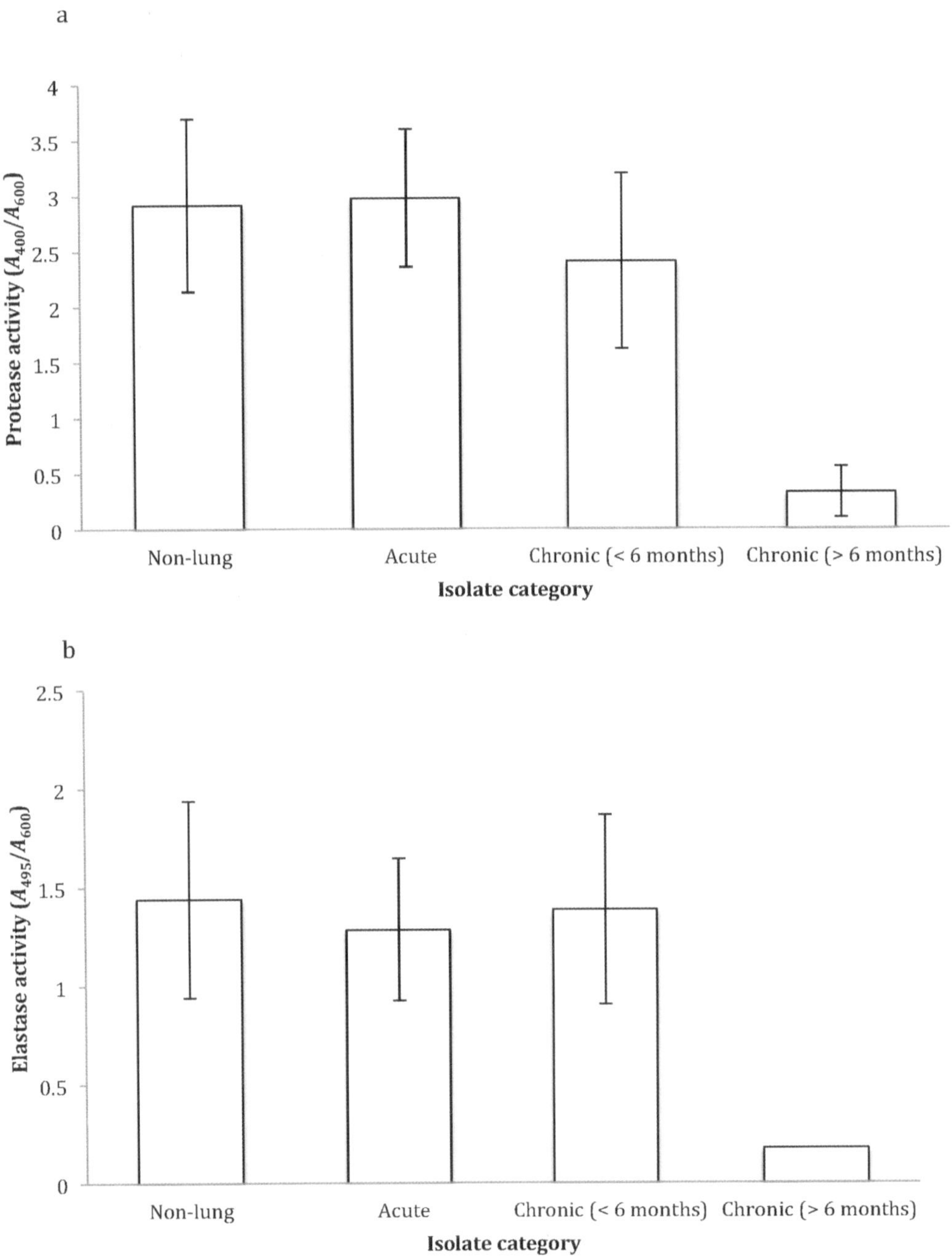

Figure 4. The production of ezymes protease (a) and elastase (b) of the four *P. aeruginosa* isolate categories. Protease and elastase activity calculated as A_{440}/A_{600} and A_{495}/A_{600}, respectively. Data shown as untransformed averages of five replicates per isolate per category ±SE.

trait across the four isolate categories. We merged data that showed no significant differences in production across categories, naïve to chronic (confirmed by Tukey's HSD (honestly significant difference) test); Figure 1) and repeated the above analysis on merged data sets. When the merged data resulted in only two categories, we performed a t-test to check for significant differences, and no OH tests would be required in such cases. To correct for multiple comparisons being applied to the same dataset, the Bonferroni correction was applied to all analyses, with each test on exo-product traits requiring P-values of $P<0.0125$ (0.05/4 tests) and each test of signal molecule production requiring $P<0.0125$ (0.05/4 tests).

Binomial GLMs were used to check whether there is a significant representation of siderotypes I, II or III in each isolate category. All analysis was implemented in R statistical software (http://www.R-project.org) (Summary of all tests and significance levels reported in Figure 1).

Results

Secretion of exo-products

There was a significant negative correlation between the production of pyoverdin, and stage of infection, with the least productive strains isolated from patients with chronic infections

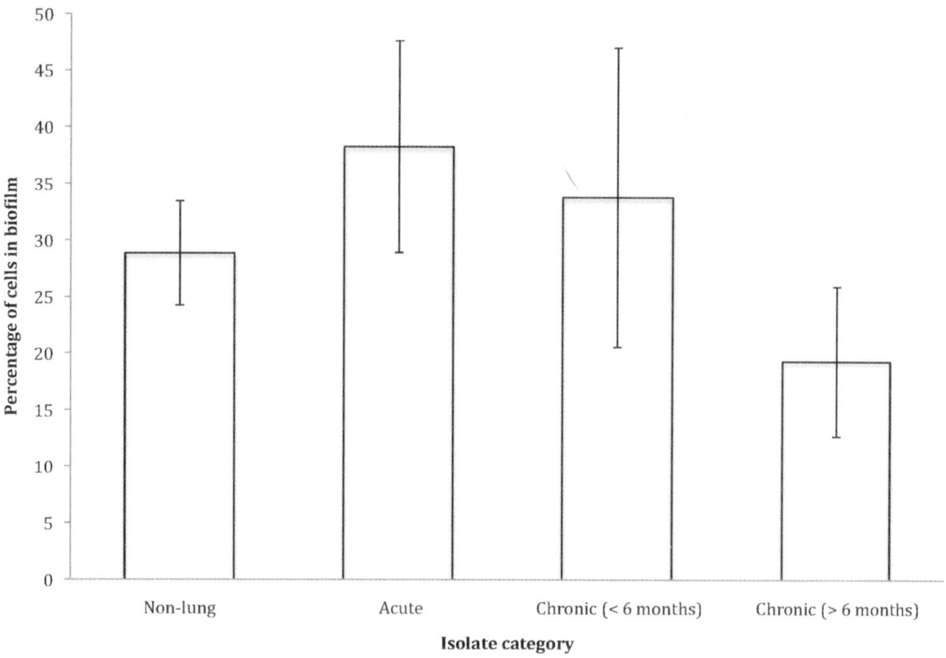

Figure 5. The percentage of cells in microtitre culture existing in biofilm of the four *P. aeruginosa* isolate categories. Data shown as untransformed averages of five replicates per isolate per category ±SE.

(>6 months) (OH test: $F_{(1,\ 3)} = 18.415$, $P = P = 0.000014 <$ Bonferroni (0.0125) Figure 1, Figure 2). Pyocyanin production was not significantly correlated with duration of infection (Figure 1, Figure 3). OH test (ln transformed): $F_{(1,\ 3)} = 4.92$, $P = 0.01 >$ Bonferroni (0.0125)). Both protease and elastase production were significantly reduced with increasing duration of infection (Figure 1, Figures 4a and 4b): protease – Kruskall Wallis $\chi^2 = 12.85$, $p = 0.005 <$ Bonferroni (0.0125); elastase - OH test (exp transformed), $F_{(1,\ 3)} = 6.96$, $p = 0.003$, Bonferroni (0.0125).

Biofilm Formation

There was no significant difference in the proportion of cells in biofilm, relative to growing in suspension, across categories (OH test (ln transformed): $F_{(1,\ 3)} = 1.37$, $P = 0.29 >$ Bonferroni (0.05) Figure 1, Figure 5), suggesting that the propensity of cells to form biofilm is not reduced with duration of infection.

Communication

We found evidence for reduced production of two out of four quorum sensing signal molecules that we assayed with increased duration of infection (Figure 1, Figure 6a–6d): 3-oxo-C_{12}-HSL showed a significantly negative trend with increased duration of infection when assayed using LC/MS (ordered heterogeneity test P<,0.001 Bonferroni (0.0125)). We also found that PQS was significantly reduced in strains isolated from chronic infections (>6 months) relative to isolates in the other three categories ($t = 4.386$, $p = 0.0006$, Bonferroni (0.0125). In contrast, C_4-HSL showed no trend and the production of C_7-HHQ in strains isolated from patients with chronic infections (>6 months) was significantly greater than isolates from other categories ($t = 2.27$, $P = 0.0002$, Bonferroni (0.0125); Figure 1).

Discussion

We examined a range of social traits in *P. aeruginosa* strains isolated from outside and inside the lungs of cystic fibrosis patients that were estimated to have been infected for different lengths of time. We found that: (1) pyoverdin, total protease and elastase production were reduced with increased duration of infection (Figures 1, 2, and 3); (2) the ability of cells to form biofilm showed no significant change with increased duration of infection (Figure 5); and (3) while the production of the QS signals 3-oxo-C12-HSL and PQS declined with increased duration of infection (Figures 6a and 6c), the production of C4-HSL did not change and HHQ increased (Figure 6b and 6d). Overall, these results suggest that a number of *P. aeruginosa* social traits, but not all, are lost over time, during the lung infections of cystic fibrosis patients. These changes could occur as a result of evolution within a lineage, or by displacement of one by another lineage – for example, chronic infections of >6 months are typically caused by one of two strains known to be transmissible between patients in the Danish CF community [22] (Table S1 in File S1).

The extent to which cooperative traits are vulnerable to exploitation is expected to depend on several factors and these factors are likely to vary widely between traits. For example, the ability of one cell to exploit a public good produced by another cell will depend on the diffusion distance of the molecule, the spatial structuring of the environment, and the ability of cells to produce exo-products which can only be utilised by cells of the same genotype. Specificity is likely to vary between traits: it has been shown that members of different species benefit from information obtained from signalling systems, the production of beta-lactamases. On the other hand, it has been shown that strains of *P. aeruginosa* produce pyoverdin molecules which produce iron-complexes that can only be taken up by cells of the same strain. High levels of diversifying selection at *pvd* syntheses loci are consistent with the possibility that this is a mechanism to prevent exploitation. Evidently, therefore, it is extremely challenging to make predictions about whether a population of cooperative bacteria is vulnerable to invasion by cheats. We would argue, however, that the possibility that interspecific competitive dynamics are at least partially responsible for the phenotypic patterns

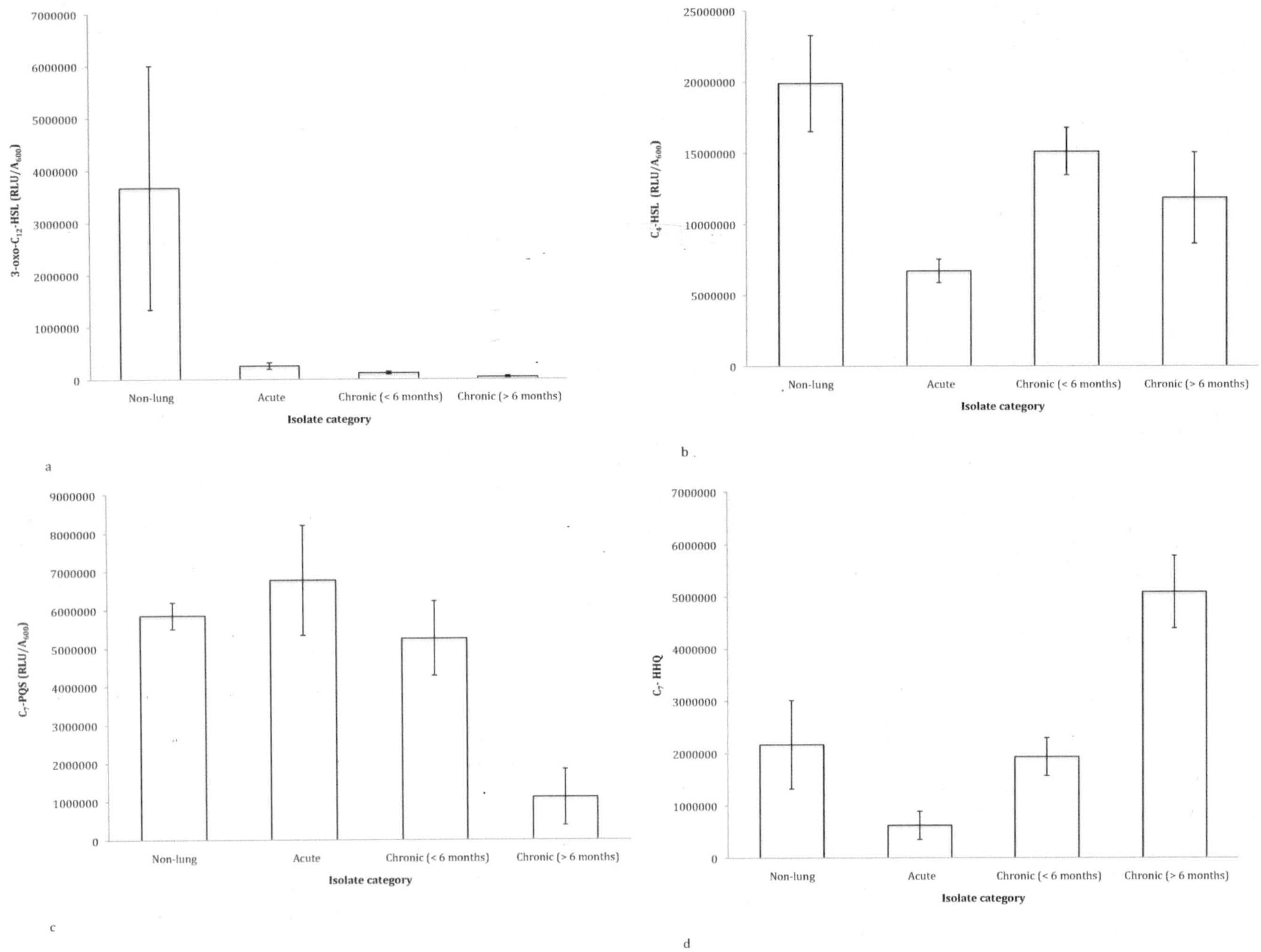

Figure 6. Relative production of (a) 3-oxo-C12-HSL and (b) C_4-HSL (c) PQS and (d) C_7-HHQ interpreted from LC/MS peak readings. Data shown as untransformed averages of single replicates per isolate per category ±SE.

described in this paper is important to consider. No natural population of organisms has yet been discovered to have evolved entirely in response to its environment, without the additional influence of intra- and inter-specific interactions.

In interpreting our observations, it is important to consider that the traits we measured are unlikely to vary independently from one another. Many of the trends we observed suggest the accumulation of *lasR* QS mutants with increasing duration of infection, a finding in common with previous studies [17,18,24]. We found a decrease in total protease, elastase and the autoinducer 3-oxo-C_{12}-HSL, the production of which are absent or greatly reduced in *lasR* mutants [47,48]. We also noted a decrease in PQS and an increase in HHQ. Again an accumulation of *lasR* mutants could explain these results. The production of HHQ is regulated by the *pqsABCDE* operon and conversion of HHQ into PQS is via PqsH, which is under the control of LasR [49]. We did not observe a trend in production of either the *rhl* QS signal molecule C_4-HSL or the *rhl*-dependent phenazine pyocyanin. It is known that activity of the *rhl*-system is only delayed in a *lasR* mutant and both C4-HSL and pyocyanin have been shown to be produced in the absence of LasR [50,51]. Complex interactions between loci emphasises the importance of studying phenotypic as well as genetic patterns as the presence or absence of a gene may not necessarily effect phenotype and therefore exposure to selection [52].

A remaining challenge is to characterise the selective environment experienced by bacterial cells living in the lung environment. It is likely that the phenotypes of bacterial cells living inside the lung are largely determined by selection for antibiotic resistance, but the lung is a complex environment with multiple niches, which change during the course of an infection [22]. It is clear, however, that not all of the patterns we observed in this study are easily explained by adaptation alone. For example, production of the iron-chelator, pyoverdin, is predicted to decrease with availability of free iron in the environment, but we find that pyoverdin production is relatively high in isolates from acute infections where iron levels have been shown to be highest [53]. Similarly, production of the QS signal molecule PQS is specifically involved in evasion of the immune system by triggering defence mechanisms against polymorphonuclear phagocytes, and suppressing the activation of T-cells [54] but we find that PQS is reduced with duration of infection. Competition between cooperative and cheating strains, selecting for mutations that reduce investment in cooperative behaviours, could provide an additional explanation for observed changes in behaviour.

A primary aim of research into the behaviour of *P. aeruginosa* in the CF lung is to improve treatment strategies. Potentially the most important difference between a community shaped by adaptation to the lung and a community shaped by social interactions is the effect on transmission between patients. Cheats are expected to be poor at establishing a novel infection but have resistance to invasion from wild-type cooperative strains that will quickly be exploited. The highly transmissible Liverpool Epidemic Strains LES, has been characterised as having highly up-regulated quorum sensing systems but show similar patterns of down-regulation in strains isolated from chronic infections [55]. This suggests that cheating could reduce transmission but also raises questions about where highly transmissible strains originate from and how they are able to persist in populations dominated by QS mutants that have been shown to be competitively superior in the lab [3]. Taking social interactions into account could not only help explain the phenotypes observed in chronic infections but also why infections seem to be initiated by highly cooperative strains.

Supporting Information

File S1 Supporting information includes list of isolates in Table S1 and section on siderotype analysis. Data from siderotype analysis presented in Figure S1. Section 1: Categorisation of *P. aeruginosa* isolates; Table S1. Section 2: Results of siderotype analysis; Figure S1.

Acknowledgments

We thank Niels Høiby for the supply of clinical isolates.

Author Contributions

Conceived and designed the experiments: NJ KF SPD SAW ASG. Performed the experiments: NJ PDS MG LAS RP. Analyzed the data: NJ MG. Contributed reagents/materials/analysis tools: SM KF SPD HKJ SAW ASG. Wrote the paper: NJ SM KF SPD PDS MG HKJ LAS RP SAW ASG.

References

1. Nadell C, Xavier J, Foster K (2009) The sociobiology of biofilms. FEMS Microbiology Reviews 33: 206–224.
2. West SA, Diggle SP, Buckling A, Gardner A, Griffins AS (2007) The social lives of microbes. Annual Review of Ecology Evolution and Systematics 38: 53–77.
3. Diggle SP, Griffin AS, Campbell GS, West SA (2007) Cooperation and conflict in quorum-sensing bacterial populations. Nature 450: 411–U417.
4. Jiricny N, Diggle SP, West SA, Evans BA, Ballantyne G, et al. (2010) Fitness correlates with the extent of cheating in a bacterium. Journal of Evolutionary Biology 23: 738–747.
5. Griffin AS, West SA, Buckling A (2004) Cooperation and competition in pathogenic bacteria. Nature 430: 1024–1027.
6. Rumbaugh KP, Diggle SP, Watters CM, Ross-Gillespie A, Griffin AS, et al. (2009) Quorum Sensing and the Social Evolution of Bacterial Virulence. Current Biology 19: 341–345.
7. Buckling A, Harrison F, Vos M, Brockhurst MA, Gardner A, et al. (2007) Siderophore-mediated cooperation and virulence in *Pseudomonas aeruginosa*. Fems Microbiology Ecology 62: 135–141.
8. Govan J, Deretic V (1996) Microbial pathogenesis in cystic fibrosis: mucoid *Pseudomonas aeruginosa* and *Burkholderia cepacia*. MIcrobiological Reviews 60: 539–574.
9. Köhler T, Buckling A, van Delden C (2009) Cooperation and virulence of clinical *Pseudomonas aeruginosa* populations. Proceedings of the National Academy of Sciences of the United States of America 106: 6339–6344.
10. Rumbaugh KP, Trivedi U, Watters C, Burton-Chellew MN, Diggle SP, et al. (2012) Kin selection, quorum sensing and virulence in pathogenic bacteria. Proceedings of the Royal Society B - Biological Sciences 279: 3584–3588.
11. Lee B, Haagensen JAJ, Ciofu O, Andersen JB, Hoiby N, et al. (2005) Heterogeneity of biofilms formed by nonmucoid *Pseudomonas aeruginosa* isolates from patients with cystic fibrosis. Journal of Clinical MIcrobiology 43: 5247–5255.
12. De Vos D, De Chial M, Cochez C, Jansen S, Tümmler B, et al. (2001) Study of pyoverdine type and production by *Pseudomonas aeruginosa* isolated from cystic fibrosis patients: prevalence of type II pyoverdine isolates and accumulation of pyoverdine-negative mutations. Archives of Microbiology 175: 384–388.
13. Hancock R, Mutharia L, Chan L, Darveau R, Speert D, et al. (1983) *Pseudomonas aeruginosa* isolates from patients with cystic fibrosis: a class of serum-sensitive, nontypable strains deficient in lipopolysaccharide O side chains. Infection and Immunity 42: 170–177.
14. Spencer DH, Kas A, Smith E, Raymond C, Sims EH, et al. (2003) Whole-genome sequence variation among multiple isolates of *Pseudomonas aeruginosa*. Journal of Bacteriology 185: 1316–1325.
15. Römling U, Fiedler B, Bosshammer J, Grothues D, Greipel J, et al. (1994) Spidemiology of chronic *Pseudomonas aeruginosa* infection in cystic fibrosis. Journal of Infectious Diseases 170: 1616–1621.
16. Carlsson M, Shukla S, Petersson A, Segelmark M, Hellmark T (2011) Pseudomonas aeruginosa in cystic fibrosis: pyocyanin negative strains are associated with BPI-ANCA and progressive lung disease. Journal of Cystic Fibrosis 10: 265–271.
17. Salunkhe P, Smart C, Morgan J, Panagea S, Walshaw M, et al. (2005) A cystic fibrisos epidemic strain of *Pseudomonas aeruginosa* displays enhanced virulence and antimicrobial resistance. Journal of Bacteriology 187: 4908–4920.
18. Smith E, Buckley D, Wu Z, Saephimmachak C, Hoffman L, et al. (2006) Genetic adaptation by *Pseudomonas aeruginosa* to the airways of cystic fibrosis patients. Proceedings of the National Academy of Sciences of the United States of America 103: 8487–8492.
19. Wilder C, Allada G, Schuster M (2009) Instantaneous within-patient diversity of *Pseudomonas aeruginosa* quorum-sensing populations from cystic fibrosis lung infections. Infection and Immunity 77: 5631–5639.
20. Lee B, Schjerling C, Kirkby N, Hoffmann N, Borup R, et al. (2011) Mucoid *Pseudomonas aeruginosa* isolates maintain the biofilm formation capacity and the gene expression profiles during the chronic lung infection of CF patients. APMIS 119: 263–274.
21. Hogardt M, Heesemann J (2013) Microevolution of *Pseudomonas aeruginosa* to a chronic pathogen of the cystic fibrosis lung. Current Topics in Microbiology and Immunology 358: 91–118.
22. Folkesson A, Jelsbak L, Yang L, Krogh Johansen H, Ciofu O, et al. (2012) Adaptation of *Pseudomonas aeruginosa* to the cystic fibrosis airway: an evolutionary perspective. Nature Reviews Microbiology 10: 841–851.
23. Yang L, Holm Rau M, Yang L, Høiby N, Molin S, et al. (2011) Bacterial adaptation during chronic infection revealed by independent component analysis of transcriptomic data. BMC Evolutionary Biology 11: 184.
24. Yang L, Marvig R, Damkiær S, Workman C, Holm Rau M, et al. (2011) Evolutionary dynamics of bacteria in a human host environment. Proceedings of the National Academy of Sciences of the United States of America 108: 7481–7486.
25. Harrison F, Browning LE, Vos M, Buckling A (2006) Cooperation and virulence in acute *Pseudomonas aeruginosa* infections. BMC Biology 4: 21.
26. D'Argenio D, Manhong W, Hoffman L, Kulasekara H, Déziel E, et al. (2007) Growth phenotypes of *Pseudomoas aeruginosa lasR* mutants adapted to the airways of cystic fibrosis patients. Molecular Microbiology 64: 512–533.
27. Rainey PB, Rainey K (2003) Evolution of cooperation and conflict in experimental bacterial populations. Nature 425: 72–74.
28. Klockgether J, Munder A, Neugebauer J, Davenport C, Stanke F, et al. (2010) Genome diversity of *Pseudomonas auruginosa* PA01 laboratory strains. Journal of Bacteriology 192: 1113–1121.
29. Holloway B (1955) Genetic recombination in *Pseudomonas aeruginosa*. Journal of General Microbiology 13: 572–581.
30. Holloway B (1975) Genetic organization of *Pseudomonas*. In: Clarke P, Richmond M, editors. Genetics and biochemistry of *Pseudomonas*. London: John Wiley & Sons Ltd.
31. Johansen H, Norregard L, Gotzche P, Pressler T, Koch C, et al. (2004) Antibody response to Pseudomonas aeruginosa in cystic fibrosis – a marker of therapeutic success? Pediatric Pulmonology 37: 427–432.
32. Hansen S, Rau M, Johansen H, Ciofu O, Jelsbak L, et al. (2012) Evolution and diversification of *Pseudomonas aeruginosa* in the paranasal sinuses of cystic fibrosis children have implications for chronic lung infection. . ISME 12: 31–45.
33. Rau M, Hansen S, Johansen H, Thomsen L, Workman C, et al. (2010) Early adpative developments of *Pseudomonas aeruginosa* after the transition from life in the environment to persistent colonization in the airways of human cystic fibrisos hosts. Environmental Microbiology 12: 1643–1658.
34. Jelsbak L, Johansen H, Frost A-L, Thøgeren R, Thomsen L, et al. (2007) Molecular epidemiology and dynamics of *Pseudomonas aeruginosa* populations in lungs of cystic fibrosis. Infection and Immunity 75: 2214–2224.
35. Hurlbert SH (1984) Pseudoreplication and the design of ecological field experiments. Ecological Monographs 54: 187–211.
36. Schwyn B, Neilands JB (1987) Universal chemical assay for the detection and determination of siderophores. Analytical Biochemistry 160: 47–56.
37. Meyer J, Neely A, Stintzi A, Georges C, IA H (1996) Pyoverdin is essential for virulence of *Pseudomonas aeruginosa*. Infection and immunity 64: 518–523.
38. Ankenbauer R, Srioyosachati S, Cox C (1985) Effects of siderophores on the growth of *Pseudomonas aeruginosa* in human serum and transferrin. Infection and Immunity 49: 132–140.

39. Bodilis J, Ghysels B, Ossayande J, Mattijs S, Pirnay J, et al. (2009) Distribution and evolution of ferri-pyoverdine receptors in *Pseudomonas aeruginosa*. Environmental Microbiology 11: 2123–2135.
40. Essar D, Eberly L, Hadero A, Crawford I (1990) Identification and characterization of genes for a second anthranilate synthase in *Pseudomonas aeruginosa*: interchangeability of the two anthranilate synthases and evolutionary implications. Journal of Bacteriology 172: 884–900.
41. Kurachi M (1958) Studies on the biosynthesis of pyocyanine. II. Isolation and determination of pyocyanine. Bulletin of the Institute for Chemical Research, Kyoto University 36.
42. Ayora S, Gotz F (1994) Genetic and biochemical properties of an extracellular neutral metalloprotease from *Staphylococcus hyicus* subsp. *hyicus*. Molecular and General Genetics 242: 421–430.
43. Hentzer M, Riedel K, Rasmussen T, Heydorn A, Andersen J, et al. (2002) Inhibition of quorum sensing in *Pseudomonas aeruginosa* biofilm bacteria by halogenated furanone compound. Microbiology 148: 87–102.
44. Ohman DE, Cryz S, Iglewski B (1980) Isolation and characterization of *Pseudomonas aeruginosa* PAO mutant that produces altered elastase. Journal of Bacteriology 142: 836–842.
45. Ortori C, Atkinson S, Chhabra S, Cámara M, Williams P, et al. (2007) Comprehensive profiling of N-acylhomoserine lactones produced by *Yersinia* pseudotuberculosis using liquid chromatography coupled to hybrid quadrupole-linear ion trap mass spectrometry. Analytical and Bioanalytical Chemistry 387: 497–511.
46. Ortori C, Dubern J, Chhabra S, Cámara M, Hardie K, et al. (2011) Simultaneous quantitative profiling of N-acyl-L-homoserine lactone and 2-alkyl-4(1H)-quinolone families of quorum-sensing signaling molecules using LC-MS/MS. Analytical and Bioanalytical Chemistry 399: 497–511.
47. Passador L, Cook J, Gambello M, Rust L, Iglewski BH (1993) Expression of *Pseudomonas aeruginosa* virulence genes requires cell-to-cell communication. Science 260: 1127–1130.
48. Gambello M, Kaye S, Iglewski BH (1993) LasR of *Pseudomonas aeruginosa* is a transcriptional activator of the alkaline protease gene (apr) and an enhancer of exotoxin A expression. Infection and Immunity 61: 1180–1184.
49. Dubern J, Diggle SP (2008) Quorum sensing by 2-alkyl-4-quinolines in *Pseudomonas aeruginosa* and other bacterial species. Molecular Biosystems 4: 882–888.
50. Diggle SP, Winzer K, Chabra S, Worrall K, Cámara M, et al. (2003) The *Pseudomonas aeruginosa* quinolone signal molecule overcomes the cell density-dependency of the quorum sensing hierarchy, regulates rhl-dependent genes at the onset of stationary phase and can be produced in the absence of LasR. Molecular Microbiology 50: 29–43.
51. Dekimpe V, Déziel E (2009) Revisiting the quorum-sensing hierarchy in *Pseudomonas aeruginosa*: the transcriptional regulator RhlR regulates LasR-specific factors. Microbiology 155: 712–723.
52. Barrett R, Hoekstra H (2011) Molecular spandrels: tests of adaptation at the genetic level. Nature Reviews Genetics 12: 767–780.
53. Reid D, Carroll V, O'May C, Champion A, Kirov S (2007) Increased airway iron as a potential factor in the persistence of *Pseudomonas aeruginosa* infection in cystic fibrosis. European Respiratory Journal 30: 286–292.
54. Fletcher M, Heeb S, Chhabra S, Diggle SP, Williams P, et al. (2010) 2-alkyl-4(1H)-quinolone signalling in *Pseudomonas aeruginosa*. In: Ramos J, Filloux A, editors. Molecular microbiology, infection and biodiversity. London: Springer. pp. 29–57.
55. Mowatt E, Paterson S, Fothergill J, Wright E, Ledson M, et al. (2011) *Pseudomonas aeruginosa* population diversity and turnover in cystic fibrosis chronic infections. American Journal of Respiratory and Critical Care Medicine 183: 1674–1679.

6

Lipoxin A_4 Stimulates Calcium-Activated Chloride Currents and Increases Airway Surface Liquid Height in Normal and Cystic Fibrosis Airway Epithelia

Valia Verrière[1]⁹, Gerard Higgins[1,4]⁹, Mazen Al-Alawi[1,3], Richard W. Costello[3], Paul McNally[4], Raphaël Chiron[2], Brian J. Harvey[1], Valérie Urbach[1,4]*

1 Department of Molecular Medicine, RCSI Education and Research Centre, Beaumont Hospital, Dublin, Ireland, **2** CRCM, Montpellier, France, **3** Department of Respiratory Medicine, Beaumont Hospital, Dublin, Ireland, **4** National Children's Research Centre, Our Lady's Children's Hospital Crumlin, Dublin, Ireland

Abstract

Cystic Fibrosis (CF) is a genetic disease characterised by a deficit in epithelial Cl^- secretion which in the lung leads to airway dehydration and a reduced Airway Surface Liquid (ASL) height. The endogenous lipoxin LXA_4 is a member of the newly identified eicosanoids playing a key role in ending the inflammatory process. Levels of LXA_4 are reported to be decreased in the airways of patients with CF. We have previously shown that in normal human bronchial epithelial cells, LXA_4 produced a rapid and transient increase in intracellular Ca^{2+}. We have investigated, the effect of LXA_4 on Cl^- secretion and the functional consequences on ASL generation in bronchial epithelial cells obtained from CF and non-CF patient biopsies and in bronchial epithelial cell lines. We found that LXA_4 stimulated a rapid intracellular Ca^{2+} increase in all of the different CF bronchial epithelial cells tested. In non-CF and CF bronchial epithelia, LXA_4 stimulated whole-cell Cl^- currents which were inhibited by NPPB (calcium-activated Cl^- channel inhibitor), BAPTA-AM (chelator of intracellular Ca^{2+}) but not by CFTRinh-172 (CFTR inhibitor). We found, using confocal imaging, that LXA_4 increased the ASL height in non-CF and in CF airway bronchial epithelia. The LXA_4 effect on ASL height was sensitive to bumetanide, an inhibitor of transepithelial Cl^- secretion. The LXA_4 stimulation of intracellular Ca^{2+}, whole-cell Cl^- currents, conductances and ASL height were inhibited by Boc-2, a specific antagonist of the ALX/FPR2 receptor. Our results provide, for the first time, evidence for a novel role of LXA_4 in the stimulation of intracellular Ca^{2+} signalling leading to Ca^{2+}-activated Cl^- secretion and enhanced ASL height in non-CF and CF bronchial epithelia.

Editor: James L. Kreindler, Abramson Research Center, United States of America

Funding: This work was funded by the French National Institute of Health (INSERM), the Centre Hospitalier Universitaire (CHU) of Montpellier, the French Cystic Fibrosis Association (Vaincre La Mucoviscidose), a Career Enhancement and Mobility Programme Marie Curie Fellowship, the Higher Education Authority of Ireland under the Programme for Research in Third Level Institutions (PRTLI) Cycle 4 and the National Biophotonics and Imaging Platform, Ireland. The funders had no role in study design, data collection and analysis, decision to publish, or preparation of the manuscript.

Competing Interests: The authors have declared that no competing interests exist.

* E-mail: valerie.urbach@ncrc.ie

⁹ These authors contributed equally to this work.

Introduction

Cystic fibrosis is caused by the mutation of the gene coding for the Cystic Fibrosis Transmembrane conductance Regulator (CFTR), a cyclic AMP-dependent Cl^- channel. The major clinical features of CF are chronic pulmonary disease, exocrine pancreatic insufficiency and male infertility [1,2]. The lung disease is the main cause of morbidity and mortality in CF. The airway epithelium of patients with CF fails to transport Cl^- and water, resulting in a reduced ASL height and impaired mucociliary clearance. The hyper-absorption of Na^+ observed in the CF bronchial epithelium may further exacerbate the dehydration of the ASL. It is generally accepted that the dehydration of the airway lumen favours chronic infection and inflammation leading to progressive destruction of the lung [3]. Identification of agents, particularly natural endogenous biologicals, which stimulate alternative non-CFTR Cl^- secretory pathways and promote ASL hydration and recovery of optimal ASL height are likely to be of therapeutic benefit in improving mucociliary clearance in patients with CF.

The levels of LXA_4 in the airways have been reported to be decreased in patients with CF [4]. Lipoxins are bioactive lipids derived from omega-6 polyunsaturated fatty acids and play important roles in various biological functions [5]. The endogenous lipoxin A_4 (LXA_4: 5S,6R,15S-trihydroxy-7,9,13-trans-11-eicosatetraenoic acid) is produced at inflammatory sites from the interaction of lipoxygenase activities of several cell types including leukocytes, platelets and epithelial cells. $LXA_4$is one member of the newly identified lipid molecules playing a role in ending/resolving the inflammatory process by modulating neutrophilic inflammation, clearing apoptotic PMN and inhibiting the production of pro-inflammatory cytokines [6]. The deficit in LXA_4 levels in CF airways could be a contributing factor in chronic airway inflammation which characterises these patients.

Very little is known about the role of LXA_4 in the lung beyond its anti-inflammatory effects. We have previously shown that normal human bronchial epithelial cells are a biological target for LXA_4. The receptor for LXA_4 (ALX/FPR2) is expressed in the bronchial epithelial cell line 16HBE14o- and LXA_4 stimulates an intracellular Ca^{2+} mobilisation in these cells [7]. Intracellular Ca^{2+} is a major regulator of Cl^- transport and the stimulation of epithelial Cl^- secretion would be of major therapeutic benefit in CF to restore efficient airway clearance. We have investigated the effect of LXA_4 on epithelial Cl^- secretion and its functional consequences on ASL height using bronchial epithelial cells obtained from CF and non-CF patient biopsies and in a variety of bronchial epithelial cell lines commonly used as models for CF ion transport and immunological studies.

Results

LXA_4 Effects on Intracellular Ca^{2+} in Normal and CF Bronchial Epithelial Cells

LXA_4 induced a rapid increase of intracellular Ca^{2+} in all human airway epithelial cell types tested. These results are summarised in typical records obtained in Nuli-1 and CuFi-3 cell lines (figure 1A) and NHBE and CFBE primary cultures (Figure 1B) and on corresponding histograms (Figure 1C). There was no significant difference in the maximum increase in calcium induced by LXA_4 (100 nM) between non-CF and CF bronchial epithelial cell lines (Figure 1A and 1C). However the maximum increase obtained in CF bronchial epithelial primary culture (CFBE) was significantly higher than in non-CF (NHBE) bronchial epithelial primary cultures (Figure 1B and 1C). The kinetics of the Ca^{2+} responses were markedly different between CF and non-CF cells. In the non-CF bronchial epithelial cells (NHBE primary cultures and Nuli-1 cell line), the intracellular Ca^{2+} rise induced by LXA_4 was fast and transient with a recovery to basal values within 2 to 5 min (Figure 1C). In contrast, in the CF bronchial epithelial cells (CFBE primary cultures and CuFi cell lines), LXA_4 induced a slower increase in Ca^{2+} and a delayed (or absent) recovery toward basal values (Figure 1C). Thus the total amount of Ca^{2+} mobilised in the cytosol upon LXA_4 exposure was higher in CF cells than in non-CF bronchial epithelial cells.

In order to investigate the origin of the calcium signal induced by LXA_4, we tested the effect of LXA_4 on intracellular Ca^{2+} mobilization in the absence of extracellular Ca^{2+} in non-CF and CF airway epithelial cells. The results presented in Figure 1A show that in Nuli-1 cells bathed in an external Ca^{2+}-free solution, the response to LXA_4 was not different from control conditions (plain line). In Nuli-1 cells, there was no significant difference in the maximum Ca^{2+} increase obtained after LXA_4 exposure with or without external Ca^{2+} (F340/F380 : control 8.49±0.48 and external Ca^{2+}-free 8.57±0.32) and in the value measured 2 min after the peak (5.22±0.43 in control condition and 5.89±0.36 in external Ca^{2+}-free ($n=4$, $p>0.1$)). These results indicate that in normal airway epithelial cells, LXA_4 generates a calcium signal mainly due to the release of Ca^{2+} from intracellular stores rather than Ca^{2+} entry. As shown in Figure 1A, there was no difference in the maximum Ca^{2+} increase in CuFi-3 cells obtained after LXA_4 exposure with or without external Ca^{2+} (F340/F380: control 8.76±0.55 and external Ca^{2+}-free: 8.99±0.49 ($n=4$, $p>0.1$)). However, in external Ca^{2+}-free medium, the calcium response to LXA_4 in CuFi-3 cells was more transient with a rapid recovery to basal values. The F340/F380 ratio values obtained 2 min after the peak Ca^{2+} response were 7.17±0.43 in control conditions and 2.29±0.46 ($n=4$, $p<0.05$) in an external Ca^{2+}-free solution. Taken together, these results suggest that, in CF airway epithelia, in addition to the Ca^{2+} mobilisation from intracellular stores, LXA_4 also stimulates Ca^{2+} entry and this response is absent in non-CF bronchial epithelial cells (Figure 1A).

Role of the ALX/FPR2 Receptor in the Calcium Response to LXA_4

The role of the ALX /FPR2 receptor in the Ca^{2+} response to LXA_4 was investigated using the specific inhibitor, Boc-2 (Figure 2). The effect of LXA_4 (100 nM) on intracellular Ca^{2+} was completely abolished after treatment with Boc-2 (10 μM) in both NuLi-1 ($n=5$) and CuFi-3 ($n=4$) cells (figure 2A and 2B). However, ATP (100 μM), a known stimulator of intracellular Ca^{2+} mobilisation via purinergic receptor stimulation, produced a Ca^{2+} signal in cells treated with Boc-2 (Figure 2A). These results support the involvement of the ALX/FPR2 receptor in the Ca^{2+} signalling response to LXA_4.

LXA_4 Effects on Whole-cell Currents in Non-CF and CF Bronchial Epithelial Cells

Since intracellular Ca^{2+} is a regulator of Cl^- transport and we have shown that LXA_4 we regulates Ca^{2+}, we investigated the effect of LXA_4 on ion transport using whole cell patch-clamp recording techniques. The whole-cell current-voltage relationships were obtained from whole-cell patch-clamp recordings in non-CF (NHBE primary culture and Nuli-1 cell line) and CF (CFBE primary culture and CuFi-3 cell line) human bronchial epithelial cells.

As shown from the current-voltage curves (Figure 3 and 4) and in Table 1, the whole-cell currents under control conditions were outwardly rectified in non-CF and CF cell lines and in primary airway epithelial cells. The reversal potentials (E_{rev}) obtained in the cell lines (E_{rev} Nuli-1 = −23.8±3.2 mV, E_{rev} CuFi-3 = −21. ±3.6 mV) and primary cultures (E_{rev} NHBE = −22.4±3.9 mV and E_{rev} CFBE = −22.4±1.9 mV) indicate that Cl^- ($E_{Cl} = -39$ mV) is the main charge carrier under these conditions (Table 1).

LXA_4 exposure stimulated the whole-cell currents in non-CF and CF airway epithelial cell lines and in normal and CF primary cultures, in a time-dependent and dose-dependent manner, as illustrated in Figure 3 and Figure 4, respectively.

Typical whole-cell current-voltage relationship in NHBE and CFBE primary cultures recorded over variable duration of LXA_4 (100 nM) exposure illustrate the time-dependence of the response (Figure 3A and 3B). The statistical significance of the time dependence of current responses have been investigated in non-CF and CF airway epithelial cell lines and primary cultures as shown in Figure 3C. The maximum stimulatory effect on the inward conductance (for outward flux of Cl^- from the cell) in non-CF airway epithelial cells (Nuli-1 and NHBE) was obtained after 10 min exposure to LXA_4 and declined thereafter to control levels (Figure 3C). In CF airway epithelial cells (CuFi-3 and CFBE), the increased inward conductance induced by LXA_4 was sustained without recovery to basal values over the 15 min period of observation (Figure 3C).

The dose dependence of the response to LXA_4 was investigated in the non-CF and CF cell lines. The stimulatory effect of LXA_4 on membrane conductance was found to be dose-dependent as illustrated on the typical whole-cell current-voltage relationship obtained from Nuli-1 and CuFi-3 cell lines upon exposure to different LXA4 concentrations (figure 4A and 4B). In both cell lines, significant responses were observed at concentrations as low as 1 pM and the maximum response achieved at 10 nM LXA_4 (Figure 4C).

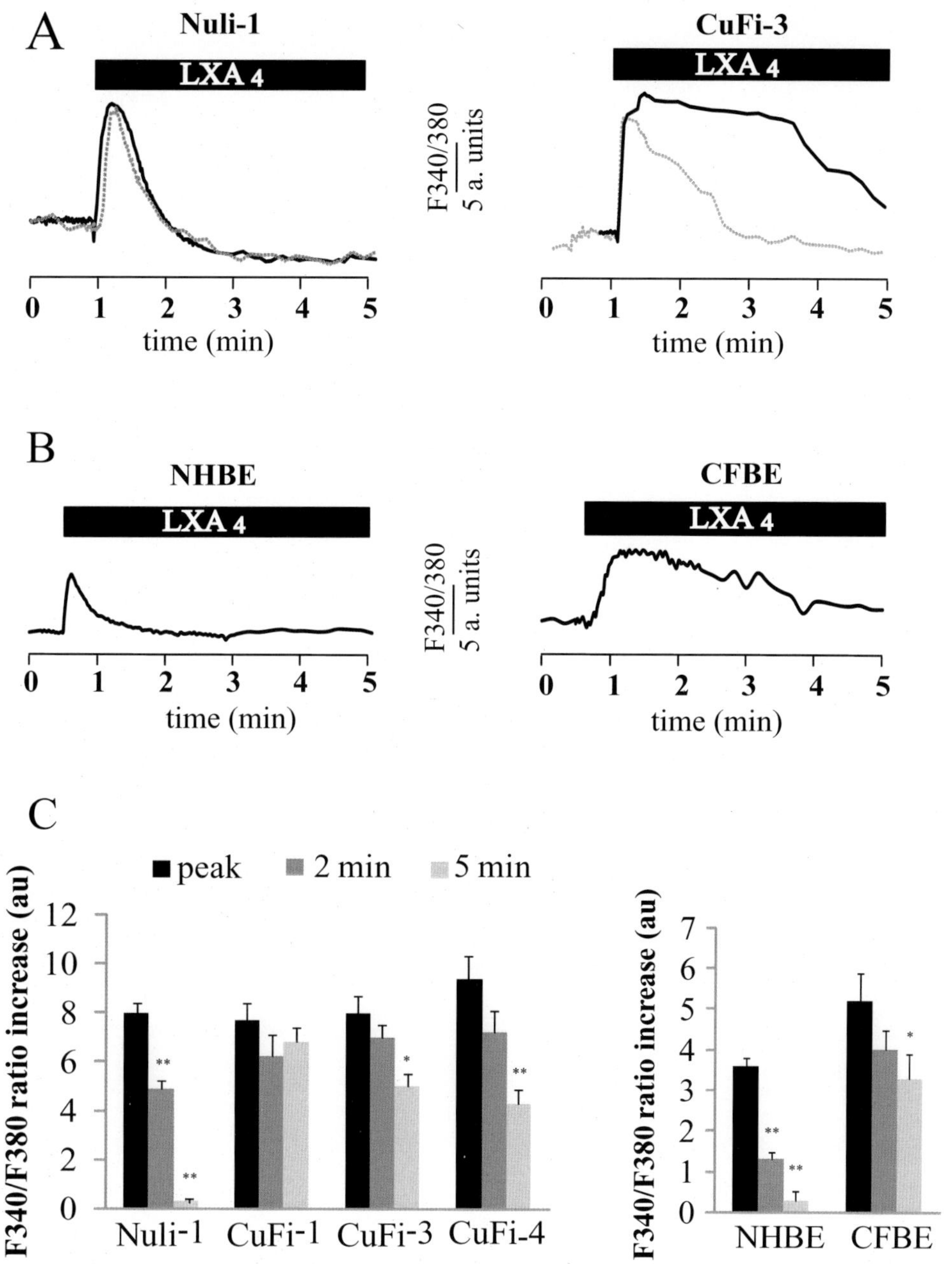

Figure 1. LXA_4 effect on intracellular Ca^{2+} activity in non-CF and CF bronchial epithelial cells. (A) Typical effect of LXA_4 (100 nM) on the cytosolic Ca^{2+} (ratio F340/F380) measured in Nuli-1 and CuFi-3 cell lines in control (plain line) and in external Ca^{2+} -free conditions (dotted line). (B) Typical effect of LXA_4 (100 nM) on the cytosolic Ca^{2+} in normal and CF primary cultures of bronchial epithelial cells (NHBE and CFBE). (C) Mean values of the maximum increase in Ca^{2+} (peak) and measured 2 and 5 minutes after the peak, in Nuli-1 (n = 6), CuFi-1 (n = 6), CuFi-3 (n = 6), CuFi-4 (n = 4) cell lines and in NHBE (n = 4) and CFBE (n = 4) bronchial epithelial cells in primary culture (* $p<0.05$, ** $p<0.01$).

As reported in Table 1, the inward and outward conductances were significantly increased by LXA_4 (100 nM, 10 min) without any change in the reversal potential in all cell types studied including primary cultures of CF and non-CF bronchial epithelia and CF and non-CF cell lines.

Role of the ALX/FPR2 Receptor in the Whole Cell Conductance Responses to LXA_4

The inhibitory effect of the Boc-2 antagonist on calcium responses to LXA_4 indicate a role for the ALX/FPR2 receptor in transducing LXA_4 responses in airway epithelial cells. This is also true for lipoxin effects on membrane ionic currents where treatment of Nuli-1 and CuFi-3 cells with Boc-2 (10 μM) completely abolished the stimulatory effect of LXA_4 on the whole-cell current. As indicated in figure 4C, Boc-2 did not affect the basal inward conductance but significantly prevented the increase in inward conductance induced by LXA_4 (Figure 4C).

Role of Intracellular Ca^{2+} in the Whole-cell Conductance Responses to LXA_4

The role of intracellular Ca^{2+} in the LXA_4 induced whole-cell currents was evaluated using BAPTA-AM in the patch pipette as a

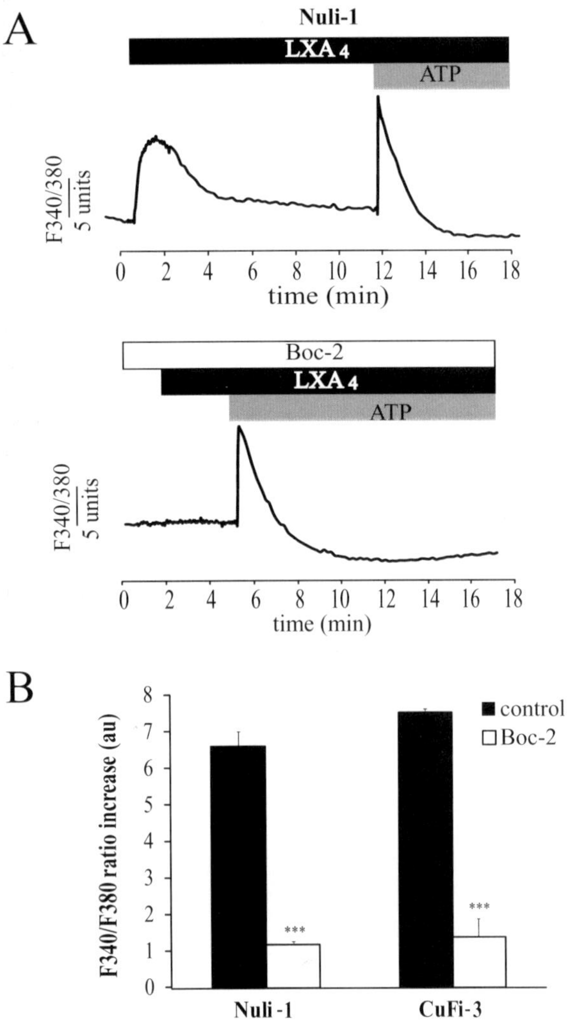

Figure 2. Effect of Boc-2 on the intracellular Ca^{2+} signal induced by LXA_4. (A) Representative effect of LXA_4 (100 nM) and ATP (100 μM) on cytosolic Ca^{2+} (ratio F340/F380) in NuLi-1 cells in control conditions (upper panel) and after 24 hours of pre-treatment with Boc-2 (10 μM) a specific inhibitor of ALX/FPR2 (lower panel). (B) Mean values corresponding to the effect of Boc-2 on the Ca^{2+} response to LXA_4 in Nuli-1 (n = 5) and in CuFi-3 (n = 4) cell lines (*** $p<0.001$).

chelator of intracellular Ca^{2+}. Under these conditions of low intracellular Ca^{2+}, the basal whole-cell conductances remained unchanged, whereas the lipoxin-stimulated currents were absent in BAPTAM-treated cell. The use of BAPTA-AM demonstrated the absolute requirement for an increase in intracellular calcium levels to transduce the effect of LXA_4 on whole-cell inward conductance in both NuLi-1 cells and in CuFi-3 cells (Figure 4C).

LXA_4 Effect on Cl^- Secretion

The contribution of Cl^- channels to the LXA_4 induced current, was tested using chloride ion channel inhibitors; NPPB (calcium-activated Cl^- channel inhibitor) and CFTR-inh172 (CFTR Cl^- channel inhibitor), and recording their effect on membrane current and conductance responses to LXA_4 in CF and non-CF cells (Figure 5). Pre-treatment of CFBE primary cultured cells for 2 min with NPPB (1 μM) prior to LXA_4 exposure, completely inhibited the stimulatory effect of LXA_4 on whole-cell current ($p>0.5$, n = 3). Furthermore, the addition of NPPB (1 μM) 10 min after exposure to LXA_4 (100 nM), immediately inhibited the whole-cell currents in non-CF and CF cells. Figure 5A illustrates a typical experiment performed in NHBE primary cells showing the inhibitory effect of NPPB treatment after LXA4 stimulation of the whole cell currents. A summary of the inhibitory effects of NPPB on inward conductance in the CF and non-CF primary cultures, and CF cell line (CuFi-3) are presented in figure 5A. As an additional proof for the role of Cl^- channels in driving the LXA_4 induced current, we found that in the absence of an electrochemical driving force for chloride ions (equimolar Cl^- replacement in the bath and patch pipette), LXA_4 did not produce a change in whole-cell current in any of the cell types tested (data not shown).

The specific CFTR inhibitor, CFTR-inh172, had no effect of CFTR-inh172 on basal or LXA_4-stimulated membrane current and conductance in CFBE and CuFi-3 cells (data not shown), consistent with the absence of functional CFTR. Moreover, the CFTR inhibitor did not affect the stimulation of the whole-cell current by LXA_4 in NuLi-1 cells (Figure 5B). When Nuli-1 cells were pre-treated with CFTR-inh172 (5 μM), subsequent LXA_4 exposure stimulated the outward and inward conductances by 2.1±0.15 fold and 2.5±0.14 fold (n = 3), respectively (Figure 5B). These results indicate that the stimulatory effect of LXA_4 on whole-cell current and conductance in non-CF and CF bronchial cells is mainly due to activation of NPPB-sensitive Cl^- channels and does not involve CFTR channels.

LXA_4 Effects on Airway Surface Liquid Height

The consequence of LXA_4 stimulation of Cl^- channels and transepithelial Cl^- secretion on ASL height was investigated in the cell lines (Nuli-1, CuFi-1 and CuFi-3) and in primary cultures of non-CF and CF airway epithelial cells grown on permeable supports under an air/liquid interface. The ASL measurements were carried out after a period of 24 hours exposure to apical fluid (8 μl of PBS) to allow fluid absorption/secretion and ASL height to reach a steady state. Under control conditions (without LXA_4), the non-CF epithelia from NuLi-1 cell and primary cultures displayed a continuous unbroken ASL layer (*not shown*) whereas CF epithelia from cell lines and primary cultures presented a disrupted and thinner ASL layer (figure 6). Exposure to LXA_4 (100 nM, 15 min) increased the ASL height in both non-CF and CF cell lines and primary cultures (figure 6). LXA_4 treatment produced a maximum ASL height increase from 7.25±0.07 μm (n = 6) to 9.9±0.1 μm (n = 6) in Nuli-1 epithelia ($p<0.001$) and from 4.6±0.20 μm (n = 6) to 11.1±0.20 μm (n = 6) in CuFi-1 epithelia ($p<0.001$), and from 6.4±0.1 μm (n = 6) to 9.5±0.2 μm (n = 6) in CuFi-3 epithelia ($p<0.001$) and from 4.9±0.32 μm (n = 9) to 9.8±0.10 μm (n = 9) in CFBE primary cultures ($p<0.001$). The ASL height response to LXA_4 obtained in CFBE primary cultures from 3 different CF patients was found to be robust and similar to the ASL response obtained in CuFi-1 differentiated cells. In all of the CF bronchial epithelia, the disrupted appearance of the ASL layer was absent following LXA_4 treatment (Figure 6 B, C, D).

Role of Cl^- Transport in the ASL Height Responses to LXA_4

The Na/K/2Cl co-transporter inhibitor bumetanide was used to investigate the contribution of Cl^- secretion to the generation of the ASL. Bumetanide (1 μM) treatment significantly decreased the basal ASL height (control 7.25±0.07 μm, bumetanide 5.9±0.1 μm ($p<0.001$, n = 6)) in NuLi-1 monolayers but had no significant effect on ASL height in CuFi-1 epithelia (control 4.6±0.1 μm, bumetanide 4.82±0.10 μm ($p>0.5$, n = 6)), in CuFi-3 epithelia (control 6.4±0.1 μm, bumetanide 6.3±0.3 μm ($p>0.5$, n = 6)) and in CFBE (control 4.9±0.32 μm, bumetanide

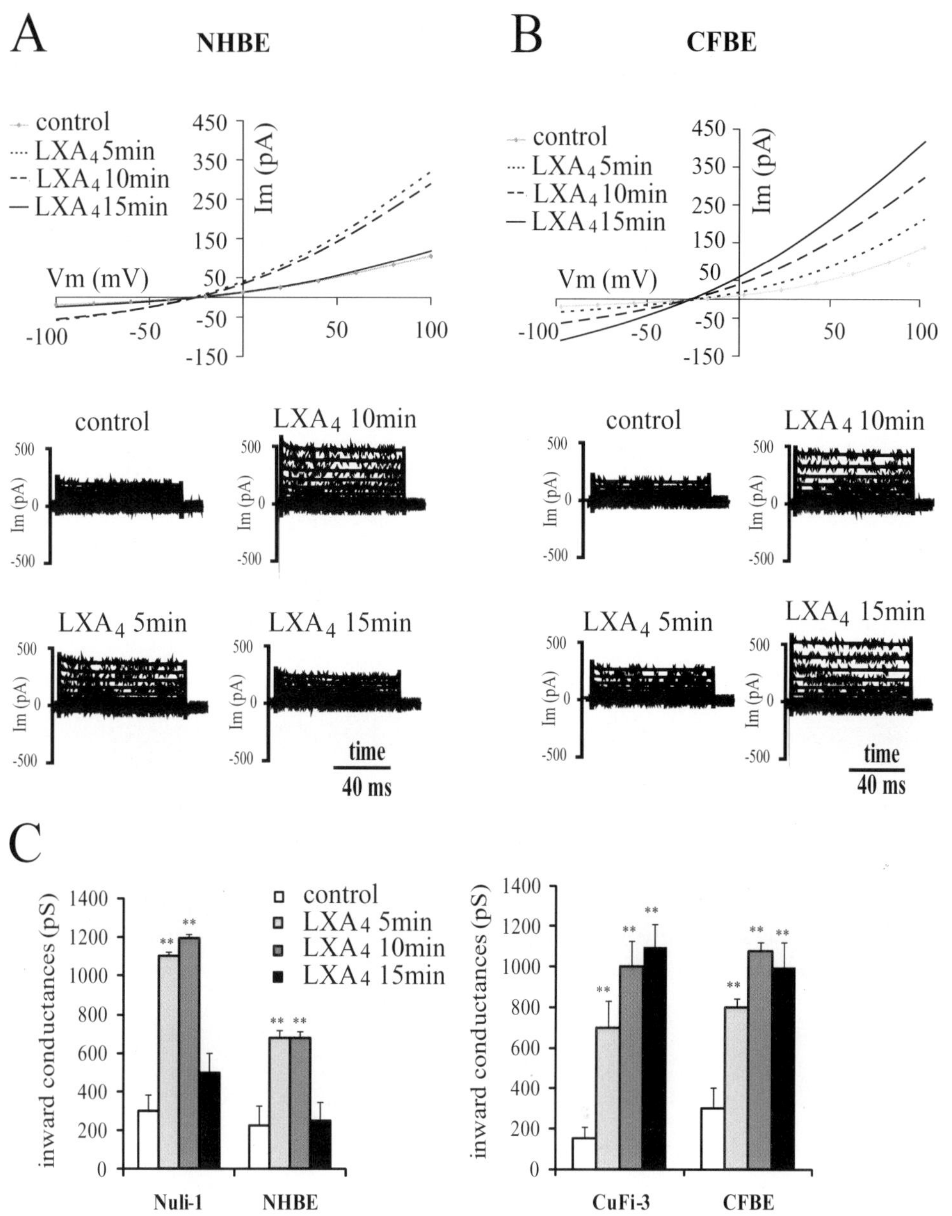

Figure 3. Time dependency of the effect of LXA_4 on whole-cell currents in normal and CF bronchial epithelial cells in primary culture. Typical I-V relationships and corresponding current records obtained before and after 5, 10 and 15 min exposure to LXA_4 (100 nM) in NHBE (A) and CFBE (B) isolated bronchial epithelial cells in primary culture. (C) Mean values corresponding to the time dependency of the LXA_4 effect onwhole cell inward conductances in Nuli-1 (n = 8) and in CuFi-3 (n = 4) cell lines and NHBE (n = 8) and CFBE (n = 6) primary cultures (**$p<0.01$).

4.9±0.25 µm ($p>0.5$, n = 8)). These data indicate that Cl^- secretion contributes to the generation of the basal ASL height in the non-CF epithelium. Furthermore, bumetanide (1 µM) significantly abolished the ASL height increase induced by LXA_4 in cell types tested. The ASL height measured after LXA_4 exposure in the presence of bumetanide was significantly decreased in NuLi-1 (5.6±0.11 µm, n = 5, $p<0.05$), in CuFi-1 (4.86±0.1 µm, n = 6, $p<0.001$) and in CuFi-3 (6.2±0.1 µm, n = 6, $p<0.001$) cell lines and in CFBE primary cultures (4.7±0.2 µm, n = 9, $p<0.001$) compared to LXA_4 alone (Figure 6). Taken together, these results demonstrate that the stimulatory effect of LXA_4 on ASL height mainly involves Ca^{2+}-dependent Cl^- secretion via NPPB-sensitive channels in both CF and non-CF epithelia grown from cell lines and primary cultures.

Role of the ALX/FPR2 Receptor in the ASL Height Responses to LXA_4

We tested the effect of the ALX/FPR2 receptor antagonist Boc-2 on the ASL height response to LXA_4. Boc-2 significantly reduced the effect of LXA_4 on ASL height in Nuli-1, CuFi-1 and CuFi-3 bronchial epithelial cell lines and CFBE primary cultures without affecting the basal ASL height (Figure 6). These data support the conclusion that the LXA_4 receptor ALX/FPR2 mediates the effect of LXA_4 on airway surface liquid height as well

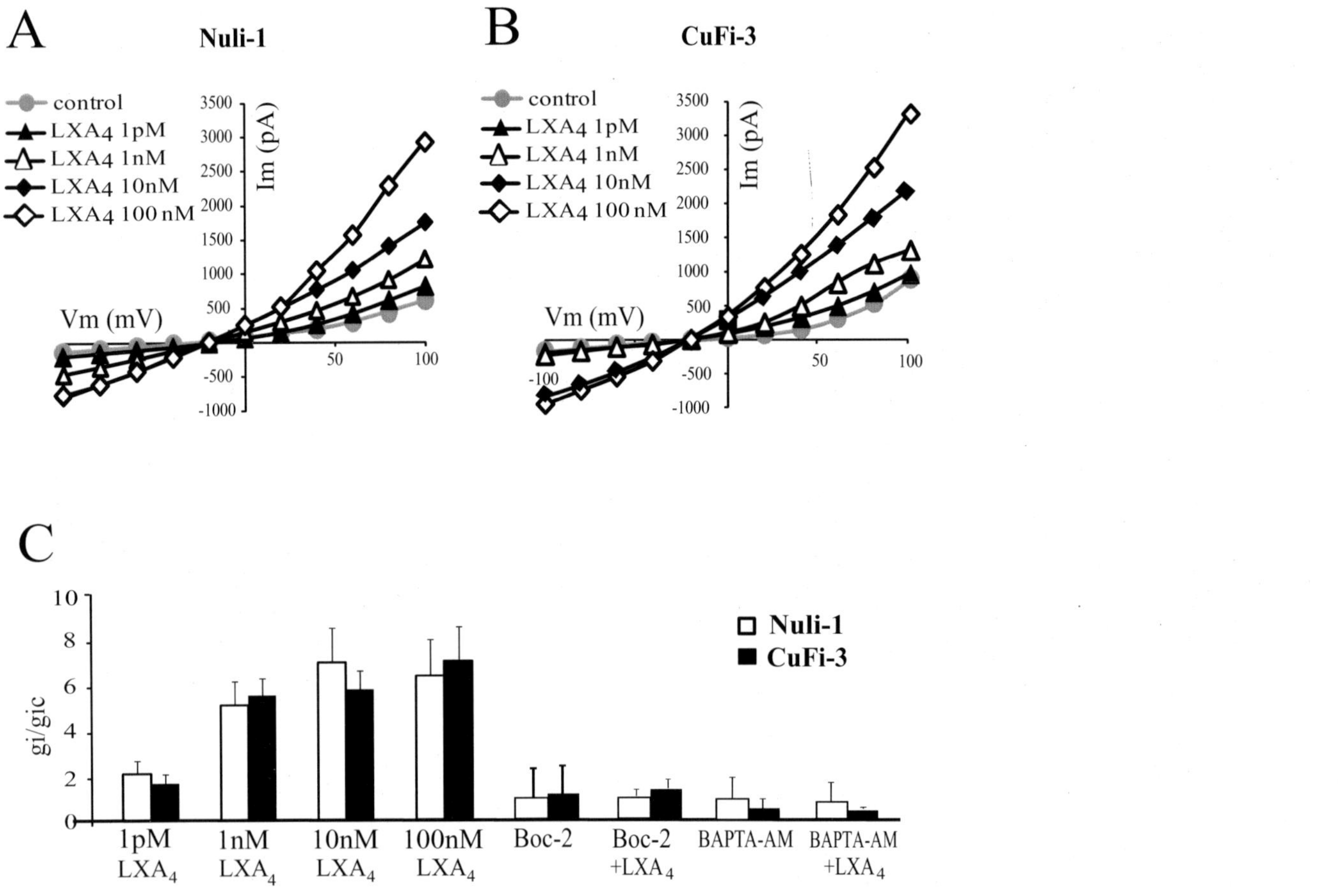

Figure 4. Dose dependency of the effect of LXA_4 on whole-cell currents of normal (Nuli-1) and CF (CuFi-3) bronchial epithelial cell lines. Typical I-V relationships obtained before and after 10 min exposure to 1 pM (n = 6 Nuli-1, n = 6 CuFi-3), 1 nM (n = 4 Nuli-1, n = 4 CuFi-3), 10 nM (n = 3 Nuli-1, n = 3 CuFi-3) and 100 nM (n = 6 Nuli-1, n = 6 CuFi-3) LXA_4 in Nuli-1 (A) and CuFi-3 (B) cell lines. (C) Mean inward conductance changes normalized to control values (gi/gic obtained without LXA_4) as a function of LXA_4 concentration in Nuli-1 (open bars) and CuFi-3 (black bars) cells in control conditions and obtained upon exposure to Boc-2 (10 µM) alone (10 min, 100 nM, n = 4 Nuli-1, n = 4 CuFi-3) or with Boc-2 (10 µM) and LXA_4 (10 min, 100 nM, n = 6 Nuli-1, n = 6 CuFi-3) and after BAPTA-AM pre-treatment alone (n = 6 Nuli-1, n = 6 CuFi-3) or with BAPTA-AM and LXA_4 (10 min, 100 nM, n = 4 Nuli-1, n = 6 CuFi-3).

Table 1. Mean outward (G_{out}) and inward (G_{in}) conductances and reversal potentials (E_{rev}) measured in non CF and CF airway epithelial cells in primary culture and NuLi-1 and CuFi-3 cell lines in control conditions and stimulated by LXA_4 (100 nM, 10 min).

		G_{out} (pS)	G_{in} (pS)	E_{rev} (mV)	n
NHBE	Control	612.2±165.2	227.7±99.3	−22.4±3.9	16
	LXA_4	1742±147.2	676±36.6	−21.4±5.8	13
CFBE	Control	855.4±192.9	302.9±100.4	−22.4±1.9	8
	LXA_4	3187.5±172.1	1078.14±43.4	−23.8±3.1	8
NuLi-1	Control	622.1±168.9	298.7±85.5	−23.8±3.2	8
	LXA_4	1365.1±75.8	1192±24.2	−22.9±3.7	6
CuFi-3	Control	979.6±146.8	150±61.36	−21.7±3.6	5
	LXA_4	2156.5±232.7	999±132.97	−24.7±4.0	5

as on calcium mobilization and Cl^- secretion in bronchial epithelium.

Discussion

This is the first study to report a novel effect of the endogenous lipoxin LXA_4 to stimulate an increase in Airway Surface Liquid height, by enhancing Ca^{2+} activated Cl^- transport in bronchial epithelial cells obtained from patients with CF and non-CF patients and in airway cell lines.

In the healthy lung, the ASL forms a thin layer of fluid on the surface of the bronchial epithelium which allows cilia to beat effectively [8]. Maintenance of an optimal ASL height for ciliary beat is crucial for the efficacy of mucociliary clearance [8–12]. Bronchial epithelial ion transport regulates the ASL height, mainly by generating osmotic gradients which provide the driving force for transepithelial water movement [13]. In CF, the lack of functional CFTR leads to a reduced ASL height, resulting in an impaired mucociliary clearance that promotes chronic bacterial infection of the airways [3]. In a previous study, we reported that LXA_4 stimulated an intracellular Ca^{2+} mobilization in a normal human airway epithelial cell line 16HBE14o- [7]. Here, we tested the hypothesis that LXA_4 induces a Ca^{2+} signal to drive an

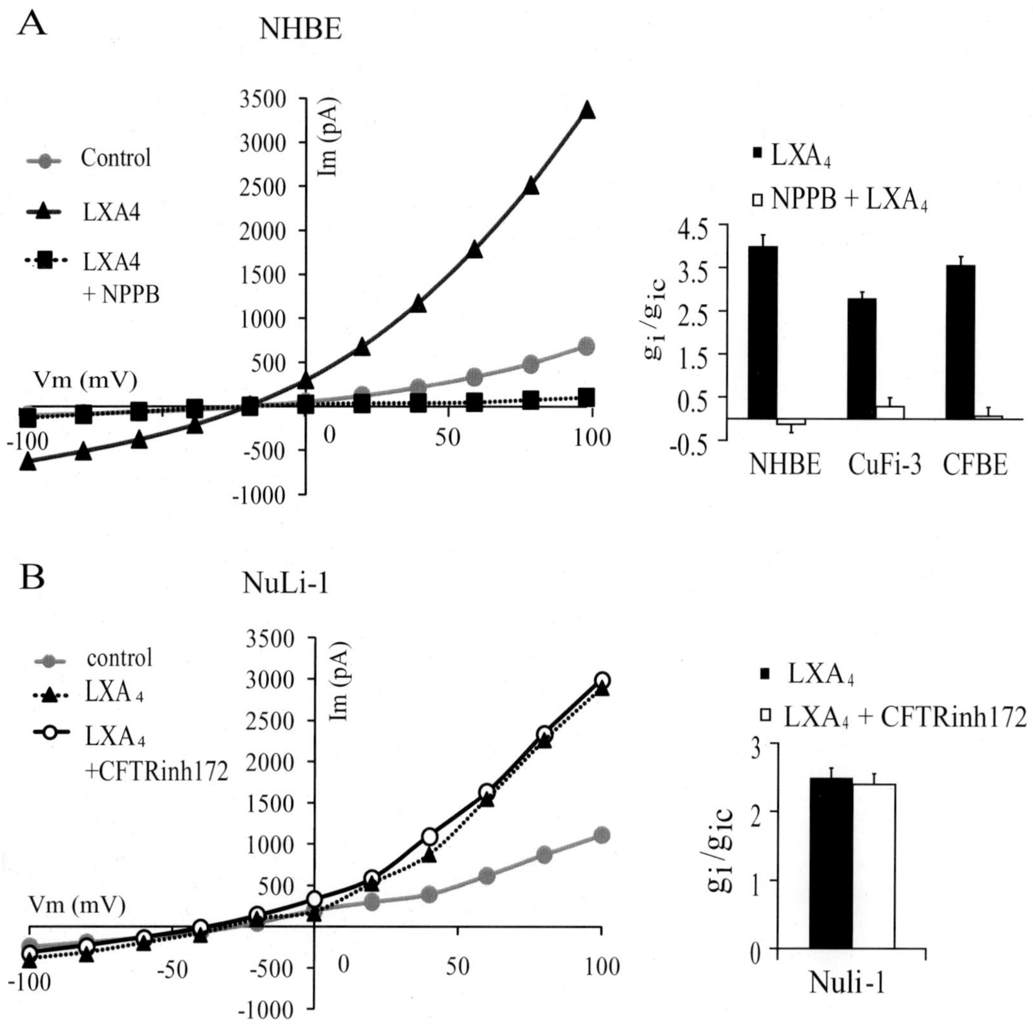

Figure 5. Effects of Cl⁻ channel inhibitors on whole-cell currents stimulated by LXA_4. (A) Representative I-V relationship of the effect of NPPB (1 μM) after the stimulation of primary cultures of bronchial epithelial cells with LXA_4 (100 nM). Corresponding histogram of the inhibitory effect of NPPB on the inward conductance obtained in non-CF primary NHBE cells (n = 4), CuFi-3 cells (n = 3) and CF primary CFBE cells (n = 3) after stimulation with LXA_4 (100 nM, 10 min). (B). Typical I-V relationships of the effect of LXA_4 (100 nM) obtained in NuLi-1 cells after treatment with the CFTR channel inhibition CFTR-inh172 (5 mM) and histogram showing the absence of inhibitory effect in Nuli-1 cells (n = 3).

increased Cl^- secretion and ASL height in CF epithelium. Lipoxin A_4 thus stimulates a compensatory calcium-activated chloride secretory mechanism which overcomes the lack of CFTR mediated Cl^- transport and enhances airway lumen hydration.

Other studies have shown that LXA_4 exerts biological actions on human airway epithelial cells, with a maximal effect observed at 100 nM. LXA_4 (100 nM) inhibited IL-8 production by airway epithelial cells [14], stimulated an intracellular Ca^{2+} signaling [7], increased Z0–1 expression and transepithelial electrical resistance [15], and enhanced epithelial repair after an acid injury [16]. We report here, novel effects of LXA_4 on ion and fluid transport in normal and CF bronchial epithelia.

Our studies show that LXA_4 induces an intracellular Ca^{2+} mobilization in normal and CF epithelia. The Ca^{2+} response to LXA_4 involves signal transduction via the ALX/FPR2 receptor, since the FPR2 receptor antagonist Boc-2 inhibited the LXA_4 effect. This result supports our previous study which suggested that the Ca^{2+} signal induced by LXA_4 was mediated by the ALX/FPR2 receptor since the Ca^{2+} response to LXA_4 was only obtained in the 16HBE14o- airway epithelial cell line that express the receptor whereas LXA_4 did not produce any Ca^{2+} response in the A549 cell line which does not express ALX/FPR2 [7].

Our results indicate that in non-CF airway epithelial cells, LXA_4 generates a rapid and transient calcium signal mainly arising from the release of Ca^{2+} from intracellular stores and not as a result of increased Ca^{2+} entry since the calcium signal was not affected by the removal of external Ca^{2+}. This is in agreement with our previous findings showing that the Ca^{2+} mobilization induced by LXA_4 was generated from thapsigargin sensitive stores [7]. In contrast, in CF airway epithelial cells, the duration of the Ca^{2+} signal induced by LXA_4 was greater than in non-CF cells. Although, in CF cells, the removal of external calcium did not affect the maximum peak calcium increase, the calcium response to LXA_4 became more transient. These results suggest that, in CF airway epithelial cells, in addition to the calcium release from intracellular stores, LXA_4 also stimulates calcium entry which leads to an overall larger calcium mobilisation than in normal airway epithelial cells. The observed differences reported in the

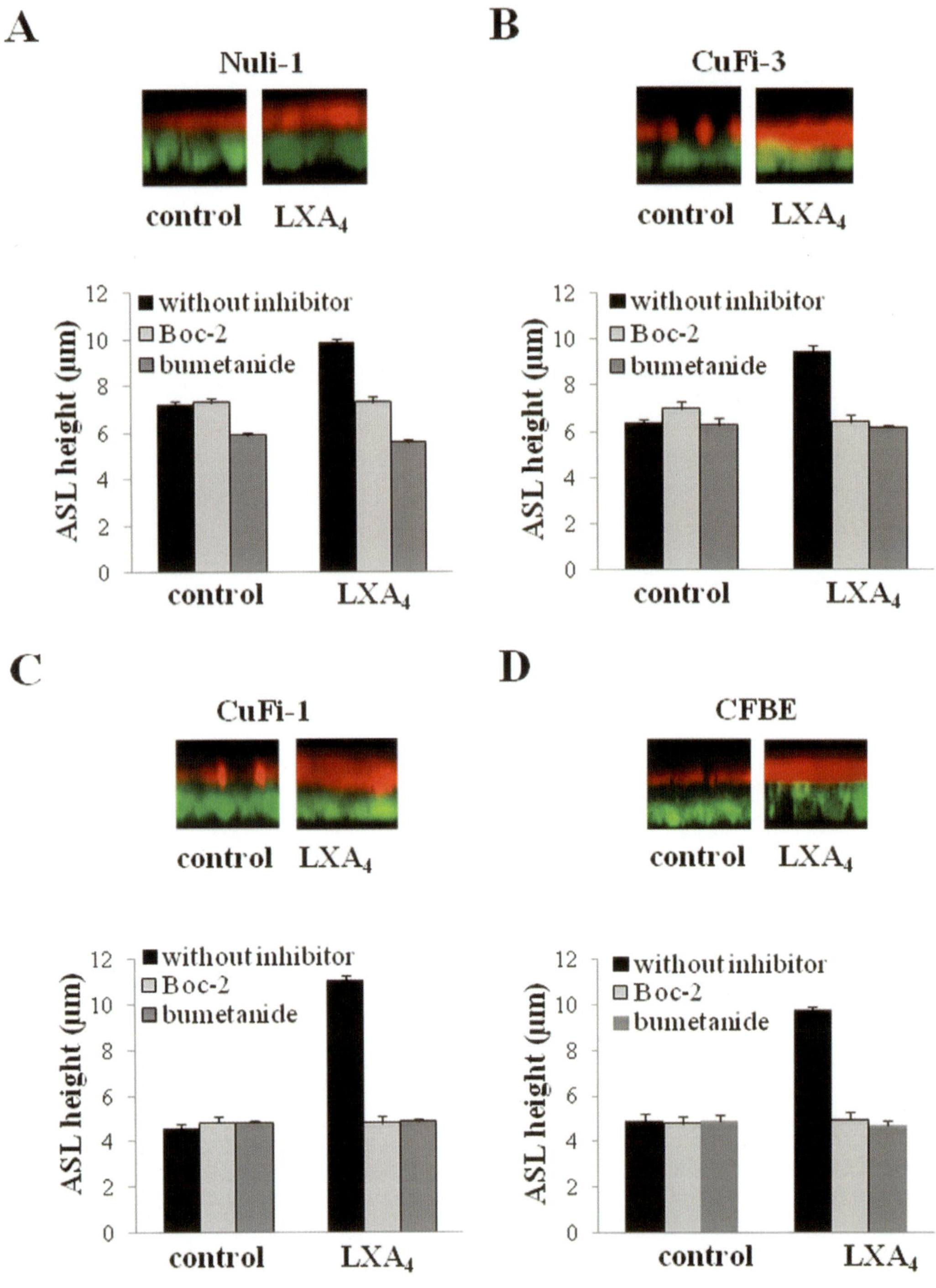

Figure 6. LXA_4 (100 nM) effects on airway surface liquid height in NuLi-1 (A), CuFi-3 (B) and CuFi-1 epithelial cell line (C) and CFBE primary cultures (D). Epithelial cells were stained with calcein green, and the ASL labelled with dextran-conjugated Texas red™ fluorochrome. For each cell preparation, typical z-plane confocal sections showing ASL responses to LXA_4 (top) and mean ASL height changes (bottom) in control conditions or following LXA_4 (100 µM) exposure in NuLi-1,CuFi-3, CuFi-1 and CFBE epithelia treated or not with Boc-2 (10 µM) and with bumetanide (10 µM).

literature between the Ca^{2+} signal obtained upon agonist exposure in CF and non-CF airway epithelial cells are controversial. Some authors reported that expression of either CFTR or ΔF508CFTR in airway epithelial cells had no effect on intracellular Ca^{2+} [17]. However, our results are in accordance with the demonstration that Ca^{2+} signaling is abnormal in CF airway epithelial cells and that correction of the abnormal trafficking of ΔF508CFTR protein restored intracellular Ca^{2+} homeostasis [18]. Recent reports also indicate that intracellular Ca^{2+} signals induced by pro-inflammatory mediators are increased in CF airway epithelia compared to non-CF due to an expansion of the apical endoplasmic reticulum Ca^{2+} stores in CF airway epithelial cells [19]. This finding is consistent with several studies showing that the nasal transepithelial electrical potential responses to agents that promote an intracellular Ca^{2+}mobilization and Ca^{2+}-dependent Cl^- conductance were higher in CF patients than in normal subjects [20–23].

Intracellular Ca^{2+} regulates several epithelial functions including ion transport, mucin secretion, and ciliary beat frequency which constitute a primary mode of a non-specific cleansing process and lung protection. Our results indicate that the Ca^{2+} signal induced by LXA_4 is coupled to an increased Cl^- secretion in CF epithelium. LXA_4 stimulated the whole-cell current and conductance in non-CF and CF epithelial cells. The inhibitory effect of BAPTA-AM used as a chelator of intracellular Ca^{2+} demonstrated the essential role of Ca^{2+} in the stimulation of the whole-cell currents by LXA_4. The sensitivity of basal and stimulated whole-cell currents to NPPB or Cl^- substitution, underscores the major contribution of Cl^- secretion to the generation of the whole-cell current. These results agree with our previous report indicating that LXA_4 stimulated a Ca^{2+}-activated transepithelial Cl^- secretion in non-CF bronchial epithelial cells [7]. Since we found that LXA_4 stimulation of the whole-cell currents was present in CF airway epithelia (in which CFTR is not functionally expressed), LXA_4 most probably affects Cl^- channels other than CFTR. In addition, we found that the duration of the LXA_4 effect on whole-cell currents was different between non-CF and CF cells, with a transient current increase in non-CF cells compared to CF cells where the current increase was more sustained. One explanation may be that the time course of the effect of LXA_4 on the Cl^- currents is directly related to the time course of the intracellular calcium change induced by LXA_4. Therefore, the greater and sustained effect of LXA_4 on whole-cell currents in CF cells could be related to the long lasting Ca^{2+} signal obtained in CF airway epithelial cells. Finally, the ineffectiveness of CFTR inh-172 on the LXA_4 stimulated whole-cell currents indicates that the effect of LXA_4 on Cl^- secretion is not mediated by CFTR activation. This conclusion is strengthened by the observation that bumetanide reduces further the ASL height compared to Boc-2 treatment in Nuli-1 cells but not in CuFi-3 cells where functional CFTR is absent. If LXA_4 had stimulated CFTR and Ca^{2+}-dependent Cl^- channels together we would expect equivalent inhibition of ASL height by Boc-2 and bumetanide in Nuli-1 cells.

We have described a novel stimulatory effect of LXA_4 on Cl^- secretion which produces an increased ASL height in both normal and CF epithelia. The CF bronchial epithelia generate a thinner ASL layer than non-CF airway epithelia. This finding is consistent with the diminished ASL in CF airways reported in the literature [12]. In addition, we observed that in control conditions, the non-CF epithelial monolayers showed a continuous ASL layer whereas in CuFi-1, CuFi-3 cell lines and CFBE primary cultures the liquid layer was disrupted. The gaps in the airway surface liquid layer result from localised de-hydration of the ASL. Following LXA_4 exposure in CF bronchial epithelia, the ASL height significantly increased and appeared uniform. The inhibitory effect of bumetanide indicates that the effect of LXA_4 on ASL height is mainly dependent on stimulation of transpithelial Cl^- transport. However, we cannot exclude the possibility that LXA_4 can also exert its action to increase ASL height through the inhibition of ENaC activity which is known to be stimulated in CF airway and down-regulated by increased intracellular Ca^{2+}.

An important outcome of this work is the comparable results found for LXA_4 effects on ASL height in cell lines and primary CF cultures. We have demonstrated that using thin film airway liquid cell culture techniques, the NuLi and CuFi cell lines provide a robust model of airway liquid dynamics. Although ASL volume measurements have been published for the Calu-3 airway cell line [24], it is important to distinguish between ASL volume and height measurements and their meaning for effective mucociliary clearance. ASL height is the relevant physiological parameter as it determines the effective beating of cilia which must be covered to an optimal height with ASL. The volume of ASL on the other hand may change without revealing the true optimal ASL height covering the cilia but instead may reflect flooding of the airways which would also render cilia beat inefficient for mucocilary clearance. Although the use of primary airway epithelia tissue is the ideal for research in CF, the access to patient tissue samples, particularly children with CF and 'normal' non-CF controls as in our study, is non-trivial. The use of particular airway cell lines such as NuLi and CuFi which in our hands display normal and CF airway epithelium phenotype to secrete a thin ASL and mucus provides an additional validated cell model for CF research where human tissue samples are rare and difficult to obtain for research purposes.

Taken together, our results provide evidence for a novel role of LXA_4 in stimulating Ca^{2+} activated Cl^- secretion and ASL generation in CF and non-CF airway epithelium. Thus LXA_4 or its stable analogues may provide a novel therapeutic strategy to rehydrate the CF airway by modulating ion transport and airway surface liquid height via pathways which bypass defective CFTR. Our findings also indicate that the reduced levels of LXA_4 observed in CF patients may be an additional contributory mechanism by which mucociliary clearance is diminished in CF airways.

Materials and Methods

Cell Culture

For the primary culture of human bronchial epithelium, the cells were obtained from bronchial brushing specimens obtained from 6 children (<6 years old) with CF and 5 non-CF controls through the SHIELD CF study (Study of Host Immunity and Early Lung Disease in CF). The children with CF were homozygous for the Phe508del mutation. Local ethics committee approval for the study was granted and written informed consent obtained. Bronchial epithelium brushings were washed and incubated for two hours at room temperature with 250 µg/ml amphotericin B in Phosphate Buffer Saline (PBS) without calcium and magnesium. After centrifugation, the pellet was collected and re-suspended in 500 µl of Bronchial Epithelium Basal Medium (BEBM, Clonetics, BioWhittaker, San Diego, USA) supplemented with 0.5 µg/ml human recombinant epidermal growth factor, 7.5 mg/ml bovine pituitary extract, 0.5 mg/ml epinephrine, 10 mg/ml transferrin, 5 mg/ml insulin, 0.1 µg/ml retinoic acid, 6.5 µg/ml triiodothyronine, and 50 mg/ml gentamicin (BD, Erembodegem, Belgium) and 250 µg/ml amphotericin B (BD, Erembodegem, Belgium). The explants were plated in a 24 well plate (Nunc, Roskilde, Denmark) previously coated with a fibronectin/collagen solution and incubated at 37°C in a humidified 5% CO_2 atmosphere. Twenty four hours after seeding, the volume of media was adjusted to 400 µl. The cells were cultured under these conditions for six to nine days (confluence close to 70%) before splitting. Fibroblasts were removed by 1 minute treatment with trypsin EDTA (Gibco, Invitrogen, Paisley, UK). Epithelial cells referred in this paper as NHBE (non-CF bronchial epithelial cells) and CFBE (CF bronchial epithelial cells) were then trypsinised and re-suspended after centrifugation, in supplemented BEBM. The cells were seeded at 2500–4000 cells/cm^2 in flasks (BD, Erembodegem, Belgium).

NuLi-1, CuFi-1, CuFi-3, and CuFi-4 cells were kindly donated by Prof Zabner,University of Iowa, USA. The NuLi-1 cell line was derived from human airway epithelium of normal genotype, whereas CuFi-1, Cufi-3 and CuFi-4 cell lines were derived from CF patients with Δ508/Δ508, R553X/Δ508, and G551D/Δ508 genotypes respectively. The cell lines were transformed with a RT component of telomerase and human papillomavirus type 16 E6 and E7 genes [25]. Cells were initially grown to confluency in flasks using BEBM with EGF, hydrocortisone, bovine pituitary extract, transferin, bovine insulin, triiodothyronine, epinephrine, retinoic acid, penicillin-streptomycin (0.025 μg/ml), gentamicin (0.05 ng/ml), and amphotericin (25 μg/ml).

Airway epithelial cells were plated at 2×10^6 cells/cm^2 on Millicell hanging cell culture inserts (Millipore, Billerica, USA) for ASL height measurements. All inserts were pre-coated with collagen type VI and grown in BEGM medium until confluence was achieved. Once cell confluence was confirmed under visual inspection, the medium was switched to DMEM/F-12 (Invitrogen, Auckland, New Zealand) to aid cell differentiation. This medium was supplemented with Ultroser G (2%, Pall Biospera, Cergy-Saint-Christophe, France), which enhances ion transport [25], and penicillin-streptomycin (0.025 μg/ml), gentamicin (0.05 ng/ml), and amphotericin (25 μg/ml). Medium at the apical aspect was aspirated every 3–4 days until the establishment of an air-liquid interface. The basolateral culture medium was replaced every 2–3 days. After 4–6 weeks growth, the cells formed a polarised confluent monolayer with a high transepithelial electrical resistance (TER) of >700 Ω/cm^2.

Intracellular Calcium Imaging

Intracellular Ca^{2+} was measured by epifluorescence microscopy as previously described [26]. The human airway epithelial cells were cultured on fibronectin-collagen coated (for primary culture cells) and on collagen VI coated (for NuLi-1 and CuFi-1 cells) glass bottom dishes (WPI, Stevenage, UK) for 6 days until 70% of confluence was reached. Cells were loaded with 5 μM of the Ca^{2+} -sensitive fluorescent probe fura-2-acetoxy-methyl ester (fura 2-AM, Invitrogen, Auckland, New Zealand) for 30 min, in the dark, at room temperature (22°C) and were then washed twice in HEPES-buffered Krebs-Henseleit solution (140 mM NaCl, 5 mM KCl, 2 mM CaCl2, 1 mM $MgCl_2$, 10 mM HEPES, pH 7.4, 280–290 mOsmol). The glass bottom dishes covered with the fura 2-AM loaded epithelial cell monolayer were mounted on the stage of an inverted microscope equipped for epi-fluorescence (TE-300, Nikon, Badhoeve Dorp, Netherlands). Intracellular Ca^{2+} imaging was performed using the Metafluor Imaging System (Universal Imaging Corporation). The cell preparation was excited alternatively with monochromatic light at 340 and 380 nm using an Optoscan monochromator (Cairn Research Ltd, Kent, UK). The emission fluorescence produced after fura 2-AM excitation was filtered at 512 nm. The emitted light image was detected using a Photometrics CoolSNAP-fx video camera (Roper Scientific, Evry, France) coupled to the microscope. The fluorescence obtained at each excitation wavelength (F340 and F380) depended upon the level of Ca^{2+} binding to fura 2-AM. The results are given as ratiometric data (F340/F380), or as amplitude of variation compared to the basal ratio level (ΔF340/F380).

Whole-cell Patch-clamp Recording

Freshly isolated epithelial cells obtained from 4 non-CF patients and from 3 CF patients (genotype: ΔF508/ΔF508) and from the NuLi-1 and CuFi-3 cell lines were used for patch-clamp experiments. The CuFi-1 cells were not used for patch-clamp experiments since we could not reach a Giga ohm seal with these cells. Cells were patch-clamped at room temperature (25°C) on an inverted microscope (TE-300, Nikon, Badhoeve Dorp, Netherlands). Patch-pipettes were prepared from soda glass (Vitrex, Modulhom, Herlev, Denmark), pulled on a programmable puller (P80/PC, Sutter Instrument Company, USA). The whole-cell configuration was obtained from cell-attached mode after breaking the patch membrane by applying a brief negative pressure in the patch pipette. Whole-cell currents were amplified (Axopatch 200B, Axon instrument, CA) and digitized using a 16-bit data converter (Digidata 1322A, Axon instrument, CA) following low pass filtering at 5 Khz and sampled in real-time. Whole-cell current voltage (IV) relationships were analysed using Clampfit software (Axon instrument, CA).

The patch pipette was filled with a "high K^+ solution" at pH = 7.2, 290 mosm: 110 mM K-gluconate, 20 mM NaCl, 1.2 mM KH_2PO_4, 3.46 mM, 3mM KH_2PO_4, 5 mM EGTA, 6 mM HEPES, 2.78 mM CaCl2, pH = 7.2 adjusted with KOH. The bathing solution had the following composition: 140 mM NaCl, 5 mM KCl, 6 mM Hepes, 2 mM $CaCl_2$, 1.2 mM KH_2PO_4, 1.2 mM $MgSO_4$ and pH = 7.4. The Nernst potentials between the patch pipette and bath for K^+ and for Cl^- were −77 mV and −39 mV, respectively. The access resistance (*Ra*) was determined by fitting the current transients produced by a 5mV voltage pulse with a single exponential. The measured *Ra* was 5.43±0.08Ω (n = 40).

For experiments performed in "low internal calcium", cells were bathed in Kreb's solution and the patch pipette contained 100 nM $CaCl_2$ with 5 mM EGTA and 10 μM BAPTA-AM. In these conditions the free Ca^{2+} has been estimated at 1 pM using the free software WEBMAXC http://www.stanford.edu/cpatton/webmaxc/webmaxcS.htm.

Airway Surface Liquid (ASL) Height Measurements

ASL height was measured using a protocol adapted from Tarran *et al.* (10), using live-cell confocal fluorescence microscopy. To label the ASL, 8 μl PBS containing 1 mg/ml Texas red®-dextran (10 kD; Invitrogen, Auckland, New Zealand) was added to the apical surface of the well-differentiated airway epithelium. The epithelial cells were stained using Calcein-AM (5 μM, Invitrogen, Auckland, New Zealand) dissolved in medium culture for 30 minutes and introduced to the basolateral compartment of the insert. The Fluorinet™ electronic fluid Perfluorocarbon-72 (FC-72, 3M, St Paul, USA) was added to the apical compartment of the insert at a volume of 0.5 ml. Perfluorocarbon-72 is immiscible with the ASL and was used to prevent ASL evaporation on transferring the inserts from the incubator to the microscope stage and during the confocal scanning experiments. Epithelia were Z-scanned using a Zeiss LSM 510 Meta using a 40X objective. For each culture insert, 3 different microscope fields randomly chosen were XZ scanned. In each microscope field, the ASL height was measured using the Zeiss LSM Image analyser software (Carl Zeiss MicroImaging GmbH, Germany) in 9 separate regions randomly determined and then averaged. This method of quantification was carried out after blind analysis performed by multiple users. The n values referred to the number of culture inserts tested in a given condition.

Drugs

The lipoxin LXA_4 was purchased from Calbiochem. Aliquots of LXA_4 solution (100 μM) in ethanol were stored at −80°C to avoid degradation of the molecule. The peptide Boc-Phe-Leu-Phe-Leu-Phe (Boc-2) (Phoenyx pharmaceutical, Belmont, USA) was used as specific inhibitor of the ALX/FPR2 receptor (11). For these latter experiments, cells were pre-incubated with 10^{-5} M Boc-2 for 24 hours at 37°C. BAPTA-AM (10 μM, Molecular probes, Leiden, Netherlands) was used to chelate intracellular Ca^{2+} (12). The 5-Nitro-2-(3-phenylpropylamino) benzoic acid (NPPB, Sigma, USA) used at 1 μM is an inhibitor of Ca^{2+}-activated Cl^- channels (13). CFTRinh-172 an antagonist of the CFTR channel and bumetanide an inhibitor of the NKCC1 co-transporter were supplied by Sigma (14).

Data Analysis

The intracellular Ca^{2+} variations were measured as the difference between the mean F340/F380 ratio during the 2 min prior to exposure to LXA_4 and the ratio measured at the peak of the Ca^{2+} response and 2 and 5 min after the peak. In each experiment, the mean ratio was obtained from all cells in the microscopic field. In whole-cell patch-clamp experiments, conductances were determined by linear regression of the current-voltage relationship obtained in n cells. For the ASL height measurements, three confocal image acquisitions were performed on each culture insert and nine regions of interest were analysed in the acquisition field using the LSM image browser (Zeiss). Values were loaded in an Excel spreadsheet and averaged. Mean value were obtained from n independent experiments. The experiments were repeated under the same conditions on a minimum of three different cell passages. Data are presented as the mean ± S.E.M. of n experiments. Measures of statistical significance were obtained using the Student's t test for paired data. A p value <0.05 was deemed to be significant. All statistical operations were performed using Excel software (Microsoft).

Author Contributions

Conceived and designed the experiments: VU BJH VV. Performed the experiments: VV GH MA. Analyzed the data: VU BJH VV. Contributed reagents/materials/analysis tools: RWC RC PM. Wrote the paper: VU BJH.

References

1. Boat TF, Cheng PW (1989) Epithelial cell dysfunction in cystic fibrosis: implications for airways disease. Acta Paediatr Scand Suppl 363: 25–29; discussion 29–30.
2. Mickle JE, Macek M, Fulmer-Smentek SB, Egan MM, Schwiebert E, et al. (1998) A mutation in the cystic fibrosis transmembrane conductance regulator gene associated with elevated sweat chloride concentrations in the absence of cystic fibrosis. Hum Mol Genet 7: 729–735.
3. Davis PB, Drumm M, Konstan MW (1996) Cystic fibrosis. Am J Respir Crit Care Med 154: 1229–1256.
4. Karp CL, Flick LM, Park KW, Softic S, Greer TM, et al. (2004) Defective lipoxin-mediated anti-inflammatory activity in the cystic fibrosis airway. Nat Immunol 5: 388–392.
5. Serhan CN, Takano T, Gronert K, Chiang N, Clish CB (1999) Lipoxin and aspirin-triggered 15-epi-lipoxin cellular interactions anti-inflammatory lipid mediators. Clin Chem Lab Med 37: 299–309.
6. Parkinson JF (2006) Lipoxin and synthetic lipoxin analogs: an overview of anti-inflammatory functions and new concepts in immunomodulation. Inflamm Allergy Drug Targets 5: 91–106.
7. Bonnans C, Mainprice B, Chanez P, Bousquet J, Urbach V (2003) Lipoxin A4 stimulates a cytosolic Ca2+ increase in human bronchial epithelium. J Biol Chem 278: 10879–10884.
8. Wanner A, Salathé M, O'Riordan TG (1996) Mucociliary clearance in the airways. Am J Respir Crit Care Med 154: 1868–1902.
9. Boucher RC (1994) Human airway ion transport. Part one. Am J Respir Crit Care Med 150: 271–281.
10. Boucher RC (1994) Human airway ion transport. Part two. Am J Respir Crit Care Med 150: 581–593.
11. Boucher RC (1999) Molecular insights into the physiology of the 'thin film' of airway surface liquid. J Physiol 516 (Pt 3): 631–638.
12. Boucher RC (2004) New concepts of the pathogenesis of cystic fibrosis lung disease. Eur Respir J 23: 146–158.
13. Boucher RC (2003) Regulation of airway surface liquid volume by human airway epithelia. Pflugers Arch 445: 495–498.
14. Bonnans C, Gras D, Chavis C, Mainprice B, Vachier I, et al. (2007) Synthesis and anti-inflammatory effect of lipoxins in human airway epithelial cells. Biomed Pharmacother 61: 261–267.
15. Grumbach Y, Quynh NV, Chiron R, Urbach V (2009) LXA4 stimulates ZO-1 expression and transepithelial electrical resistance in human airway epithelial (16HBE14o-) cells. Am J Physiol Lung Cell Mol Physiol 296: L101–108.
16. Bonnans C, Fukunaga K, Levy MA, Levy BD (2006) Lipoxin A(4) regulates bronchial epithelial cell responses to acid injury. Am J Pathol 168: 1064–1072.
17. Hybiske K, Fu Z, Schwarzer C, Tseng J, Do J, et al. (2007) Effects of cystic fibrosis transmembrane conductance regulator and DeltaF508CFTR on inflammatory response, ER stress, and Ca2+ of airway epithelia. Am J Physiol Lung Cell Mol Physiol 293: L1250–1260.
18. Antigny F, Norez C, Cantereau A, Becq F, Vandebrouck C (2008) Abnormal spatial diffusion of Ca2+ in F508del-CFTR airway epithelial cells. Respir Res 9: 70.
19. Ribeiro CM (2006) The role of intracellular calcium signals in inflammatory responses of polarised cystic fibrosis human airway epithelia. Drugs R D 7: 17–31.
20. Knowles MR, Clarke LL, Boucher RC (1991) Activation by extracellular nucleotides of chloride secretion in the airway epithelia of patients with cystic fibrosis. N Engl J Med 325: 533–538.
21. Willumsen NJ, Boucher RC (1989) Activation of an apical Cl- conductance by Ca2+ ionophores in cystic fibrosis airway epithelia. Am J Physiol 256: C226–233.
22. Grubb BR, Vick RN, Boucher RC (1994) Hyperabsorption of Na+ and raised Ca(2+)-mediated Cl- secretion in nasal epithelia of CF mice. Am J Physiol 266: C1478–1483.
23. Paradiso AM, Ribeiro CM, Boucher RC (2001) Polarized signaling via purinoceptors in normal and cystic fibrosis airway epithelia. J Gen Physiol 117: 53–67.
24. Scheckenbach KE, Losa D, Dudez T, Bacchetta M, O'Grady S, et al. (2011) Prostaglandin E_2 regulation of cystic fibrosis transmembrane conductance regulator activity and airway surface liquid volume requires gap junctional communication. Am J Respir Cell Mol Biol. 44(1): 74–82.
25. Zabner J, Karp P, Seiler M, Phillips SL, Mitchell CJ, et al. (2003) Development of cystic fibrosis and noncystic fibrosis airway cell lines. Am J Physiol Lung Cell Mol Physiol 284: L844–854.
26. Urbach V, Harvey BJ (2001) Rapid and non-genomic reduction of intracellular [Ca(2+)] induced by aldosterone in human bronchial epithelium. J Physiol 537: 267–275.

7

Stationary Phase-Specific Virulence Factor Overproduction by a *lasR* Mutant of *Pseudomonas aeruginosa*

Matthew T. Cabeen*

Department of Molecular and Cellular Biology, Harvard University, Cambridge, Massachusetts, United States of America

Abstract

Secreted virulence factors of the human pathogen *Pseudomonas aeruginosa* are often under quorum sensing control. Cells lacking the quorum-sensing regulator LasR show reduced virulence factor production under typical laboratory conditions and are hypo-virulent in short-term animal infection models, yet *lasR* mutants are frequently associated with long-term infection in cystic fibrosis patients. Here, I show that in stationary-phase or slow-growth conditions, *lasR* cells continuously and strongly produce the important virulence factor pyocyanin while wild-type cells do not. Pyocyanin overproduction by *lasR* cells is permitted by loss of repression by RsaL, a LasR-dependent negative regulator. *lasR* cells also contribute pyocyanin in mixed cultures, even under "cheating" conditions where they depend on their wild-type neighbors for nutrients. Finally, some clinical *P. aeruginosa* isolates with *lasR* mutations can overproduce pyocyanin in the laboratory. These results imply that slow-growing clinical populations of *lasR* cells in chronic infections may contribute to virulence by producing pyocyanin under conditions where *lasR*$^{+}$ cells do not.

Editor: Tom Coenye, Ghent University, Belgium

Funding: This work was funded by the BASF (www.basf.com) Advanced Research Initiative at Harvard University, Grant 5366005-01. The funders had no role in study design, data collection and analysis, decision to publish, or preparation of the manuscript.

Competing Interests: This work was funded by the BASF (www.basf.com) Advanced Research Initiative at Harvard University, Grant 5366005-01. This does not alter the author's adherence to PLOS ONE policies on sharing data and materials.

* E-mail: cabeen@fas.harvard.edu.

Introduction

Pseudomonas aeruginosa is a common opportunistic bacterial pathogen that causes human infections in a variety of clinical situations [1] but is especially important in cystic fibrosis lung infections [2]. Many of the numerous virulence factors produced by *P. aeruginosa* are under the control of quorum sensing, which uses diffusible autoinducer molecules as a way to monitor cell density [3]. Specific genes are thus activated when bacterial cell population density, and hence autoinducer concentration, exceeds a threshold. *P. aeruginosa* has at least three quorum-sensing systems, with distinct autoinducer molecules and partially overlapping regulons, that are hierarchically arranged. The Las system is the first to become activated, and it in turn stimulates additional systems known as Rhl and PQS, which additionally regulate each other (Fig. 1) [3]. Finally, pyocyanin, a phenazine small molecule and virulence factor, acts as a terminal signaling factor in the quorum-sensing cascade [4]. Consistent with this hierarchy, inactivation of LasR, the regulatory protein of the Las quorum-sensing system, has been reported to severely attenuate quorum sensing, the production of quorum-regulated factors, and virulence in typical laboratory culture and in short-term animal models [5,6,7,8,9,10,11].

Decreased quorum sensing can permit *lasR* mutants to become social cheaters that gain a growth advantage by utilizing quorum-regulated "public goods" (including virulence factors) produced by nearby wild-type cells rather than producing their own [12,13]. Cheating was thus proposed as one reason [13] why *lasR* mutants are detected in highly chronic human infections such as those occurring in cystic fibrosis patients [14]. Consistent with this idea, *lasR* mutant cells outcompeted co-infected wild-type cells and lowered overall virulence in a murine burn-infection model, consistent with their being non-producing cheaters [11]. However, recent work has revealed that cells lacking LasR function can in fact accomplish quorum sensing by employing the Rhl and PQS systems [15,16]. Without activation by LasR, the quorum response is substantially delayed, but it appears to resemble the wild-type response in terms of gene expression and virulence factor synthesis [15]. Such LasR-independent virulence factor production is another potential explanation for why *lasR* mutants may not reduce overall virulence in long-term cystic fibrosis infections. In accord with this idea, the presence of *lasR* mutant cells has been correlated with disease progression and declining lung function in cystic fibrosis patients [17].

Pyocyanin is one of the most important quorum-regulated virulence factors of *P. aeruginosa*. It has numerous toxic effects on host tissues at such infection sites as the respiratory epithelium, where its toxicity is thought to be related to the generation of reactive oxygen species when pyocyanin is oxidized [18]. Pyocyanin is under the control of the Rhl and PQS systems and can accordingly be produced even in the absence of LasR after a delay [15]. As with the presence of *lasR* mutants, high levels of sputum pyocyanin have been associated with advanced infection in cystic fibrosis patients [19]. Pyocyanin also serves as an antibiotic thanks to its redox activity, can act as a terminal electron

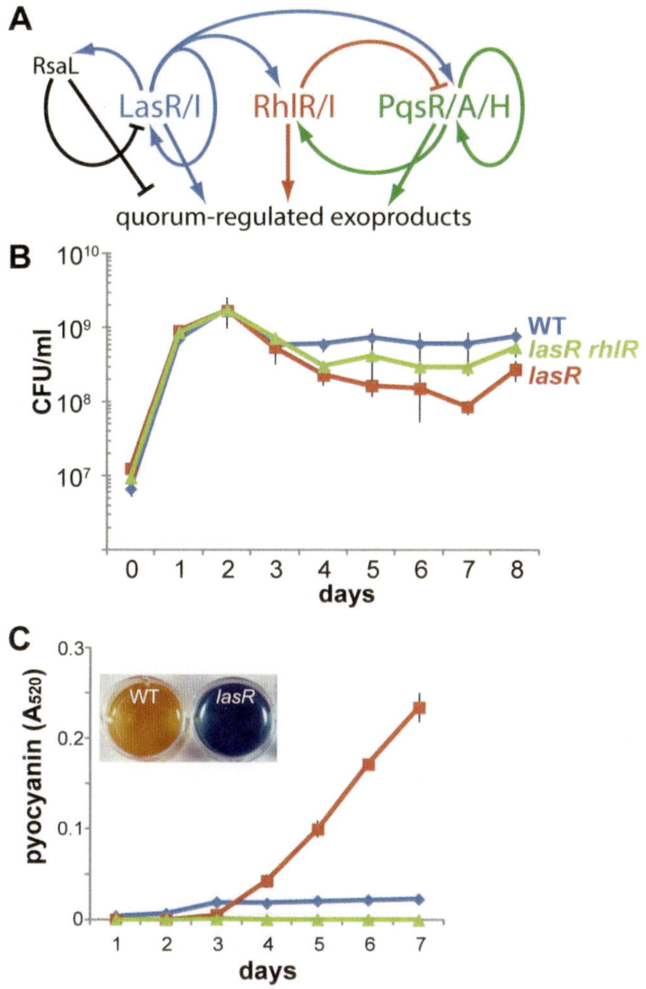

Figure 1. A *lasR* mutant overproduces pyocyanin under stationary-phase culture conditions. A. A simplified diagram showing some of the regulatory pathways linking the three quorum-sensing systems of *P. aeruginosa* and exoproduct synthesis. Each system and its regulatory pathways is color coded. B. Plot of the number of live cells (colony-forming units) in static cultures of strains with wild-type (WT) PA14 (MTC772), PA14 *lasR* (MTC774), and PA14 *lasR rhlR* (MTC797) backgrounds in LB at 25°C. C. Pyocyanin quantification in static cultures of wild-type (WT) PA14 (MTC1), PA14 *lasR* (MTC390), and PA14 *lasR rhlR* (MTC626) in LB at 25°C. The inset image shows the appearance of the cultures in a 12-well plate after 7 d. All plots show the mean ± standard deviation of 3 biological replicates.

acceptor for *P. aeruginosa*, and is a terminal signaling molecule in the quorum-sensing cascade [4]. It is therefore useful for monitoring quorum-sensing activity in *P. aeruginosa*, especially given its bright blue color when oxidized.

Most previous laboratory studies of *P. aeruginosa* quorum sensing have observed bacteria exponentially growing in shaking culture. Under such conditions, wild-type quorum-sensing behaviors begin during late exponential phase and continue into stationary phase, while LasR-independent behaviors do not begin to appear until the onset of stationary phase, between 8 and 24 h [15]. However, most bacterial cells in nature are not growing in optimal laboratory-like conditions. Instead, pathogens often form biofilms during infection [20]. The physiology of slowly growing bacteria resembles that of bacteria growing in biofilms [21], and *P. aeruginosa* expresses the stationary-phase sigma factor RpoS both in clinical sputum samples [22] and in continuously fed biofilms in vitro [23]. Indeed, one reason for the treatment resistance of cells growing in biofilms is their relatively slow growth [24]. Therefore, I reasoned that slow-growing or stationary-phase cells maintained in longer-term culture might manifest phenotypes that reflect their behavior in a more physiologically relevant state. Here, I report that wild-type and *lasR* cells exhibit clearly distinct yet complementary stationary-phase phenotypes. Moreover, wild-type/*lasR* mixtures can collaborate to enact behaviors inaccessible to the individual strains.

Materials and Methods

Routine bacterial culture

Pseudomonas aeruginosa and *Escherichia coli* strains were routinely cultured on LB Lennox solid (1.5% agar) and liquid media at 37°C. Culture stocks were stored in 25% glycerol at -80°C, and fresh plates were grown for each experiment. The following antibiotics were used for selection/maintenance for *P. aeruginosa*; the maintenance concentration was used for *E. coli* culture: gentamycin (75/15 μg/ml) and tetracycline (75/25 μg/ml). Irgasan (25 μg/ml) was used as an *E. coli*-specific selective agent. *P. aeruginosa* strains are listed in Table 1. *E. coli* strains are listed in Table S1 in File S1, plasmids are listed in Table S2 in File S1, and primer sequences are listed in Table S3 in File S1.

Specialized media

M63 medium contained 100 μM (13.6 g/L) KH_2PO_4, 15.14 mM (2 g/L) $(NH_4)_2SO_4$, and 0.36 μM (0.1 mg/L) $FeSO_4{\cdot}H_2O$. A 5X salts stock was adjusted to pH 7.0 with KOH before autoclaving. To make the final medium, the 5X stock was mixed with 0.2% casamino acids and 0.5% glycerol from 20% and 50% sterile stocks, respectively, and adjusted to 1X with sterile H_2O.

M9 medium was based on a salt solution of 12.8 g/L $NaHPO_4{\cdot}7H_2O$, 3 g/L KH_2PO_4, 0.5 g/L NaCl, 1 g/L NH_4Cl. A 5X salts stock was prepared and autoclaved. To make the final medium, the 5X stock was mixed with 2 mM $MgSO_4$ and 0.1 mM $CaCl_2$ from sterile 1M stocks, the appropriate carbon sources (sodium caseinate was added from a 10% autoclaved stock), and was adjusted to 1X with sterile H_2O.

SCFM medium was made as described by Palmer *et al.* [25] and was prepared and used freshly, as it displayed a short shelf life.

Specialized culture conditions

Static cultures of *P. aeruginosa* were grown in 4-ml volumes in 12-well microtiter plates, in 2-ml volumes in 24-well plates, or in 200-μl volumes in 96-well plates. A 1% volume of stationary-phase LB starter culture (OD_{600}~2-3), adjusted to OD_{600} = 1.0, was used for inoculation (hence, the starting OD_{600} was equivalent to 0.01). Pure autoinducer molecules (3OC12-HSL, C4-HSL, and PQS; Sigma) were added from 100 mM stocks in DMSO, and equivalent volumes of DMSO were used for controls.

Reporter assays

Luminescent *lux* reporter strains were grown in static 200-μL LB cultures in 96-well microtiter plates. The cultures were inoculated at an initial OD_{600} of 0.01 (from starter cultures diluted to OD_{600} = 1.0) and grown at 25°C and 40% relative humidity. At daily time points, the luminescence values of the plate were read with a BioTek Synergy 2 plate reader. Data were collected using BioTek Gen5 software. At the same time points, static cultures with isogenic backgrounds, bearing an empty reporter and prepared identically, were taken, vortexed to disperse cells

Table 1. Strains used in this study.

Strain	Alias	Relevant genotype or description	Source or reference
P. aeruginosa			
MTC1		PA14	
MTC63		PA14 Δ*phz*	[4]
MTC390		PA14 Δ*lasR*	This study
MTC498		PA14 Δ*rsaL*	This study
MTC500		PA14 Δ*rsaL* Δ*lasI*	This study
MTC537		PA14 Δ*pqsA*	This study
MTC556		PA14 Δ*rhlI* Δ*pqsA*	This study
MTC625		PA14 Δ*lasR* Δ*rhlI*	This study
MTC626		PA14 Δ*lasR* Δ*rhlR*	This study
MTC628		PA14 Δ*lasR* Δ*pqsA*	This study
MTC637		PA14 Δ*lasR attB::CTX-1-aacC1* ($Gent^R$)	This study
MTC723		PA14 *attB::CTX-1-*P_{lasB}*-lux*	This study
MTC725		PA14 *attB::CTX-1-*P_{phzA1}*-lux*	This study
MTC733		PA14 *attB::CTX-1-*P_{hcnA}*-lux*	This study
MTC735		PA14 *attB::CTX-1-*P_{rhlA}*-lux*	This study
MTC737		PA14 *attB::CTX-1-*P_{rsaL}*-lux*	This study
MTC745		PA14 Δ*lasR attB::CTX-1-*P_{lasB}*-lux*	This study
MTC747		PA14 Δ*lasR attB::CTX-1-*P_{phzA1}*-lux*	This study
MTC755		PA14 Δ*lasR attB::CTX-1-*P_{hcnA}*-lux*	This study
MTC757		PA14 Δ*lasR attB::CTX-1-*P_{rhlA}*-lux*	This study
MTC759		PA14 Δ*lasR attB::CTX-1-*P_{rsaL}*-lux*	This study
MTC772		PA14 *attB::CTX-1-lux*	This study
MTC774		PA14 Δ*lasR attB::CTX-1-lux*	This study
MTC789		PA14 Δ*lasR* Δ*rhlR attB::CTX-1-*P_{lasB}*-lux*	This study
MTC790		PA14 Δ*lasR* Δ*rhlR attB::CTX-1-*P_{phzA1}*-lux*	This study
MTC794		PA14 Δ*lasR* Δ*rhlR attB::CTX-1-*P_{hcnA}*-lux*	This study
MTC795		PA14 Δ*lasR* Δ*rhlR attB::CTX-1-*P_{rhlA}*-lux*	This study
MTC797		PA14 Δ*lasR* Δ*rhlR attB::CTX-1-lux*	This study
MTC838		PA14 Δ*lasR* Δ*ambB*	This study
MTC842		PA14 Δ*lasR* Δ*phoB*	This study
MTC949		PA14 Δ*lasR* Δ*rhlI* Δ*pqsA*	This study
0007-2	CF1	*lasR* wild type (confirmed by sequencing)	[17]
0022-1	CF2	$lasR_{179C>T}$ (W60STOP identified by sequencing)	[17]
0024-5	CF3	*lasR* wild-type (identified by sequencing)	[17]
0029-1	CF4	$lasR_{557T>G}$ (Q186P identified by sequencing)	[17]
0053-2	CF5	$lasR_{520G>A}$ (P174S identified by sequencing)	[17]
0063-6	CF6	$lasR\Delta_{350-362}$ (deletion and frameshift identified by sequencing)	[17]

(effective dispersion was verified by phase-contrast microscopy) and serially diluted to obtain colony-forming unit (CFU) counts. The resulting CFU counts were then used to normalize the luminescence values of their respective reporter strains.

Pyocyanin extraction and quantification

Pyocyanin was extracted from the supernatants of liquid cultures by adding an equal volume of chloroform ($CHCl_3$) and vigorously vortexing. The lower, pyocyanin-containing organic layer was then taken and vortexed with an equal volume of 0.2 M HCl. The pink pyocyanin-containing aqueous layer was taken, and its absorbance at 520 nm (A_{520}) was read in a BioTek Synergy 2 plate reader.

For some experiments, pyocyanin was quantified directly in culture supernatants by reading the absorbance at 691 nm as previously described [19]. Sterile medium was used as a blank.

Cheating experiments

For cheating experiments, PA14 cells or mixtures of PA14 or PA14 *phz* cells with *lasR* cells were grown in liquid M9 medium (6 mL) containing 1% casein at 25°C in a tube roller. Pyocyanin was quantified as described above. The fraction of *lasR* cells within

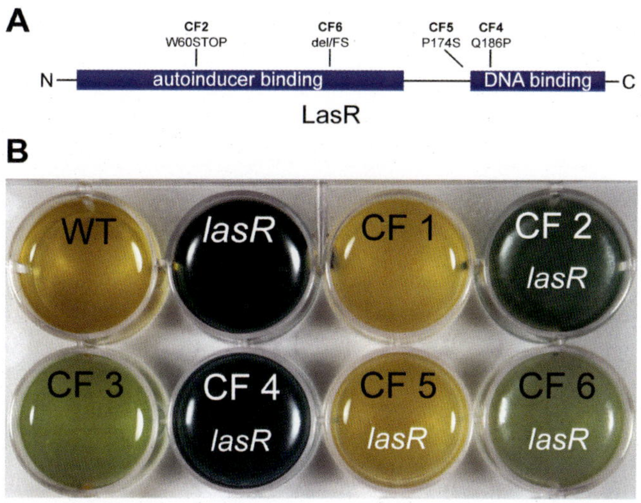

Figure 6. Clinical *lasR* isolates can overproduce pyocyanin. A. Locations of mutations in the LasR protein detected by sequencing. The mutations are in clinical isolates from Ref. 17. B. Appearance of static LB cultures of PA14 and *lasR* laboratory strains and of clinical isolates (CF1-6) [17] with and without *lasR* mutations. The cultures were grown for 12 days at 25°C to allow weaker phenotypes to develop.

Supporting Information

File S1 This file contains Tables S1–S3 and Figure S1–S4. Table S1, *Escherichia coli* strains used in this study. Table S2, Plasmids used in this study. Table S3, Primer sequences used in this study. Figure S1, Pyocyanin production in static culture. Figure S2, Pyocyanin production by *lasR* cells after overnight regrowth. Figure S3, LasR-independent pyocyanin production does not depend on AmbB or PhoB. Figure S4, Growth of wild-type PA14 or lasR cells in M9 medium with added casamino acids or casein.

Acknowledgments

I gratefully acknowledge my postdoctoral advisor Richard Losick, in whose laboratory this work was performed, for invaluable advice about the experiments in this study and during the preparation of the manuscript and for giving me the opportunity to publish on my own. I also thank Stephen Lory and Debbie Yoder-Himes for valuable advice and for supplying strains and vectors. I received clinical isolates from Jane Burns. Thanks to Marvin Whiteley, Karine Gibbs and Christine Jacobs-Wagner for comments on an earlier version of the paper and to Roberto Kolter, Quincey Justman, Peter Girguis and Thomas Norman for helpful discussions. M.T.C. is a Merck Fellow of the Jane Coffin Childs Foundation for Medical Research.

Author Contributions

Conceived and designed the experiments: MTC. Performed the experiments: MTC. Analyzed the data: MTC. Contributed reagents/materials/analysis tools: MTC. Wrote the paper: MTC.

References

1. Driscoll JA, Brody SL, Kollef MH (2007) The epidemiology, pathogenesis and treatment of *Pseudomonas aeruginosa* infections. Drugs 67: 351–368.
2. Lyczak JB, Cannon CL, Pier GB (2002) Lung infections associated with cystic fibrosis. Clin Microbiol Rev 15: 194–222.
3. Rutherford ST, Bassler BL (2012) Bacterial quorum sensing: its role in virulence and possibilities for its control. Cold Spring Harb Perspect Med 2.
4. Dietrich LE, Price-Whelan A, Petersen A, Whiteley M, Newman DK (2006) The phenazine pyocyanin is a terminal signalling factor in the quorum sensing network of *Pseudomonas aeruginosa*. Mol Microbiol 61: 1308–1321.
5. D'Argenio DA, Wu M, Hoffman LR, Kulasekara HD, Deziel E, et al. (2007) Growth phenotypes of *Pseudomonas aeruginosa* lasR mutants adapted to the airways of cystic fibrosis patients. Mol Microbiol 64: 512–533.
6. Hentzer M, Wu H, Andersen JB, Riedel K, Rasmussen TB, et al. (2003) Attenuation of *Pseudomonas aeruginosa* virulence by quorum sensing inhibitors. EMBO J 22: 3803–3815.
7. Pesci EC, Pearson JP, Seed PC, Iglewski BH (1997) Regulation of *las* and *rhl* quorum sensing in *Pseudomonas aeruginosa*. J Bacteriol 179: 3127–3132.
8. Schuster M, Lostroh CP, Ogi T, Greenberg EP (2003) Identification, timing, and signal specificity of *Pseudomonas aeruginosa* quorum-controlled genes: a transcriptome analysis. J Bacteriol 185: 2066–2079.
9. Smith RS, Iglewski BH (2003) *P. aeruginosa* quorum-sensing systems and virulence. Curr Opin Microbiol 6: 56–60.
10. Wagner VE, Bushnell D, Passador L, Brooks AI, Iglewski BH (2003) Microarray analysis of *Pseudomonas aeruginosa* quorum-sensing regulons: effects of growth phase and environment. J Bacteriol 185: 2080–2095.
11. Rumbaugh KP, Diggle SP, Watters CM, Ross-Gillespie A, Griffin AS, et al. (2009) Quorum sensing and the social evolution of bacterial virulence. Curr Biol 19: 341–345.
12. Diggle SP, Griffin AS, Campbell GS, West SA (2007) Cooperation and conflict in quorum-sensing bacterial populations. Nature 450: 411–414.
13. Sandoz KM, Mitzimberg SM, Schuster M (2007) Social cheating in *Pseudomonas aeruginosa* quorum sensing. Proc Natl Acad Sci U S A 104: 15876–15881.
14. Smith EE, Buckley DG, Wu Z, Saenphimmachak C, Hoffman LR, et al. (2006) Genetic adaptation by *Pseudomonas aeruginosa* to the airways of cystic fibrosis patients. Proc Natl Acad Sci U S A 103: 8487–8492.
15. Dekimpe V, Deziel E (2009) Revisiting the quorum-sensing hierarchy in *Pseudomonas aeruginosa*: the transcriptional regulator RhlR regulates LasR-specific factors. Microbiology 155: 712–723.
16. Diggle SP, Winzer K, Chhabra SR, Worrall KE, Camara M, et al. (2003) The *Pseudomonas aeruginosa* quinolone signal molecule overcomes the cell density-dependency of the quorum sensing hierarchy, regulates rhl-dependent genes at the onset of stationary phase and can be produced in the absence of LasR. Mol Microbiol 50: 29–43.
17. Hoffman LR, Kulasekara HD, Emerson J, Houston LS, Burns JL, et al. (2009) *Pseudomonas aeruginosa lasR* mutants are associated with cystic fibrosis lung disease progression. J Cyst Fibros 8: 66–70.
18. Rada B, Leto TL (2013) Pyocyanin effects on respiratory epithelium: relevance in *Pseudomonas aeruginosa* airway infections. Trends Microbiol 21: 73–81.
19. Hunter RC, Klepac-Ceraj V, Lorenzi MM, Grotzinger H, Martin TR, et al. (2012) Phenazine content in the cystic fibrosis respiratory tract negatively correlates with lung function and microbial complexity. Am J Respir Cell Mol Biol 47: 738–745.
20. Bjarnsholt T, Alhede M, Alhede M, Eickhardt-Sørensen SR, Moser C, et al. (2013) The in vivo biofilm. Trends in microbiology 21: 466–474.
21. Fux CA, Costerton JW, Stewart PS, Stoodley P (2005) Survival strategies of infectious biofilms. Trends Microbiol 13: 34–40.
22. Foley I, Marsh P, Wellington EM, Smith AW, Brown MR (1999) General stress response master regulator *rpoS* is expressed in human infection: a possible role in chronicity. J Antimicrob Chemother 43: 164–165.
23. Xu KD, Franklin MJ, Park CH, McFeters GA, Stewart PS (2001) Gene expression and protein levels of the stationary phase sigma factor, RpoS, in continuously-fed *Pseudomonas aeruginosa* biofilms. FEMS Microbiol Lett 199: 67–71.
24. Mah TF, O'Toole GA (2001) Mechanisms of biofilm resistance to antimicrobial agents. Trends Microbiol 9: 34–39.
25. Palmer KL, Aye LM, Whiteley M (2007) Nutritional cues control *Pseudomonas aeruginosa* multicellular behavior in cystic fibrosis sputum. J Bacteriol 189: 8079–8087.
26. Navarro Llorens JM, Tormo A, Martinez-Garcia E (2010) Stationary phase in gram-negative bacteria. FEMS Microbiol Rev 34: 476–495.
27. Jensen V, Lons D, Zaoui C, Bredenbruch F, Meissner A, et al. (2006) RhlR expression in *Pseudomonas aeruginosa* is modulated by the *Pseudomonas* quinolone signal via PhoB-dependent and -independent pathways. J Bacteriol 188: 8601–8606.
28. Deziel E, Lepine F, Milot S, He J, Mindrinos MN, et al. (2004) Analysis of *Pseudomonas aeruginosa* 4-hydroxy-2-alkylquinolines (HAQs) reveals a role for 4-hydroxy-2-heptylquinoline in cell-to-cell communication. Proc Natl Acad Sci U S A 101: 1339–1344.
29. Gallagher LA, McKnight SL, Kuznetsova MS, Pesci EC, Manoil C (2002) Functions required for extracellular quinolone signaling by *Pseudomonas aeruginosa*. J Bacteriol 184: 6472–6480.

30. Lee J, Wu J, Deng Y, Wang J, Wang C, et al. (2013) A cell-cell communication signal integrates quorum sensing and stress response. Nat Chem Biol.
31. Rampioni G, Schuster M, Greenberg EP, Bertani I, Grasso M, et al. (2007) RsaL provides quorum sensing homeostasis and functions as a global regulator of gene expression in *Pseudomonas aeruginosa*. Mol Microbiol 66: 1557–1565.
32. de Kievit T, Seed PC, Nezezon J, Passador L, Iglewski BH (1999) RsaL, a novel repressor of virulence gene expression in *Pseudomonas aeruginosa*. J Bacteriol 181: 2175–2184.
33. Rampioni G, Polticelli F, Bertani I, Righetti K, Venturi V, et al. (2007) The *Pseudomonas* quorum-sensing regulator RsaL belongs to the tetrahelical superclass of H-T-H proteins. J Bacteriol 189: 1922–1930.
34. Dandekar AA, Chugani S, Greenberg EP (2012) Bacterial quorum sensing and metabolic incentives to cooperate. Science 338: 264–266.
35. Van Delden C, Pesci EC, Pearson JP, Iglewski BH (1998) Starvation selection restores elastase and rhamnolipid production in a *Pseudomonas aeruginosa* quorum-sensing mutant. Infect Immun 66: 4499–4502.
36. Alvarez-Ortega C, Harwood CS (2007) Responses of *Pseudomonas aeruginosa* to low oxygen indicate that growth in the cystic fibrosis lung is by aerobic respiration. Mol Microbiol 65: 153–165.
37. Worlitzsch D, Tarran R, Ulrich M, Schwab U, Cekici A, et al. (2002) Effects of reduced mucus oxygen concentration in airway *Pseudomonas* infections of cystic fibrosis patients. J Clin Invest 109: 317–325.
38. Rampioni G, Schuster M, Greenberg EP, Zennaro E, Leoni L (2009) Contribution of the RsaL global regulator to *Pseudomonas aeruginosa* virulence and biofilm formation. FEMS Microbiol Lett 301: 210–217.

8

Influenza A(H1N1)pdm09 and Cystic Fibrosis Lung Disease

Hanna Renk[1]*, Nicolas Regamey[2], Dominik Hartl[1]

1 University Children's Hospital, Eberhard-Karls-University, Tuebingen, Germany, **2** Department of Paediatrics, Inselspital and University of Bern, Bern, Switzerland

Abstract

Background: To systematically assess the literature published on the clinical impact of Influenza A(H1N1)pdm09 on cystic fibrosis (CF) patients.

Methods: An online search in PUBMED database was conducted. Original articles on CF patients with Influenza A(H1N1)pdm09 infection were included. We analyzed incidence, symptoms, clinical course and treatment.

Results: Four surveys with a total of 202 CF patients infected by Influenza A(H1N1)pdm09 were included. The meta-analysis showed that hospitalisation rates were higher in CF patients compared to the general population. While general disease symptoms were comparable, the clinical course was more severe and case fatality rate (CFR) was higher in CF patients compared to asthmatics and the general population.

Conclusions: Evidence so far suggests that CF patients infected with Influenza A(H1N1)pdm09 show increased morbidity and a higher CFR compared to patients with other chronic respiratory diseases and healthy controls. Particularly, CF patients with advanced stage disease seem to be more susceptible to severe lung disease. Accordingly, early antiviral and antibiotic treatment strategies are essential in CF patients. Preventive measures, including vaccination as well as hygiene measures during the influenza season, should be reinforced and improved in CF patients.

Editor: Marco Idzko, University Hospital Freiburg, Germany

Funding: The authors have no support or funding to report.

Competing Interests: The authors have declared that no competing interests exist.

* E-mail: Hanna.Renk@med.uni-tuebingen.de

Introduction

Influenza A (H1N1)pdm09

A new Influenza A(H1N1) virus subtype with a large antigenic difference to the previously encountered seasonal A(H1N1) viruses was detected for the first time in Mexico in April 2009 [1]. The virus rapidly spread around the world and in June 2009 the first influenza pandemic of the twenty-first century was declared [2]. Today, in the post-pandemic period, the Influenza A(H1N1)pdm09 virus has adopted the properties of a seasonal influenza virus [3]. Several countries have already experienced seasonal outbreaks during the last few years, but since the Influenza A(H1N1)pdm09 virus has now become one of the seasonal strains of influenza viruses it has lost public interest [4–7]. However, at the beginning of 2013, the Influenza A(H1N1)pdm09 virus launched a remarkable "comeback" in some regions like the Middle East, Northern Africa and some European countries, e.g. Germany. Influenza A(H1N1)pdm09 was the predominant laboratory confirmed subtype in Europe in the 2013 winter season [8].

Influenza A(H1N1)pdm09, first isolated in 2009, is a reassortment between four different viruses: North American swine influenza, Eurasian swine influenza, avian influenza and human influenza. The virus is transmitted by direct contact with infected individuals, contaminated objects or by inhalation of virus-laden aerosols. The incubation period is 1.5–3 days. Influenza A(H1N1)pdm09 differs in pathogenic mechanisms, epidemiological features and virulence from previous seasonal influenza A viruses. In contrast to other influenza viruses, the pdm09 subtype lacks mutations which are responsible for high pathogenicity. Replication of the virus takes longer and the level of pulmonary replication is higher than in other seasonal influenza viruses [9,10].

Incidence rates of Influenza A(H1N1)pdm09 in adults and children with influenza-like illnesses (ILI) were reported to be 33% and 36%, respectively during the pandemic [11,12]. Contrary to expectations during the pandemic, Influenza A(H1N1)pdm09 caused only relatively mild disease in the general population. Main symptoms of infection were fever and cough in around 80% of patients, followed by dyspnea, fatigue and myalgias, headache, sore throat and gastrointestinal symptoms [13]. Hospitalization rates ranged between 7–20% at the beginning of the pandemic [14]. Younger age groups, including patients with chronic respiratory diseases such as CF patients, were particularly affected by the Influenza A(H1N1)pdm09 virus during the 2009 pandemic. In seasonal influenza (eg H3N2 and H1N1) hospitalization rates among children and adults aged between 18 and 64 years were lower than in Influenza A(H1N1)pdm09. Vice versa, among elderly persons hospitalization rates were lower in Influenza A(H1N1)pdm09 than in seasonal influenza strains [15]. 90% of all deaths occurred in persons <65 years and the highest hospitalization rates were found in children <5 years of age [16,17]. Ethnic minorities and children with pre-existing disorders were disproportionately affected [17]. Risk factors for severe course included age <5 years or ≥65 years, obesity, underlying neurological diseases, diabetes, cardiovascular disease, chronic kidney or liver disease, immunosuppression and/or pregnancy [18,19]. In a large observational study in England during the pandemic period, overall childhood mortality rate was 6 per million population. Children with severe pre-existing disorders such as chronic neurological, gastrointestinal or respiratory disease accounted for 64% of deaths [17].

Bacterial coinfection was the cause of death of many individuals with Influenza A(H1N1)pdm09. In lung tissue specimens from fatal cases, bacterial coinfection occurred in 22/77 (29%) patients [20]. Furthermore in a prospective Canadian study, bacterial coinfection was confirmed by positive culture in 259/681 (38%) of adult ICU admissions [21]. The most common pathogens isolated from respiratory cultures in critically ill children with Influenza A(H1N1)pdm09 were *Staphylococcus aureus* (including *MRSA*) (39%), *Pseudomonas species* (16%), *Streptococcus pneumoniae* (8%), *Haemophilus influenzae* (7%) and *Streptococcus pyogenes* (4%) [22]. Thus, secondary bacterial infection is a leading cause of severe course and death in Influenza A(H1N1)pdm09 virus infection. Influenza A(H1N1)pdm09 related death was reported in 7% and 5.3% of patients hospitalized with ILI and PCR confirmed infection [18,19]. Case fatality rate (CFR) of Influenza A(H1N1)pdm09 infection in the general population was overestimated at the beginning of the pandemic and finally ranged 2.9 to 7-fold lower than in seasonal influenza infections from 1990–1999 [23]. Contrarily to the early expectations, CFR of Influenza A(H1N1)pdm09 infection was retrospectively calculated only around 0.04% to 0.05% [24,25].

Cystic fibrosis

Cystic fibrosis (CF) is the most common autosomal recessive inherited lethal metabolic disorder of the white population with an incidence of about 1 in 2000–3000 live births [26,27]. The disease is caused by a mutation in the *cystic fibrosis transmembrane conductance regulator gene (CFTR)* resulting in a dysfunctional protein of the apical membrane of epithelial cells [28]. This protein serves as a cAMP-regulated chloride channel. Lack or dysfunction leads to ineffective chloride secretion and increased absorption of water from the respiratory tract. Consequently, mucociliary clearance is impaired and viscous mucus is present, which in turn favors chronic bacterial colonization of the airways and pulmonary inflammation. Chronic pulmonary disease accounts for most of the morbidity and mortality in CF. Airway obstruction, infection with typical pathogens including *Staphylococcus aureus*, *Haemophilus influenza* and *Pseudomonas aeruginosa*, and inflammation lead to progressive deterioration of pulmonary function [29]. Cough, increased sputum production and dyspnea are the most prominent signs of pulmonary manifestations of the disease.

Epithelial cells also are affected by reduced or defective *CFTR* activity in other organs, which leads to mucinous obstruction of various secretory glands. Pancreatic insufficiency, intestinal obstruction, liver damage and infertility may occur. Since the identification of the *CFTR* gene in 1989, the life expectancy of CF patients has continuously increased, due to improved treatment. Nowadays, the average life expectancy of CF patients in countries of the western world adds up to 40 years [30].

Recently, viral respiratory infections in CF were given more and more attention [31,32]. In pediatric and adult CF patients the risk of pulmonary exacerbations as well as length and frequency of hospitalizations were found to be increased by viral respiratory infections. Additionally, viral respiratory infections in CF patients have been shown to be associated with deterioration of pulmonary function and predispose to secondary bacterial infection [33–35]. It does not seem that CF patients are affected more frequently by viral respiratory infections than the general population, but the clinical consequences are worse. The rate of symptomatic respiratory illnesses was significantly higher in CF patients than in their healthy siblings [36]. It was also shown that children with CF were affected longer and more severely by viral respiratory disease [37]. Viral respiratory infection in general and especially RSV and Influenza might have serious consequences for CF patients [38].

Currently, little is known about short-term morbidity and disease progression associated with recently detectable viruses such as newly recognized rhinovirus subtypes, human metapneumovirus (hMPV) and coronaviruses. In particular, the impact of the Influenza A(H1N1)pdm09 virus on CF patients is unclear. In this study, we aimed at describing the impact of the Influenza A(H1N1)pdm09 pandemic on CF patients based on a retrospective data analysis of the currently available literature. We wished to answer the following questions: What impact did the Influenza A(H1N1)pdm09 pandemic have on the CF population and what impact of the Influenza A(H1N1)pdm09 virus has to be expected in the future for CF patients? What recommendations for prevention and treatment of CF patients with Influenza A(H1N1)pdm09 infection can be given according to the current knowledge?

Methods

We performed a systematic literature search in PUBMED for original articles from 2009 to 2013, describing the effects of Influenza A(H1N1)pdm09 infection on CF patients. All published articles since the onset of the Influenza A (H1N1)pdm09 pandemic in April 2009 were extracted. The search term was "cystic fibrosis [MeSH] and H1N1 influenza", generating 16 results. Case reports, non-clinical studies and publications dealing just with H1N1 vaccination or pharmacokinetics of Oseltamivir were excluded. The search yielded four original articles from four different countries, all published in English language. Two surveys had been conducted as multicenter studies. All studies were designed retrospectively and data collection was based on questionnaires as well as web-based in the two multicenter studies. Incidence (i.e. incidence of the illness), symptoms, treatment and clinical course (i.e. hospitalization, ICU treatment, death) of Influenza A (H1N1)pdm09 infection in CF patients were analyzed from 06/2009 to 04/2010. Out of the four studies and their supplements the following data were recorded: name of first author, journal, country and year of publication, period of analysis, number, age and characteristics of Influenza A(H1N1)pdm09 positive CF patients (eg *Pseudomonas* colonization, percent predicted forced expiratory volume in one second (FEV1% pred.), vaccination status), symptoms associated with Influenza A(H1N1)pdm09 infection, treatment and clinical course. Mean values of the frequency of clinical symptoms in the different studies were calculated. Similar symptom groups were summarized.

Clinical course was not described consistently in the four studies, therefore "mild course" was defined as outpatient treatment, "moderate course" as hospitalization without complications and "serious course" as intensive care treatment, mechanical ventilation, or death due to complications. In addition, conclusions and recommendations of the authors regarding

Influenza A(H1N1)pdm09 infection in CF patients were summarized.

Results of the literature review

The four studies included in the meta-analysis are summarized in Table 1. Two studies were performed as multicenter surveys, one Europe-wide, the other one confined to Italy. The two single-center studies were conducted in England and Australia. A total of 5429 subjects with CF were included in the four studies, and Influenza A (H1N1)pdm09 infection was confirmed by PCR in 202 of them (3.7%). The European study by Viviani et al. was the largest, including 110 patients [39].

Incidence. attributable to Influenza A(H1N1)pdm09 ranged from 2.3% in the Europe-wide multicenter study (0% to 9.4% depending on the center) to 4.4% in the Australian study by Nash et al. [40]. In the Italian study by Colombo et al., the proportion of patients who were tested positive for Influenza A(H1N1)pdm09 (53%) was based only on CF patients with ILI, and therefore incidence was not calculable [41].

Patient characteristics. The mean age of the 202 Influenza A(H1N1)pdm09-positive patients ranged from 13 to 22 years in the four studies. The majority of the patients were infected chronically with *Pseudomonas aeruginosa*. In two studies, a rate of pancreatic insufficiency of 85–90% was reported. The pulmonary status was described by mean FEV1% pred. in all studies and ranged between 51% and 69%. Due to the lack of general availability of the Influenza A(H1N1)pdm09 vaccine until the end of 2009, immunization data of Influenza A(H1N1)pdm09 vaccination were not documented in the Australian and the English study. The two multicenter studies reported an Influenza A(H1N1) vaccination rate of 8.8% and 13.2%, respectively in CF patients.

Symptomatology. Fever occurred in nearly all cases (90–100%), increased cough and sputum production were consistently the most common symptoms. Dyspnea, sore throat, headache, myalgia, arthralgia, fatigue and gastrointestinal symptoms occurred in only 50% of cases or less. Rarely hemoptysis (in 4.5%) was reported. In Figure 1, each symptom is compared with frequency of symptoms in asthmatics and subjects with no comorbidities infected by Influenza A(H1N1)pdm09 from a US study by McKenna [13].

Treatment. In all studies Oseltamivir was used exclusively for antiviral therapy. In the two multicenter trials approximately 80% of patients were treated with Oseltamivir and antibiotic treatment was administered in 66% and 68%, respectively. In the two other studies, all patients received Oseltamivir and antibiotics were given in 75% and 100% of cases, respectively.

Clinical course. There was no consistent description of the clinical course of Influenza A(H1N1)pdm09 infection in CF patients in the four studies. Mild course (outpatient treatment) occurred in 86/202 (43%); moderate course (hospitalization without complications) in 100/202 (49%) and severe course (intensive care treatment or death) in 16/202 (8%) (Figure 2). Mortality rates (2.7% and 4.4%, respectively) were available only from the two multicenter trials.

Recommendations and conclusions. from the four studies are summarized in headwords in Table 1. Principal points of prevention and treatment of Influenza A(H1N1)pdm09 infection in CF patients mentioned by the authors included vaccination, infection control measures and the rapid onset of aggressive antiviral and antibiotic treatment.

Discussion

Our search revealed that, surprisingly, there are only few data on CF patients infected with Influenza A(H1N1)pdm09 in the literature. Merely four studies could be identified, and data were only available from the pandemic in 2009/2010.

Incidence

Incidence of Influenza A(H1N1)pdm09 in the four studies was not consistently described. Results of the multicenter Europe-wide survey of Viviani et al. [39] and the studies of Nash et al. [40] and France et al. [42] refer to the total CF population, regardless of symptoms of ILI. Incidence of Influenza A(H1N1)pdm09 infection ranged from 2.3 to 4.4% in these studies. However, Colombo et al. specifically referred to CF patients with ILI and 68/127 (53%) patients were tested positive for Influenza A(H1N1)pdm09 [41]. This rate is remarkably increased compared to the general population with ILI, where 36% of patients in a pediatric and 34% in an adult emergency room were proven positive during the pandemic [11,12]. Pecavar et al. used a similar study period and case definition of ILI compared to Colombo's data in italian CF patients [11,41]. Although local differences, like a higher amount of circulating virus in the Italian centers, is a possible reason for the difference, these data suggest that CF patients may have an increased susceptibility to the Influenza A(H1N1)pdm09 virus, at least during the pandemic period. However, to verify this, additional evidence needs to be collected during future influenza seasons.

Patient characteristics

Particularly CF patients in advanced stages of the disease seem susceptible to Influenza A(H1N1)pdm09 infection. The mean of FEV1% pred., which is a prognostic factor for progression of pulmonary disease, was poor (50 to 70%) in the analyzed studies. On average, patients aged up to 22 years have a higher FEV1% pred. [43]. Consequently, reported CF patients infected by Influenza A(H1N1)pdm09, often had poor pulmonary conditions. One may conclude that patients in advanced stages of CF suffer the most from increased Influenza A(H1N1)pdm09 mediated incidence, like it has already been described for viral respiratory infections in CF patients in general [36]. However, it is possible that only centers with severely affected patients reported their cases and thus reporting bias also provides an explanation for the increased incidence.

Symptomatology

The clinical presentation of Influenza A(H1N1)pdm09 infection differed only slightly from the symptomatology in the general population and from asthmatics. The main symptom of infection was fever in 92–100%, followed by cough, sore throat and other symptoms characteristic for common viral respiratory infections. However, increased sputum production was found to predominate and rarely hemoptysis was present in CF patients with Influenza A(H1N1)pdm09 compared to the general population and asthmatics [13,18].

Treatment

Early antiviral therapy and, if appropriate, antibiotic coverage in CF patients are crucial for the treatment of Influenza A(H1N1)pdm09 infection. Antiviral treatment with Oseltamivir was performed in all of the analyzed studies. Early start of treatment during the first three days of disease reduces viral shedding and thus is not only of therapeutic use, but also contributes to infection control [44].

Table 1. Characteristics, treatment and outcome of Influenza A(H1N1)pdm09-infected CF patients.

Country	Inf A(H1N1)pdm09 infection in CF patients			Characteristics of CF patients infected with Inf A(H1N1)pdm09 (%)				Treatment (%)	Outcome (%)			Conclusion/Recommendation	Ref
	N[1]	*Age*[2]	*Incidence* (%)*	*P. aerug.*	*Pancreatic*	*FEV1*	*Vacc*	*Oseltamivir*	*Hospital*	*ICU*[4] *or*	*CFR*[5]		
				//	*Insufficiency*	*pred*[3]		*//*	*admission*	*ventilation*			
				B. cepacia				*Antibiotics*					
				coinfection									
Europe#	110	13	2.3*	n.r.	84	69	8.8	81/66	48	5.4	2.7	awareness,	[39]
								81//66					
												infection control,	
												vaccination campaign	
Italy#	68	15	53**	48.5//8.8	89.7	53	13.2	82//68	69	1.5 ventilation	4.4	annual vaccination in	[41]
				48.5//8.8									
										13.2 on oxygen		adult CF patients	
Australia	11	22	4.4*	100//1	n.r.	66	n.av.	100//75	63	n.r.	n.r.	prompt	[42]
				100//1									
												commencement of	
												oseltamivir and	
												antibiotic therapy	
UK	13	22	4*	100//n.r.	n.r.	51.4	n.r.	100//100	69	0	n.r.	generally mild illness	[40]
					n.r.			100//100					
												in CF,	
												potentially more	
												virulent pandemic in	
												the future	

[1]Number of Influenza A(H1N1)pdm09 positive CF patients.
[2]Mean age (years).
[3]Mean of all CF patients studied.
[4]Intensive care unit.
[5]Case fatality rate.
#multicenter surveys;
*incidence of Inf A(H1N1)pdm09 infections in CF patients.
**incidence of Inf A(H1N1)pdm09 infections relating to CF patients with influenza-like illness.
(ILI); n.r. – not reported; Vacc – Vaccination coverage; P. aerug. = Pseudomonas aeruginosa; B. cepacia = Burkholderia cepacia.

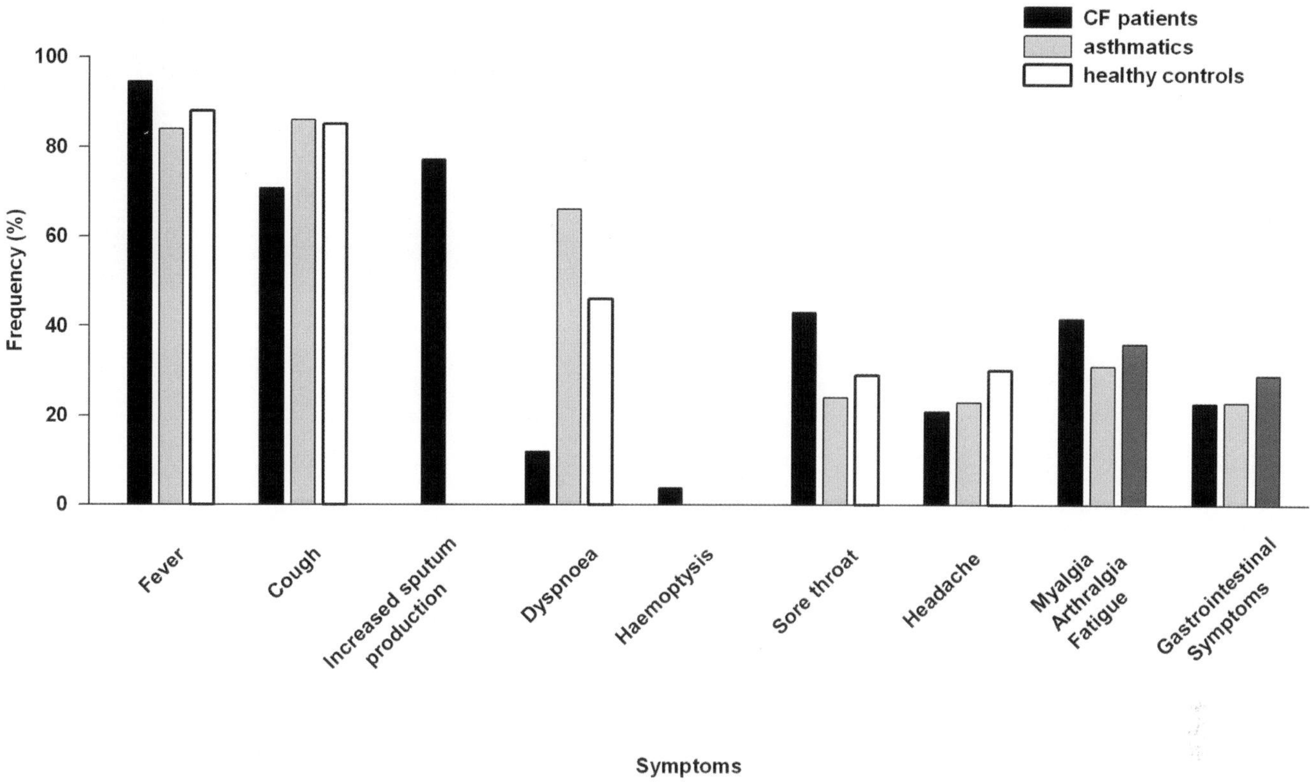

Figure 1. Symptoms of Influenza A(H1N1)pdm09 infection in CF, asthmatics and healthy controls. Frequency of presenting symptoms in CF patients, asthmatics and healthy controls from four studies of Influenza A(H1N1)pdm09 infection in CF patients [39–42], and a study of asthmatics and healthy controls [13] during the 2009 pandemic.

Antibiotics were administered in 66–100% of infected CF patients. During former and during the 2009 influenza pandemic, bacterial coinfection caused substantial morbidity and mortality in healthy individuals and in patients with comorbidities [45,46]. In this context, CF patients, frequently colonized with *Pseudomonas aeruginosa* and other pathogens, seem to be at high risk for pulmonary exacerbation and fatal course from bacterial coinfection during an influenza outbreak. Therefore, adequate initiation of appropriate antibiotic treatment, like it was done in the analyzed studies, is important. However, currently there is no consensus of optimal mode of antibiotic therapy (single or combination) as well as its duration in CF patients [47].

Clinical course

Approximately 50–70% of all CF patients tested positive required hospitalization. This high rate in CF patients compared to the general population (hospitalization rate 7–20%) should be interpreted with caution, though [13]. For medical staff confronted with CF patients experiencing a H1N1 infection, the need for hospitalization was difficult to estimate at the beginning of the pandemic phase due to lack of experience with the clinical course of the disease. This likely resulted in excess hospitalizations, especially in patients with comorbidities. Therefore, the high hospitalization rate in CF patients may in fact not correspond to a more severe course of the disease.

In general, patients with comorbidities, especially chronic respiratory diseases, were at particular risk for severe course and complications of Influenza A(H1N1)pdm09 infection [19]. Collectively, clinical course in the four studies was worse in CF patients compared to the general population. More than half of all CF patients (57%) showed a moderate or severe course of disease, requiring hospitalization or even ICU treatment (Figure 2). These data are consistent with previous studies, reporting a three-fold increase for ICU admission or fatal course in patients with chronic lung disease (other than asthma) infected by Influenza A(H1N1)pdm09 [18,19]. Accordingly, CF lung disease, in contrast to asthma, is likely to represent a clinical risk factor for severe disease course in Influenza A(H1N1)pdm09 infection [48]. A possible explanation for this might be that CF patients generally do not suffer more often from viral infections than non-CF individuals, but with worse clinical consequences. Thus CF patients with viral respiratory infections are prone to exacerbations and severe course [36,37,49,50].

Consistently, the case fatality rate of the two multicenter trials of Viviani et al. and Colombo et al. was increased. A total of 6/4825 CF patients died from Influenza A(H1N1)pdm09 infection, representing a case fatality rate (CFR) of 3.5% (2.7% and 4.4% in each study) [39,41]. Assuming that this CFR reflects the population related mortality rate of CF patients infected by Influenza A(H1N1)pdm09, it is higher than the CFR of 0.05% in the general population [17,25].

Pathophysiological mechanisms

Explaining the increased respiratory morbidity in CF patients towards viral infection are unclear. Several mechanisms have been proposed.

First an alteration of the inflammatory response of CF airway epithelium on virus infection compared to healthy controls has been discussed. On the one hand, increased inflammatory response of CF airway epithelial cells was shown with parainflu-

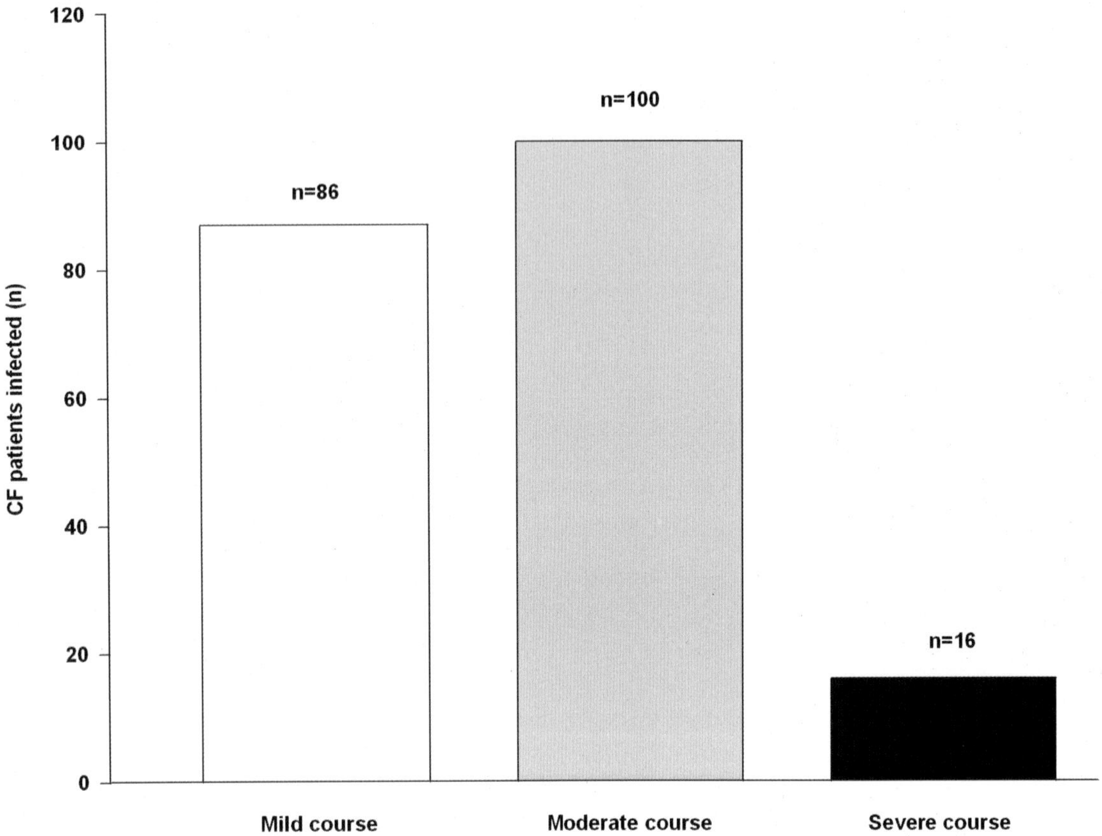

Figure 2. Clinical course of Influenza A(H1N1)pdm09 infection in CF patients. Number of CF patients with mild, moderate or severe course of Influenza A(H1N1)pdm09 infection in the analyzed studies [39–42]. Mild course: outpatient treatment. Moderate course: hospitalization without complications. Serious course: intensive care treatment, mechanical ventilation, or death.

enza virus 3 and influenza A infection [51,52]. CF airway epithelial cells of children also showed a greater IL-8 neutrophilic response after exposure to human rhinovirus than airway epithelial cells of healthy controls in vitro [53]. Thus dysregulation in the innate response of CF airway epithelial cells upon viral infection is possible. Airway inflammation, slower clearance of virus, increased severity and prolonged inflammation may be the consequence of an exaggerated immune response [53]. On the other hand, in a recent study, rhinovirus infection results were vice versa. A lower inflammatory response and increased cell death were found in rhinovirus infected CF airway epithelium, suggesting a greater susceptibility of CF airway epithelium towards viral toxic effects [54].

Second, impaired control of viral replication provides a possible mechanism for increased respiratory morbidity of CF patients. Replication of human rhinovirus (serotype 14 and 1b) and human parainfluenzavirus was increased in airway epithelial cells of CF children compared to control subjects [51,53]. In influenza infection antiviral response was compromised and apoptotic response reduced. This may lead to higher viral titers as well as a longer time of viral residence and proliferation. Increased viral replication in airway epithelial cells may facilitate a more severe course of viral respiratory illness in CF patients.

A possible explanation is that specific antiviral host defense mechanisms may be compromised by viral respiratory infection. Impairment of antiviral pathways mediated by high–level NO synthesis and IFN/STAT 1 suggests that airway epithelial cells in CF may allow increased viral replication and increased production of proinflammatory cytokines compared to healthy subjects. This results in a higher degree of airway inflammation and severe respiratory symptoms as it was shown for human parainfluenza-virus infection in CF children [51]. In BAL specimens of CF children with rhinovirus infection, a 100 fold higher viral load was detected compared to healthy children. Higher viral load was negatively associated with production of antiviral mediators. Possibly, impaired production of antiviral mediators in CF patients leads to a high viral burden in the lower airways and may particularly occur in the context of CF exacerbations [50].

Finally, viral respiratory infection may trigger pulmonary exacerbation by interaction with bacterial pathogens. In vitro, RSV serves as a coupling agent between airway epithelial cells and *P. aeruginosa* and enhances its adherence to these cells. Thereby, RSV facilitates bacterial colonization (eg with *P. aeruginosa*) [55]. Moreover there is evidence that viral superinfection leads to oxidative stress, followed by dispersal of planktonic bacteria from biofilm matrix. Planktonic bacteria may interact with basolateral receptors in the airway epithelium and stimulate an intense inflammatory response through increased chemokine responses [56].

Prevention and recommendations

Especially patients in advanced stages of CF, who often have to visit health care facilities, are prone to an Influenza A(H1N1)pdm09 infection with severe course. Therefore, infection control in facilities that care for CF patients is of particular importance. The two main pillars of prevention are vaccination and improvement of hygiene measures. Data on effectiveness of the vaccine in CF patients are scarce and specific immune responses to influenza vaccination in CF patients with advanced disease are not known. Nevertheless, vaccination is strongly recommended by health authorities throughout the world. On the one hand, coverage with the monovalent pandemic vaccine in CF patients was reported to be high but differed markedly between countries [57]. On the other hand, the clinical problem is that the overall acceptance of seasonal influenza vaccination particularly in healthcare workers is poor [58,59]. In the face of future influenza seasons, efforts to increase vaccination rates in healthcare personnel and close contacts are crucial. Thereby, incidence and serious complications in CF patients might be reduced through herd immunity. Particular attention should be paid on the implementation of hygiene measures in public and private life as well as in hospital settings. Information of CF patients on hygiene and infection control measures e.g. in advance to the influenza season should be performed and combined with influenza vaccination. Furthermore, pneumococcal vaccine provides protection for CF patients from secondary bacterial infection due to *Streptococcus pneumoniae.*

Limitations of this meta-analysis

This meta-analysis is subject to several limitations. First, there is a certain bias and limited comparability of data due to different methods of analysis and retrospective design of the studies. Second, reporting bias has to be considered in all four surveys. Particularly centers that experienced only mild cases were possibly less likely to participate in the study than those who experienced severe cases. Physicians' awareness and reporting behavior may have influenced data collection and was not assessed. Furthermore different local situations and heterogeneity of the CF population (e.g. children or young adults, different stages of disease) bear further bias. Another caveat relates to the symptoms of disease, which were not consistently described. There is also a lack of systematic assessment of disease severity, which may affect comparability of data. Additionally, calculation of the CFR in the CF population analyzed in these four studies certainly bears a higher inaccuracy than calculations in the general population. However, as diagnosis of Influenza A(H1N1)pdm09 infection was verified by PCR in all studies, a high reliability of the viral detection data and thus a distinct case definition can be assumed.

Summary

Influenza A(H1N1)pdm09 infection had substantial effects on CF patients during the 2009 pandemic. CF patients seemed to have an increased susceptibility to the virus compared to the general population. Initial clinical symptoms of Influenza A(H1N1)pdm09 infection in CF patients were similar to the general population, beside a significantly increased sputum production. Particularly, patients in advanced stages of CF lung disease were prone to severe course of disease (e.g. ICU admission or death). Early administration of antiviral treatment and antibiotic coverage are crucial. Vaccination and infection control measures should be of public interest at the beginning of an influenza season. However, the impact of Influenza A(H1N1)pdm09 on the CF population in the post-pandemic period remains poorly understood.

Author Contributions

Conceived and designed the experiments: HR NR DH. Performed the experiments: HR. Analyzed the data: HR. Contributed reagents/materials/analysis tools: HR NR DH. Wrote the paper: HR NR DH.

References

1. CDC (2009) Swine influenza A (H1N1) infection in two children–Southern California, March–April 2009. MMWR Morb Mortal Wkly Rep 58: 400–402.
2. Chan M (2009) World now at the start of 2009 influenza pandemic - Statement to the press by WHO Director-General Dr Margaret Chan. WHO Media centre.
3. WHO (2013) Epidemiological and virological situation update of the 2012/2013 influenza season in the WHO European Region. WHO Europe Publications. Available: http://www.euro.who.int/__data/assets/pdf_file/0010/184690/Epi-and-virological-update-of-the-2012-13-influenza-season-in-the-WHO-EURO-EuroFlu-data-week-40,2012-to-week-04,2013.pdf.
4. Canada PHAo Public Health Agency of Canada. Flu Watch – January 30 to 5 Febrary, 2011 (week 05).
5. Inamasu T, Sudo K, Kato S, Deguchi H, Ichikawa M, et al. (2012) Pandemic influenza virus surveillance, Izu-Oshima Island, Japan. Emerg Infect Dis 18: 1882–1885.
6. Lopez L, Bandaranayake D, Huang QS (2011) Influenza surveillance in New Zealand 2010. Wellington: Institute of Environmental Science and Research Ltd.
7. Mytton OT, Rutter PD, Donaldson LJ (2012) Influenza A(H1N1)pdm09 in England, 2009 to 2011: a greater burden of severe illness in the year after the pandemic than in the pandemic year. Euro Surveill 17.
8. WHO (2013) Influenza update N° 182. 182: 3–4. Available: http://www.who.int/influenza/surveillance_monitoring/updates/2013_04_02_surveillance_update_182.pdf.
9. Munster VJ, de Wit E, van den Brand JM, Herfst S, Schrauwen EJ, et al. (2009) Pathogenesis and transmission of swine-origin 2009 A(H1N1) influenza virus in ferrets. Science 325: 481–483.
10. Itoh Y, Shinya K, Kiso M, Watanabe T, Sakoda Y, et al. (2009) In vitro and in vivo characterization of new swine-origin H1N1 influenza viruses. Nature 460: 1021–1025.
11. Pecavar B, Nadrah K, Papst L, Cec V, Kotar T, et al. (2011) Clinical characteristics of adult patients with influenza-like illness hospitalized in general ward during Influenza A H1N1 pandemic 2009/2010. Wien Klin Wochenschr 123: 662–667.
12. Lera E, Worner NT, Sancosmed M, Fabregas A, Casquero A, et al. (2011) Clinical and epidemiological characteristics of patients with influenza A (H1N1) 2009 attended to at the emergency room of a children's hospital. Eur J Pediatr 170: 371–378.
13. McKenna JJ, Bramley AM, Skarbinski J, Fry AM, Finelli L, et al. (2013) Asthma in patients hospitalized with pandemic influenza A(H1N1)pdm09 virus infection-United States, 2009. BMC Infect Dis 13: 57.
14. Institute RK (2009) Epidemiologisches Bulletin. October 12, 2009/Nr. 41: 409.
15. Yang L, Wang XL, Chan KP, Cao PH, Lau HY, et al. (2012) Hospitalisation associated with the 2009 H1N1 pandemic and seasonal influenza in Hong Kong, 2005 to 2010. Euro Surveill 17.
16. Bautista E, Chotpitayasunondh T, Gao Z, Harper SA, Shaw M, et al. (2010) Clinical aspects of pandemic 2009 influenza A (H1N1) virus infection. N Engl J Med 362: 1708–1719.
17. Sachedina N, Donaldson LJ (2010) Paediatric mortality related to pandemic influenza A H1N1 infection in England: an observational population-based study. Lancet 376: 1846–1852.
18. Myles PR, Semple MG, Lim WS, Openshaw PJ, Gadd EM, et al. (2012) Predictors of clinical outcome in a national hospitalised cohort across both waves of the influenza A/H1N1 pandemic 2009–2010 in the UK. Thorax 67: 709–717.
19. Jain S, Kamimoto L, Bramley AM, Schmitz AM, Benoit SR, et al. (2009) Hospitalized patients with 2009 H1N1 influenza in the United States, April–June 2009. N Engl J Med 361: 1935–1944.
20. CDC (2009) Bacterial coinfections in lung tissue specimens from fatal cases of 2009 pandemic influenza A (H1N1) - United States, May–August 2009. MMWR Morb Mortal Wkly Rep 58: 1071–1074.
21. Muscedere J, Ofner M, Kumar A, Long J, Lamontagne F, et al. (2013) The Occurrence and Impact of Bacterial Organisms Complicating Critical Care Illness Associated with Influenza A(H1N1) infection. Chest.
22. Randolph AG, Vaughn F, Sullivan R, Rubinson L, Thompson BT, et al. (2011) Critically ill children during the 2009–2010 influenza pandemic in the United States. Pediatrics 128: e1450–1458.
23. Hadler JL, Konty K, McVeigh KH, Fine A, Eisenhower D, et al. (2010) Case fatality rates based on population estimates of influenza-like illness due to novel H1N1 influenza: New York City, May–June 2009. PLoS One 5: e11677.

24. Nishiura H (2010) The virulence of pandemic influenza A (H1N1) 2009: an epidemiological perspective on the case-fatality ratio. Expert Rev Respir Med 4: 329–338.
25. Presanis AM, De Angelis D, Hagy A, Reed C, Riley S, et al. (2009) The severity of pandemic H1N1 influenza in the United States, from April to July 2009: a Bayesian analysis. PLoS Med 6: e1000207.
26. WHO (2013) Genes and human disease: Monogenic diseases - Cystic Fibrosis. Genomic resource centre. Available: http://www.who.int/genomics/public/geneticdiseases/en/index2.html#CF.
27. Mehta G, Macek M Jr, Mehta A (2010) Cystic fibrosis across Europe: EuroCareCF analysis of demographic data from 35 countries. J Cyst Fibros 9 Suppl 2: S5–S21.
28. Riordan JR, Rommens JM, Kerem B, Alon N, Rozmahel R, et al. (1989) Identification of the cystic fibrosis gene: cloning and characterization of complementary DNA. Science 245: 1066–1073.
29. Rosenstein BJ, Zeitlin PL (1998) Cystic fibrosis. Lancet 351: 277–282.
30. Rowe SM, Miller S, Sorscher EJ (2005) Cystic Fibrosis. New England Journal of Medicine 352: 1992–2001.
31. Burns JL, Emerson J, Kuypers J, Campbell AP, Gibson RL, et al. (2012) Respiratory viruses in children with cystic fibrosis: viral detection and clinical findings. Influenza Other Respi Viruses 6: 218–223.
32. Hoek RA, Paats MS, Pas SD, Bakker M, Hoogsteden HC, et al. (2013) Incidence of viral respiratory pathogens causing exacerbations in adult cystic fibrosis patients. Scand J Infect Dis 45: 65–69.
33. Wat D (2003) Impact of respiratory viral infections on cystic fibrosis. Postgrad Med J 79: 201–203.
34. van Ewijk BE, van der Zalm MM, Wolfs TF, van der Ent CK (2005) Viral respiratory infections in cystic fibrosis. J Cyst Fibros 4 Suppl 2: 31–36.
35. Stelzer-Braid S, Johal H, Skilbeck K, Steller A, Alsubie H, et al. (2012) Detection of viral and bacterial respiratory pathogens in patients with cystic fibrosis. J Virol Methods 186: 109–112.
36. Wang EE, Prober CG, Manson B, Corey M, Levison H (1984) Association of respiratory viral infections with pulmonary deterioration in patients with cystic fibrosis. N Engl J Med 311: 1653–1658.
37. van Ewijk BE, van der Zalm MM, Wolfs TF, Fleer A, Kimpen JL, et al. (2008) Prevalence and impact of respiratory viral infections in young children with cystic fibrosis: prospective cohort study. Pediatrics 122: 1171–1176.
38. Wat D, Doull I (2003) Respiratory virus infections in cystic fibrosis. Paediatric Respiratory Reviews 4: 172–177.
39. Viviani L, Assael BM, Kerem E (2011) Impact of the A (H1N1) pandemic influenza (season 2009–2010) on patients with cystic fibrosis. J Cyst Fibros 10: 370–376.
40. Nash EF, Whitmill R, Barker B, Rashid R, Whitehouse JL, et al. (2011) Clinical outcomes of pandemic (H1N1) 2009 influenza (swine flu) in adults with cystic fibrosis. Thorax 66: 259.
41. Colombo C, Battezzati PM, Lucidi V, Magazzu G, Motta V, et al. (2011) Influenza A/H1N1 in patients with cystic fibrosis in Italy: a multicentre cohort study. Thorax 66: 260–261.
42. France MW, Tai S, Masel PJ, Moore VL, McMahon TL, et al. (2010) The month of July: an early experience with pandemic influenza A (H1N1) in adults with cystic fibrosis. BMC Pulm Med 10: 8.
43. Taylor-Robinson D, Whitehead M, Diderichsen F, Olesen HV, Pressler T, et al. (2012) Understanding the natural progression in %FEV1 decline in patients with cystic fibrosis: a longitudinal study. Thorax 67: 860–866.
44. Ling LM, Chow AL, Lye DC, Tan AS, Krishnan P, et al. (2010) Effects of early oseltamivir therapy on viral shedding in 2009 pandemic influenza A (H1N1) virus infection. Clin Infect Dis 50: 963–969.
45. Morens DM, Taubenberger JK, Fauci AS (2008) Predominant role of bacterial pneumonia as a cause of death in pandemic influenza: implications for pandemic influenza preparedness. J Infect Dis 198: 962–970.
46. Rice TW, Rubinson L, Uyeki TM, Vaughn FL, John BB, et al. (2012) Critical illness from 2009 pandemic influenza A virus and bacterial coinfection in the United States. Crit Care Med 40: 1487–1498.
47. Doring G, Flume P, Heijerman H, Elborn JS (2012) Treatment of lung infection in patients with cystic fibrosis: current and future strategies. J Cyst Fibros 11: 461–479.
48. Nguyen-Van-Tam JS, Openshaw PJ, Hashim A, Gadd EM, Lim WS, et al. (2010) Risk factors for hospitalisation and poor outcome with pandemic A/H1N1 influenza: United Kingdom first wave (May–September 2009). Thorax 65: 645–651.
49. Ramsey BW, Gore EJ, Smith AL, Cooney MK, Redding GJ, et al. (1989) The effect of respiratory viral infections on patients with cystic fibrosis. Am J Dis Child 143: 662–668.
50. Kieninger E, Singer F, Tapparel C, Alves MP, Latzin P, et al. (2012) High rhinovirus burden in lower airways of children with cystic fibrosis. Chest.
51. Zheng S, De BP, Choudhary S, Comhair SA, Goggans T, et al. (2003) Impaired innate host defense causes susceptibility to respiratory virus infections in cystic fibrosis. Immunity 18: 619–630.
52. Xu W, Zheng S, Goggans TM, Kiser P, Quinones-Mateu ME, et al. (2006) Cystic fibrosis and normal human airway epithelial cell response to influenza a viral infection. J Interferon Cytokine Res 26: 609–627.
53. Sutanto EN, Kicic A, Foo CJ, Stevens PT, Mullane D, et al. (2011) Innate inflammatory responses of pediatric cystic fibrosis airway epithelial cells: effects of nonviral and viral stimulation. Am J Respir Cell Mol Biol 44: 761–767.
54. Kieninger E, Vareille M, Kopf BS, Blank F, Alves MP, et al. (2012) Lack of an exaggerated inflammatory response on virus infection in cystic fibrosis. Eur Respir J 39: 297–304.
55. Van Ewijk BE, Wolfs TF, Aerts PC, Van Kessel KP, Fleer A, et al. (2007) RSV mediates Pseudomonas aeruginosa binding to cystic fibrosis and normal epithelial cells. Pediatr Res 61: 398–403.
56. Chattoraj SS, Ganesan S, Jones AM, Helm JM, Comstock AT, et al. (2011) Rhinovirus infection liberates planktonic bacteria from biofilm and increases chemokine responses in cystic fibrosis airway epithelial cells. Thorax 66: 333–339.
57. Patria MF, Longhi B, Esposito S (2013) Influenza vaccination in children with cystic fibrosis. Expert Rev Vaccines 12: 415–420.
58. Hollmeyer H, Hayden F, Mounts A, Buchholz U (2012) Review: interventions to increase influenza vaccination among healthcare workers in hospitals. Influenza Other Respi Viruses.
59. Bohmer MM, Walter D, Falkenhorst G, Muters S, Krause G, et al. (2012) Barriers to pandemic influenza vaccination and uptake of seasonal influenza vaccine in the post-pandemic season in Germany. BMC Public Health 12: 938.

9

Stenotrophomonas maltophilia Virulence and Specific Variations in Trace Elements during Acute Lung Infection: Implications in Cystic Fibrosis

Arianna Pompilio[1,2]⁹, Domenico Ciavardelli[1,3]⁹, Valentina Crocetta[1,2], Ada Consalvo[1], Roberta Zappacosta[2], Carmine Di Ilio[1,2], Giovanni Di Bonaventura[1,2]*

1 Clinical Microbiology Unit, Center of Excellence on Aging, "G. d'Annunzio" University Foundation, Chieti, Italy, **2** Department of Experimental and Clinical Sciences, School of Medicine, "G. d'Annunzio" University, Chieti, Italy, **3** School of Engineering, Architecture and Motor Science, "Kore" University, Enna, Italy

Abstract

Metal ions are necessary for the proper functioning of the immune system, and, therefore, they might have a significant influence on the interaction between bacteria and host. Ionic dyshomeostasis has been recently observed also in cystic fibrosis (CF) patients, whose respiratory tract is frequently colonized by *Stenotrophomonas maltophilia*. For the first time, here we used an inductively mass spectrometry method to perform a spatial and temporal analysis of the pattern of changes in a broad range of major trace elements in response to pulmonary infection by *S. maltophilia*. To this, DBA/2 mouse lungs were comparatively infected by a CF strain and by an environmental one. Our results showed that pulmonary ionomic profile was significantly affected during infection. Infected mice showed increased lung levels of Mg, P, S, K, Zn, Se, and Rb. To the contrary, Mn, Fe, Co, and Cu levels resulted significantly decreased. Changes of element concentrations were correlated with pulmonary bacterial load and markers of inflammation, and occurred mostly on day 3 post-exposure, when severity of infection culminated. Interestingly, CF strain – significantly more virulent than the environmental one in our murine model - provoked a more significant impact in perturbing pulmonary metal homeostasis. Particularly, exposure to CF strain exclusively increased P and K levels, while decreased Fe and Mn ones. Overall, our data clearly indicate that *S. maltophilia* modulates pulmonary metal balance in a concerted and virulence-dependent manner highlighting the potential role of the element dyshomeostasis during the progression of *S. maltophilia* infection, probably exacerbating the harmful effects of the loss of CF transmembrane conductance regulator function. Further investigations are required to understand the biological significance of these alterations and to confirm they are specifically caused by *S. maltophilia*.

Editor: Gunnar F Kaufmann, The Scripps Research Institute and Sorrento Therapeutics, Inc., United States of America

Funding: The present work was supported by a grant from University of Chieti-Pescara ("ex-60%"), and by a grant from Fondazione per la Ricerca sulla Fibrosi Cistica - Onlus, Verona (Italy). The funders had no role in study design, data collection and analysis, decision to publish, or preparation of the manuscript.

Competing Interests: The authors have declared that no competing interests exist.

* E-mail: gdibonaventura@unich.it

⁹ These authors contributed equally to this work.

Introduction

Stenotrophomonas maltophilia is a Gram-negative opportunistic pathogen especially in hospitalized or compromised patients where infection is associated to high mortality and morbidity [1,2]. *S. maltophilia* has recently emerged as one of the most frequently found bacteria in cystic fibrosis (CF) patients [3,4].

Despite increased *S. maltophilia* isolation from CF patients, its potential for pathogenicity remains undetermined because of conflicting clinical results from studies investigating the correlation between the presence of this microorganism and lung damage [5,6]. However, in a series of studies we found evidences highly suggestive for the pathogenetic role of *S. maltophilia* in CF patients [7–13]. This microorganism is in fact able to grow as biofilms – sessile communities inherently resistant to antibiotics - not only on abiotic surfaces [7–10], but also on CF-derived epithelial monolayer [11], probably as a consequence of a selective adaptation to CF airways [12]. Furthermore, in a model of acute respiratory infection we observed that *S. maltophilia* significantly contributes to the inflammatory process resulting in compromised respiratory function and death [13].

It is well known that during an infectious process, along with immune system activation, a sequential series of alterations in metabolism occurs, including changes in trace element balance [14–16]. In fact, the host's acute response to infection generally includes increased synthesis of metal-binding proteins and a concomitant flux of trace elements between blood and tissues [16]. Metal ions are necessary for the proper functioning of the immune system, and, therefore, they might have a significant influence on the interaction between bacteria and host.

Ionic dyshomeostasis has also recently been observed in CF patients. Sputum and lavage fluid from CF patients infected with *P. aeruginosa* contain high concentrations of calprotectin [17], whose antimicrobial properties are mediated by the chelation of zinc [18], and increased total iron and iron-binding proteins levels [19,20]. Gray et al. [19] suggested a relationship between high concentrations of total zinc and iron and airways inflammation both in CF and non-CF bronchiectasis, with longitudinal changes being observed in CF patients.

Although changes in some essential and non-essential trace elements have been previously described for some bacterial and parasitic pathogens [15,21,22], to the best of our knowledge no efforts have been made to evaluate the impact of *S. maltophilia* infection on trace element levels.

The main objective of the present study was, therefore, to evaluate the changes of a broad range of trace elements during the course of acute *S. maltophilia* lung infection. Moreover, we wanted to study whether these changes were associated to bacterial virulence.

To this, DBA/2 mouse lungs were comparatively infected by a strain collected from CF patient (Sm111), and one collected from an environmental source (C39). Mice were monitored during 7 days post-exposure (p.e.) for weight and health, pulmonary bacterial clearance, dissemination of infection, lung damage, and cytokine expression. Changes in trace elements were assessed, in both lungs and bronchoalveolar lavage (BAL), by Inductively Coupled Plasma Mass Spectrometry (ICP-MS) analysis, previously evaluated for its pre-analytical and analytical performances.

For the first time, here we demonstrated that *S. maltophilia* significantly affects the element profiles of both pulmonary tissue and BAL, and that these alterations strictly depend on bacterial virulence.

Methods

Ethics statement

This study was carried out in strict accordance with the recommendations in the Guide for the Care and Use of Laboratory Animals of the National Institute of Health. The protocol was approved by the Animal Care Committee of "G. d'Annunzio" University of Chieti-Pescara (Permit Number: 1989/09). Efforts were made to minimize suffering. Particularly, all surgery was performed under anaesthesia and animals were humanely euthanized when they showed clinical signs suggestive for moribund condition [23].

S. maltophilia strains and growth conditions

Two *S. maltophilia* strains were used in all experiments: Sm111 strain, repeatedly isolated during a 2-years period from the sputum of a CF patient; and C39 strain, isolated from wastewater. Bacteria were stored at -80°C until use.

To prepare infectious doses for mice exposure, each *S. maltophilia* strain was grown under agitation (130 rpm) in 200 ml of Trypticase soy broth (OxoidSpA; Garbagnate M.se, Milan, Italy) at 37°C for 16 h, then harvested by centrifugation (4000 rpm, 10 min, 4°C). Pellets were then washed twice and resuspended in cold 1% PBS (Sigma-Aldrich Srl, Milan, Italy). Cell density was adjusted to about 1.0×10^{11} CFU/ml, and 8 ml of this suspension were nebulized in challenge procedure.

Mouse model of acute lung infection

i) Mice. Eight-week-old male (n = 100; mean weight $\pm$ SD: 22.6$\pm$1.3 g) specific-pathogen-free DBA/2N inbred mice (Charles River Laboratories Italia, Calco, Italy) were used in all experiments. Animals were randomly assigned to each group (n = 10 mice), housed, bred and maintained in polycarbonate HEPA-filtered cages with a 12-h light/dark cycle, with *ad libidum* access to sterile acidified water and irradiated diet.

ii) Exposure to *S. maltophilia*. To simulate an airborne lung infection, a "home-made" aerosol dispersal system housed in a biosafety cabinet was used, as previously described [13]. Briefly, mice were exposed to nebulized inoculum for 60 min, followed by 5 min for cloud decay, and finally exposed for 5 min to UV irradiation for decontamination. As a control, mice were treated in the same way but exposed to PBS only.

iii) Experimental lay-out. Ten mice were allocated for each group (infected, and control uninfected mice) at each time point (days 1, 3, and 7 p.e.). Following infection, both groups were monitored daily for weight and behaviour, considering them to be unwell when a >10% weigh loss or ill appearance (ruffled coats, huddled position, lack of retreat in handler's presence) were observed.

On days 1, 3, and 7 p.e., mice were intraperitoneally anesthetized by Avertin 10 mg/ml (Sigma-Aldrich), then sacrificed by exanguation. Mice were observed for macroscopic pulmonary damage, according to the "four-point scoring system" proposed by Johansen et al. [24], then subjected to BAL. Mice were then perfused *in situ* with 0.9% NaCl via the heart. At each time point considered, in each group 8 animals were randomly selected to be undergone to bacterial count, cytokines measurement, and ICP-MS analysis, while the remaining 2 mice were assigned to histological analysis. At each time point, spleen was also collected and homogenized in sterile saline for evaluating bacterial dissemination.

Microbiological assays

i) Lungs homogenization. For each mouse, both lungs were pooled and then homogenized (24000 g/min, 15 sec) - on ice in 2 ml of sterile saline containing protease inhibitors (cOmplete, EDTA-free; Roche Diagnostic SpA, Milan, Italy) and phenylmethanesulfonyl fluoride (PMSF; Sigma-Aldrich) - using an homogenizer (Ultra Turrax T8; Ika-Werke GmbH & Co. KG, Germany).

ii) Evaluation of pulmonary bacterial load and infection dissemination. Bacterial load was assessed in both lung homogenate and BAL samples by plating, in triplicate, 10-fold serial dilutions of each sample on Mueller-Hinton agar (Oxoid). Following 24 h-incubation at 37°C, the number of CFU was counted, then normalized according to the wet weight of lungs, averaged, and compared between groups. The initial bacterial deposition in the lungs was also assessed in homogenized lungs collected 1 h p.e. Dissemination of infection was evaluated, by viable count, in spleen samples collected at each time point considered.

iii) Cytokine measurements. Lung homogenates were centrifuged (1500×g, 4°C, 10 min), then supernatants were collected for measurement of cytokine levels (IFN-γ, MIP-2 IL-6, and TNF-α) by an ELISA system (R&D Systems Inc; Minneapolis, USA), according to the manufacturer's recommendations. The detection limit for IFN-γ, IL-6, TNF-α, and MIP-2 was <2.0, equal to 1.6, <5.1, and <1.5 pg/ml, respectively.

iv) Histopathological analysis. Following perfusion, lungs were immediately fixed in 10% neutral buffered formalin at RT. Each lung was then sectioned along its longitudinal axis obtaining tissue 3 μm-thickness sections from dorsal lung surfaces, throughout the entire tissue block and at regular intervals of 50 μm. Sections were stained with hematoxylin-eosin. The degree of inflammation was scored by using of "five-point system" proposed by Dubin et al. [25]. Ten fields/lung were evaluated at low (10×), and high (63×) magnification. Histopathological evaluation was performed blindly respect to the origin of the samples.

ICP-MS analysis

i) Chemicals and reagents. Nitric acid (69%) and S stock (Na_2SO_4, 1000 mg/l, H_2O) solutions were purchased from Romil

(Cambridge, UK), while P stock solution (H_3PO_4, 1000 mg/l, H_2O) was from Merck (Darmstadt, Germany). The multi-element calibration standard stock solution (Mg, Ca, Mn, Fe, Co, Cu, Zn, Se, Rb, and Sr at 10 mg/l; 2% HNO_3), the tuning solution (Li, Y, Ce, and Tl at 10 mg/l; 2% HNO_3), and the internal standard stock solution (Sc, Ge, and Y at 10 mg/l; 1% HNO_3) were purchased from Agilent Technologies (Tokyo, Japan). Stock solutions and samples were diluted by deionised H_2O with a specific resistance of 18.2 MΩ cm (Milli-Q system, Millipore, Watford, Hertfordshire, UK).

ii) ICP-MS operating conditions. ICP-MS analysis was performed by a 7500A ICP mass spectrometer (Agilent Technologies) fitted with an ASX-510 auto-sampler (Cetac Technologies, Omaha, NE), a peristaltic pump, a Babington nebulizer, and a Scott spray chamber (Agilent Technologies) as previously described [26,27]. A detailed description of ICP-MS operating conditions can be found in Data S1.

iii) Samples. Lungs and BAL samples collected on days 1, 3, and 7 p.e. from both perfused sham-exposed (controls) and *S. maltophilia*-exposed mice were analysed by ICP-MS. Briefly, lung samples were homogenized, freeze-dried by using a Modulyo freeze-dryer (ThermoSavant, USA), accurately weighted by an AX26 DeltaRange^{TM} balance (Mettler-Toledo, Greifensee, Switzerland), and then quantitatively transferred in sterile 15 ml-polystyrene tubes (BD Falcon, BD Biosciences, Franklin Lakes, NJ). Samples were dissolved in 0.8 ml of 65% (v/v) HNO_3 (Romil) and 0.2 ml of 30% (v/v) H_2O_2 at 75°C for 5 h. The samples were diluted 1:20 with 18 MΩ cm H_2O, then analysed for Mg, P, S, K, Ca, V, Cr, Mn, Fe, Co, Cu, Zn, Se, and Rb. BAL samples were centrifuged and supernatants stored at −80°C until assayed. Samples were diluted 1:10 in 18 MΩ cm deionised H_2O and analysed for the same elements with exception of P, S, and K. Quantification was performed using the standard addition method and internal standard correction. Three spike levels were made on the basis of the specific element concentration. Samples showing evident blood contaminations were excluded. Limit of detection (LOD), limit of quantitation (LOQ), calibration functions, repeatability, trueness, and recovery function of ICP-MS analysis were assessed as reported in Data S1.

Statistical analysis

All assays were carried out in triplicate and repeated on two different occasions. Differences among groups were evaluated using two-tailed Student's t test (to compare the element concentrations measured in both perfused and not perfused lung tissues) or one-way analysis of variance (ANOVA) followed by Tukey's multiple comparison *post-hoc* for parametric data (to evaluate the main effects on trace element levels of p.e. time and group, as well as the interaction between these factors), Kruskal-Wallis test followed by Dunn's multiple comparison *post-hoc* for nonparametric data, and chi-square test for percentages.

3×3 factor ANOVA followed by Tukey's multiple comparison *post-hoc* test was performed in order to evaluate the main effects of post-exposure time (1, 3, 7 days p.e.) and exposure to PBS, *S. maltophilia* SM111 or C39 strains, as well as the interaction between these factors and element concentrations in lung and BAL.

The assumption of homoscedasticity was verified by Levene test. Alignment and ranking were performed for heteroscedastic data before two-way ANOVA by using the ART web software available at http://faculty.washington.edu/aimgroup/proj/art/artweb [28].

Principal component analysis (PCA) was performed following the autoscaling of data that were normalized at mean = 0 and SD = 1. Significance of correlations between elements and markers of infection was evaluated by Spearman correlation analysis of the combined data derived from the infected and control mice using MetaboAnalyst statistical analysis module [29]. Multiple testing corrections were performed by calculating the false discovery rate (FDR). Statistical analysis was performed by GraphPad 6.0 (GraphPad Software Inc., San Diego, CA, USA), Statistica 6.0 (Statsoft, Tulsa, OK), and XLStat (Microsoft, USA) software. Statistical significance was set at 95% confidence level.

Results

Clinical mice response to *S. maltophilia* acute lung infection

i) Mice health and weight. The changes in body weight of infected and control mice over 7 days monitored, expressed as percentages of initial body weights, are shown in Figure 1A.

Compared to unexposed mice, the mean weight of mice infected by CF Sm111 strain showed to be significantly reduced from day 2 through day 7 p.e., whereas mice infected by environmental C39 strain significantly lost their body weight from day 2 through day 4 p.e. only ($p<0.01$).

With regard to strain type, Sm111-infected mice showed a mean body weight significantly lower than C39-infected ones from day 3 through day 7 p.e. (day 3: 80.6 vs 90.9%; day 4: 83.9 vs 93%; day 5: 87.7 vs 98.6%; day 6: 90.0 vs 97.7%; day 7: 96.3 vs 101%; $p<0.05$, except than for day 5, $p<0.01$). Mice infected with CF Sm111 strain lost more than 10% of their body weight from day 1 through day 6 p.e., and they did not completely regain weight during the period monitored. Contrarily, mice infected with environmental C39 strain showed a reduction higher than 10% on day 2 p.e. only, completely regaining weight on day 5 p.e. Control mice lost up to 5% of their body weight during the period monitored.

Contrary to control mice, infected ones usually showed symptoms suggestive for illness (slow responsiveness, and piloerection) from day 1 through day 7 p.e., regardless of strain tested.

ii) Infection clearance, dissemination, and mortality. Bacterial load was comparatively evaluated in lung tissue homogenates 1 h, and 1, 3, and 7 days p.e. Results, normalized to the wet lung weight and expressed as CFU/g, are summarized in Figure 1B.

The pulmonary deposition of *S. maltophilia* observed following 1 h p.e. was comparable for both strains (3.5 ± 1.1 vs $6.3\pm3.9\times10^7$ CFU/g, for Sm111 and C39 strains, respectively). Although bacterial load decreased from day 0 through day 7 p.e. regardless of strain tested, Sm111-infected mice retained significantly higher bacterial concentrations, regardless of time point considered (Sm111 vs C39: $4.1\pm2.8\times10^6$ vs $1.9\pm1.1\times10^4$ CFU/g, $5.0\pm7.7\times10^4$ vs $1.8\pm3.5\times10^3$ CFU/g, and $5.4\pm10.1\times10^3$ vs 2.8 ± 5.4 CFU/g, on days 1, 3, and 7 p.e., respectively; $p<0.001$) (Figure 1B). Control mice were negative for *S. maltophilia* at any time point.

To evaluate the invasiveness of *S. maltophilia*, we carried out microbiological analysis of spleen homogenates. The percentage of spleens positive for *S. maltophilia* was significantly higher in mice exposed to Sm111, compared to those infected with C39 (90 vs 10%, and 40 vs 0%, on days 1 and 3 p.e., respectively; $p<0.001$), although the bacterial counts were generally very low at each time point. On day 7 p.e., no spleens were positive for *S. maltophilia*, regardless of strain tested. Spleens from control mice were negative for *S. maltophilia*.

No mice were euthanized since signs suggestive for "moribund" status were not observed up to day 7 p.e. [23]. One *S. maltophilia*

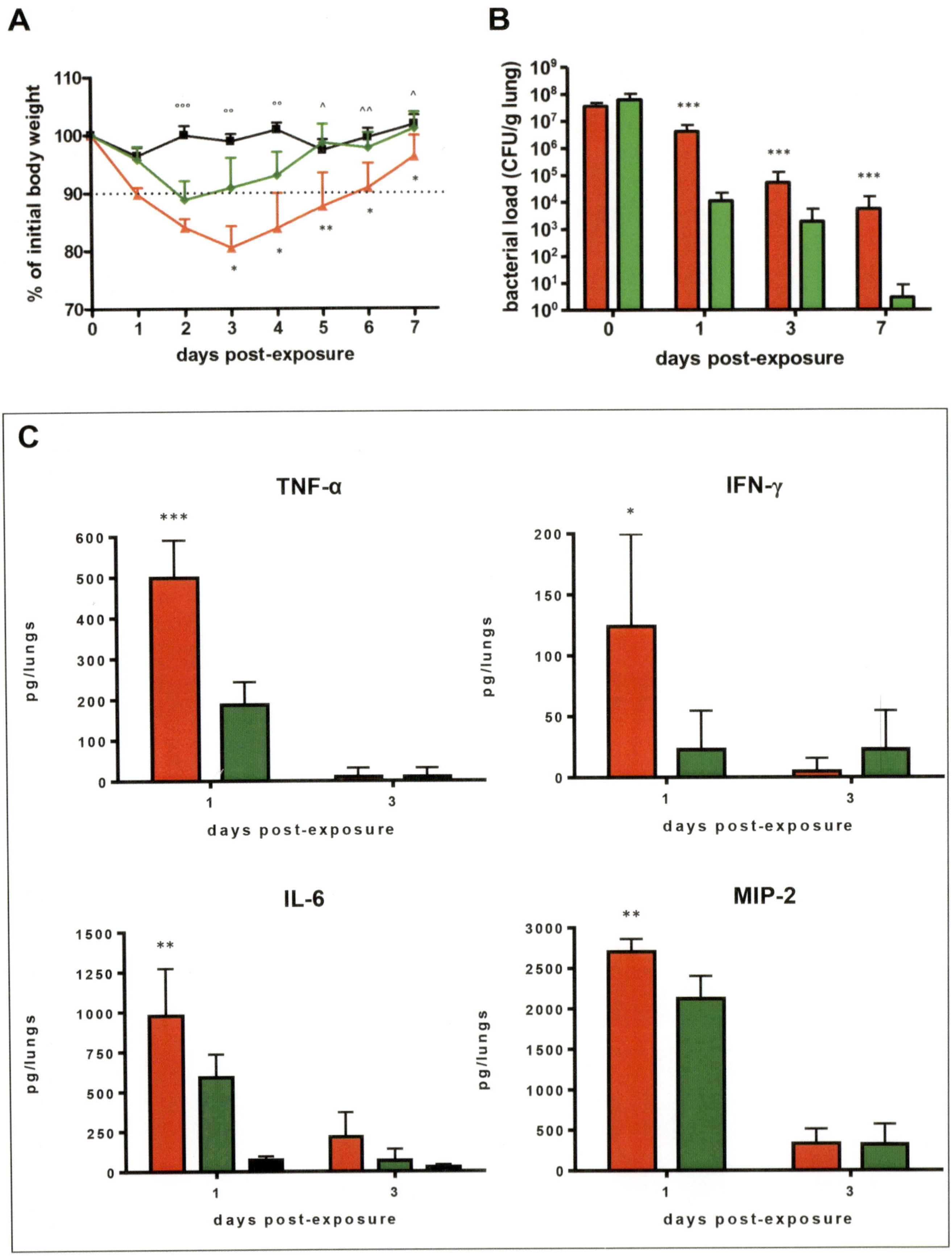
A
110
100
90
80
70
% of initial body weight
0 1 2 3 4 5 6 7
days post-exposure
B
bacterial load (CFU/g lung)
10^9
10^8
10^7
10^6
10^5
10^4
10^3
10^2
10^1
10^0
0 1 3 7
days post-exposure
C
TNF-α
pg/lungs
days post-exposure
IFN-γ
IL-6
MIP-2

Figure 1. *S. maltophilia* acute lung infection in DBA/2 mice: weight, bacterial clearance, and cytokine levels. DBA/2 mice (n = 100) were exposed on day 0 to aerosolized *S. maltophilia* (CF Sm111 strain, red line or bars; environmental C39 strain, green line or bars) or PBS only (controls; black line or bars). A) Mice weight variations during the course of infection. The dotted line shows a 10% weight loss with regard to mean body weight before infection. Results were expressed as means + SDs. * $p<0.05$, ** $p<0.01$ for Sm111 vs C39; °°° $p<0.001$, °° $p<0.01$ for ctrl vs Sm111 and C39; ^ $p<0.05$, ^^ $p<0.01$ for ctrl vs Sm111, chi-square test. B) Kinetic of DBA/2 mouse lung bacterial clearance. Following 1 h (day 0), and on days 1, 3, and 7 p.e. lungs were homogenized, then cultured for bacterial counts. Results were normalized to the lung wet weight (CFU/g) and shown as means + SDs. *** $p<0.001$ Sm111 vs C39, ANOVA followed by Tukey's multiple comparison *post-hoc* test. C) Cytokine levels measured in lung homogenates. Cytokines were assayed by ELISA on days 1, and 3 p.e. both in control and *S. maltophilia*-infected mice. Results were expressed as total content of cytokines in both lungs (pg/lungs) and shown as means + SDs. No detectable TNF-α, IFN-γ, and MIP-2 levels were found in lungs of control mice. * $p<0.05$, ** $p<0.01$, *** $p<0.001$, Sm111 vs C39, ANOVA followed by Tukey's multiple comparison *post-hoc* test.

Sm111-infected mouse died on day 3 p.e. This animal couldn't be humanely euthanized because it died during the night. Mortality was not observed in control mice.

iii) Cytokine levels. Pulmonary TNF-α, IFN-γ, IL-6 and MIP-2 levels were assayed, in infected and control mice, on days 1 and 3 p.e., and results are reported in Figure 1C.

On day 1 p.e., all cytokines tested were found at levels significantly higher in Sm111-infected mice lungs than in C39-infected ones: TNF-α (498.8±92.4 vs 187.0±56.2 pg/lungs, respectively; $p<0.001$), IFN-γ (123.9±75.7 vs 22.7±31.8 pg/lungs, respectively; $p<0.05$); IL-6 (977.2±297.6 vs 590.0±145.8 pg/lungs, respectively; $p<0.05$), MIP-2 (2703.4±157.3 vs 2124.6±279.8 pg/lungs, respectively; $p<0.01$).

To the contrary, no difference in pulmonary levels of all cytokines assayed were found among groups on day 3 p.e. Therefore, pulmonary levels at day 7 p.e. were not assessed.

In control mice, none of the cytokines tested were detectable at the time points tested, except for IL-6 whose levels were significantly lower than those measured in infected mice, regardless of strain or time point considered (72.5±23.0 pg/lungs, and 26.9±15.0 pg/lungs on days 1 and 3 p.e., respectively; $p<0.001$).

iv) Macroscopic lung pathology. Macroscopic DBA/2 mouse lung damage, assessed by using the "four-point scoring system" [24], is summarized in Figures 2A and 2C.

At each time point monitored, *S. maltophilia*-infected lungs showed to be significantly more damaged compared to unexposed ones, regardless of strains considered (median scores, day 1 p.e.: 2.5 and 2 vs 1; day 3 p.e.: 3 and 2 vs 1; day 7 p.e.: 2 and 2 vs 1, for Sm111- and C39-exposed vs control mice, respectively; $p<0.05$).

Particularly, on days 1 and 7 p.e. infected lungs of both Sm111- and C39-exposed mice showed comparable damage (hyperemia and edema), although Sm111-exposed ones exhibited larger actelectasis, and consolidation. To the contrary, on day 3 p.e. Sm111-infected lungs were found to be significantly ($p<0.05$) more damaged than C39-infected ones, showing numerous abscesses, large atelectasis, and hemorrhage.

Control mice showed a score of 1 (normal lungs) throughout the study-period.

v) Lung histopathology. Histologic examination was carried out on lungs of both untreated and infected mice on days 1, 3 and 7 p.e. Representative sections illustrating lung inflammation for each group are shown in Figure 2B. In lungs of infected mice, we constantly observed a robust neutrophilic airway inflammation, irrespective of bacterial strain considered. However, Sm111-infected mice showed a more prominent area of inflammation than C39 mice did (60% vs 20%; $p<0.001$). Inflammation also involved in succession alveolar walls and sacs, and caused an increased septal thickening, oedema, and obliteration of most of alveolar spaces. Generally, lungs of untreated mice showed no evidence of inflammation. Necroscopy of Sm111-infected mouse died on day 3 p.e. revealed a marked neutrophilic inflammation involving about 90% of the alveolar compartment.

Microscopic DBA/2 mouse lung damage was also assessed by using a "five-point scoring system" [25], and results are summarized in Figure 2D. On day 1 p.e. no differences were observed among groups, all showing a median score of 1, suggestive for a normal lung. On day 3 p.e., although *S. maltophilia*-infected lungs showed a score significantly higher compared to unexposed control ones, damage caused by CF Sm111 strain resulted to be significantly higher than environmental C39 did (median score: 3.5 and 1.5 vs 0, for Sm111-, C39-exposed, and control mice, respectively; $p<0.05$).

This trend was also observed on day 7 p.e., when C39-exposed mice showed the same score of control mice (median score: 2.0, 1, and 1, for Sm111-, C39-exposed, and control mice, respectively; $p<0.05$).

Changes in lung element profiles caused by *S. maltophilia* infection are dependent on strain and time

The analytical performances of ICP-MS element profiling of lung tissues fulfilled the requirement of quantitative analysis providing suitable sensitivity and accuracy for several analysed elements, although particular attention should be paid to remove blood contamination from lung tissue. A detailed description of analytical figures of merit and the effect of perfusion on pulmonary trace elements recovery by ICP-MS are shown in Data S1, Table S1, and Figure S1.

Differences in major trace, and ultra-trace elements observed in lung tissue samples collected on days 1, 3, and 7 days p.e. to *S. maltophilia* or PBS (sham-exposed mice) are shown in Figure 3.

Two-factor ANOVA showed significant differences for all trace elements among groups considered, with the exception of Ca. Compared to sham-exposed mice, *S. maltophilia*-infected ones showed significantly higher pulmonary levels of Mg, P, S, K, Zn, Se, and Rb regardless of *S. maltophilia* strain. On the contrary, Mn, Fe, Co, and Cu concentrations were significantly reduced (Figure 3).

However, *S. maltophilia* strains tested exhibited markedly different behaviours. Particularly, Sm111 CF strain induced greater alterations compared to the environmental C39 strain, significantly increasing, on day 3 p.e., lung levels of Mg, S, K, Cu, Se, and Rb (mean ± SD, Mg: 532±62 vs 364±57 ng/mg; S: 7680±435 vs 6115±673; K: 9370±1133 vs 5582±958; Cu: 5.9±0.8 vs 4.6±0.4; Se: 1.8±0.2 vs 1.5±0.1; Rb: 10±1 vs 6±1, respectively; $p<0.05$) (Figure 3).

Furthermore, exposure to CF Sm111 strain significantly decreased Fe levels, while increased P levels on day 3 p.e., compared to controls (mean ± SD, Fe: 128±15 vs 194±33 ng/mg; P: 12674±1441 vs 9215±1635, respectively; $p<0.05$) (Figure 3). These effects were not observed in mice infected with C39 strain.

The unsupervised multivariate analysis by PCA shown in Figure 4 suggested that changes in element concentrations

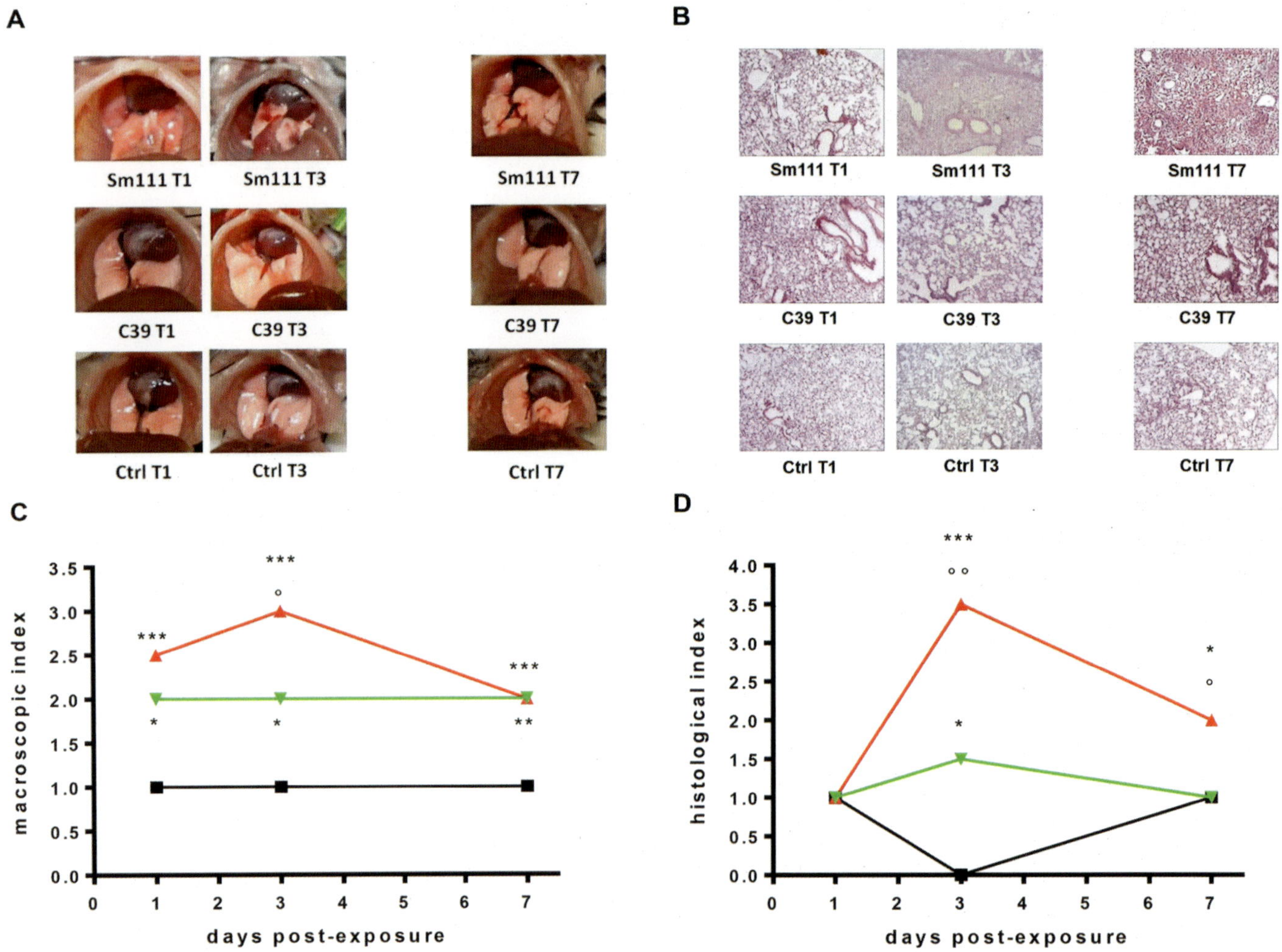

Figure 2. Assessment of lung damage in DBA/2 lung following infection with *S. maltophilia*. Lung damage was macroscopically and histologically assessed in DBA/2 mice (n = 18) on days 1, 3, and 7 p.e. to *S. maltophilia* (Sm111 CF strain, red line; C39 environmental strain, green line), or PBS only (control; black line). A–C) Macroscopic examination. A) Photographs of control and infected mouse lungs are representative for lung damage observed at each time point (days 1, 3, and 7 p.e.) in 8 mice per group. C) Lung damage was assessed by using "four-point scoring system" [24], and results are shown as median values. B–D) Histological assessment. B) Lung sections were stained with hematoxylin-eosin and ten fields/lung were observed at low (10×), and high (63×) magnification. For each group, only one representative microscopic field was reported. Since there were no significant differences in the degree of inflammation at any of the time point when evaluating the left and the right lung separately, the data were pooled and considered representative for both lungs. Mean percentage of tissue area characterized by the presence of neutrophilic infiltrate: 60% (Sm111-infected mice) vs 20% (C39-infected mice) ($p<0.001$, chi-square test.). D) Lung damage was quantified by using the "five-point scoring system" [25], and results are shown as median histopatological index. *** $p<0.001$, ** $p<0.01$, * $p<0.05$ vs ctrl; °° $p<0.01$, ° $p<0.05$ Sm111 vs C39; Kruskall-Wallis followed by Dunn's multiple comparison *post-hoc* test.

provoked by *S. maltophilia* infection were dependent on time p.e., and that these differences were higher on day 3 p.e. (Figure 4B).

Spearman correlation coefficient analysis showed significant correlations among analysed elements (Table 1), suggesting that changes of lung element concentrations in response to *S. maltophilia* infection are clustered in specific patterns. Particularly, Co levels were negatively correlated to Mg, S, and Zn levels ($p<0.01$).

Strain-specific correlations among elements were also observed (Figure 4D; Table S2). Particularly, in Sm111-infected mice P was positively correlated to Mg, Se, and Rb levels, while Cu levels with Rb and K ones. A negative relationship instead was observed between P and Co, and between Mn and pulmonary bacterial load. In contrast, exposure to C39 strain resulted in a direct correlation between Ca and both Co and Cu levels.

Changes in lung element concentrations correlate with the severity of infection

In order to tentatively investigate the biological significance of lung metal dyshomeostasis caused by *S. maltophilia* infection, we further evaluated the existence of a correlation between changes in lung element concentrations and markers for the severity of the infection, as assessed by pulmonary bacterial load (CFU/lung) and pro-inflammatory cytokine levels.

Overall, Spearman correlation analysis showed that several elements significantly correlated with pulmonary bacterial load (Table 1). Particularly, Mg, P, S, K, Zn, Se, and Rb levels positively correlated with bacterial load ($p<0.001$). To the contrary, Mn, Co, and Cu negatively correlated with CFU/lung ($p<0.001$ for Co; $p<0.05$ for Mn and Cu).

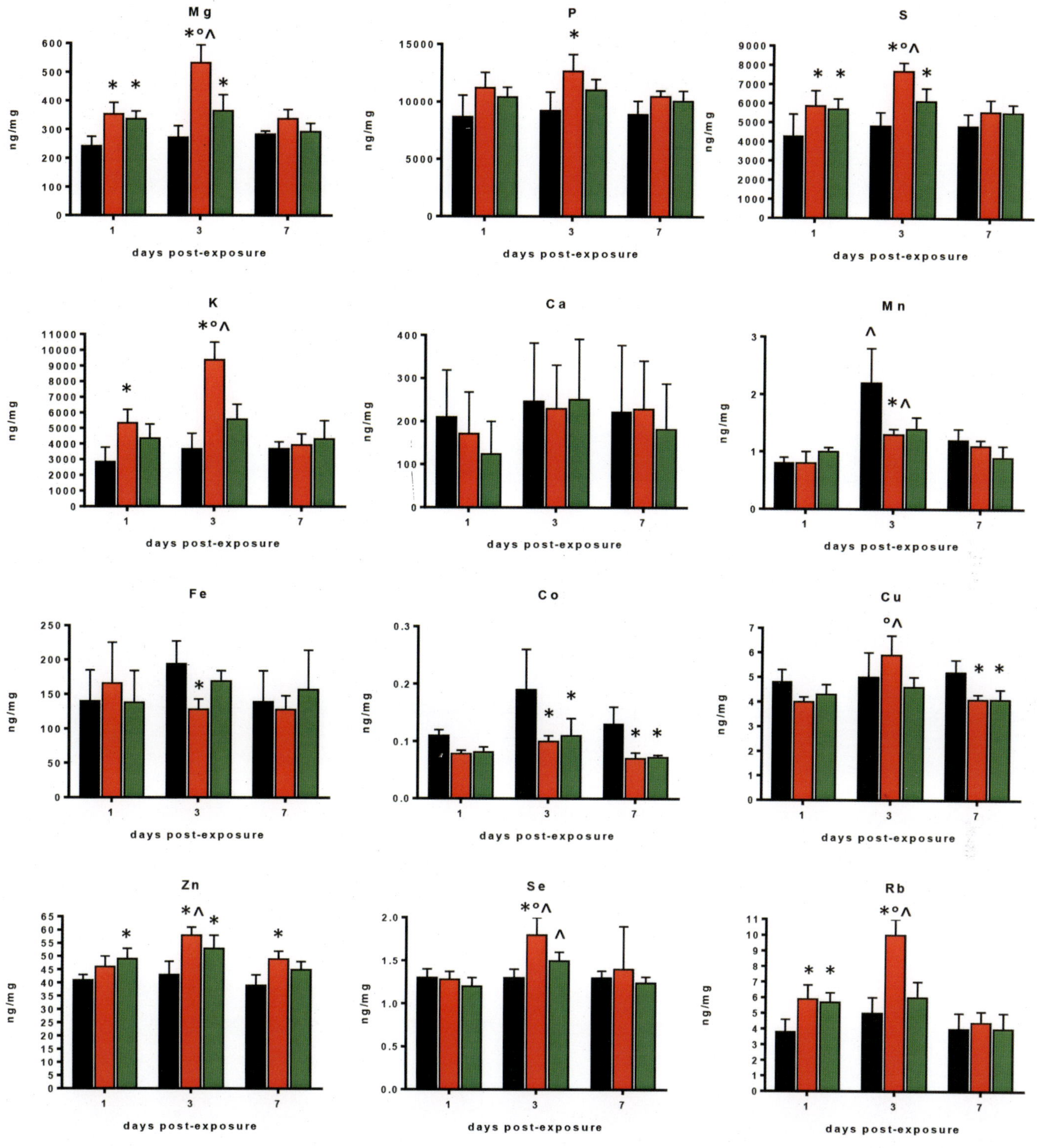

Figure 3. Changes in element profiles observed in lung tissues of control and *S. maltophilia*-infected DBA/2N mice. Amount of each element was assessed - on days 1, 3, and 7 p.e. to *S. maltophilia* (Sm111 CF strain, red bars; C39 environmental strain, green bars)or PBS only (controls, black bars) - by ICP-MS analysis in lung homogenates from DBA/2 mice (n = 10 each group). Results are expressed as ng of element for mg of lung tissue (dry weight), and graphed as means + SDs. * $p<0.05$, vs control mice; ° $p<0.05$, vs C39 strain; ^ $p<0.05$, between days p.e.; two-way ANOVA followed by Tukey's post-hoc test.

Statistically significant correlations were also found with cytokine levels (Table 1). Particularly, Mn, Co, and Cu levels were negatively correlated with all cytokines tested ($p<0.001$). To the contrary, Mg, P, S, and Zn levels were positively correlated to MIP-2 levels ($p<0.001$).

On the other hand, specific changes induced by exposure to C39 strain involved mainly cytokines. S and Zn levels were

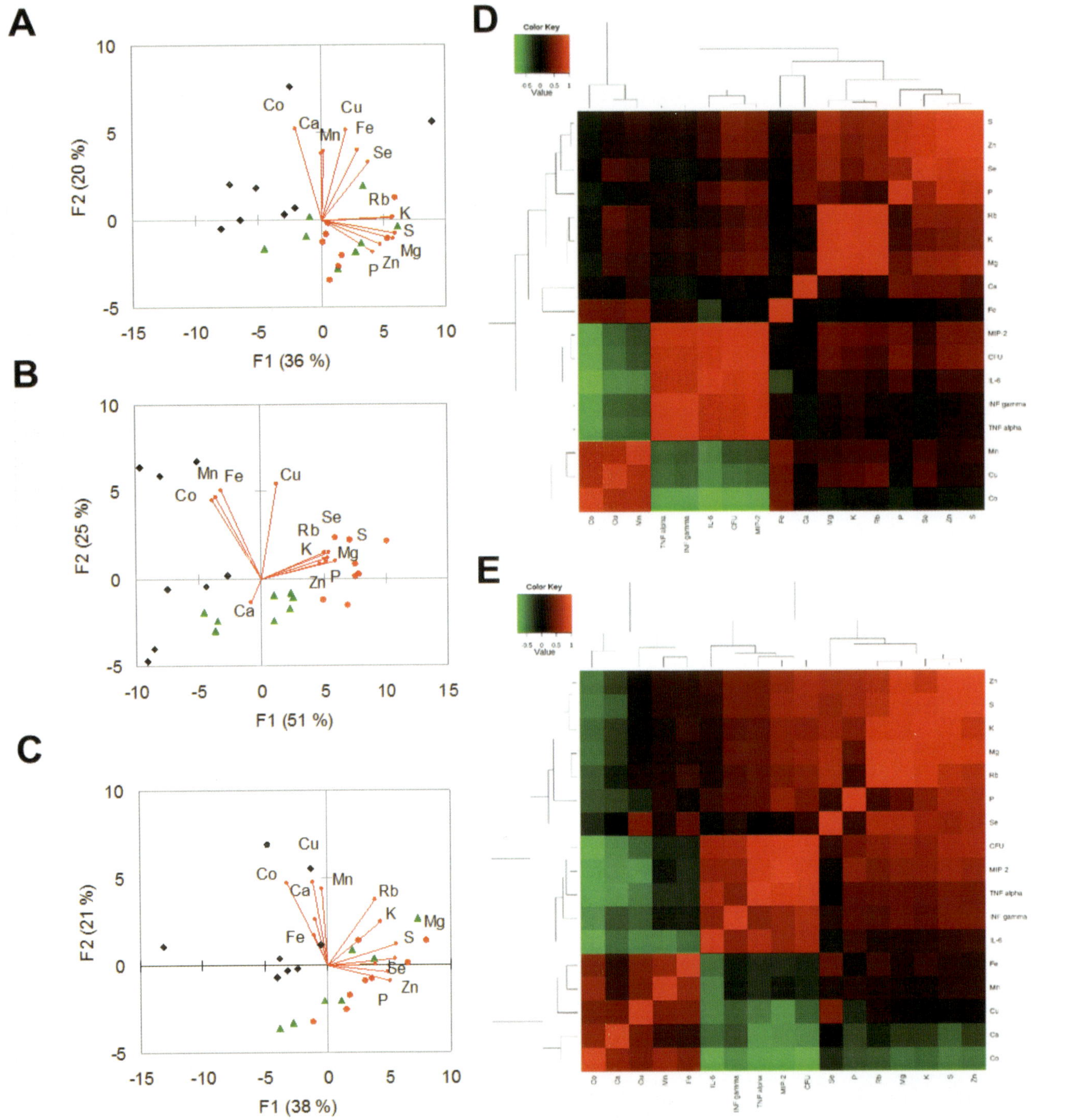

Figure 4. Trace elements, bacterial load, and cytokine levels observed in lung tissue of *S. maltophilia*-infected DBA/2N mice. A–C) Score and loading plots obtained by Principal Component Analysis. These plots show PC1 vs PC2summarizing 56%, 76%, and 59% of the variation among lung samples collected on days 1 (A), 3 (B), and 7 (C) p.e. to *S. maltophilia* (Sm111 CF strain, red circles; C39 environmental strain, green triangles) or PBS only (controls, black rhombi). The amounts of variance explained by each PC are shown in parentheses. D–E) Correlation maps. The heatmaps show the unsupervised hierarchical clustering of lung elements, bacterial counts in lung homogenate (CFU), and cytokines assessed using Spearman's correlation in response to *S. maltophilia* infection by Sm111 CF (D) or C39 (E) strain. Direct and inverse correlations are shown in red and green, respectively. Correlation and cluster analysis were performed using MetaboAnalyst statistical analysis module [29].

positively correlated to IFN-γ and TNF-α levels, while MIP-2 levels were directly correlated with K and Rb levels (Figure 4E; Table S3). To the contrary, a negative relationship was observed between Ca levels and both MIP-2, TNF-α, IL-6 levels, and pulmonary bacterial load.

Changes in BAL element profiles caused by *S. maltophilia* infection are dependent on strain and time

To investigate the differences in ionomic profile between lung and BAL samples, the ICP-MS method developed for lung tissue

Table 1. Correlations among trace elements, cytokines, and bacterial load observed in lung tissue from control and *S. maltophilia*-exposed DBA/2N mice.

Variable	Mg	P	S	K	Ca	Mn	Fe	Co	Cu	Zn	Se	Rb	IFN-γ	TNF-α	IL-6	MIP-2	CFU/lung
Mg	**1**																
P	**0,567*****	**1**															
S	**0,786*****	**0.791*****	**1**														
K	**0,823*****	**0.539*****	**0.745*****	**1**													
Ca	0,052	0.020	0.005	−0.041	**1**												
Mn	0,123	0.043	0.045	0.027	**0.309*****	**1**											
Fe	−0.055	−0.091	0.089	0.011	0.028	**0.274***	**1**										
Co	**−0.287***	−0.205	**−0.282***	−0.201	**0.250***	**0.655*****	**0.264****	**1**									
Cu	**0.243***	0.010	0.171	**0.331****	0.211	**0.383****	0.180	**0.474*****	**1**								
Zn	**0.749*****	**0.754*****	**0.868*****	**0.590*****	0.117	0.118	0.049	**−0.292***	0.158	**1**							
Se	**0.576*****	**0.539*****	**0.699*****	**0.498*****	0.205	0.155	0.231	−0.081	**0.448*****	**0.685*****	**1**						
Rb	**0.838*****	**0.451*****	**0.684*****	**0.906*****	0.033	0.091	−0.036	−0.123	**0.451*****	**0.592*****	**0.506*****	**1**					
IFN-γ	0.176	0.110	0.178	0.199	−0.191	**−0.372***	0.067	**−0.679*****	**−0.395***	0.180	−0.019	0.168	**1**				
TNF-α	0.111	0.101	0.155	0.142	−0.299	**−0.474****	−0.007	**−0.710*****	**−0.510****	0.165	−0.133	0.123	**0.818*****	**1**			
IL-6	0.230	0.246	0.247	0.208	−0.184	**−0.587****	−0.286	**−0.802*****	**−0.534****	0.258	−0.010	0.212	**0.760*****	**0.863*****	**1**		
MIP-2	**0.365***	**0.379***	**0.418***	0.359	−0.252	**−0.364***	−0.103	**−0.752*****	**−0.558****	**0.418***	0.049	0.322	**0.789*****	**0.898*****	**0.860*****	**1**	
CFU/lung	**0.531*****	**0.612*****	**0.611*****	**0.442*****	−0.083	**−0.281***	−0.116	**−0.455*****	**−0.271***	**0.576*****	**0.271***	**0.438*****	**0.753*****	***	**0.808*****	**0.920*****	**1**

Spearman coefficients calculated for significant correlations are shown in bold: * $p<0.05$, ** $p<0.01$, *** $p<0.001$. Correlations between pulmonary bacterial load (CFU/lung) and element concentrations were assessed by combining data sets from lung collected on days 1, 3, and 7 p.e. to PBS or *S. maltophilia* (Sm111 and C39 strains). Correlations between element concentrations and cytokines levels were calculated by combining data sets from lung collected on days 1 and 3 p.e. to PBS or *S. maltophilia* (Sm111 and C39 strains).

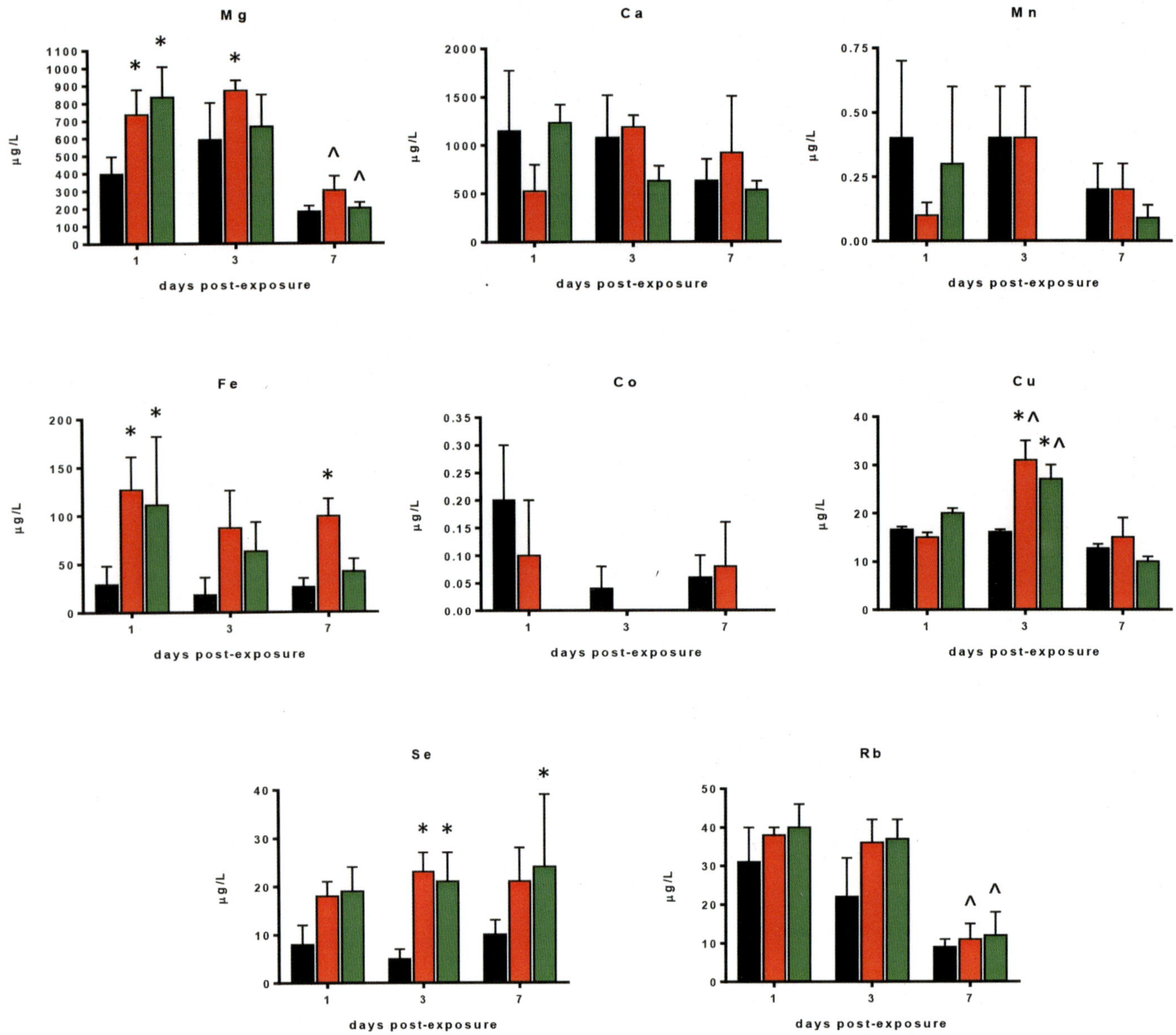

Figure 5. Changes in element profiles observed in BAL samples of control and *S. maltophilia*-infected DBA/2N mice. Amount of each element was assessed - on days 1, 3, and 7 p.e. to *S. maltophilia* (Sm111 CF strain, red bars; C39 environmental strain, green bars)or PBS only (controls, black bars) - by ICP-MS analysis in BAL from DBA/2 mice (n = 10 each group). Results are expressed as μg of element for liter of BAL, and graphed as means + SDs. * $p<0.05$, vs control mice. ^ $p<0.05$, between days post-exposure; two-way ANOVA followed by Tukey's post-hoc test.

was tentatively applied to measure trace element levels in BAL samples obtained before collecting lung samples. However, spike recovery experiments indicated the presence of a significant systematic error affecting ICP-MS analysis of BAL (data not shown). This is probably due to increased Na and Cl concentrations in BAL compared to lung samples, thus leading to higher matrix effect. The standard addition method with internal standard correction was, therefore, applied instead of external standard method. The sensitivity of the method was suitable for analysis of several elements with exception of Zn that was quantifiable only in few samples. In particular, Zn concentrations were not detectable in mice exposed to PBS and C39 strain. In contrast, Zn was measured in BAL collected on day 3 p.e. to Sm111 strain (21±4 μg/l).

The differences in trace elements found in BAL samples collected on days 1, 3, and 7 p.e. to *S. maltophilia*, or PBS (sham exposed mice) are shown in Figures 5–6.

Two-way ANOVA showed significant differences in Mg, Fe, Cu, Se, and Rb levels among study groups. Particularly, *S. maltophilia*-infected mice showed increased pulmonary Mg, Fe, Cu, Se, and Rb levels compared to sham-exposed control mice (Figure 5).

Univariate data analysis and PCA indicated that changes in BAL ionomic profiles depended on strain and time (Figure 5; Figures 6A–B–C). In fact, Sm111 strain only caused higher Mg and Fe levels on days 3 and 7 p.e., respectively, compared to control mice (Mg: 871±58 vs 590±212 μg/l, Fe: 99±18 vs 26±9 μg/l, respectively) (Figure 5; Figure 6B). On the other hand, C39 strain increased Se levels on day 7 p.e. (24±15 vs 10±3 μg/l,

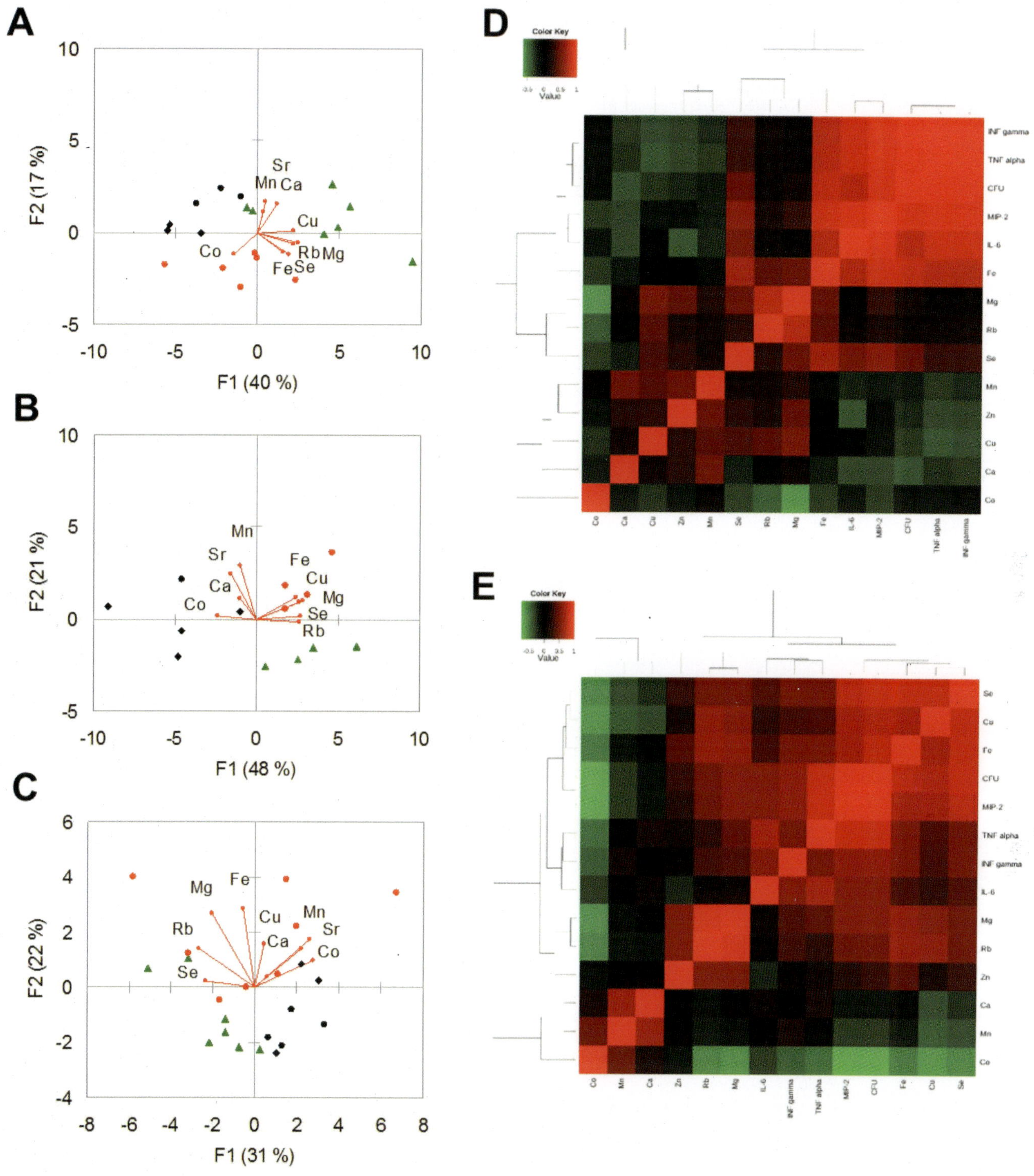

Figure 6. Trace elements, bacterial load, and cytokine levels observed in BAL samples of *S. maltophilia*-infected DBA/2N mice. A–C) Score and loading plots obtained by Principal Component Analysis. These plots show PC1 vs PC2 summarizing 57%, 69%, and 53% of the variation among BAL samples collected on days 1 (A), 3 (B), and 7 (C) p.e. to *S. maltophilia* (Sm111 CF strain, red circles; C39 environmental strain, green triangles) or PBS only (controls, black rhombi). The amounts of variance explained by each PC are shown in parentheses. D–E) Correlation maps. The heatmaps show the unsupervised hierarchical clustering of BAL elements, bacterial counts in lung homogenate (CFU), and pulmonary cytokines assessed using Spearman's correlation in response to *S. maltophilia* infection by Sm111 CF (D) or C39 (E) strain. Direct and inverse correlations are shown in red and green, respectively. Correlation and cluster analysis were performed using MetaboAnalyst statistical analysis module [29].

Table 2. Correlations among trace elements found in BAL from control and *S. maltophilia*-exposed DBA/2N mice.

Variable	Mg	Ca	Mn	Fe	Co	Cu	Zn	Se	Rb	IFN-γ	TNF-α	IL-6	MIP-2	CFU/lung
Mg	**1**													
Ca	**0.393****	**1**												
Mn	0.079	**0.535*****	**1**											
Fe	**0.529*****	0.114	0.057	**1**										
Co	**−0.304***	−0.005	**0.385****	−0.170	**1**									
Cu	**0.681*****	**0.366****	0.154	**0.386****	−0.127	**1**								
Zn	**0.474*****	**0.295***	**0.294***	0.115	−0.155	**0.500*****	**1**							
Se	0.226	−0.200	**−0.358****	**0.506*****	**−0.487*****	0.083	0.090	**1**						
Rb	**0.925*****	0.221	−0.030	**0.435****	−0.259	**0.561*****	**0.385****	0.174	**1**					
IFN-γ	0.103	−0.201	0.103	**0.698*****	−0.058	−0.232	−0.278	0.237	0.098	**1**				
TNF-α	0.117	−0.095	−0.061	**0.701*****	−0.118	−0.270	−0.288	0.223	0.081	**0.832*****	**1**			
IL-6	0.100	−0.072	0.063	**0.633*****	−0.126	−0.107	−0.316	0.331	0.024	**0.790*****	**0.859*****	**1**		
MIP-2	0.287	−0.215	−0.145	**0.770*****	−0.347	0.024	−0.114	**0.507****	0.197	**0.806*****	**0.897*****	**0.847*****	**1**	
CFU/lung	**0.553*****	−0.031	−0.028	**0.785*****	−0.186	**0.399****	0.122	**0.410****	**0.444****	**0.776*****	**0.819*****	**0.804*****	**0.931*****	**1**

Spearman rank correlation coefficients were calculated and significant correlations are shown in bold: * $p<0.05$, ** $p<0.01$, *** $p<0.001$. Correlations between pulmonary bacterial load (CFU/lung) and element concentrations were assessed by combining data sets from lung collected on days 1, 3, and 7 p.e. to PBS or *S. maltophilia* (Sm111 and C39 strains). Correlations between element concentrations and cytokines levels were calculated by combining data sets from BAL collected on days 1 and 3 p.e. to PBS or *S. maltophilia* (Sm111 and C39 strains).

respectively (Figure 5; Figure 6C). Furthermore, we found that Mg and Ca positively correlated with Cu and Zn, Fe positively correlated with Mn and Cu, while Co inversely correlated with Fe and Se regardless to the *S. maltophilia* strain (Table 2). These correlations were also found following the analysis for each *S. maltophilia* strain (Figures 6D–E; Table S4; Table S5), with minor differences.

Changes in BAL element concentrations correlate with the severity of infection

As well as for lung samples, we evaluated relationship between the changes in BAL element levels and markers for the severity of the infection.

Regardless of strain considered, Spearman correlation analysis showed that several elements significantly correlated with pulmonary bacterial load or cytokine levels (Table 2). In particular, we found that Mg, Cu, and Rb positively correlated with bacterial load (CFU/lung). We also found a direct correlation between Se and both bacterial load and MIP-2, and between Fe and all markers of infection.

Furthermore, *S. maltophilia* strains significantly differed for correlation between elements and bacterial load or citokines (Tables S3–S4). Particularly, in Sm111-infected mice, Fe levels were positively correlated to all considered markers of infection, while Se levels correlated with bacterial load ($p<0.001$), IL-6 ($p<0.05$), and MIP-2 ($p<0.001$) concentrations (Figure 6D; Table S4).

With regard to C39 strain, bacterial load was positively correlated to Mg ($p<0.01$), Fe ($p<0.01$), Cu ($p<0.01$), Se ($p<0.001$), and Rb ($p<0.01$), while a negative relationship instead was observed with Co concentrations ($p<0.01$) (Figure 6E; Table S5). Referring to cytokines, Fe and Se levels were positively correlated to IFN-γ, TNF-α, and MIP-2 levels. A positive correlation with MIP-2 levels only was found for Mg ($p<0.01$), Cu ($p<0.01$), and Rb ($p<0.05$) levels. To the contrary, a negative

Table 3. Correlations between elements in lung tissue and BAL from control and *S. maltophilia*-exposed DBA/2N mice.

	BAL							
	Element	**Mg**	**Ca**	**Mn**	**Fe**	**Cu**	**Se**	**Rb**
	Mg	**0.294***°	−0.047	−0.052	**0.376****	**0.390****	**0.394****	0.176
	Ca	−0.067	0.043	0.180	−0.045	0.167	−0.142	−0.123
	Mn	−0.081	0.033	**0.273***°	**−0.277***	0.084	−0.148	−0.154
LUNG	**Fe**	−0.005	−0.070	0.148	**−0.319***°	−0.207	−0.138	−0.003
	Cu	−0.184	0.074	0.234	**−0.463*****	0.091	**−0.415****	−0.216
	Se	0.202	0.194	0.239	0.243	**0.372****	0.228	0.052
	Rb	0.259	−0.014	0.009	0.179	**0.316***	0.127	0.175

Spearman correlation coefficients were calculated and significant correlations are shown in bold: * $p<0.05$, ** $p<0.01$, *** $p<0.001$.
° Significant correlation between lung tissue and BAL levels for the same element.

relationship was observed between Co levels and MIP-2, and TNF-α levels ($p<0.01$, and $p<0.05$; respectively).

BAL element concentrations correlate with lung element levels

In order to assess whether BAL element alterations may correlate to lung metal dyshomeostasis, we assessed the correlation between the ionomic profiles found in lung and BAL samples.

We found a significant direct correlation between Mg levels measured in the lung and those in BAL. The same correlation was found for Mn (Table 3). To the contrary, Fe levels measured in lung and BAL samples were inversely correlated (Table 3).

With regard to strain type, exposure to CF Sm111 strain was associated to a positive correlation for Mg, Mn, and Se, while a negative correlation was observed for Fe (Spearman correlation coefficient: 0.346, 0.410, 0.404, and −0.357, respectively; $p<0.05$) (Table S6; Figure S2). On the contrary, exposure to environmental C39 strain caused a positive correlation for Co only (Spearman correlation coefficient: 0.568; $p<0.001$) (Table S7).

Discussion

Although changes in plasma concentrations of several trace elements during various infections have been reported [14–16,21,22], the information on the concomitant changes in trace element balance in the target tissues of the infectious organism is limited. The assessment of local availability of trace elements in an infected tissue could be important since being part of systems regulating basic cell functions and essential to immune cell function, they might affect infection outcome.

In this study, for the first time we used ionomic approach to perform a spatial and temporal analysis of the pattern of changes in a broad range of both essential and non-essential trace elements in response to pulmonary infection by *S. maltophilia*. To this, ICP-MS was carried out, in both lung and BAL samples, to assess changes in ionomic profiles provoked, throughout 7 days, by *S. maltophilia* in a mouse model of acute lung infection we recently described [13].

The main finding of the present study was that pulmonary element profile is significantly affected by *S. maltophilia* infection, depending on post-exposure time and bacterial strain.

Increased lung levels of Mg, P, S, K, Zn, Se, and Rb were observed. In contrast, Mn, Fe, Co, and Cu levels were significantly decreased in lungs following exposure to *S. maltophilia*. The most consistent response to infection was, however, observed with Mg, S, and Co since their levels significantly changed regardless of strain tested and with greater persistence.

To tentatively correlate the observed changes in trace elements with the severity of lung infection, it is worthy of note that, as suggested by PCA analysis, most relevant changes in element concentrations caused by *S. maltophilia* infection occurred on day 3 p.e., that is when the severity of infection - in terms of body weight loss and lung damage - culminated in our murine model.

Furthermore, levels of all trace elements - except than for Fe, Ca, and Se - were significantly correlated with pulmonary bacterial load, thus suggesting that the observed changes are due to the host redistribution of elements in response to infection. On the other hand, it is improbable that these changes reflect bacterial ion content, considering that the contribution of bacterial biomass to samples tested is probably negligible.

Although the biological significances of these alterations are far to be completely understood and surely requires further investigations, some speculations can be made on the bases of our findings.

The increase in Zn, Mg, and Se levels is probably involved in the immunological host response, macrophage recruitment, and neutrophil infiltration, as suggested by the positive correlation we found with bacterial concentration and MIP-2 levels.

Zinc is a nutritional component necessary to the normal development and maintenance of immunologic functions related to T lymphocytes [29], and its levels in the host are increased during inflammation [30,31]. There is increasing evidence suggesting that the host actively sequesters Zn during infection to hinder microbial growth. Consistent with our results, increased Zn in host tissues and fluids during *P. aeruginosa* chronic infection and inflammation has been reported [19,32,33]. Particularly, Gray et al. [19] recently found sputum Zn levels significantly higher in CF and non-CF bronchiectasis compared with chronic obstructive pulmonary disease and healthy control, while Griese et al. [33] observed higher Zn levels in exhaled air condensate of CF patients.

The increased Zn levels we observed may be consequence of a passive release by neutrophils, since they are rich in this element [34]. Gray et al. [19] observed higher sputum Zn levels correlated with calprotectin, MPO, and IL-8. Accordingly, we found that levels of Zn and MIP-2, a chemoattractant for neutrophils both *in vitro* and *in vivo* [35], were positively correlated. Furthermore, we observed most of lung tissue area was characterized by the presence of an abundant neutrophilic infiltrate, especially in the case of Sm111 strain-infected mice. A contribution to higher Zn levels could be also result from circulation during inflammation.

Similarly to Zn, Mg and Se are as well modulators of the immune system and increased levels in infected tissue have been reported [29,36]. Increased Se concentrations could be related to the accumulation of immune cells and up-regulation of selenoproteins, particularly those with antioxidant function [37]. To the contrary, higher Mg levels in infected tissues cannot be completely explained on the basis of immune cell infiltrate, as suggested by the positive correlation with MIP-2 levels we observed. In fact, several studies reported that immune and anti-inflammatory responses are stimulated by Mg deficiency, and decreased serum Mg levels have been related to immune cells proliferation [38].

Necrotizing inflammation we observed during *S. maltophilia* infection is very likely the cause for higher Rb levels, since this element is mainly deposited intracellularly.

In partial agreement with previous results [31], *S. maltophilia* infection also caused significant reduction of Co and Cu lung levels, furtherly corroborated by the negative correlation found between these elements and pulmonary bacterial load. Interestingly, all markers of infection we considered were negatively correlated to Co and Cu levels, thus suggesting an efflux/recruitment of these elements from lung tissue in response to the bacterial infection.

In order to individuate the presence of ionomic profiles specifically associated to *S. maltophilia* virulence, changes in trace elements provoked in DBA/2N mice by Sm111 strain, isolated from a CF patient chronically infected, were comparatively evaluated to those observed following exposure to C39 strain, isolated from wastewater.

Our murine model of acute lung infection clearly showed that Sm111 CF strain was significantly more virulent than the environmental one, probably reflecting an adaptive behaviour of the microorganism during chronic infection that enables it to survive to the environmental stresses that are likely to be encountered within the habitat of the CF lung [12].

Particularly, Sm111 strain showed to be more efficient in persisting and invading murine airways, thus allowing dissemination of infection. Exposure to Sm111 also caused a lung damage significantly more severe than C39 did, as suggested by both macroscopic and histological examinations, and higher pro-inflammatory effects, as showed by cytokine pulmonary levels measurement.

It is interesting to highlight that the differential element profiles showed that *S. maltophilia* Sm111 CF strain significantly differed from C39 environmental one in pulmonary trace elements dyshomeostasis. Particularly, lung levels of Mg, S, K, Cu, Se, and Rb were significantly increased by Sm111 CF strain on day 3 p.e., compared to C39 strain.

It is worthy of note that exposure to Sm111 CF strain exclusively increased P and K lung levels, while decreased Fe and Mn ones. Manganese is another important trace metal required in numerous cellular processes, including metabolism and oxidative stress defense [39]. A recent work has demonstrated that in addition to Zn, vertebrates sequester Mn and Fe both intracellularly and extracellularly to protect themselves against infections [40]. Our results are consistent with these findings, although Sm111 CF strain probably provoked Fe and Mn dyshomeostasis by different mechanisms since only Mn levels negatively correlated with all markers of infection considered.

Correlation analysis among elements, and between elements and markers of infection also showed the existence of relationships shared by both strains, while others resulted to be exclusive for one strain only.

Taken together, our findings clearly suggest the existence of complex interactions among elements, and that *S. maltophilia* infection modulates lung metal balance in a concerted and strain-dependent manner. Essential trace elements are not only important for the host immune defense but also for microorganisms. Some elements - such as Zn, Cu, Mn, and Fe - are in fact essential components of many proteins and co-factors in enzymatic reactions [41,42]. However, above certain concentrations, they can be also toxic to bacterial cells. Maintenance of intracellular homeostasis of metal ions is, therefore, crucial for survival of bacteria, and therefore they have developed several systems to monitor and control trace element levels, especially in certain environments as they can modulate the expression of genes necessary for colonization and virulence [43–47]. In this regard, some trends in trace elements we observed might significantly increase *S. maltophilia* virulence and, probably, its ability in establishing infection in CF lung. It has in fact reported that in *S. maltophilia* increased concentrations of Mg caused higher resistance levels to aminoglycosides, penicillins, quinolones, and cotrimoxazole [48]. Furthermore, RNase activity of *S. maltophilia* resulted to be inhibited by Co, while stimulated by Mg [49].

That said, the extensive flow of trace elements, in response to bacterial infection, is also aimed at affecting virulence potential of invading microorganisms. In that regard, the concerted changes in some trace elements we observed – namely, increased Zn levels, decreased Fe levels, and constant Ca levels – might represent a combined host defense against infection, since under these conditions haemolytic activity of *S. maltophilia* is significantly inhibited [50]. Further studies have to be performed using an adequate number of strains to fully evaluate the contribution of these changes to pathogenesis, and whether they were associated to virulence degree or, rather, related to the biological inter-strain variability.

During the course of most infections, an extensive adjustment in host metabolism occurs and trace elements are simultaneously redistributed, carried by acute-phase metal-binding proteins (i.e. Fe-binding ferritin, and the Cu-binding ceruloplasmin), among organs/compartments involved by the disease process [51]. Therefore, the ionomic profile of BAL samples was also assessed and comparatively evaluated with that observed in lung homogenates.

Spearman correlation coefficients analysis showed that, during *S. maltophilia* infection, lung and BAL levels were positively related in the case of Mg and Mn. On the contrary, increased Fe levels in BAL were associated to a simultaneous decrease of this element in the lung.

Iron is an essential micronutrient for both microbial pathogens and their mammalian hosts. Changes in Fe availability and distribution have significant effects on pathogen virulence and on the immune response to infection [52]. In agreement with our findings, increased Fe levels in sputum have been described in CF patients [20], possibly contributing to the proliferation of bacteria [53]. The inverse relationship we observed between lung and BAL Fe levels might, therefore, be an adaptive response intended to deprive invading pathogens of iron.

On the other hand, it is also possible to hypothesize that *S. maltophilia* might affect Fe efflux from tissues by competing with host for iron uptake, particularly ferrous iron. In this regard, the major route for bacterial ferrous iron uptake, namely Feo (Ferrous iron-transport) system, has been recently characterized also in *S. maltophilia* [54]. This hypothesis is further supported by the significant positive correlation we observed, in BAL samples, between Fe levels and bacterial load. In accordance to this trend, lung Fe levels also inversely correlated with bacterial load, even if did not reach the significance.

Stratifying for strain type, trends observed for Fe, Mg, and Mn were observed in CF Sm111 strain-infected mice only, also with addition of a positive correlation for Se. To the contrary, exposure to environmental C39 strain caused a positive correlation between compartments for Co levels only.

It is also interesting to note that Sm111 CF strain showed a more significant effect and a higher degree of correlation between Fe levels and bacterial load observed in BAL samples, thus suggesting its higher iron scavenging ability compared with the environmental isolate.

These findings support our previous hypothesis that - during *S. maltophilia* infection - Mg, Mn, and Fe lung dyshomeostasis are regulated by different and strain-dependent mechanisms. Particularly, our results were highly suggestive for an association between virulence and the specific recruitment of Mg, Mn, and Se, from lung parenchyma toward epithelial surface. Evaluation of these elements in BAL samples could be, therefore, helpful in assessing *S. maltophilia* virulence and, consequently, lung damage.

This may be of particular interest in CF research field. In fact, an adequate assessment of cytology and protein biomarkers (i.e. cytokines, chemokines) in sputum is critical for understanding and managing CF, as well as other inflammatory lung diseases. In this regard, several studies have focused on measurement of cytokines to assess levels of airways inflammation. Accordingly, we observed that *S. maltophilia* pulmonary concentration and cytokines (IL-6, MIP-2, IFN-γ, and TNF-α) expression were significantly correlated. The fluid phase of the induced sputum also contains nonorganic elements that might be considered as marker of lung pathophysiology, thus allowing more reliable measurement of inflammation in the airway compared to cytokines whose activity is significantly affected by protease activity in sputum [55]. However, our findings suggested that BAL ionomic profile did not exactly reflect lung physiological status, in terms of trace elements profile. Therefore, BAL samples might be partially suggestive for lung dyshomeostasis and, consequently, for monitoring the development of pulmonary tissue damage during infection.

Furthermore, in CF patients, trace elements balance is also influenced by impaired chloride efflux in CF airway epithelium, the most important hallmarks of CF [19,20,33,56,57]. In particular, specific mutations of CF transmembrane conductance regulator (CFTR) significantly affected metal homeostasis *in vitro* [58]. Furthermore, dyshomeostasis of K, Zn and NO_3^- was observed in exhaled air condensate in CF patients [33], while increased levels of Cu, total Fe, and Fe-binding proteins were also found in CF sputum [19,20].

For these reasons, restoring physiological lung element balance has been proposed as a promising new therapeutic approach to CF patient. Increasing the airway surface liquid Mg concentration by aerosolized or oral Mg supplementation might improve the removal of highly viscous mucus in chronic lung disease by activating endogenous DNase activity [59]. Abdulhamid et al. [60], recently observed that oral intake of Zn reduced the number of days of oral antibiotics used to treat respiratory infections in children with CF. Supplementation of Se in CF patients has been also proposed to maintain the oxidant-antioxidant balance, so improving lung function [61].

Furthermore, trace elements might affect CFTR functionality. In this regard, Li et al. [62] recently identified extracellular pseudohalide anions – namely $Co(CN)_6^{3-}$, $Co(NO_2)_6^{3-}$, $Fe(CN)_6^{3-}$, $IrCl_6^{3-}$, and $Fe(CN)_6^{4-}$ - as increasing CFTR function.

Taken together, these observations, added to our results, further highlight the importance of a careful management of trace element balance in CF patients, especially during lung infections.

Conclusions

Our results demonstrated that ICP-MS analysis represents an useful technique to evaluate changes in host ionomic profile during pulmonary infection, in order to understand the impact infection might have on the host. This approach might be particularly relevant to the management of lung infections in CF patients for the following reasons:

i) it might inform future molecular studies on the interaction between microorganisms and the host regarding competition for specific mineral nutrients. Measurement in trace elements might in fact increase the understanding of the pathophysiological processes during pulmonary infection. This is particularly relevant for *S. maltophilia*, since bacterium-host interactions are not yet fully understood. Specifically, our findings showed that *S. maltophilia* uses the common strategy of modulating the host ionome, causing significant differences in trace elements balance, probably by direct or indirect mechanisms. The higher impact we observed on cationic homeostasis provoked by the more virulent Sm111 CF strain might be due to its adaption to a compromised environment, i.e. CF lung, and to be associated to an exacerbation of a particular step of pathogenesis.

ii) considering the potential association we observed between trace element levels and lung infection/inflammation, combined with their likely higher resistance to protease degradation compared to cytokines, trace elements could be considered as potentially robust markers of lung pathophysiology, thus offering new insight into pulmonary inflammation. Particularly, the observed changes in Mn, Mg, and Se levels in BAL samples seem to be exhaustively predictive for the severity of *S. maltophilia* lung infection. Therefore, their measurement in sputum might have potential diagnostic and prognostic usefulness.

iii) it might be valuable in defining/designing disease management strategies in CF patients. Control of CF disease includes managing nutritional status, as well as using of therapeutic modulators of CFTR function. Therefore, the observed adverse effect caused by *S. maltophilia* infection on trace elements status emphasizes the importance of careful monitoring and, if necessary, supplementation of oligoelements during therapy in CF patients concomitantly suffer from infections. This might otherwise jeopardise the outcome of treatment in the patient.

Further studies are warranted to confirm that changes in ionomic profile we observed are specifically caused by *S. maltophilia*, rather than they represent a consequence of infection-induced changes in host metabolism.

Supporting Information

Data S1 Methods and Results.

Figure S1 Effect of perfusion on pulmonary trace elements recovery by ICP-MS. Lungs of DBA/2 mice (n = 10) lungs were collected following perfusion with 0.9% NaCl (green bars). Control mice (n = 10) were not perfused (red bars). Results are means + SDs. * $p<0.05$, ** $p<0.01$ vs perfused lungs, two tailed Student's t-test.

Figure S2 Correlation between Mg, Fe, and Se levels quantified in lung and BAL samples from *S. maltophilia*-infected DBA/2N mice. A, B, C) mice infected with CF Sm111 strain; D, E, F) mice infected with environmental C39 strain. Significance of correlations was assessed by Spearman correlation analysis. p values were: 0.039, 0.033, and 0.002 for Mg (A), Fe (B), and Se (C), respectively; 0.381, 0.492, and 0.850 for Mg (D), Fe (E), and Se (F), respectively (see also Tables S6 and S7).

Table S1 ICP-MS analysis of mouse lung tissue: analytical figures of merit. The m/z measured for quantification, the internal standard (IS), the values of limit of detection (LOD) and limit of quantization (LOQ), the external calibration functions, precision and trueness are shown. Spike levels were: 20, 50, and 200 µg/l for Mg; 300, 500, and 1000 µg/l for P, S, and K; 20, 50, and 100 µg/l for Ca and Fe; 5, 20, and 100 µg/l for Cu and Rb; and 1, 5, and 10 µg/l for Mn, Co, and Se. [a] µg/l (µg/g); [b] µg/l; [c] CI = confidence interval, 95% confidence level; [d] 95% confidence level; [e] Coefficient of variation (%); [f] Standard deviation; [g] Relative standard deviation (%).

Table S2 Correlations among elements, cytokines, and bacterial load observed in lung tissue of DBA/2N mice exposed to PBS or CF Sm111 *S. maltophilia* strain. Spearman rank correlation coefficients were calculated on data collected on days 1, 3, and 7 p.e. Significant correlations are shown in bold. * $p<0.05$, ** $p<0.01$, *** $p<0.001$.

Table S3 Correlations among elements, cytokines, and bacterial load observed in lung tissue of DBA/2N mice exposed to PBS or environmental C39 *S. maltophilia* strain. Spearman rank correlation coefficients were calculated on data collected on days 1, 3, and 7 p.e. Significant correlations are shown in bold. * $p<0.05$, ** $p<0.01$, *** $p<0.001$.

Table S4 Correlations among elements, cytokines, and bacterial load observed in BAL from DBA/2N mice exposed to PBS or CF

Sm111 *S. maltophilia* strain. Spearman rank correlation coefficients were calculated on data collected on days 1, 3, and 7 p.e. Significant correlations are shown in bold. * $p<0.05$, ** $p<0.01$, *** $p<0.001$.

Table S5 Correlations among elements, cytokines, and bacterial load observed in BAL from DBA/2N mice exposed to PBS or environmental C39 *S. maltophilia* strain. Spearman rank correlation coefficients were calculated on data collected on days 1, 3, and 7 p.e. Significant correlations are shown in bold. * $p<0.05$, ** $p<0.01$, *** $p<0.001$.

Table S6 Correlations among elements observed in lung tissue and BAL from DBA/2N mice exposed to PBS or CF Sm111 *S. maltophilia* strain. Spearman rank correlation coefficients were calculated on data collected on days 1, 3, and 7 p.e. Significant correlations are shown in bold. * $p<0.05$, ** $p<0.01$, *** $p<0.001$.

Table S7 Correlations among elements observed in lung tissue and BAL from DBA/2N mice exposed to PBS or environmental C39 *S. maltophilia* strain. Spearman rank correlation coefficients were calculated on data collected on days 1, 3, and 7 p.e. Significant correlations are shown in bold. * $p<0.05$, ** $p<0.01$, *** $p<0.001$.

Acknowledgments

We would like to thank Francesca Petrelli for her technical assistance. We greatly appreciate Ersilia Fiscarelli (CF Microbiology Laboratory, CF Center of the "Bambino Gesù" Hospital, Rome, Italy) and Veronika Holà (Masarykovy University, Brno, Czech Republic) for providing CF and environmental *S. maltophilia* strains, respectively.

Author Contributions

Conceived and designed the experiments: DC AP GDB. Performed the experiments: AP VC AC RZ. Analyzed the data: DC AP VC AC GDB. Contributed reagents/materials/analysis tools: DC CDI RZ GDB. Wrote the paper: DC AP CDI GDB.

References

1. Brooke JS (2012) *Stenotrophomonas maltophilia*: an emerging global opportunistic pathogen. Clin Microbiol Rev 25: 2–41.
2. Samonis G, Karageorgopoulos DE, Maraki S, Levis P, Dimopoulou D, et al. (2012) *Stenotrophomonas maltophilia* infections in a general hospital: patient characteristics, antimicrobial susceptibility, and treatment outcome. PLoS One 7:e37375.
3. Davies JC, Rubin BK (2007) Emerging and unusual gram-negative infections in cystic fibrosis. Semin Respir Crit Care Med 28: 312–321.
4. Ciofu O, Hansen CR, Høiby N (2013) Respiratory bacterial infections in cystic fibrosis. Curr Opin Pulm Med 19: 251–258.
5. Goss CH, Ott K, Aitken ML, Rubenfeld GD (2002) Detecting *Stenotrophomonas maltophilia* does not reduce survival of patients with cystic fibrosis. Am J Respir Crit Care Med 166: 356–361.
6. Karpati F, Malmborg AS, Alfredsson H, Hjelte L, Strandvik B (1994) Bacterial colonisation with *Xanthomonas maltophilia* a retrospective study in a cystic fibrosis patient population. Infection 22: 258–263.
7. Di Bonaventura G, Spedicato I, D'Antonio D, Robuffo I, Piccolomini R (2004) Biofilm formation by *Stenotrophomonas maltophilia*: modulation by quinolones, trimethoprim-sulfamethoxazole, and ceftazidime. Antimicrob Agents Chemother 48: 151–160.
8. Di Bonaventura G, Stepanović S, Picciani C, Pompilio A, Piccolomini R (2007) Effect of environmental factors on biofilm formation by clinical *Stenotrophomonas maltophilia* isolates. Folia Microbiol (Praha) 52: 86–90.
9. Di Bonaventura G, Prosseda G, Del Chierico F, Cannavacciuolo S, Cipriani P, et al. (2007) Molecular characterization of virulence determinants of *Stenotrophomonas maltophilia* strains isolated from patients affected by cystic fibrosis. Int J Immunopathol Pharmacol 20: 529–537.
10. Pompilio A, Piccolomini R, Picciani C, D'Antonio D, Savini V, et al. (2008) Factors associated with adherence to and biofilm formation on polystyrene by *Stenotrophomonas maltophilia*: the role of cell surface hydrophobicity and motility. FEMS Microbiol Lett 287: 41–47.
11. Pompilio A, Crocetta V, Confalone P, Nicoletti M, Petrucca A, et al. (2010) Adhesion to and biofilm formation on IB3-1 bronchial cells by *Stenotrophomonas maltophilia* isolates from cystic fibrosis patients. BMC Microbiol 10: 102.
12. Pompilio A, Pomponio S, Crocetta V, Gherardi G, Verginelli F, et al. (2011) Phenotypic and genotypic characterization of *Stenotrophomonas maltophilia* isolates from patients with cystic fibrosis: genome diversity, biofilm formation, and virulence. BMC Microbiol 11:159.
13. Di Bonaventura G, Pompilio A, Zappacosta R, Petrucci F, Fiscarelli E, et al. (2010) Role of excessive inflammatory response to *Stenotrophomonas maltophilia* lung infection in DBA/2 mice and implications for cystic fibrosis. Infect Immun 78: 2466–2476.
14. Corbin DB, Seeley EH, Raab A, Feldmann J, Miller MR, et al. (2008) Metal chelation and inhibition of bacterial growth in tissue abscesses. Science 319: 962–965.
15. Edvinsson M, Frisk P, Molin Y, Hjelm E, Ilbäck NG (2008) Trace element balance is changed in infected organs during acute *Chlamydophila pneumoniae* infection in mice. Biometals 21: 229–237.
16. Beisel WR (2004) Metabolic response of the host to infections. In: Feigin RD, Demmler GJ, Cherry JD, Kaplan SL, Textbook of pediatric infectious diseases, vol 1. Saunders, Philadelphia. pp. 62–77.
17. MacGregor G, Gray RD, Hilliard TN, Imrie M, Boyd AC, et al (2008) Biomarkers for cystic fibrosis lung disease: application of SELDI-TOF mass spectrometry to BAL fluid. J Cyst Fibros 7: 352–358.
18. Lusitani D, Malawista SE, Montgomery RR (2003) Calprotectin, an abundant cytosolic protein from human polymorphonuclear leukocytes, inhibits the growth of *Borrelia burgdorferi*. Infect Immun 71: 4711–4716.
19. Gray RD, Duncan A, Noble D, Imrie M, O'Reilly DS, et al. (2010) Sputum trace metals are biomarkers of inflammatory and suppurative lung disease. Chest 137: 635–641.
20. Stites SW, Plautz MW, Bailey K, O'Brien-Ladner AR, Wesselius LJ (1999) Increased concentrations of iron and isoferritins in the lower respiratory tract of patients with stable cystic fibrosis. Am J Respir Crit Care Med 160: 796–801.
21. Amini M, Nahrevanian H, Khatami S, Farahmand M, Mirkhani F, et al. (2009) Biochemical association between essential trace elements and susceptibility to *Leishmania* major in BALB/c and C57BL/6 mice. Braz J Infect Dis 13: 83–85.
22. Culha G, Sangün MK (2007) Serum levels of zinc, copper, iron, cobalt, magnesium, and selenium elements in children diagnosed with *Giardia intestinalis* and *Enterobiosis vermicularis* in Hatay, Turkey. Biol Trace Elem Res 118: 21–26.
23. Toth LA (2000) Defining the moribund condition as an experimental endpoint for animal research. ILAR J 41:72–79.
24. Johansen HK, Espersen F, Pedersen SS, Hougen HP, Rygaard J, et al. (1993) Chronic *Pseudomonas aeruginosa* lung infection in normal and athymic rats. APMIS 101: 207–225.
25. Dubin PJ, Kolls JK (2007) IL-23 mediates inflammatory responses to mucoid *Pseudomonas aeruginosa* lung infection in mice. Am J Physiol Lung Cell Mol Physiol 292: 519–528.
26. Ciavardelli D, Consalvo A, Caldaralo V, Di Vacri ML, Nisi S, et al. (2012) Characterisation of element profile changes induced by long-term dietary supplementation of zinc in the brain and cerebellum of 3xTg-AD mice by alternated cool and normal plasma ICP-MS. Metallomics 4: 1321–1332.
27. Ciavardelli D, Ammendola S, Ronci M, Consalvo A, Marzano V, et al. (2011) Phenotypic profile linked to inhibition of the major Zn influx system in *Salmonella enterica*: proteomics and ionomics investigations. Mol Biosyst 7(3): 608–619.
28. Wobbrock JO, Findlater L, Gergle D, Higgins JJ (2011) The Aligned Rank Transform for Nonparametric Factorial Analyses Using Only ANOVA Procedures. Proceedings of CHI 2011 Conference on Human Factors in Computing Systems 1:143–146.
29. Xia J, Wishart DS (2011) Web-based inference of biological patterns, functions and pathways from metabolomic data using MetaboAnalyst. Nat Protoc 6: 743–760.
30. Shankar AH, Prasad AS (1998) Zinc and immune function: the biological basis of altered resistance to infection. Am J Clin Nutr 68: 447S–463S.
31. Milanino R, Marrella M, Gasperini R, Pasqualicchio M, Velo G (1993) Copper and zinc body levels in inflammation: an overview of the data obtained from animal and human studies. Agents Actions 39: 195–209.
32. Thurnham DI, Mburu AS, Mwaniki DL, De Wagt A (2005) Micronutrients in childhood and the influence of subclinical inflammation. Proc Nutr Soc 64: 502–509.
33. Griese M, Noss J, Schramel P (2003) Elemental and ion composition of exhaled air condensate in cystic fibrosis. J Cyst Fibros 2: 136–142.
34. Milne DB, Ralston NV, Wallwork JC (1985) Zinc content of cellular components of blood: methods for cell separation and analysis evaluated. Clin Chem 31: 65–69.
35. Wolpe SD, Sherry B, Juers D, Davatelis G, Yurt RW, et al. (1989) Identification and characterization of macrophage inflammatory protein 2. Proc Natl Acad Sci USA 86: 612–616.

36. McKenzie RC, Rafferty TS, Beckett GJ (1998) Selenium: an essential element for immune function. Immunol Today 19: 342–345.
37. Rahmanto AS, Davies MJ (2012) Selenium-containing amino acids as direct and indirect antioxidants. IUBMB Life 64: 863–871.
38. Tam M, Gómez S, González-Gross M, Marcos A (2003) Possible roles of magnesium on the immune system. Eur J Clin Nutr 57: 1193–1197.
39. Jakubovics NS, Jenkinson HF (2001) Out of the iron age: new insights into the critical role of manganese homeostasis in bacteria. Microbiology 147: 1709–1718.
40. Kehl-Fie TE, Skaar EP (2010) Nutritional immunity beyond iron: a role for manganese and zinc. Curr Opin Chem Biol 14: 218–224.
41. Pfeiffer J, Guhl J, Waidner B, Kist M, Bereswill S (2002) Magnesium uptake by CorA is essential for viability of the gastric pathogen Helicobacter pylori. Infect Immun 70: 3930–3934.
42. Rink L, Haase H (2007) Zinc homeostasis and immunity. Trends Immunol 28: 1–4.
43. Abrantes MC, Lopes Mde F, Kok J (2011) Impact of manganese, copper and zinc ions on the transcriptome of the nosocomial pathogen *Enterococcus faecalis* V583. PLoSOne 6: e26519.51.
44. Nielubowicz GR, Smith SN, Mobley HL (2010) Zinc uptake contributes to motility and provides a competitive advantage to *Proteus mirabilis* during experimental urinary tract infection. Infect Immun 78: 2823–2833.
45. Gode-Potratz CJ, Chodur DM, McCarter LL (2010) Calcium and iron regulate swarming and type III secretion in *Vibrio parahaemolyticus*. J Bacteriol 192: 6025–6038.
46. Foster SL, Richardson SH, Failla ML (2001) Elevated iron status increases bacterial invasion and survival and alters cytokine/chemokine mRNA expression in Caco-2 human intestinal cells. J Nutr 131: 1452–1458.
47. Papp-Wallace KM, Maguire ME (2006) Manganese transport and the role of manganese in virulence. Annu Rev Microbiol 60: 187–209.
48. Felegie TP, Yu VL, Rumans LW, Yee RB (1979) Susceptibility of *Pseudomonas maltophilia* to antimicrobial agents, singly and in combination. Antimicrob Agents Chemother 16: 833–837.
49. Arella M, Sylvestre M (1979) Production of an extracellular ribonuclease by *Pseudomonas maltophilia*. Can J Microbiol 25: 321–328.
50. Figueirêdo PM, Furumura MT, Santos AM, Sousa AC, Kota DJ, et al (2006) Cytotoxic activity of clinical *Stenotrophomonas maltophilia*. Lett Appl Microbiol 43: 443–449.
51. Ilbäck NG, Glynn AW, Wikberg L, Netzel E, Lindh U (2004) Metallothionein is induced and trace element balance changed in target organs of a common viral infection. Toxicology 199: 241–250.
52. Wang L, Cherayil BJ (2009) Ironing out the wrinkles in host defense: interactions between iron homeostasis and innate immunity. J Innate Immun 1: 455–464.
53. Reid DW, Withers NJ, Francis L, Wilson JW, Kotsimbos TC (2002) Iron deficiency in cystic fibrosis: relationship to lung disease severity and chronic *Pseudomonas aeruginosa* infection. Chest 121: 48–54.
54. Su YC, Chin KH, Hung HC, Shen GH, Wang AH, et al. (2010) Structure of *Stenotrophomonas maltophilia* FeoA complexed with zinc: a unique prokaryotic SH3-domain protein that possibly acts as a bacterial ferrous iron-transport activating factor. Acta Crystallogr Sect F Struct Biol Cryst Commun 66: 636–642.
55. Pizzichini E, Pizzichini MM, Efthimiadis A, Evans S, Morris MM, et al. (1996) Indices of airway inflammation in induced sputum: reproducibility and validity of cell and fluid-phase measurements. Am J Respir Crit Care Med 154: 308–317.
56. Cuthbert AW (1991) Cystic fibrosis. 4. Abnormalities of airway epithelial function and the implications of the discovery of the cystic fibrosis gene. Thorax 46: 124–130.
57. Gupta A, Eastham KM, Wrightson N, Spencer DA (2007) Hypomagnesaemia in cystic fibrosis patients referred for lung transplant assessment. J Cyst Fibros 6: 360–362.
58. Ciavardelli D, D'Orazio M, Pieroni L, Consalvo A, Rossi C, et al. (2013) Proteomic and ionomic profiling reveals significant alterations of protein expression and calcium homeostasis in cystic fibrosis cells. Mol Biosyst 9: 1117–1126.
59. Rosenecker J, Naundorf S, Rudolph C (2009) Airway surface liquid contains endogenous DNase activity which can be activated by exogenous magnesium. Eur J Med Res 14: 304–308.
60. Abdulhamid I, Beck FW, Millard S, Chen X, Prasad A (2008) Effect of zinc supplementation on respiratory tract infections in children with cystic fibrosis. Pediatr Pulmonol 43: 281–287.
61. Wood LG, Fitzgerald DA, Lee AK, Garg ML (2003) Improved antioxidant and fatty acid status of patients with cystic fibrosis after antioxidant supplementation is linked to improved lung function. Am J Clin Nutr 77: 150–159.
62. Li MS, Cowley EA, Linsdell P (2012) Pseudohalide anions reveal a novel extracellular site for potentiators to increase CFTR function. Br J Pharmacol 167: 1062–1075.

MicroRNA-21 is Induced by Rapamycin in a Model of Tuberous Sclerosis (TSC) and Lymphangioleiomyomatosis (LAM)

Anil J. Trindade[❡], **Douglas A. Medvetz**[❡], **Nicole A. Neuman, Faina Myachina, Jane Yu, Carmen Priolo, Elizabeth P. Henske***

Division of Pulmonary and Critical Care Medicine, Brigham and Women's Hospital and Harvard Medical School, Boston, Massachusetts, United States of America

Abstract

Lymphangioleiomyomatosis (LAM), a multisystem disease of women, is manifest by the proliferation of smooth muscle-like cells in the lung resulting in cystic lung destruction. Women with LAM can also develop renal angiomyolipomas. LAM is caused by mutations in the tuberous sclerosis complex genes (*TSC1* or *TSC2*), resulting in hyperactive mammalian Target of Rapamycin (mTOR) signaling. The mTOR inhibitor, Rapamycin, stabilizes lung function in LAM and decreases the volume of renal angiomyolipomas, but lung function declines and angiomyolipomas regrow when treatment is discontinued, suggesting that factors induced by mTORC1 inhibition may promote the survival of TSC2-deficient cells. Whether microRNA (miRNA, miR) signaling is involved in the response of LAM to mTORC1 inhibition is unknown. We identified Rapamycin-dependent miRNA in LAM patient angiomyolipoma-derived cells using two separate screens. First, we assayed 132 miRNA of known significance to tumor biology. Using a cut-off of >1.5-fold change, 48 microRNA were Rapamycin-induced, while 4 miRs were downregulated. In a second screen encompassing 946 miRNA, 18 miRs were upregulated by Rapamycin, while eight were downregulated. Dysregulation of miRs 29b, 21, 24, 221, 106a and 199a were common to both platforms and were classified as candidate "RapamiRs." Validation by qRT-PCR confirmed that these microRNA were increased. miR-21, a pro-survival miR, was the most significantly increased by mTOR-inhibition ($p<0.01$). The regulation of miR-21 by Rapamycin is cell type independent. mTOR inhibition promotes the processing of the miR-21 transcript (pri-miR-21) to a premature form (pre-miR-21). In conclusion, our findings demonstrate that Rapamycin upregulates multiple miRs, including pro-survival miRs, in TSC2-deficient patient-derived cells. The induction of miRs may contribute to the response of LAM and TSC patients to Rapamycin therapy.

Editor: Alfons Navarro, University of Barcelona, Spain

Funding: Funding for this project came from NIH-T32 HL007633-27 (AJT) and the LAM Foundation (EPH). The funders had no role in study design, data collection and analysis, decision to publish, or preparation of the manuscript.

Competing Interests: The authors have declared that no competing interests exist.

* E-mail: ehenske@partners.org

❡ These authors contributed equally to this work.

Introduction

Lymphangioleiomyomatosis (LAM) is a devastating multi-system disease that almost exclusively affects women and can result in end-stage lung disease. LAM is characterized by the diffuse proliferation of smooth muscle-like cells (LAM cells) that express melanocyte lineage proteins. In the lungs, LAM cells can lead to small airway obstruction, blockage of lymphatic vessels leading to the formation of chylous pleural effusions, and cystic parenchymal destruction which is believed to be due to the release of matrix metalloproteinases and other catabolic enzymes [1,2]. LAM occurs in two forms: in association with germline mutations in the tuberous sclerosis complex (TSC) genes, and in women who do not have tuberous sclerosis (sporadic LAM). The majority of women with TSC-LAM and about 40% of women with sporadic LAM have renal angiomyolipomas, which are benign tumors consisting of smooth muscle, fat and dysplastic vasculature. Angiomyolipoma cells have many similarities to LAM cells and may arise from a common progenitor cell [3]. LAM cells from women with sporadic LAM can carry somatic mutations in the *TSC2* gene, which is a tumor suppressor gene that regulates the mammalian Target of Rapamycin (mTOR) [4,5,6,7,8].

mTOR is a kinase that integrates cellular and environmental cues, including growth factor activity and glucose levels, to regulate cell growth and proliferation. mTOR exists in two distinct complexes: mTOR complex 1 (mTORC1), which includes Raptor, and mTOR complex 2, which includes Rictor [9,10]. Recent clinical trials of allosteric mTORC1-inhibitors such as Sirolimus (Rapamycin) in women with LAM have been promising in that they confer a partial reduction in angiomyolipoma volume and stabilization of lung function [11,12]. However, upon cessation of therapy lung function decline resumes and angiomyolipomas regrow, suggesting that allosteric mTORC1 inhibitors exert a cytostatic but not cytotoxic effect.

MicroRNA (miRNA or miRs) are small RNA molecules that regulate gene expression, primarily by affecting transcript stability. Many miRNA have their own promoter regions and undergo transcription in a tightly regulated manner. Mature miRNA form a RNA-induced silencing complex (RISC) with chaperone proteins, binding to the 3′ untranslated region of mRNA to either promote transcript degradation or repress protein translation. Over 1000 miRNA species have been identified, each with the ability to regulate hundreds of genes; moreover the 3′UTR of individual genes can recognize multiple miRNAs and mRNAs of differing abundance can "compete" for miRNA binding and consequent silencing [13].

Given the increasing evidence that microRNA participate in the pathogenesis of malignancies, inflammatory bowel disease, cardiomyopathies, and lung diseases including asthma, pulmonary hypertension and idiopathic pulmonary fibrosis [14,15,16,17,18], we explored whether dysregulated miRNA expression is associated with mTORC1 activity in LAM and TSC. We utilized TSC2-deficient LAM patient-derived cells with hyperactive mTORC1 and two different miRNA screens to identify "RapamiRs"-miRNA that are modulated by the mTORC1-inhibitor, Rapamycin. Using qRT-PCR, we confirmed the dysregulation of six miRs by Rapamycin and focused our attention on miR-21, which is a known "oncomiR." Interestingly, miR-21 induction by Rapamycin appears to be TSC2-independent.

Our results demonstrate that Rapamycin promotes the expression of several miRNA species, which we term "RapamiRs," in cellular models of LAM. Of the RapamiRs identified in our screens, miR-21, which has pro-survival effects in many cell types, is the most strongly induced by Rapamycin. To our knowledge, this is the first unbiased identification of mTORC1-dependent miRNA in human cells. Manipulation of pro-survival mTORC1-dependent miRNA may prove to be a valuable adjunct to Rapamycin therapy for TSC and LAM patients. RapamiRs may also have relevance to the broad range of human diseases that are associated with activation of mTORC1, including the majority of human malignancies.

Results

High-throughput screening identifies Rapamycin-dependent microRNA

To determine whether Rapamycin regulates miRNA, we performed two unbiased miRNA screens using LAM patient-derived 621-101 cells as an *in vitro* model of LAM (Tables 1, 2). These cells were derived from the angiomyolipoma of a woman with the sporadic form of LAM and carry bi-allelic inactivation of the *TSC2* gene [19]. An identical TSC2 mutation (R611Q) was present in this patient's pulmonary LAM cells [5]. 621-101 cells, cultured in DMEM containing 10% FBS, were treated with the allosteric mTOR inhibitor, Rapamycin (20 nM, 24 hours) or with vehicle control (DMSO). Isolated RNA was applied to a Signosis microRNA platform which assays 132 cancer-specific human miRNA by ligating two complementary tagged DNA probes to each target miRNA and hybridizing the complexes to a nitrocellulose membrane. Each target is assayed in duplicate and normalized to the expression of RNU48, a small nucleolar RNA molecule commonly used for normalization of miRNA levels [20]. The western blot in **Figure 1A** shows the level of phospho-S6 downregulation with rapamycin treatment. Nineteen miRNA were induced more than 2-fold, with miRs- 29b, 22, 26a, 199b and 181a being most highly increased. Four miRs - 375, 488, 142-5p, and 368 - were downregulated (**Figure 1B**). These results point toward a previously unknown miR-regulated signaling network downstream of mTORC1 with the potential to impact the expression of hundreds of mRNA in a cell-type dependent manner. We termed these Rapamycin-dependent miRs "RapamiRs."

To further investigate this putative RapamiR network, we performed a second, broader screen using the Exiqon platform, which incorporates locked-nucleic acid technology to increase probe-target specificity. This platform assays 946 human miRNA in quadruplet, including all known human miRNA listed in miRBase (version 15.0, http://mirbase.org/). A pool of three biological replicates was used for each sample. Results were normalized to RNU44. Interestingly, only 18 miRNAs were upregulated >1.5-fold (**Figure 2**), versus 19 miRNA upregulated >2 fold and 48 upregulated >1.5 fold in the Signosis array (Figure 1), despite the fact that the Signosis array contained fewer miRNA. miRs 29b, 31, 29a, 222 and 300 were among the most strongly induced miRNA using the Exiqon platform; 8 miRs were downregulated >1.5 fold.

Upregulation of miRNA 29b, 21, 24, 221, 106a and 199a was common to both the Signosis and Exiqon platforms. Of the miRs assayed in the Exiqon array that were not included in the Signosis array, Rapamycin promoted a >1.5-fold induction of miR-31, 222, 300, 1973, 886-5p, 886-3p, 23 and 214 and a >1.5-fold repression of miRs 210, 451, 513 and 1275.

The miRs that were dysregulated in both screens (miRs- 29b, 21, 24, 221, 106a and 199a) were included in a set selected for qRT-PCR confirmation. We also included miR-31 and miR-210, which were among the twelve miRNA dysregulated in the Exiqon array but not included in the Signosis array. miR-31, which was upregulated by Rapamycin, is anti-tumorigenic, preventing metastasis in models of breast cancer [21,22], and miR-210, which was downregulated by Rapamycin, is a well-described hypoximiR [23,24,25]. HypoximiRs are upregulated during hypoxia and have been shown to promote angiogenesis and smooth muscle proliferation. We first confirmed that similar levels of RapamiRs were observed using either RNU44 or RNU48 to normalize miRNA expression (**Figure 3A**). Three different biological replicates were used for the confirmation studies and miRNA expression was normalized to RNU48. MiRNA 21, 24, 31 and 221 were induced by Rapamycin >1.5-fold, consistent with the array results, with miR-21 being the most highly induced (**Figure 3B**). MiR-210 was decreased >1.5-fold, again consistent with the array results (Figure 3B).

Rapamycin induces miR-21 expression in multiple TSC2-deficient cell types and miR-21 expression may be TSC2-independent

To identify whether miR-21 is regulated by Rapamycin and/or TSC2 in other cell lines, tuberin (TSC2) was stably downregulated in C3H-10T1/2 mouse pre-pericyte fibroblasts with a lentiviral shRNA vector (**Figure 4A**). Cells were cultured in DMEM containing 10% FBS and treated with Rapamycin (20 nM) or control for 24 hours. Rapamycin increased miR-21 levels approximately 2-fold in both tuberin-deficient and control shRNA cells (**Figure 4B**), but unexpectedly no decrease in miR-21 was observed in the cells with tuberin downregulation despite the increased phosphorylation of ribosomal protein S6, a downstream target of mTORC1. Next, we utilized Tsc2-null mouse embryonic fibroblasts and ELT3 cells (Tsc2-null cells from an Eker rat uterine leiomyoma), which are established cellular models of TSC [26,27,28] compared to HEK293 and A549 cells, which express TSC2. Cells were cultured in DMEM containing 10% FBS and treated with Rapamycin (20 nM, 24 h) versus vehicle control. The human cells were normalized to RNU44, murine cells to snoRNA202, and rat cells to U87. miR-21 was induced >1.5-fold ($p<0.05$, $n = 3$) by Rapamycin in each of these cell lines (**Figure 4C**). These results further confirm that miR-21 is induced

Table 1. Rapamycin-regulated miRNA in LAM patient-derived cells identified by the Signosis Array (Fold Change >1.5).

miRNA	Fold Change (Rapa 24 h/ DMSO	miRNA	Fold Change (Rapa 24 h/ DMSO)	miRNA	Fold Change (Rapa 24 h/ DMSO)
miR-29b	4.47	miR-206	2.21	miR-10a	1.63
miR-22	2.99	miR-224	1.97	miR-136	1.62
miR-26a	2.95	miR-125a	1.95	miR-182	1.62
miR-199b	2.93	miR-106b	1.92	miR-188	1.62
miR-181a	2.82	miR-154	1.88	miR-221	1.60
miR-30b	2.69	miR-9	1.87	miR-34a	1.59
miR-19a	2.64	miR-21	1.85	miR-181d	1.58
miR-125b	2.52	miR-204	1.85	miR-20a	1.57
miR-137	2.48	miR-9-1	1.83	miR-10b	1.57
miR-181b	2.47	Let-7b	1.80	miR-126	1.57
miR-181c	2.47	miR-140	1.76	miR-30c	1.56
miR-30a-5p	2.47	miR-106a	1.74	miR-131	1.56
miR-17-3p	2.44	miR-30a-3p	1.72	miR-17-5p	1.53
miR-197	2.30	miR-24	1.71	miR-368	0.67
miR-199a	2.30	miR-135b	1.70	miR-142-5p	0.65
miR-183	2.29	miR-141	1.70	miR-488	0.56
miR-18a	2.23	miR-19b	1.70	miR-375	0.54
miR-95	2.21				

by Rapamycin in different cell lineages and species and suggest that the regulation of miR-21 may be TSC2-independent.

Rapamycin regulates miR-21 levels independently of AKT signaling

TSC2-null cells display feedback inhibition to the PI3K/AKT signaling pathway via hyperactivation of mTORC1 [29,30]. When TSC2-null cells are treated with Rapamycin this feedback inhibition is released and AKT is phosphorylated and activated. To determine whether Rapamycin regulates miR-21 expression via an AKT-dependent mechanism, we treated 621-101 cells with Rapamycin and the AKT inhibitor MK2206 (Selleckchem, Catalog No. S1078) (**Figure 5**). In Figure 5A (lanes 1–2), western blot analysis was performed to confirm that p-AKT levels are

Table 2. Rapamycin-regulated miRNA in LAM patient-derived cells identified by the Exiqon Array (Fold Change >1.5, normalized to RNU44).

microRNA	Expression Change (Rapamycin/DMSO)	microRNA	Expression Change (Rapamycin/DMSO)
miR-29b	2.65	miR-1274	0.67
miR-31	2.64	miR-210	0.67
miR-29a	2.15	miR-451	0.64
miR-222	2.14	miR-1285	0.62
miR-300	2.13	miR-1308	0.62
miR-21	2.07	miR-1908	0.58
miR-1973	1.97	miR-513a-5p	0.43
miR-221	1.91	miR-1275	0.42
miR-886-5p	1.86		
miR-24	1.82		
miR-574	1.73		
miR-106a	1.62		
let-7d	1.57		
mir-886-3p	1.55		
miR-23b	1.53		
miR-214	1.53		

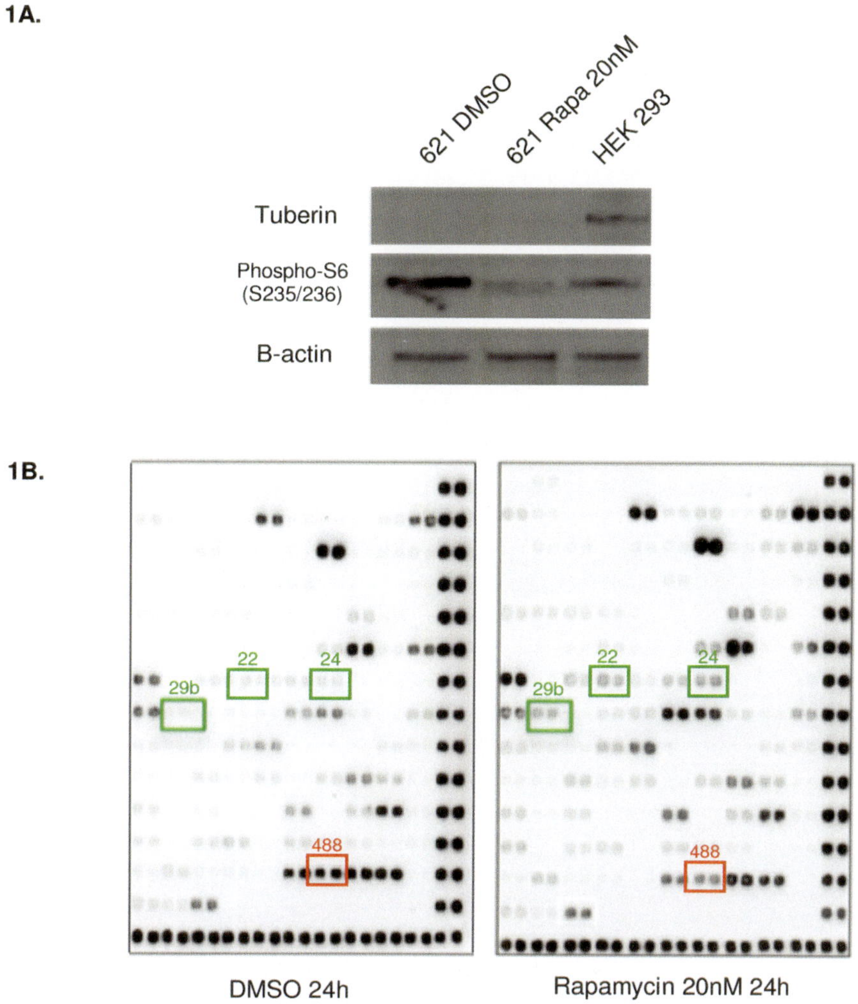

Figure 1. Rapamycin regulates miRNA in TSC2-deficient LAM patient angiomyolipoma-derived cells. A) Western blot demonstrating that Rapamycin inhibits phosphorylation of ribosomal protein S6 (S235/236) in TSC2-deficient 621-101 cells. **B**) Signosis miRNA microarray identifies Rapamycin-dependent miRNA; boxed dots display an induction of miR-22, 24, and 29b (in green) and a decrease in miR-488 (in red) amongst others by Rapamycin. The array assays cancer-specific miRNA in duplicate.

elevated in 621-101 cells treated with Rapamycin (20 nM, 24 h) compared to DMSO treated cells. Additionally, we confirmed that MK2206 (10 nM, 24 h) inhibited AKT phosphorylation at S473 when 621-101 cells were treated with Rapamycin and MK2206. In Figure 5B, we analyzed miR-21 levels in the same 621-101 cell samples used for western blot. miR-21 levels were upregulated by Rapamycin and unaffected by AKT inhibition (compare blue bar to purple bar). These results indicate that miR-21's regulation by Rapamycin is AKT-independent in 621-101 cells.

Rapamycin potentiates the post-transcriptional processing of pri-miR-21

MiRNA biogenesis is a tightly regulated process, with key enzyme complexes participating in transcription and processing at three major junctions (**Figure 6A**). Post-transcriptional processing is a key mechanism to controlling miRNA levels [31]. The regulation of miR-21, in particular, has been well-characterized, with Davis and colleagues demonstrating that TGF-beta and Smad signaling induces a Drosha-mediated post-transcriptional processing of pri-miR-21 to induce miR-21 expression [32]. To determine whether Rapamycin influences the processing of pri-miR-21, we treated 621-101 cells, cultured in DMEM containing 10% FBS, with Rapamycin (20 nM) or DMSO for 24 hours and assayed the expression of pri-miR-21, pre-miR-21 and miR-21 using qRT-PCR. Rapamycin significantly induced pre-miR-21 and miR-21 at 24-hours, but did not affect expression of pri-miR-21 (**Figure 6B**). This result suggests that Rapamycin potentiates the DROSHA-mediated processing of pri-miR-21.

Discussion

The landmark Multicenter International LAM Efficacy of Sirolimus (MILES) Trial, a randomized, placebo controlled trial in 89 women with sporadic or TSC-associated LAM, demonstrated that Rapamycin (an allosteric mTOR inhibitor) stabilized lung function during one year of therapy; discontinuation of therapy resulted in a rate of lung function decline similar to untreated patients [12]. These findings are consistent with results from an earlier phase I/II trial of patients with angiomyolipomas, some of who also had sporadic or TSC-associated LAM, in which Rapamycin promoted a decrease in the volume of renal angiomyolipomas by almost 50%, with regrowth to approximately

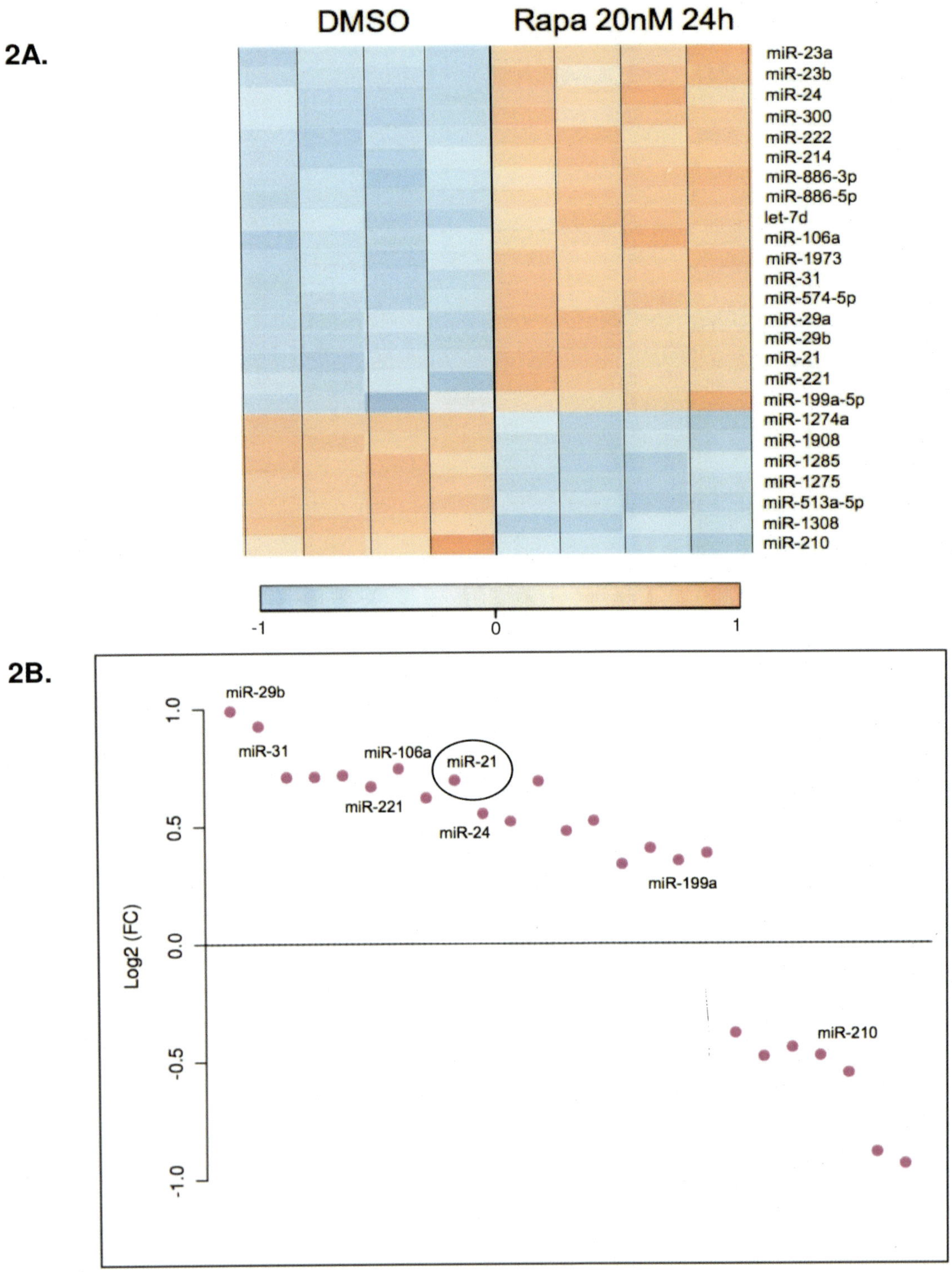

Figure 2. Exiqon miRNA microarray confirms 8 Rapamycin-dependent miRNA. 621-101 cells were treated with Rapamycin 20 nM or DMSO for 24 hours. Total RNA was isolated and applied to the Exiqon platform, which assays 946 human miRNA. **A**) Heat map of miRNA dysregulated by Rapamycin >1.5-fold, $\log_2$ scale. RNA from three biologic replicates per condition was pooled; each miRNA was assayed in quadruplet on the array. **B**) miRNA dysregulated by Rapamycin >1.5-fold (normalized to RNU44). Highlighted miRNA (except miR-31 and 210) are common to both the Exiqon and Signosis platforms. miR-21 is circled.

the original size after treatment was stopped [11]. These studies suggest that temporarily slows disease progression, but does not eradicate the TSC2-deficient LAM and angiomyolipoma cells. Therapeutic targeting of factors that promote the survival of LAM cells during Rapamycin therapy could lead to more robust and/or durable responses.

While miRNA have been studied in many human diseases, whether miRNA contribute to the therapeutic response to

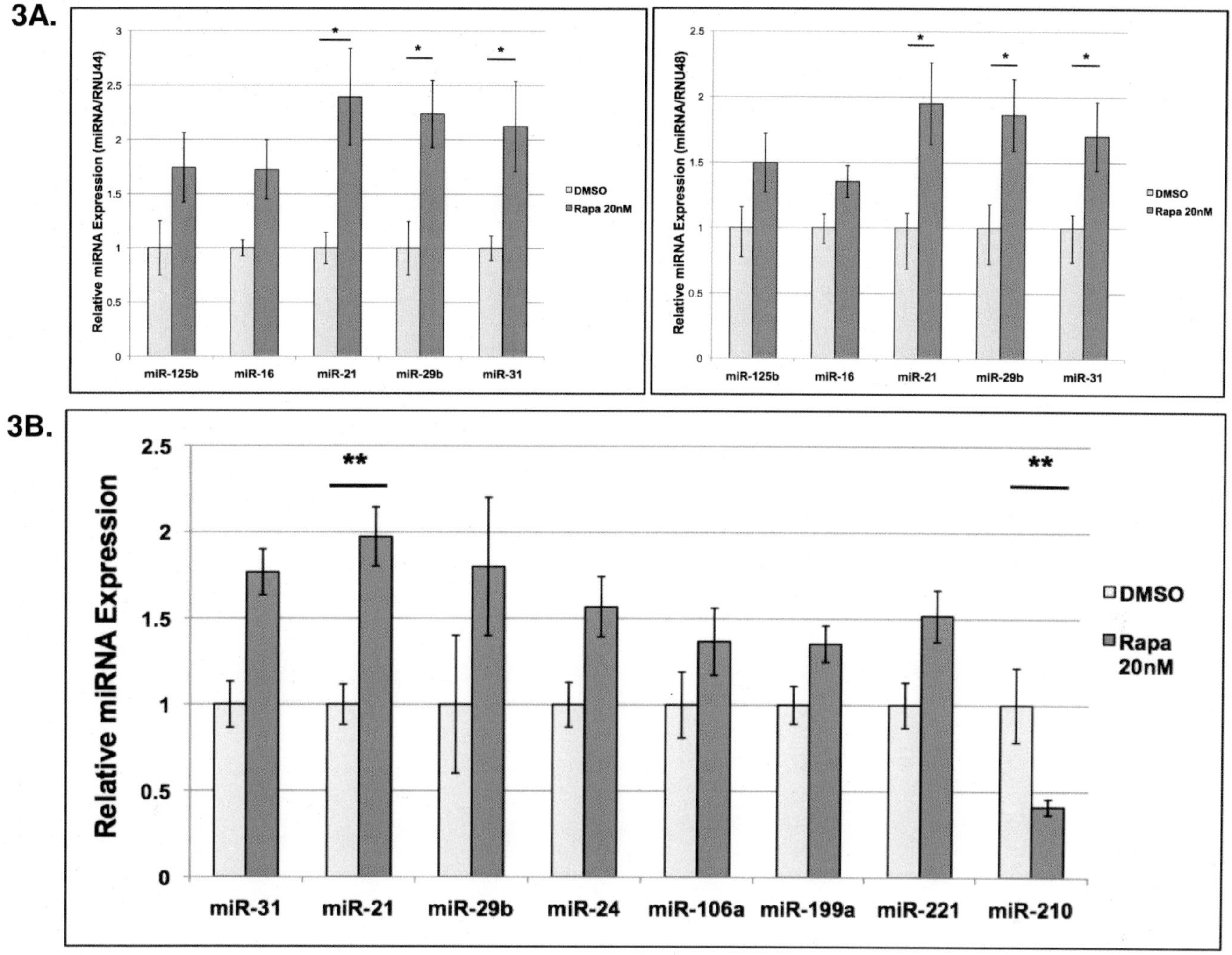

Figure 3. qRT-PCR confirmation of Rapamycin-dependent miRNA in TSC2-deficient cells. TSC2−/− cells were treated with Rapamycin 20 nM or DMSO for 24 hr and miRNA expression was assessed by qRT-PCR. **A**) miRNA expression is similar in 621-101 cells using RNU44 (left panel) or RNU48 (right panel) for normalization. **B**) miRNA expression in 621-101 cells normalized to RNU44. Highlighted results are significant using a Bonferroni correction.

Rapamycin in LAM and TSC is unknown. To address this, we performed two screens to determine whether Rapamycin impacts miRNA levels in LAM patient angiomyolipoma-derived cells. The first screen assayed 132 miRNA of known importance to cancer signaling pathways, while the second was a more comprehensive screen that assayed all 946 known miRNA listed in miRBase Version 15.0. The screens revealed a complex and previously unrecognized network of Rapamycin-regulated miRNA, which we termed "RapamiRs". Using qRT-PCR to confirm our results, we demonstrate that miR-21 is significantly induced by Rapamycin, whereas miR-210 is repressed. We further analyzed Rapamycin's effect on miR-21, demonstrating that miR-21 is induced in several different TSC2-deficient cell lines. Utilizing mouse pre-pericyte fibroblasts with stable downregulation of tuberin, we confirmed that the dysregulated expression of miR-21 is mTOR-dependent, but tuberin independent. Finally, we revealed that the induction of miR-21 expression by Rapamycin is mediated by post-transcriptional processing of the primary miR-21 transcript, as opposed to increased transcription. These studies reveal a novel regulatory network that is upregulated by Rapamycin.

We hypothesize that the upregulation of miR-21 by Rapamycin in LAM patient-derived cells impacts the therapeutic response to Rapamycin. First, miR-21 is a known "oncomiR," inhibiting multiple tumor suppressor genes, including phosphatase and tensin homolog (PTEN), programmed cell death 4 (PDCD4) and sprouty 2 (SPRY2) to promote growth, differentiation and proliferation [33,34,35,36,37]. These pro-survival effects of miR-21 may partially explain why there is a resumption of disease upon treatment discontinuation in LAM patients treated with Rapamycin. Interestingly SPRY2 has previously been shown to regulate mTORC1 signal transduction and vascularization of the lung [38]. Second, miR-21 is a known regulator of smooth muscle morphololgy, promoting a de-differentiated state marked by growth and migration, which is essential for angiogenesis [39,40]. Krymskaya and colleagues have previously demonstrated a role for regulators of smooth muscle function in the pathogenesis of LAM, identifying that RhoA is activated in TSC2-deficient cells [41,42]. Smooth muscle-like LAM cells can be identified *in vivo* in two different morphologic states, a highly proliferative "spindle shape" and a more static "epithelioid" state [43]; the pathways that regulate the phenotypic switch of LAM cells is unknown.

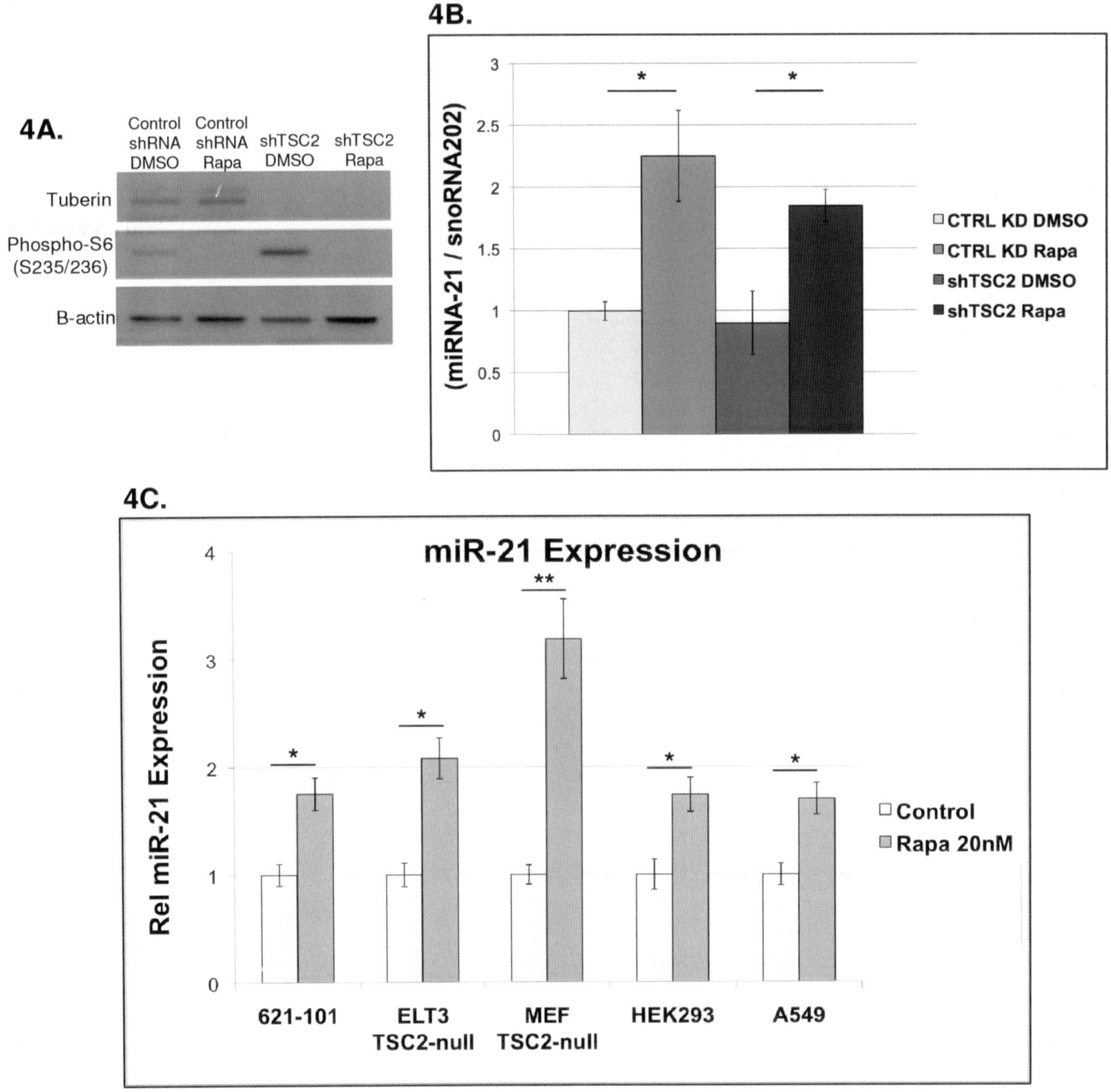

Figure 4. miR-21 is mTOR-dependent and may be TSC2-independent. A) Stable downregulation of tuberin in C3H-10T1/2 pre-pericytes results in increased phosphorylation of ribosomal protein S6, as expected. Treatment with Rapamycin (20 nM, 24 h) inhibits phosphorylation of S6. **B**) Downregulation of TSC2 in C3H-10T1/2 cells does not affect miR-21 expression. Inhibition of mTORC1 with Rapamycin induces ~2-fold increase in miR-21 expression in both control shRNA and TSC2 shRNA cells. Bars represent the mean of two biologic replicates +/− SD. * $p<0.05$. **C**) LAM patient-derived cells (621-101), TSC2-null rat uterine leiomyoma-derived cells (ELT3), TSC2-null mouse embryonic fibroblasts (MEFs), HEK293 and lung adenocarcinoma (A549) cells were treated with Rapamycin 20 nM vs Control for 24 h. Relative MiR-21 expression was determined by qRT-PCR. Human cells were normalized to RNU44, mouse cells to snora202 and rat cells to U87, which are all small nucleolar RNA molecules. For all charts, bars represent the mean of three biologic replicates +/− standard error. * $p<0.05$. ** $p<0.01$.

Third, it is possible that miR-21 induces a pro-inflammatory state that promotes the survival and metastasis of TSC2-deficient LAM cells. miR-21 is regulated by inflammatory mediators and in turn acts to promote inflammation. For example, interleukin-6 is a potent modulator of miR-21, acting via STAT3 signaling [44]. Additionally, mTORC1 has been shown to activate STAT3 signaling in mice and humans making this an intriguing link [45,46]. Moreover, miR-21 inhibits PTEN and PDCD4 to repress NF-kB signaling and IL-10, an anti-inflammatory interleukin [47]. A number of groups have identified a link between innate immunity pathways and TSC-mTOR signaling. Weichhart and colleagues have shown that TSC2-deficient cells exhibit an anti-inflammatory state via the induction of IL-10, whereas Rapamycin treatment promotes a pro-inflammatory condition by suppressing

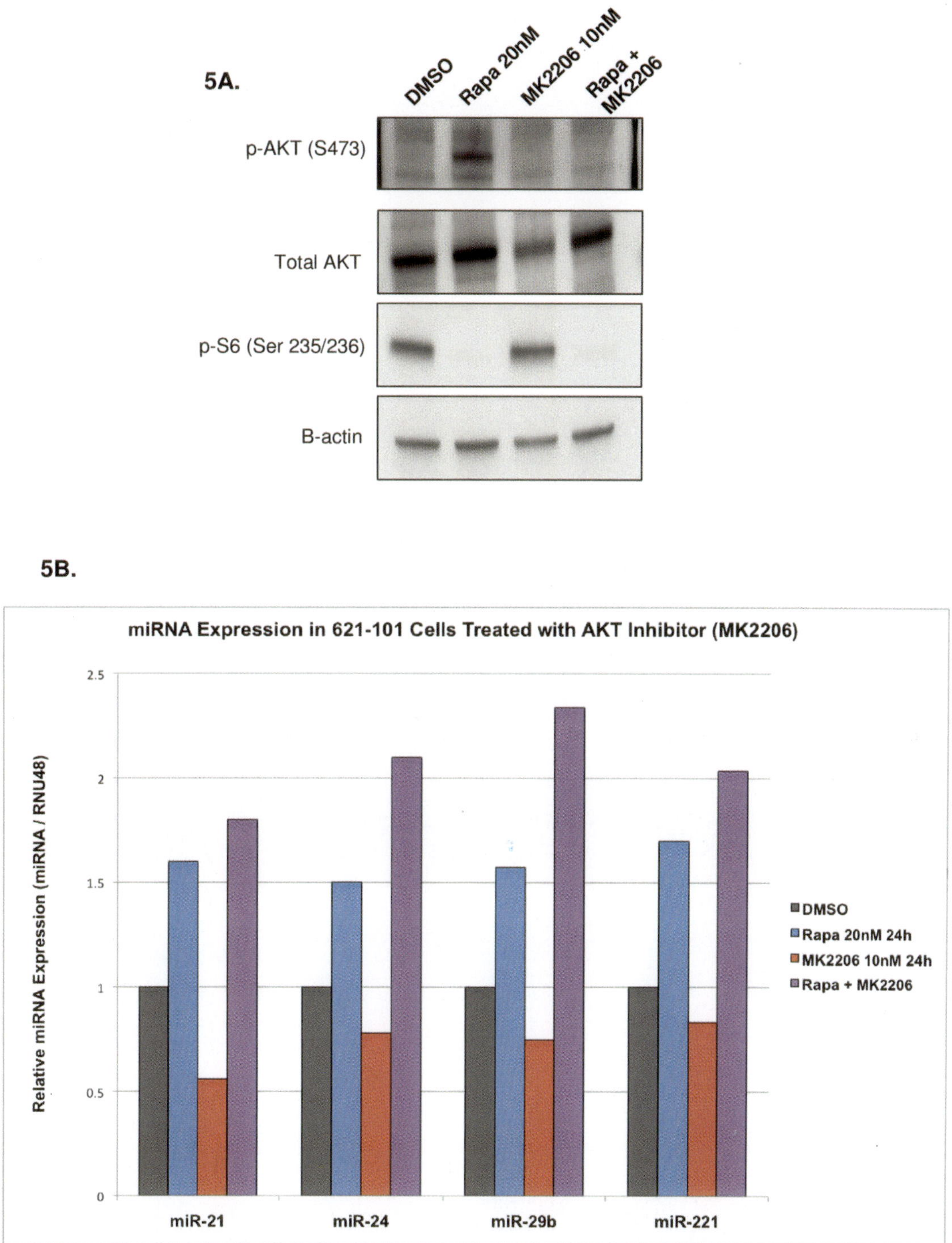

Figure 5. Rapamycin induces miR-21 expression via an AKT-independent mechanism. A) Western blot analysis of 621-101 cells treated with DMSO (lane 1), Rapamycin (20 nM, 24 h - lane 2), the AKT inhibitor MK2206 (10 nM, 24 h - lane 3), and Rapamycin and MK2206 (lane 4). Rapamycin treatment induces AKT phosphorylation at S473 and MK2206 abrogates Rapamycin's effect on phosphor-Akt. **B**) Expression of miR-21, 24, 29b, and 221 in 621-101 cells treated as in A). miR-21 levels are induced by Rapamycin, however the addition of MK2206 has no effect suggesting an AKT-independent mechanism.

IL-10 and inducing TNF-alpha, IL-6, and IL-12p40 [48]. Moss and colleagues have also contributed to the recognition of inflammatory processes underlying the pathogenesis of LAM, demonstrating that chemokines and chemokine receptors, especially CCL-2/MCP-1, are dysregulated in LAM cells and in bronchoalveolar lavage fluid obtained from LAM patients [49]. Therefore, the induction of miR-21 by Rapamycin may induce a proliferative smooth muscle morphology and contribute to a pro-inflammatory milieu.

Our identification of Rapamycin-induced miRNA reveals a novel and complex signaling network downstream of mTOR with potential therapeutic implications for women with LAM and

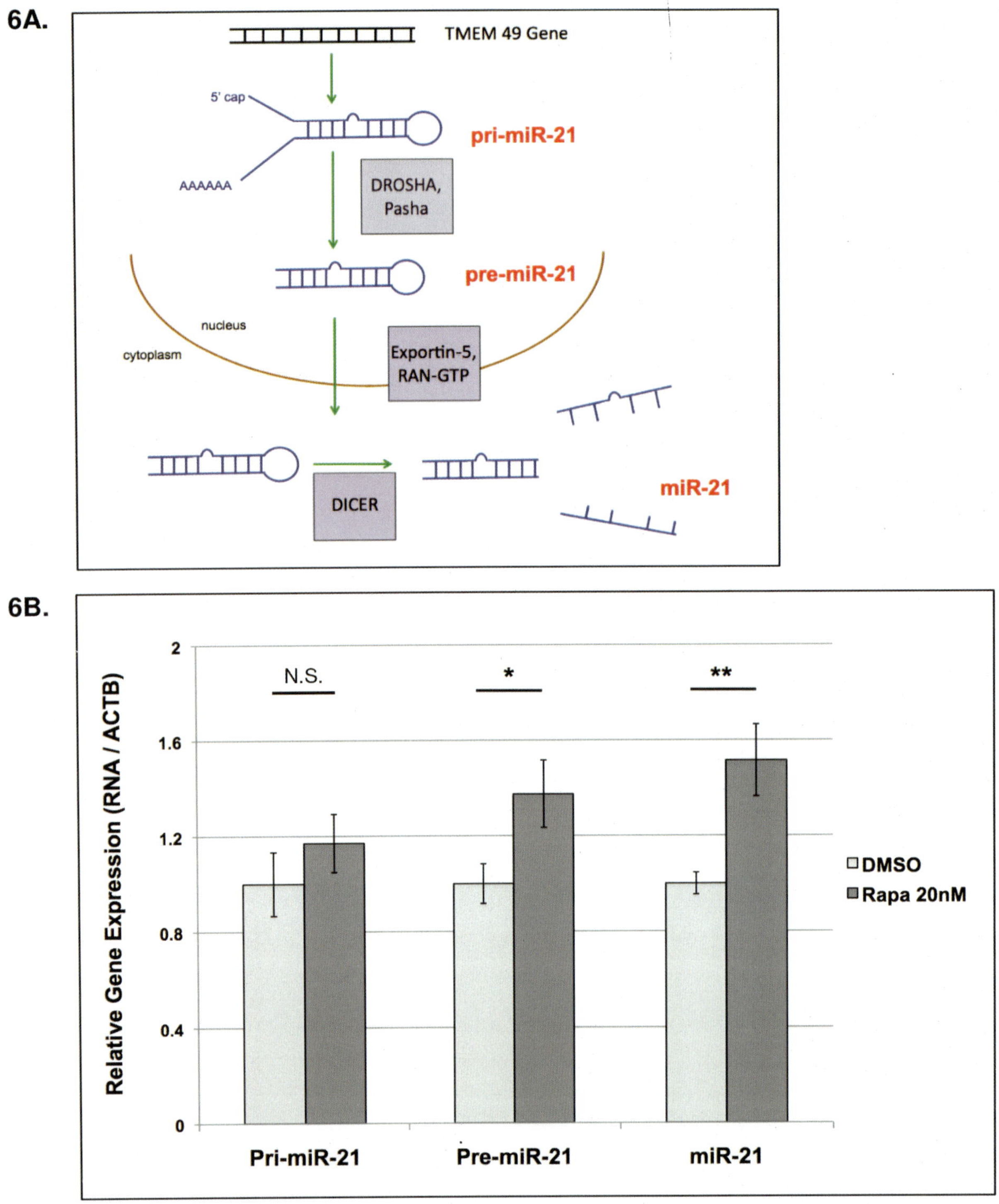

Figure 6. Rapamycin promotes the post-transcriptional processing of pre-miR-21. A) The biogenesis of mature miR-21. Pri-miR is transcribed from the intronic region of the TMEM49 gene and processed into pre-miR-21 by the Drosha/Pasha complex and further processed by Dicer to create the mature form. **B**) 621-101 cells were treated with Rapamycin 20 nM or control (DMSO) for 24 hours. Total RNA was extracted and assayed by qRT-PCR for the differential expression of pri-miR-21, pre-miR-21 and miR-21. Expression of pre-miR-21 was significantly induced by Rapamycin, whereas pri-miR-21 levels were not affected, suggesting that Rapamycin promotes the Drosha-mediated post-transcriptional processing of pri-miR-21 into pre-miR-21 at 24 hours. Bars represent the mean of three biological replicates +/− SD. * $p<0.05$, ** $p<0.01$.

patients with TSC receiving Rapamycin therapy. For example, if miR-21 induction by Rapamycin proves to be a strong pro-survival stimulus in TSC2-deficient cells cells, then suppression of miR-21 in conjunction with Rapamycin could represent an effective therapeutic strategy for TSC and LAM. Manipulation of miRNA expression is currently being studied as a therapy for malignancies and cardiomyopathies, with promising results in multiple pre-clinical models of disease [50,51]; 'antagomiRs' that suppress miRNA expression are now being tested in clinical trials. RapamiRs may also be useful as serum biomarkers of response to Rapamycin. Finally, our findings may be relevant to other diseases in which Rapamycin and its analogs are currently being used therapeutically, including cancer, for which there are currently more than 100 active cancer clinical trials using mTOR inhibitors.

Methods

Cell culture and Tsc2-downregulation

621-101 (The Rothberg Institute), Tsc2-null mouse embryonic fibroblasts (provided by Dr. David Kwiatkowski), HEK293, C3H10T1/2 cells (American Type Culture Collection) and ELT3 cells (provided by Dr. Cheryl Walker) were maintained in DMEM supplemented with 10% FBS (Sigma), Penicillin (50 units/mL) and Streptomycin (50 mg/mL); media for ELT3 cells also contained G418 (0.5 mg/mL). Lentiviral particles expressing shTSC2 were generated by transfecting HEK293T cells with plasmid DNA expressing shTSC2 (or empty vector) and lentiviral packaging particles (VSVG, PLP1, PLP2). Supernatant containing virions was applied to C3H10T1/2 cells (passage 7) for infection. C3H10T1/2 with lentiviral transfection were maintained in DMEM supplemented with 10% FBS (Sigma) with Puromycin (for selection).

Immunoblot analyses

Lysates were mixed with Laemmli Sample buffer and boiled for 10 minutes. 30 μg of sample were resolved in a 4–12% acrylamide gel and transferred to nitrocellulose membranes (Bio-Rad, Hercules, CA). The membranes were blotted overnight with rabbit anti–phospho-S235/236 S6 ribosomal protein (Cell Signaling), mouse anti-Actin (Sigma-Aldrich), or rabbit anti-Tuberin (Santa Cruz Biotechnology Inc.).

MicroRNA Screens

621-101 cells were grown in DMEM supplemented with 10% FBS until 60% confluent. Cells were then treated for 24 hours with Rapamycin (20 nM) or equal volume Dimethylsulfoxide (DMSO). Cells were washed twice with phosphate buffered saline and RNA extracted using the miRCURY RNA Isolation Kit (Exiqon). Assaying of microRNA was performed on the Signosis Cancer MicroRNA Array platform and the miRCURY LNA 5th generation microRNA microarray platform (Exiqon), which contained capture probes for all miRNAs annotated in miRBase (version 15.0; http://www.mirbase.org/).

Real-time quantitative Reverse Transcription - Polymerase Chain Reaction Analysis (qRT-PCR)

Total RNA was extracted using the miRCURY RNA Isolation Kit (Exiqon). For miRNA quantification RNA was reverse-transcribed using a Taq- ManTM microRNA reverse transcription kit, and subjected to real-time PCR using TaqManTM microRNA assay kits (Applied Biosystems). Reactions were performed in triplicate, using an Applied Biosystems Step One Plus instrument. MiRNA expression was normalized to small nuclear RNA (snRNA) RNU44 or RNU48. For quantification of pri-miR-21 and pre-miR-21, total RNA was reverse transcribed and Quantitative PCR was performed using a SYBR-green kit (Applied Biosystems). The following primers were used to assay pre-miR-21: 5′- TGTCGGGTAGCTTATCAGAC-3′ (forward), 5′- TGTCAGACAGCCCATCGACT-3′ (reverse). The following primers were used to assay pre-miR-21: 5′-TTTTGTTTTGCTTGGGAGGA-3′ (forward), 5′- AGCAGA-CAGTCAGGCAGGAT-3′ (reverse). Assays were performed using three biologic replicates and three technical replicates for each treatment condition. Assays were performed on the Applied Biosystems Step One Plus instrument. Only one PCR product was observed for each assay.

Acknowledgments

We are grateful to Augustine Choi, Mark Perrella, David Kwiatkowski and Stephen Chan for their critical comments. We thank David Kwiatkowski for providing TSC2-null MEFs and Cheryl Walker for providing ELT3 cells.

Author Contributions

Conceived and designed the experiments: AJT DAM NAN CP EPH. Performed the experiments: AJT DAM FM NAN. Analyzed the data: AJT DAM NAN FM JY CP EPH. Contributed reagents/materials/analysis tools: AJT DAM NAN FM JY CP EPH. Wrote the paper: AJT DAM.

References

1. McCormack FX (2008) Lymphangioleiomyomatosis: a clinical update. Chest 133: 507–516.
2. Henske EP, McCormack FX (2012) Lymphangioleiomyomatosis - a wolf in sheep's clothing. J Clin Invest 122: 3807–3816.
3. Finlay G (2004) The LAM cell: what is it, where does it come from, and why does it grow? Am J Physiol Lung Cell Mol Physiol 286: L690–693.
4. Astrinidis A, Khare L, Carsillo T, Smolarek T, Au KS, et al. (2000) Mutational analysis of the tuberous sclerosis gene TSC2 in patients with pulmonary lymphangioleiomyomatosis. J Med Genet 37: 55–57.
5. Carsillo T, Astrinidis A, Henske EP (2000) Mutations in the tuberous sclerosis complex gene TSC2 are a cause of sporadic pulmonary lymphangioleiomyomatosis. Proc Natl Acad Sci U S A 97: 6085–6090.
6. Smolarek TA, Wessner LL, McCormack FX, Mylet JC, Menon AG, et al. (1998) Evidence that lymphangiomyomatosis is caused by TSC2 mutations: chromosome 16p13 loss of heterozygosity in angiomyolipomas and lymph nodes from women with lymphangiomyomatosis. Am J Hum Genet 62: 810–815.
7. Sato T, Seyama K, Fujii H, Maruyama H, Setoguchi Y, et al. (2002) Mutation analysis of the TSC1 and TSC2 genes in Japanese patients with pulmonary lymphangioleiomyomatosis. J Hum Genet 47: 20–28.
8. Crooks DM, Pacheco-Rodriguez G, DeCastro RM, McCoy JP Jr, Wang JA, et al. (2004) Molecular and genetic analysis of disseminated neoplastic cells in lymphangioleiomyomatosis. Proc Natl Acad Sci U S A 101: 17462–17467.
9. Sarbassov DD, Ali SM, Kim DH, Guertin DA, Latek RR, et al. (2004) Rictor, a novel binding partner of mTOR, defines a rapamycin-insensitive and raptor-independent pathway that regulates the cytoskeleton. Curr Biol 14: 1296–1302.
10. Kim DH, Sabatini DM (2004) Raptor and mTOR: subunits of a nutrient-sensitive complex. Curr Top Microbiol Immunol 279: 259–270.
11. Bissler JJ, McCormack FX, Young LR, Elwing JM, Chuck G, et al. (2008) Sirolimus for angiomyolipoma in tuberous sclerosis complex or lymphangioleiomyomatosis. N Engl J Med 358: 140–151.
12. McCormack FX, Inoue Y, Moss J, Singer LG, Strange C, et al. (2011) Efficacy and safety of sirolimus in lymphangioleiomyomatosis. N Engl J Med 364: 1595–1606.
13. Poliseno L, Salmena L, Zhang J, Carver B, Haveman WJ, et al. (2010) A coding-independent function of gene and pseudogene mRNAs regulates tumour biology. Nature 465: 1033–1038.
14. Wu F, Zikusoka M, Trindade A, Dassopoulos T, Harris ML, et al. (2008) MicroRNAs are differentially expressed in ulcerative colitis and alter expression of macrophage inflammatory peptide-2 alpha. Gastroenterology 135: 1624–1635 e1624.
15. Sayed D, Hong C, Chen IY, Lypowy J, Abdellatif M (2007) MicroRNAs play an essential role in the development of cardiac hypertrophy. Circ Res 100: 416–424.
16. Parikh VN, Jin RC, Rabello S, Gulbahce N, White K, et al. (2012) MicroRNA-21 integrates pathogenic signaling to control pulmonary hypertension: results of a network bioinformatics approach. Circulation 125: 1520–1532.
17. Milosevic J, Pandit K, Magister M, Rabinovich E, Ellwanger DC, et al. (2012) Profibrotic Role of miR-154 in Pulmonary Fibrosis. Am J Respir Cell Mol Biol.
18. Pandit KV, Corcoran D, Yousef H, Yarlagadda M, Tzouvelekis A, et al. (2010) Inhibition and role of let-7d in idiopathic pulmonary fibrosis. Am J Respir Crit Care Med 182: 220–229.
19. Yu J, Astrinidis A, Howard S, Henske EP (2004) Estradiol and tamoxifen stimulate LAM-associated angiomyolipoma cell growth and activate both

genomic and nongenomic signaling pathways. Am J Physiol Lung Cell Mol Physiol 286: L694–700.
20. Peltier HJ, Latham GJ (2008) Normalization of microRNA expression levels in quantitative RT-PCR assays: identification of suitable reference RNA targets in normal and cancerous human solid tissues. RNA 14: 844–852.
21. Augoff K, McCue B, Plow EF, Sossey-Alaoui K (2012) miR-31 and its host gene lncRNA LOC554202 are regulated by promoter hypermethylation in triple-negative breast cancer. Mol Cancer 11: 5.
22. Koerner C, Keklikoglou I, Bender C, Woerner A, Muenstermann E, et al. (2013) microRNA-31 sensitizes human breast cells to apoptosis by direct targeting of protein kinase C epsilon (PKC{varepsilon}). J Biol Chem.
23. Bao B, Ali S, Ahmad A, Azmi AS, Li Y, et al. (2012) Hypoxia-Induced Aggressiveness of Pancreatic Cancer Cells Is Due to Increased Expression of VEGF, IL-6 and miR-21, Which Can Be Attenuated by CDF Treatment. PLoS One 7: e50165.
24. Cicchillitti L, Di Stefano V, Isaia E, Crimaldi L, Fasanaro P, et al. (2012) Hypoxia-inducible Factor 1-alpha Induces miR-210 in Normoxic Differentiating Myoblasts. J Biol Chem 287: 44761–44771.
25. Fasanaro P, Romani S, Voellenkle C, Maimone B, Capogrossi MC, et al. (2012) ROD1 is a seedless target gene of hypoxia-induced miR-210. PLoS One 7: e44651.
26. Everitt JI, Wolf DC, Howe SR, Goldsworthy TL, Walker C (1995) Rodent model of reproductive tract leiomyomata. Clinical and pathological features. Am J Pathol 146: 1556–1567.
27. Zhang H, Cicchetti G, Onda H, Koon HB, Asrican K, et al. (2003) Loss of Tsc1/Tsc2 activates mTOR and disrupts PI3K-Akt signaling through downregulation of PDGFR. J Clin Invest 112: 1223–1233.
28. Kwiatkowski DJ (2010) Animal models of lymphangioleiomyomatosis (LAM) and tuberous sclerosis complex (TSC). Lymphat Res Biol 8: 51–57.
29. Tremblay F, Marette A (2001) Amino acid and insulin signaling via the mTOR/p70 S6 kinase pathway. A negative feedback mechanism leading to insulin resistance in skeletal muscle cells. J Biol Chem 276: 38052–38060.
30. Manning BD, Logsdon MN, Lipovsky AI, Abbott D, Kwiatkowski DJ, et al. (2005) Feedback inhibition of Akt signaling limits the growth of tumors lacking Tsc2. Genes Dev 19: 1773–1778.
31. Siomi H, Siomi MC (2010) Posttranscriptional regulation of microRNA biogenesis in animals. Mol Cell 38: 323–332.
32. Davis BN, Hilyard AC, Lagna G, Hata A (2008) SMAD proteins control DROSHA-mediated microRNA maturation. Nature 454: 56–61.
33. Medina PP, Nolde M, Slack FJ (2010) OncomiR addiction in an in vivo model of microRNA-21-induced pre-B-cell lymphoma. Nature 467: 86–90.
34. Asangani IA, Rasheed SA, Nikolova DA, Leupold JH, Colburn NH, et al. (2008) MicroRNA-21 (miR-21) post-transcriptionally downregulates tumor suppressor Pdcd4 and stimulates invasion, intravasation and metastasis in colorectal cancer. Oncogene 27: 2128–2136.
35. Ma X, Kumar M, Choudhury SN, Becker Buscaglia LE, Barker JR, et al. (2011) Loss of the miR-21 allele elevates the expression of its target genes and reduces tumorigenesis. Proc Natl Acad Sci U S A 108: 10144–10149.
36. Meng F, Henson R, Wehbe-Janek H, Ghoshal K, Jacob ST, et al. (2007) MicroRNA-21 regulates expression of the PTEN tumor suppressor gene in human hepatocellular cancer. Gastroenterology 133: 647–658.
37. Sayed D, Rane S, Lypowy J, He M, Chen IY, et al. (2008) MicroRNA-21 targets Sprouty2 and promotes cellular outgrowths. Mol Biol Cell 19: 3272–3282.
38. Scott CL, Walker DJ, Cwiklinski E, Tait C, Tee AR, et al. (2010) Control of HIF-1{alpha} and vascular signaling in fetal lung involves cross talk between mTORC1 and the FGF-10/FGFR2b/Spry2 airway branching periodicity clock. Am J Physiol Lung Cell Mol Physiol 299: L455–471.
39. Wang M, Li W, Chang GQ, Ye CS, Ou JS, et al. (2011) MicroRNA-21 regulates vascular smooth muscle cell function via targeting tropomyosin 1 in arteriosclerosis obliterans of lower extremities. Arterioscler Thromb Vasc Biol 31: 2044–2053.
40. Chan MC, Hilyard AC, Wu C, Davis BN, Hill NS, et al. (2010) Molecular basis for antagonism between PDGF and the TGFbeta family of signalling pathways by control of miR-24 expression. EMBO J 29: 559–573.
41. Goncharova EA, Goncharov DA, Spaits M, Noonan DJ, Talovskaya E, et al. (2006) Abnormal growth of smooth muscle-like cells in lymphangioleiomyomatosis: Role for tumor suppressor TSC2. Am J Respir Cell Mol Biol 34: 561–572.
42. Goncharova EA, Goncharov DA, Lim PN, Noonan D, Krymskaya VP (2006) Modulation of cell migration and invasiveness by tumor suppressor TSC2 in lymphangioleiomyomatosis. Am J Respir Cell Mol Biol 34: 473–480.
43. Harari S, Torre O, Moss J (2011) Lymphangioleiomyomatosis: what do we know and what are we looking for? Eur Respir Rev 20: 34–44.
44. Shen XH, Han YJ, Zhang DX, Cui XS, Kim NH (2009) A link between the interleukin-6/Stat3 anti-apoptotic pathway and microRNA-21 in preimplantation mouse embryos. Mol Reprod Dev 76: 854–862.
45. El-Hashemite N, Kwiatkowski DJ (2005) Interferon-gamma-Jak-Stat signaling in pulmonary lymphangioleiomyomatosis and renal angiomyolipoma: a potential therapeutic target. Am J Respir Cell Mol Biol 33: 227–230.
46. Magri L, Cambiaghi M, Cominelli M, Alfaro-Cervello C, Cursi M, et al. (2011) Sustained activation of mTOR pathway in embryonic neural stem cells leads to development of tuberous sclerosis complex-associated lesions. Cell Stem Cell 9: 447–462.
47. Roy S, Sen CK (2011) MiRNA in innate immune responses: novel players in wound inflammation. Physiol Genomics 43: 557–565.
48. Weichhart T, Costantino G, Poglitsch M, Rosner M, Zeyda M, et al. (2008) The TSC-mTOR signaling pathway regulates the innate inflammatory response. Immunity 29: 565–577.
49. Pacheco-Rodriguez G, Kumaki F, Steagall WK, Zhang Y, Ikeda Y, et al. (2009) Chemokine-enhanced chemotaxis of lymphangioleiomyomatosis cells with mutations in the tumor suppressor TSC2 gene. J Immunol 182: 1270–1277.
50. Yang CH, Yue J, Pfeffer SR, Handorf CR, Pfeffer LM (2011) MicroRNA miR-21 regulates the metastatic behavior of B16 melanoma cells. J Biol Chem 286: 39172–39178.
51. Thum T, Gross C, Fiedler J, Fischer T, Kissler S, et al. (2008) MicroRNA-21 contributes to myocardial disease by stimulating MAP kinase signalling in fibroblasts. Nature 456: 980–984.

Inflammasome-Mediated IL-1β Production in Humans with Cystic Fibrosis

Anthony Tang[1], Ashish Sharma[2], Roger Jen[2], Aaron F. Hirschfeld[3], Mark A. Chilvers[3], Pascal M. Lavoie[2,3], Stuart E. Turvey[1,2,3]*

1 Department of Microbiology & Immunology, University of British Columbia, Vancouver, British Columbia, Canada, **2** Department of Experimental Medicine, University of British Columbia, Vancouver, British Columbia, Canada, **3** Department of Pediatrics, British Columbia Children's Hospital and Child & Family Research Institute, Vancouver, British Columbia, Canada

Abstract

Background: Inflammation and infection are major determinants of disease severity and consequently, the quality of life and outcome for patients with cystic fibrosis (CF). Interleukin-1 beta (IL-1β) is a key inflammatory mediator. Secretion of biologically active IL-1β involves inflammasome-mediated processing. Little is known about the contribution of IL-1β and the inflammasomes in CF inflammatory disease. This study examines inflammasome-mediated IL-1β production in CF bronchial epithelial cell lines and human patients with CF.

Results: Bronchial epithelial cell lines were found to produce negligible amounts of basal or stimulated IL-1β compared to hematopoeitic cells and they did not significantly upregulate caspase-1 activity upon inflammasome stimulation. In contrast, peripheral blood mononuclear cells (PBMCs) from both CF and healthy control subjects produced large amounts of IL-1β and strongly upregulated caspase-1 activity upon inflammasome stimulation. PBMCs from CF patients and controls displayed similar levels of caspase-1 activation and IL-1β production when stimulated with inflammasome activators. This IL-1β production was dependent on NF-κB activity and could be enhanced by priming with LPS. Finally, chemical inhibition of CFTR activity in control PBMCs and THP-1 cells did not significantly alter IL-1β or IL-8 production in response to *P. aeruginosa*.

Conclusion: Hematopoeitic cells appear to be the predominant source of inflammasome-induced pro-inflammatory IL-1β in CF. PBMCs derived from CF subjects display preserved inflammasome activation and IL-1β secretion in response to the major CF pathogen *Pseudomonas aeruginosa*. However, our data do not support the hypothesis that increased IL-1β production in CF subjects is due to an intrinsic increase in NF-κB activity through loss of CFTR function.

Editor: David M. Ojcius, University of California Merced, United States of America

Funding: This work was supported by: BC Lung Association (www.bc.lung.ca); Cystic Fibrosis Canada (www.cysticfibrosis.ca); Michael Smith Foundation For Health Research (www.msfhr.org/); Canadian Institutes For Health Research (www.cihr-irsc.gc.ca); and Child & Family Research Institute (www.cfri.ca). The funders had no role in study design, data collection and analysis, decision to publish, or preparation of the manuscript.

Competing Interests: The authors have declared that no competing interests exist.

* E-mail: sturvey@cw.bc.ca

Introduction

Cystic fibrosis is an autosomal recessive disease caused by mutations in the cystic fibrosis transmembrane conductance regulator (CFTR), which functions as a chloride ion channel. CF remains one of the most common lethal genetic diseases in populations of European descent with the current average lifespan of CF patients approximately 40 years of age [1,2]. Recurrent inflammatory pulmonary exacerbation is the primary cause of lung disease progression and ultimately, death in CF. Controlled inflammation is important for fighting infection, but in excess, it becomes destructive to host cells and to the architecture of the lungs [2,3]. In CF, airway epithelial cells have been shown to produce an exaggerated pro-inflammatory cytokine response to stimulation [4,5]. It is unclear whether this heightened inflammatory response is intrinsic to cells lacking CFTR or whether it is a result of chronic polymicrobial infection [6,7]. Regardless of this controversy, identifying and targeting relevant inflammatory mediators is a critical step in developing more specific therapeutic approaches to control inflammation and improve health outcomes in CF [8].

Interleukin-1 beta (IL-1β) is a major inflammatory mediator. Its physiological effects are diverse and potentially important to the pathogenesis of lung exacerbations in CF, including the generation of fever, the recruitment of inflammatory effector cells, the induction of other pro-inflammatory cytokines such as IL-6 and IL-8, and the shaping of T cell responses [9,10]. Following initiation of the NF-κB signaling cascade, IL-1β is produced in the cytosol as a biologically inactive full-length pro-IL-1β. Pro-IL-1β is subsequently converted into its active form by cytosolic protein complexes termed "inflammasomes." Inflammasomes assemble in response to certain cellular danger signals and mediate the auto-activation of caspase-1 [9,11], which cleaves pro-IL-1β and pro-IL-18 into their biologically active forms for secretion. Four distinct inflammasomes have been recognized. These are the

NLRP1 [12], NLRP3 [13,14], NLRC4 [15,16], and AIM2 inflammasomes [17,18], which respond to a variety of different microbial signatures and danger signals [11].

P. aeruginosa, one of the most common and clinically relevant pathogens among CF patients, activates the NLRC4 inflammasome [19,20]. Infection with *P. aeruginosa* triggers an increase in levels of IL-1β, IL-6, and IL-8 in bronchoalveolar lavage fluid (BALF) from patients with CF [21]. Inflammasome responses depend on NF-κB signaling, where NF-κB is important in both the upregulation of specific inflammasome components [22,23], as well as IL-1β expression [24,25].

Previous studies support a role for IL-1β in the pathogenesis of CF inflammatory lung disease. Levels of IL-1β are increased in BALF from CF patients with infection [21,26,27,28] and this increase has been temporally associated with a clinical response to treatment [21]. Polymorphisms in the *IL1B* gene have also been associated with varying degrees of disease severity in CF patients [29]. Murine models of CFTR dysfunction have exhibited significant increases in IL-1β expression or secretion in macrophages [30,31], and support the hypothesis that the loss of CFTR increases NF-κB activation under basal and stimulatory conditions [4,5,32,33]. Finally, replacement of chloride ions with glutamate or gluconate in cell culture media increases secretion of IL-1β in response to NLRP3 stimulation by adenosine triphosphate (ATP) [34], implying an inhibitory role for extracellular chloride in NLRP3 activation. Taken together, these data implicate the involvement of IL-1β and consequently, the inflammasomes, in CF inflammatory disease.

Results

Airway epithelial cells do not produce significant amounts of IL-1β in response to inflammasome stimulation

The inflammasomes and their respective activators examined in this study are listed in Table 1. Cells were stimulated in accordance with the schedule in Figure 1. In CF, airway epithelial cells have been shown to possess a hyper-inflammatory phenotype and produce an exaggerated pro-inflammatory cytokine response [4,5]. To determine if airway epithelial cells contribute to the increased IL-1β production in patients with CF, CF and control bronchial epithelial cell lines were stimulated with the inflammasome inducers *P. aeruginosa* strain PAO1 (PAO1) and LPS followed by ATP. IL-1β levels in cell culture supernatants were not greatly increased in either the CF or control cell lines (Fig. 2a–d), although a small increase in IL-1β production was detected in NuLi-1 and CuFi-1 cells, but not in S9 and IB3-1 cells, by 24 hours. In contrast, these airway cells were highly responsive to other inflammatory stimuli, such as recombinant IL-1β, producing large quantities of IL-8 (Fig. 2a–d inserts).

Airway epithelial cells do not significantly upregulate caspase-1 activity in response to inflammasome stimulation

To examine if inflammasome activation occurs in these airway cells, caspase-1 activity was quantified by flow cytometry. There was no significant increase upon stimulation with live PAO1 or LPS+ATP at the times examined (Fig. 3a–b). Because previous studies have indicated a role for caspase-1 in the activation of NF-κB through Toll-like receptor (TLR) signaling [35], we examined whether chemical inhibition of caspase-1 altered NF-κB-dependent IL-6 production in response to *P. aeruginosa*. However, treatment with the caspase-1 inhibitor z-YVAD-fmk (YVAD) did not decrease IL-6 secretion by airway epithelial cells (Fig. 3c).

CD14 positive monocytes from CF patients and controls show similar increases in caspase-1 activity upon inflammasome stimulation

Monocytes were identified in PBMC populations using CD14 as a phenotyping marker. CD14 positive monocytes from CF patients and healthy controls showed a significant increase in caspase-1 activation upon stimulation with LPS+ATP, PAO1, and LPS+Poly(dA:dT) (Fig. 4a) but this activation was not different between CF and control subjects (Fig. 4b).

PBMCs from CF patients do not produce increased amounts of IL-1β upon inflammasome stimulation

Previous studies have shown that the loss of CFTR results in increased NF-κB activity and pro-inflammatory cytokine secretion [4,5,32,36,37]. To further examine this relationship, PBMCs from CF patients and healthy adult controls were stimulated with PAO1, LPS+ATP, and LPS+Poly(dA:dT), to activate the NLRC4, NLRP3, and AIM2 inflammasomes, respectively. By 24 hours of stimulation, CF PBMCs did not produce increased amounts of IL-1β (Fig. 5a) or IL-8 (Fig. 5b) when compared to healthy controls. However, we did notice a transient decrease ($P<0.001$) in the amount of IL-1β produced by CF cells in response to LPS+ATP at 6 hours (data not shown). Stimulation of PBMCs with *P. aeruginosa* that lacks *exsA* (PAO1Δ*exsA*), a key regulator of type III secretion, produced three-fold less IL-1β compared to the parental PAO1 strain by 24 hours (Fig. 5a). Inflammasome stimulation without priming did not result in any IL-1β production in either CF or control PBMCs. Contrary to our hypothesis, these results indicate that PBMCs from CF patients do not display increased production of IL-1β or IL-8 with inflammasome activation nor do they suggest any increased basal or induced NF-κB activity. These results are consistent with our observation that caspase-1 activity is not different between CF and control PBMCs (Fig. 4).

Table 1. Inflammasome Activators.

INFLAMMASOME	INFLAMMASOME STIMULUS	EXOGENOUS PRIMING OF NF-κB REQUIRED?
NLRP3	ATP (Concentration: 5 mM)	Yes
NLRC4	*Pseudomonas aeruginosa* strain PAO1. (Multiplicity of Infection (MOI) = 1)	No (primed by live bacterium)
AIM2	Poly(dA:dT) (Concentration: 1 μg/ml)	Yes

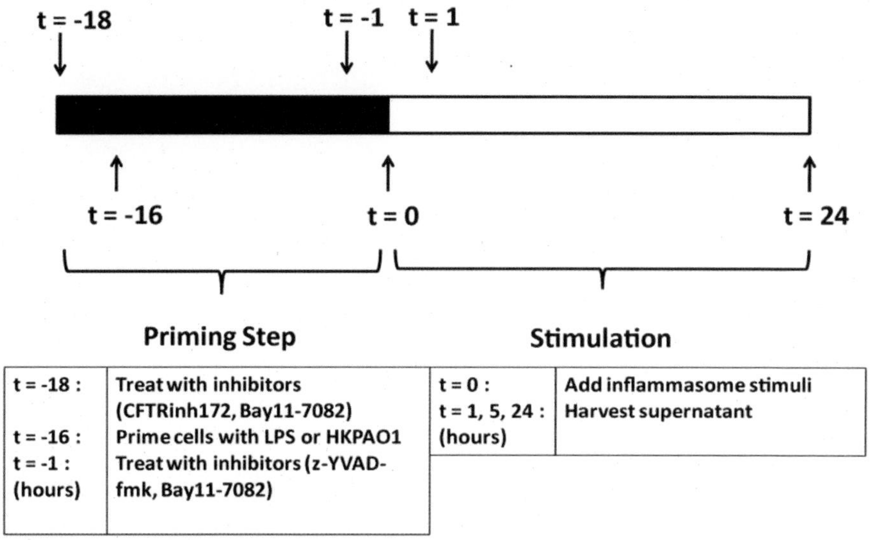

Figure 1. Cell stimulation and inhibitor schedule. Schedule outlines the timing of inhibitor addition and priming in relation to inflammasome stimulation (t = 0) for THP-1 reporter and PBMC cytokine quantification experiments. Inhibitor treatments and stimulations were carried out as described in the Materials and Methods section.

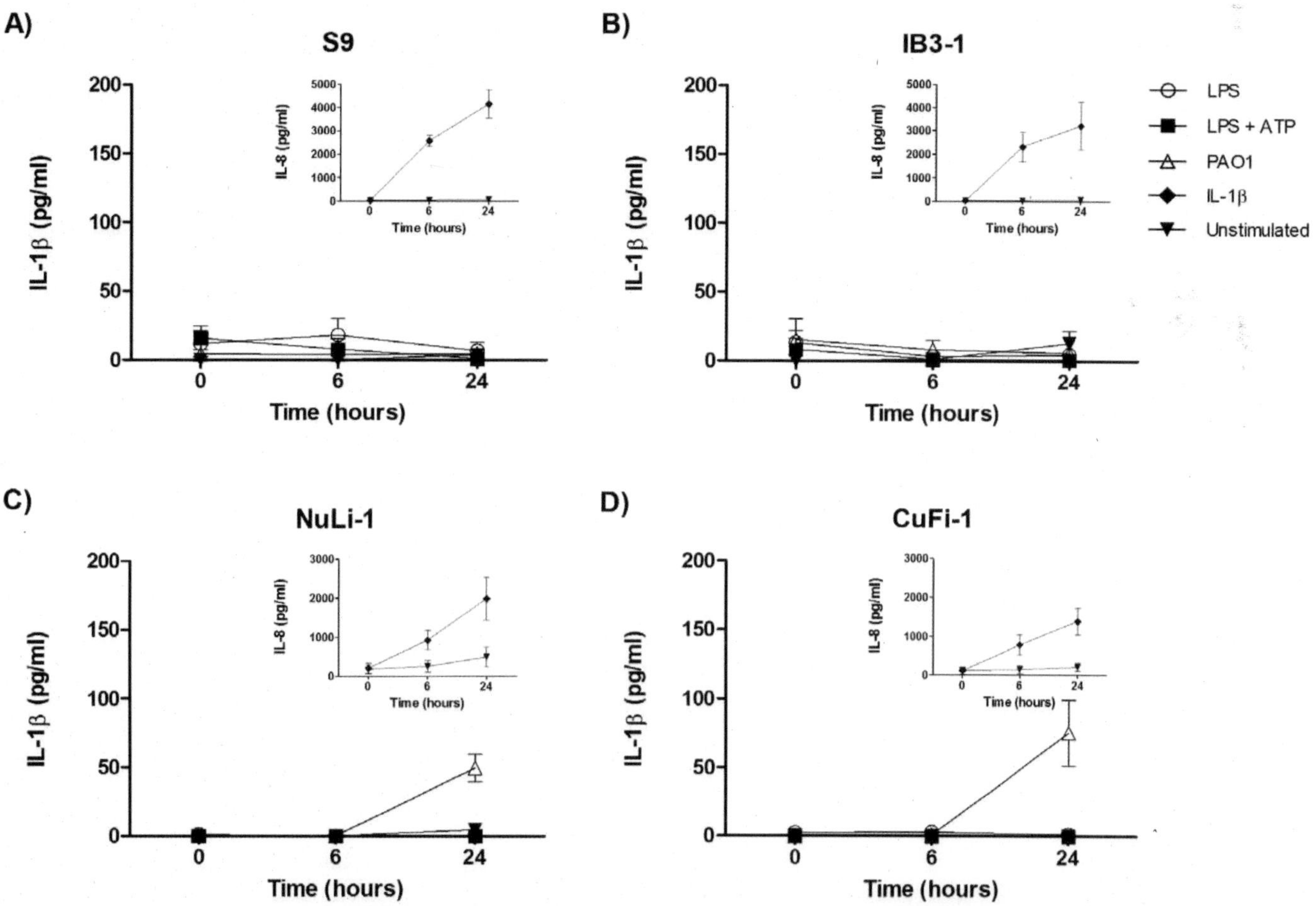

Figure 2. Airway epithelial cells do not significantly contribute to IL-1β production in response to inflammasome stimuli. Control cell lines ((A) S9, (C) NuLi-1) and their corresponding CF cell lines ((B) IB3-1, and (D) CuFi-1) cells were stimulated with *P. aeruginosa* (MOI = 10), ATP (5 mM), or IL-1β (10 ng/ml), for the indicated times (n = 3 individual experiments). Cells were primed with LPS (100 ng/ml) for 4 hours where appropriate. Cell culture supernatants were assayed for IL-1β and IL-8 production by ELISA. Insert shows IL-8 secretion in response to stimulation with IL-1β (10 ng/ml).

NF-κB activation is required for IL-1β and IL-8 responses to *P. aeruginosa*

We confirmed the dependence of PAO1-induced IL-1β and IL-8 production on NF-κB activation using THP-1 cells expressing a reporter driven by NF-κB and AP-1 response elements. We found that stimulation of primed THP-1 reporter cells with heat-killed PAO1 produced the highest levels of NF-κB/AP-1 activation (Fig. 6a) and this correlated with IL-8 secretion (Fig. 6b) but negligible amounts of IL-1β were secreted (Fig. 6c). Stimulation of primed THP-1 reporter cells with live PAO1 did not significantly increase NF-κB/AP-1 activity (Fig. 6a) or IL-8 secretion (Fig. 6b) over priming alone. However, IL-1β production was greatly augmented over primed cells stimulated with heat-killed PAO1 or unprimed cells stimulated with live PAO1 (Fig. 6c). This confirmed that NF-κB activation alone is not sufficient for maximal IL-1β secretion, but increased priming of NF-κB is capable of augmenting IL-1β production and secretion upon inflammasome stimulation. Dependency of these responses on NF-κB was confirmed by pharmacologic inhibition of NF-κB using the Bay11-7082 inhibitor of IκBα phosphorylation, which significantly reduced NF-κB/AP-1 activation ($P<0.001$) (Fig. 6d) and the subsequent production of IL-8 ($P<0.01$) (Fig. 6e) and IL-1β ($P<0.001$) (Fig. 6f) in response to both heat-killed and live PAO1. These results were also verified in CF and control PBMCs for each inflammasome examined ($P<0.001$) (Fig. 6g–h). Overall these results confirm that NF-κB is an important modulator of IL-1β production and that increased activation of NF-κB augments inflammasome-mediated production of IL-1β.

Bay11-7082 inhibits pro-IL-1β production in response to *P. aeruginosa*

In addition to inhibition of NF-κB activity, Bay11-7082 can also directly inhibit the NLRP3 inflammasome [38]. To validate its use in this study as an NF-κB inhibitor, western blots for pro-IL-1β

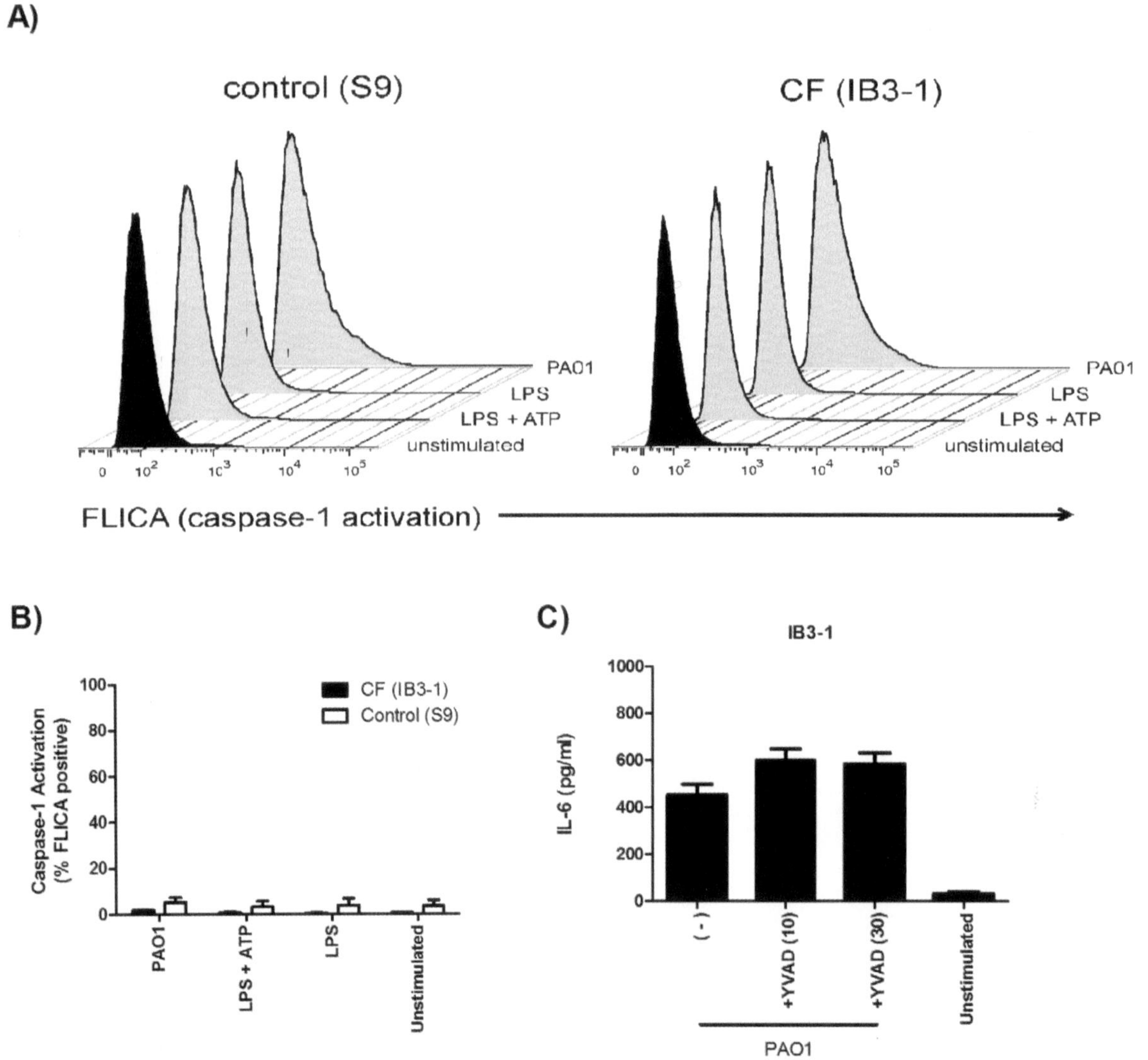

Figure 3. Airway cells do not strongly upregulate caspase-1 activity in response to inflammasome stimuli. S9 and IB3-1 cells were examined for caspase-1 activation following inflammasome stimulation with *P. aeruginosa* (MOI = 10) and ATP (5 mM). Cells were primed with LPS for 5 hours where appropriate. A representative histogram of % caspase-1-active cells is shown in (A) and the averaged values are shown in (B) (n = 3 separate experiments). (C) IB3-1 cells (5×10^4 cells/well) were pre-treated for 1 hour with increasing concentrations of z-YVAD-fmk (10–30 μM) prior to stimulation with *P. aeruginosa* (MOI = 50). Cell culture supernatants were collected after 6 hours and assayed for IL-6 by ELISA (n = 3).

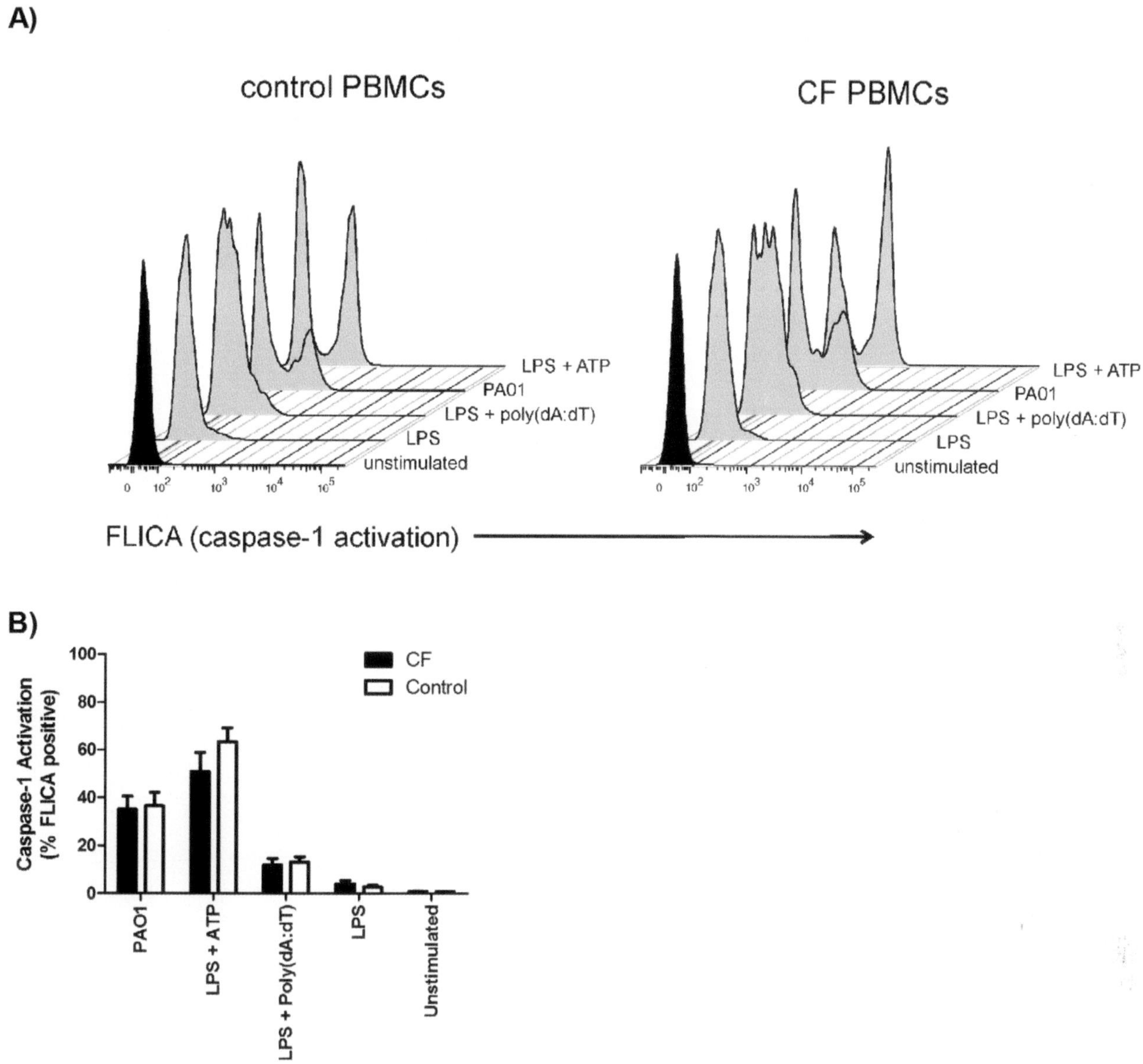

Figure 4. PBMCs from CF patients and controls show similar increases in caspase-1 activity upon inflammasome activation. PBMCs from CF patients (n = 6) and healthy controls (n = 6) were primed with LPS (10 ng/ml) for 5 hours prior to stimulation with ATP (5 mM) for 1 hour or Poly(dA:dT) (1 µg/ml) for 3 hours. PBMCs were stimulated with *P. aeruginosa* strain PAO1 for 3 hours. A representative histogram of the % caspase-1-active cells is shown in (A) with the averaged values shown in (B).

were performed alongside inhibition of CFTR activity by $CFTR_{inh}172$ in response to PAO1 at 4 hours after stimulation (Fig. 7a). Our results indicate that Bay11-7082 prevents production of pro-IL-1β whereas $CFTR_{inh}172$ does not seem to affect it. This was further corroborated by the ability Bay11-7082 to inhibit IκBα degradation at 0.5, 1, and 1.5 hours post PAO1 stimulation (Fig. 7b).

Disruption of CFTR activity does not increase IL-1β production in PBMCs and THP-1 cells

A previous study has indicated a role for chloride ion concentration in suppression of NLRP3 inflammasome activation [34]. To determine whether CFTR dysfunction alters IL-1β production, THP-1 cells and PBMCs from CF patients and healthy controls were treated with the CFTR inhibitor, $CFTR_{inh}172$, prior to simulation with live *P. aeruginosa*. Treatment with $CFTR_{inh}172$ did not alter IL-1β or IL-8 production in control subjects or CF patients (Fig. 8a–b). Similarly, IL-1β production was not different in monocyte-derived macrophages or THP-1 reporter cells treated with $CFTR_{inh}172$ (Fig. 8c–d). IL-8 (Fig. 8e) and NF-κB activity (Fig. 8f) were also unchanged in $CFTR_{inh}172$-treated THP-1 reporter cells.

Discussion

Levels of IL-1β are increased in the BALF of CF patients but the cellular source of this cytokine and its production in the context of targeted inflammasome activation are still unclear. We first studied airway epithelial cells due to their role in barrier function, proximity to infection, and ability to produce high levels of pro-inflammatory cytokines. However, we found that bronchial

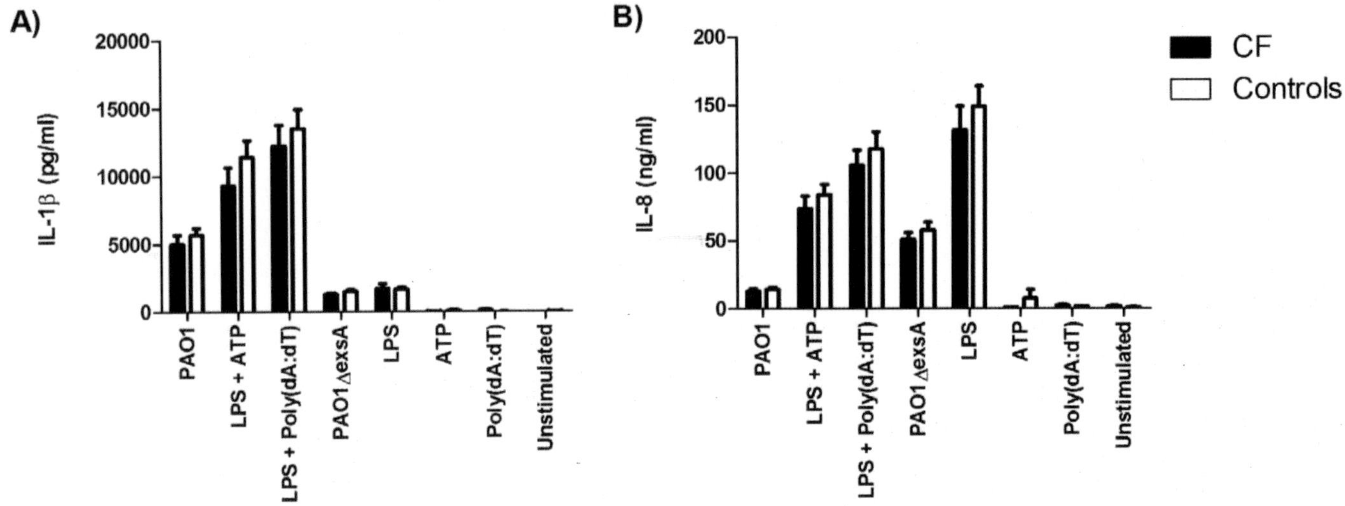

Figure 5. PBMCs from CF patients do not produce increased amounts of IL-1β. PBMCs from CF patients (n = 17–20) and healthy controls (n = 15–19) were primed with LPS (10 ng/ml) overnight and stimulated with *P. aeruginosa* PAO1 (MOI = 1), *P. aeruginosa* PAO1 lacking *exsA* (MOI = 1), ATP (5 mM), or Poly(dA:dT) (1 μg/ml) for 24 hours. *P. aeruginosa* lacking *exsA* was used as a type III secretion control in comparison with wild-type *P. aeruginosa*. Supernatants were assayed for (A) IL-1β and (B) IL-8.

epithelial cells do not produce significant amounts of IL-1β and do not show a significant increase in caspase-1 activation in response to PAO1 and LPS+ATP, in comparison to hematopoeitic mononuclear cells. Hematopoeitically-derived cells, such as monocytes and macrophages, appear to be a principal source of IL-1β. CFTR is expressed in alveolar macrophages [32,39] as well as in PBMCs at both the mRNA and protein level [40,41], and its loss is frequently associated with an augmented inflammatory phenotype.

Despite our findings indicating that bronchial epithelial cells when grown *in vitro* are unlikely to be significantly involved in the direct production of IL-1β (Fig. 2a–d), others have shown their capacity to respond to alveolar macrophage-derived IL-1β and to amplify the inflammatory response through the induction of chemokines and recruitment of inflammatory effector cells [42]. This interaction may constitute a critical component to effective host defense and diminishing the capacity of host cells to respond to IL-1β may leave the host susceptible to infections by pathogens such as *P. aeruginosa* [43]. Conversely, overproduction of IL-1β can also play a key role in chronic inflammatory responses and cause damage to the lung parenchyma [44,45].

Although we hypothesized that CF cells would secrete increased amounts of IL-1β, we found that IL-1β production in CF PBMCs was not increased upon inflammasome stimulation as compared to controls (Fig. 5a–b). This was in contrast to a previous study from our group, which showed increased IL-1β production by CF PBMCs in response to LPS [46], although this difference may be accounted for by technical issues in stimulation time and dose. Moreover, IL-1β production was not increased in CF PBMCs with inflammasome stimulation alone as would be anticipated if there were basal levels of NF-κB activation. Cells deficient in CFTR are thought to exhibit an increased basal level of NF-κB activity, which leads to increased pro-inflammatory cytokine production including an increased availability of pro-IL-1β for cleavage and secretion. This amplification of IL-1β secretion was shown by priming THP-1 monocytes and PBMCs with heat-killed *P. aeruginosa* or LPS prior to stimulation with live *P. aeruginosa*. This dramatically increased IL-1β secretion over stimulation with live *P. aeruginosa* without priming (Fig. 6c). Similarly, if CF PBMCs expressed increased basal NF-κB activity, there would be an increase in IL-1β secretion in the absence of LPS priming. However, no increase in IL-1β was observed under basal or primed conditions. Studies investigating the production of IL-1β have been somewhat inconsistent. A study by Reininger *et al.* [43] provided evidence that human bronchial epithelial cells possessing the ΔF508 CFTR mutation had a slightly reduced capacity to produce IL-1β and lacked the ability to induce an early NF-κB activation in response to *P. aeruginosa.* Conversely, a study by Kotrange *et al.* [31] found that murine bone marrow-derived macrophages expressing ΔF508-CFTR produced increased amounts of IL-1β when compared to macrophages expressing normal CFTR in response to *Burkholderia cenocepacia* K56-2. The differentiation of monocytes into macrophages may partly account for the differences observed with the study by Kotrange. Inflammasome-mediated IL-1β production by monocytes and PBMCs does differ from macrophages [47,48,49] and macrophages are found to have higher expression of CFTR over monocytes [50]. However, as monocytes and other PBMCs express CFTR [50,51] and produce large amounts of IL-1β, they are adequate models to examine the effects of CFTR function on IL-1β production. Other hematopoeitic cells may also contribute to IL-1β production. For example, neutrophil counts can be significantly increased in the lungs of CF patients [52,53,54] and may produce mature IL-1β through caspase-1 independent mechanisms [55].

The role of NF-κB activation in inflammasome activation and IL-1β secretion is not straightforward. Studies have revealed an essential role for NF-κB activation in the production of pro-IL-1β and inflammasome components such as NLRP3 [22,23]. In contrast, deletion of IKKβ, a kinase essential in NF-κB activation, increases IL-1β secretion in murine macrophages [56,57] and demonstrates a dual role for NF-κB in regulation of IL-1β. To address this uncertainty in our experiments we also quantified IL-8, an important CF cytokine and marker of NF-κB activation [58], and found no differences between CF and control subjects. Similarly, levels of intracellular pro-IL-1β in THP-1 cells were dependent on NF-κB activity and did not increase with $CFTR_{inh}172$ treatment. Subsequent treatment of THP-1 cells

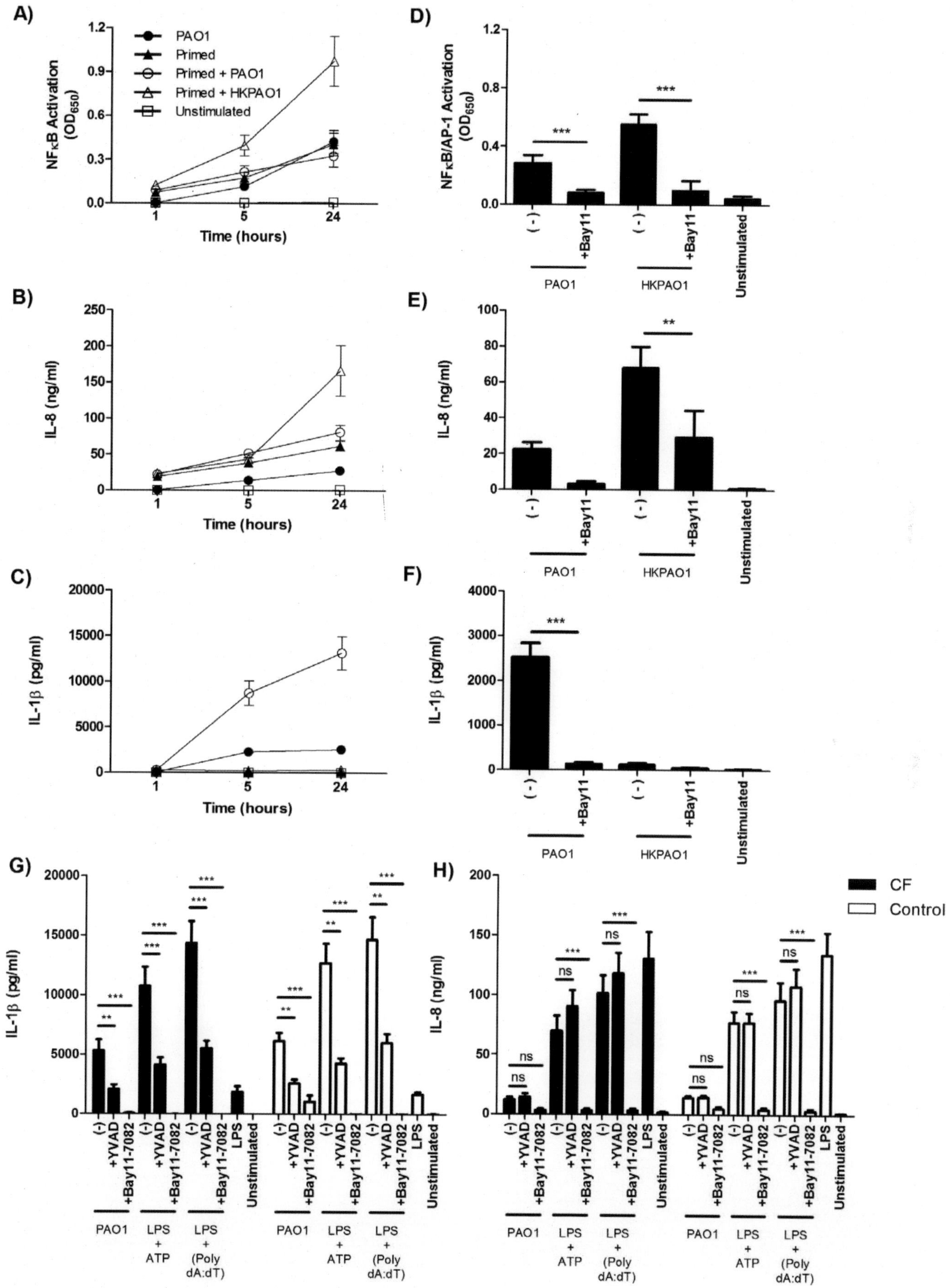

A)
PAO1
Primed
Primed + PAO1
Primed + HKPAO1
Unstimulated
NFκB Activation (OD650)
Time (hours)
B)
IL-8 (ng/ml)
Time (hours)
C)
IL-1β (pg/ml)
Time (hours)
D)
NFκB/AP-1 Activation (OD650)
(-)
+Bay11
Unstimulated
PAO1
HKPAO1
E)
IL-8 (ng/ml)
F)
IL-1β (pg/ml)
G)
IL-1β (pg/ml)
+YVAD
+Bay11-7082
LPS
Unstimulated
PAO1
LPS + ATP
LPS + (Poly dA:dT)
H)
IL-8 (ng/ml)
ns
CF
Control

Figure 6. NF-κB activation potentiates the degree of IL-1β production and secretion upon inflammasome activation. THP-1 reporter cells were primed overnight with heat-killed *P. aeruginosa* and stimulated the next day with live *P. aeruginosa* or additional heat-killed *P. aeruginosa* for the times indicated. Cell culture supernatants were assayed for (A) NF-κB/AP-1 activity, (B) IL-8, and (C) IL-1β secretion (n = 3–6 experiments). Using the same stimulation method, THP-1 reporter cells were treated with Bay11-7082 (20 μM) for 1 hour prior to priming with heat-killed PAO1 or live PAO1. Supernatants were assayed at 24 hours for (D) NF-κB/AP-1 activity, (E) IL-8, and (F) IL-1β secretion (n = 3–5). PBMCs from CF patients (n = 11–15) and controls (n = 10–13) were treated with z-YVAD-fmk (20 μM) or Bay11-7082 (10 μM) and stimulated with live PAO1 (MOI = 1), ATP (5 mM), or Poly(dA:dT) (1 μg/ml) according to the schedule in Figure 1. (G) IL-1β and (H) IL-8 levels were measured at 24 hours. Statistical analysis was performed using two way ANOVA with Bonferroni correction for multiple comparisons. *, **, and *** signify P<0.05, 0.01, and 0.001.

and PBMCs with the NF-κB inhibitor Bay11-7082 significantly inhibited both IL-1β and IL-8 secretion (Fig. 6d–h). Therefore, the IL-1β and IL-8 responses observed were both dependent upon NF-κB activation. Priming with heat-killed *P. aeruginosa*, like LPS, is unable to induce a strong IL-1β response as compared to live *P. aeruginosa* (Fig. 6c), but generated greater NF-κB/AP-1 activation (Fig. 6a) and IL-8 secretion (Fig. 6b) than live bacteria despite stimulation at equivalent MOIs. This may be indicative of the

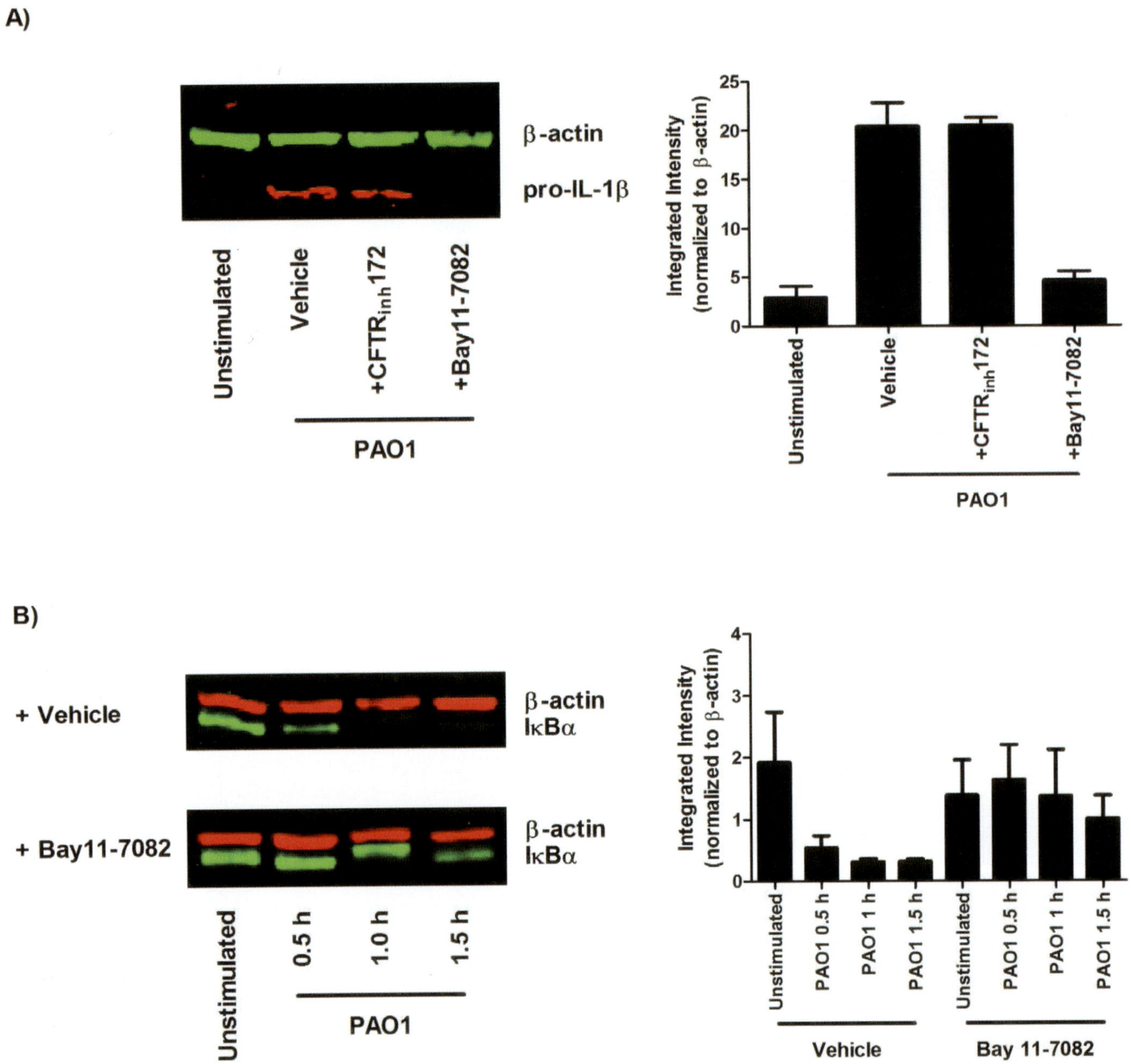

Figure 7. Bay11-7082 inhibits pro-IL-1β production in response to *P. aeruginosa*. PMA-differentiated THP-1 cells were treated with 10 μM $CFTR_{inh}172$ or 20 μM Bay11-7082 and harvested after (A) 4 hours (n = 3) or (B) 0.5, 1, and 1.5 hours (n = 3) stimulation with PAO1. One representative blot is shown with a graph of the averaged fluorescence intensity values over 3 experiments.

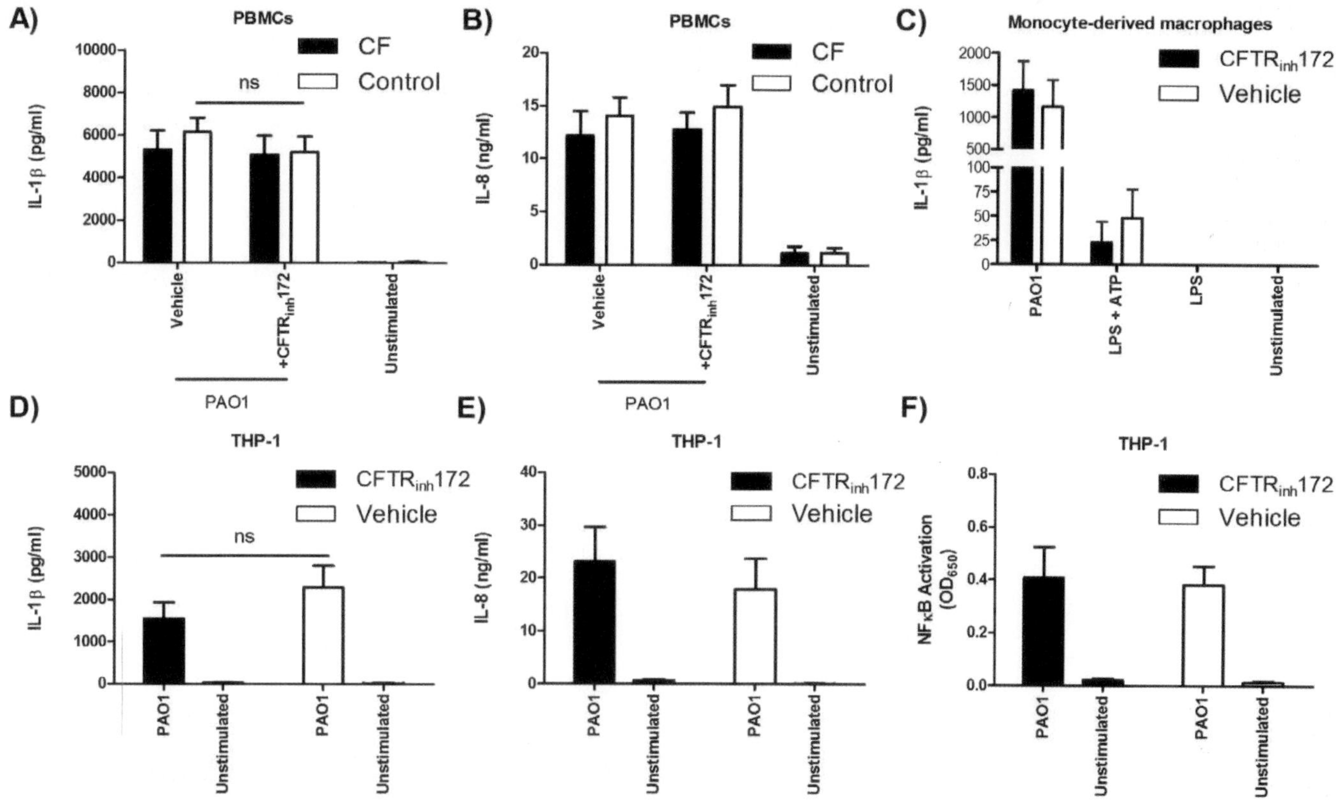

Figure 8. Disruption of CFTR activity does not increase IL-1β production in PBMCs or macrophages. PBMCs from CF patients (n = 15) and controls (n = 13) were treated with $CFTR_{inh}172$ (10 μM) for 18 hours prior to stimulation with live PAO1 (MOI = 1). (A) IL-1β and (B) IL-8 production was measured at 24 hours. (C) Monocytes from controls (n = 3) were differentiated into macrophages. Macrophages were treated with $CFTR_{inh}172$, stimulated as per monocytes, and measured for IL-1β production at 24 hours. THP-1 reporter cells were treated with $CFTR_{inh}172$ 24 hours prior to stimulation with PAO1 and measured for (D) IL-1β secretion, (E) IL-8, and (F) NF-κB/AP-1 activity at 24 hours (n = 4).

different degree and quality of the inflammatory response generated by live as opposed to dead bacteria [59].

Potential shortcomings of these experiments include its translatability to lung disease and issues related to the hypermutability of *P. aeruginosa* during the evolution of chronic infection. Although the responses measured in peripheral blood cells may not completely reflect the responses occurring in the CF lung, PBMCs have a number of useful advantages: (i) PBMCs are not subject to alterations that may emerge from long-term cell culture, cloning and immortalization, and (ii) PBMCs express a large repertoire of innate immune receptors and secrete a broad array of cytokines and chemokines allowing comprehensive analysis of the modulation of inflammatory responses by CFTR. Consideration must also be given to the nature of *P. aeruginosa* infection and genotypic changes in *P. aeruginosa* as infection progresses. *P. aeruginosa* mediates inflammasome activation through its type III secretion system (T3SS) and the NLRC4 inflammasome [19,20]. However, clones of *P. aeruginosa* established during chronic infection may accumulate mutations in virulence factors such as *exsA* [60]. By employing a deletion mutant in *exsA*, the key regulator in T3SS transcription, we confirmed that the T3SS is important for IL-1β secretion (Fig. 5a–b), and that depending on the adaptation in type III secretion, the host IL-1β response may be up or downregulated [19,60,61].

In conclusion, our data are consistent with a role for hematopoietic cells, not airway epithelial cells, as the major source of inflammasome-mediated IL-1β production in the lungs in response to ATP and *P. aeruginosa*. Furthermore, we find little evidence to support an increased IL-1β inflammatory response to NF-κB/Inflammasome stimulation in CF patients. Further studies are warranted to determine if adaptations of *P. aeruginosa* during the course of chronic lung infection alters inflammasome activation, and whether this can be correlated with disease severity in CF.

Materials and Methods

Ethics Statement

Blood samples were obtained with informed written consent from control subjects and CF patients at the BC Children's Hospital. Consent was obtained for children by their parent or legal guardian. Subjects 7 years of age and older were required to provide informed assent as well. Protocols were approved by the Clinical Research Ethics Board (H09-01192).

Cell Culture

CF (IB3-1 and CuFi-1) and control (S9 and NuLi-1) cells were obtained from the American Type Culture Collection. IB3-1 cells were derived from a patient expressing the ΔF508 and W1282X mutations and CuFi-1 were derived from a ΔF508 homozygous patient. S9 cells are IB3-1 cells that have been transfected with CFTR using an adeno-associated viral vector and NuLi-1 cells were derived from a patient possessing a wild-type CFTR genotype. THP1-XBlue cells stably express a secreted embryonic alkaline phosphatase (SEAP) reporter inducible by NF-κB and AP-1 (Invivogen). Cells were cultured as recommended by their respective suppliers using standard protocols. S9 and IB3-1 cells were cultured in basal LHC-8 (Invitrogen) supplemented with 10% (v/v) fetal bovine serum (FBS), 2 mM L-glutamine, and 1 mM sodium pyruvate. NuLi-1/CuFi-1 cells were cultured in BEBM serum-free medium (Lonza) with supplement bullet kit (EGF, hydrocortisone, bovine pituitary extract, transferrin, bovine insulin, triiodothyronine, epinephrine, retinoic acid), 2 mM L-glutamine, and 1 mM sodium pyruvate. PBMCs from CF patients and controls were cultured in RPMI-1640 (Hyclone) supplemented with 10% FBS, 2 mM L-glutamine, and 1 mM sodium pyruvate (complete RPMI). THP1-XBlue cells were cultured in complete RPMI with the addition of zeocin (100 μg/ml) to select for cells expressing the SEAP NF-κB/AP-1 reporter. Prior to stimulation, bronchial epithelial cell lines were plated in coated [62] 96-well plates (BD Biosciences) at 3×10^4 cells/well unless indicated, and allowed to adhere overnight. Plates for S9 and IB3-1 stimulations were coated in a mixture of bovine serum albumin (100 μg/ml), fibronectin (10 μg/ml), and bovine collage type I (30 μg/ml) (BD Biosciences). Plates for NuLi-1 and CuFi-1 were coated with collagen type IV (60 μg/ml) (Sigma Aldrich). PBMCs were plated in 96-well plates at a density of 1.5×10^5 cells/well in 200 μl (7.5×10^5 cells/mL). THP-1 reporter cells were differentiated into a macrophage-like phenotype using 50 ng/ml of phorbol 12-myristate 13-acetate (PMA) (Sigma Aldrich) for 24 hours at a density of 1×10^5 cells/well in 200 μl (5×10^5 cells/ml). Cells were washed with PBS and allowed to rest a further 42 hours prior to stimulation.

CF and control subject PBMCs

The diagnosis of CF was established by typical clinical features, increased sweat chloride concentrations (>60 mmol/l), and detection of CF-inducing mutations. All patients with CF were clinically stable at the time of blood donation, and we excluded any subjects who were receiving systemic corticosteroids due to potential immunomodulatory activity. Control samples were provided by healthy adult volunteers. In previously published work we have demonstrated that TLR-mediated inflammatory responses are stable in humans from birth to 60 years old [63], therefore did not age-match the CF patients and control subjects. Peripheral blood was collected in sodium heparin tubes (BD Biosciences) and PBMCs were isolated using density gradient centrifugation on Ficoll-Paque™ Plus (GE Healthcare). The layer containing PBMCs was isolated, washed twice in PBS and resuspended in complete RPMI. Cells were enumerated by trypan blue exclusion using the Countess automated cell counter (Invitrogen). For derivation of macrophages from monocytes, monocytes were allowed to adhere to plastic for 2 hours in RPMI 1640 after which non-adherent cells were removed. Monocytes were allowed to differentiate in RPMI 1640 supplemented with 10% human AB serum for 10 days.

Cell stimulation and cytokine quantification

Bronchial epithelial cells were plated and allowed to adhere overnight prior to stimulation. Bronchial epithelial cells were rested or primed with LPS for 5 hours and stimulated with live *P. aeruginosa* PAO1 or ATP for the times indicated. PBMCs and THP-1 reporter cells were either rested or primed with LPS (Invivogen) or heat-killed PAO1 overnight (16 hours). The next day the cells were challenged with live PAO1, PAO1Δ*exsA*, ATP (Invivogen), or Poly(dA:dT) (Sigma Aldrich) for the times indicated (see Fig. 1). For stimulations with Poly(dA:dT), lipofectamine LTX was used at a 1:1 (w:v) ratio of μg of DNA to μl of lipofectamine and was mixed 30 minutes prior to stimulation. The NF-κB inhibitor Bay11-7082 (Invivogen) was added to cultures 1 hour prior to priming. If no priming was involved, inhibitor was added 1 hour prior to inflammasome stimulation. The CFTR inhibitor $CFTR_{inh}172$ (Sigma Aldrich) was added to cultures 18 hours prior to inflammasome stimulation. The caspase-1 inhibitor z-YVAD-fmk (Biovision) was added to cultures 1 hour prior to inflammasome stimulation. Supernatants were collected and stored at −20°C. Cytokines released into supernatants from PBMCs stimulated with inflammasome activators were quantified using sandwich ELISA (eBioscience).

Immunoblotting

1×10^6 cells were seeded in 12-well plates, stimulated as indicated, and lysed in RIPA buffer supplemented with Halt protease and phosphatase inhibitor cocktail (Thermo Scientific). Protein concentrations were determined by Bradford assay (Thermo Scientific). Lysates were resolved by electrophoreses on 10% SDS-polyacrylamide gels and transferred onto PVDF membranes (Millipore). Blots were blocked for 1 hour at room temperature and probed overnight at 4°C for pro-IL-1β (Santa Cruz), IκBα (Cell Signaling), or β-actin (Cell Signaling). Blots were subsequently probed with fluorescently-labeled secondary antibodies, IRDye® 680 or 800CW (LI-COR Biosciences) for 1 hour. Both blocking and probing steps were carried out in tris-buffered saline (G Biosciences) containing 5% bovine serum albumin and 0.1% TWEEN 20 (Calbiochem). Blots were imaged on a LI-COR Odyssey infrared imaging system (LI-COR Biosciences) and quantified using the included analysis software.

Quantification of caspase-1 activity

Bronchial epithelial cells were plated in 6-well plates at 5×10^5 cells/well overnight. Cells were primed with LPS for 5 hours and stimulated with ATP for 1 hour or stimulated with live PAO1 for 3 hours. PBMCs were stimulated the same day as blood donation. PBMCs were seeded in a 96-well plate at a density of 4.5×10^5 cells/well (2.5×10^6 cells/ml), primed with LPS for 5 hours and then stimulated with ATP for 1 hour or Poly(dA:dT) for 3 hours or stimulated with live PAO1 for 3 hours. Caspase-1 activity was measured using FLICA (Immunochemistry Technologies), a cell-permeable fluorescent probe (FAM-YVAD-fmk) that binds active caspase-1. Cells were incubated 1 hour with FLICA at 37°C and stained with PE-Cy7-conjugated anti-CD14 antibodies (eBioscience) to identify monocytes. The gating strategy consisted of including live cells that were CD14 positive which were subsequently analyzed for the frequency of FLICA positive cells.

NF-κB/AP-1 Activity Assay

Supernatants from THP-1 reporter cells were incubated with Quanti-Blue substrate (Invivogen) at 37°C and allowed to develop for 16–18 hours. Quanti-Blue contains a substrate for alkaline phosphatase and changes in the amount of NF-κB/AP-1 activity were quantified by optical density ($\lambda = 655$) measured using a SpectraMax 384 Plus plate reader and SoftMax Pro software (Molecular Devices).

Bacterial strains

P. aeruginosa laboratory strains PAO1 and the PAO1Δ*exsA* mutant were obtained from Dr. Robert Hancock. *P. aeruginosa* strains PAO1 and PAO1Δ*exsA* were grown from overnight cultures in Luria Bertani (LB) broth and LB+streptomycin (150 μg/ml) until mid-logarithmic phase. Cells were washed once in PBS and resuspended in PBS to an optical density of 0.5 ($\lambda = 600$ nm). To prepare heat-killed bacteria, live PAO1 was resuspended in PBS to an optical density of 0.5 and heated at 60°C for 1 hour. For stimulations, live PAO1 was resuspended to an optical density of 0.5 in PBS and further diluted in culture medium prior to stimulation to achieve the desired multiplicity of infection. Heat-killed PAO1 was added in a volume equivalent to that used to achieve an MOI of 1 for live PAO1.

Statistics

All graphs display the mean ± SEM and were generated with Prism 5 (Graphpad). Statistical significance was determined by performing one or two-way ANOVA and the Bonferroni post-test where applicable.

Acknowledgments

Patients, family, and staff at the BC Children's Hospital CF Clinic for support of this research. Dr. RE Hancock for *P. aeruginosa* PAO1 and PAO1Δ*exsA* strains.

Author Contributions

Conceived and designed the experiments: AT AS. Performed the experiments: AT AS RJ. Analyzed the data: AT AS RJ AFH. Contributed reagents/materials/analysis tools: MAC PML SET. Wrote the paper: AT AFH PML SET.

References

1. O'Sullivan BP, Freedman SD (2009) Cystic fibrosis. The Lancet 373: 1891–1904.
2. Elizur A, Cannon CL, Ferkol TW (2008) Airway Inflammation in Cystic Fibrosis. Chest 133: 489–495.
3. Hamutcu R, Rowland JM, Horn MV, Kaminsky C, MacLaughlin EF, et al. (2002) Clinical Findings and Lung Pathology in Children with Cystic Fibrosis. Am J Respir Crit Care Med 165: 1172–1175.
4. Venkatakrishnan A, Stecenko AA, King G, Blackwell TR, Brigham KL, et al. (2000) Exaggerated Activation of Nuclear Factor-kappa B and Altered Ikappa B-beta Processing in Cystic Fibrosis Bronchial Epithelial Cells. Am J Respir Cell Mol Biol 23: 396–403.
5. Weber AJ, Soong G, Bryan R, Saba S, Prince A (2001) Activation of NF-kappaB in airway epithelial cells is dependent on CFTR trafficking and Cl- channel function. Am J Physiol Lung Cell Mol Physiol 281: L71–78.
6. Machen TE (2006) Innate immune response in CF airway epithelia: hyperinflammatory? American Journal of Physiology - Cell Physiology 291: C218–C230.
7. Cantin A (1995) Cystic fibrosis lung inflammation: early, sustained, and severe. Am J Respir Crit Care Med 151: 939–941.
8. Koehler DR, Downey GP, Sweezey NB, Tanswell AK, Hu J (2004) Lung inflammation as a therapeutic target in cystic fibrosis. Am J Respir Cell Mol Biol 31: 377–381.
9. Dinarello CA (2009) Immunological and Inflammatory Functions of the Interleukin-1 Family. Annual Review of Immunology 27: 519–550.
10. Weber A, Wasiliew P, Kracht M (2010) Interleukin-1 (IL-1) Pathway. Sci Signal 3: cm1-.
11. Lamkanfi M (2011) Emerging inflammasome effector mechanisms. Nat Rev Immunol 11: 213–220.
12. Martinon F, Burns K, Tschopp J (2002) The Inflammasome: A Molecular Platform Triggering Activation of Inflammatory Caspases and Processing of proIL-β. Molecular Cell 10: 417–426.
13. Agostini L, Martinon F, Burns K, McDermott MF, Hawkins PN, et al. (2004) NALP3 Forms an IL-1β-Processing Inflammasome with Increased Activity in Muckle-Wells Autoinflammatory Disorder. Immunity 20: 319–325.
14. Mariathasan S, Weiss DS, Newton K, McBride J, O'Rourke K, et al. (2006) Cryopyrin activates the inflammasome in response to toxins and ATP. Nature 440: 228–232.
15. Mariathasan S, Newton K, Monack DM, Vucic D, French DM, et al. (2004) Differential activation of the inflammasome by caspase-1 adaptors ASC and Ipaf. Nature 430: 213–218.
16. Miao EA, Alpuche-Aranda CM, Dors M, Clark AE, Bader MW, et al. (2006) Cytoplasmic flagellin activates caspase-1 and secretion of interleukin 1beta via Ipaf. Nat Immunol 7: 569–575.
17. Fernandes-Alnemri T, Yu J-W, Datta P, Wu J, Alnemri ES (2009) AIM2 activates the inflammasome and cell death in response to cytoplasmic DNA. Nature 458: 509–513.
18. Hornung V, Ablasser A, Charrel-Dennis M, Bauernfeind F, Horvath G, et al. (2009) AIM2 recognizes cytosolic dsDNA and forms a caspase-1-activating inflammasome with ASC. Nature 458: 514–518.
19. Sutterwala FS, Mijares LA, Li L, Ogura Y, Kazmierczak BI, et al. (2007) Immune recognition of Pseudomonas aeruginosa mediated by the IPAF/NLRC4 inflammasome. The Journal of Experimental Medicine 204: 3235–3245.
20. Miao EA, Ernst RK, Dors M, Mao DP, Aderem A (2008) Pseudomonas aeruginosa activates caspase 1 through Ipaf. Proceedings of the National Academy of Sciences 105: 2562–2567.
21. Douglas TA, Brennan S, Gard S, Berry L, Gangell C, et al. (2009) Acquisition and eradication of P. aeruginosa in young children with cystic fibrosis. European Respiratory Journal 33: 305–311.
22. Bauernfeind FG, Horvath G, Stutz A, Alnemri ES, MacDonald K, et al. (2009) Cutting Edge: NF-κB Activating Pattern Recognition and Cytokine Receptors License NLRP3 Inflammasome Activation by Regulating NLRP3 Expression. The Journal of Immunology 183: 787–791.
23. Kahlenberg JM, Lundberg KC, Kertesy SB, Qu Y, Dubyak GR (2005) Potentiation of Caspase-1 Activation by the P2X7 Receptor Is Dependent on TLR Signals and Requires NF-κB-Driven Protein Synthesis. The Journal of Immunology 175: 7611–7622.
24. Cogswell J, Godlevski M, Wisely G, Clay W, Leesnitzer L, et al. (1994) NF-kappa B regulates IL-1 beta transcription through a consensus NF- kappa B binding site and a nonconsensus CRE-like site. The Journal of Immunology 153: 712–723.
25. Hiscott J, Marois J, Garoufalis J, D'Addario M, Roulston A, et al. (1993) Characterization of a functional NF-kappa B site in the human interleukin 1 beta promoter: evidence for a positive autoregulatory loop. Mol Cell Biol 13: 6231–6240.
26. Bonfield T, Panuska J, Konstan M, Hilliard K, Hilliard J, et al. (1995) Inflammatory cytokines in cystic fibrosis lungs [published erratum appears in Am J Respir Crit Care Med 1996 Oct;154(4 Pt 1):following 1217]. Am J Respir Crit Care Med 152: 2111–2118.
27. Osika E, Cavaillon JM, Chadelat K, Boule M, Fitting C, et al. (1999) Distinct sputum cytokine profiles in cystic fibrosis and other chronic inflammatory airway disease. European Respiratory Journal 14: 339–346.
28. Armstrong DS, Hook SM, Jamsen KM, Nixon GM, Carzino R, et al. (2005) Lower Airway Inflammation in Infants with Cystic Fibrosis Detected by Newborn Screening. Pediatric Pulmonology 40: 500–510.
29. Levy H, Murphy A, Zou F, Gerard C, Klanderman B, et al. (2009) IL1B polymorphisms modulate cystic fibrosis lung disease. Pediatric Pulmonology 44: 580–593.
30. Meyer M, Huaux F, Gavilanes X, van den Brule S, Lebecque P, et al. (2009) Azithromycin Reduces Exaggerated Cytokine Production by M1 Alveolar Macrophages in Cystic Fibrosis. Am J Respir Cell Mol Biol. pp 2008–0155OC.
31. Kotrange S, Kopp B, Akhter A, Abdelaziz D, Abu Khweek A, et al. Burkholderia cenocepacia O polysaccharide chain contributes to caspase-1-dependent IL-1beta production in macrophages. J Leukoc Biol 89: 481–488.
32. Xu Y, Krause A, Hamai H, Harvey B-G, Worgall TS, et al. Proinflammatory Phenotype and Increased Caveolin-1 in Alveolar Macrophages with Silenced CFTR mRNA. PLoS ONE 5: e11004.
33. Bruscia EM, Zhang P-X, Ferreira E, Caputo C, Emerson JW, et al. (2009) Macrophages Directly Contribute to the Exaggerated Inflammatory Response in Cystic Fibrosis Transmembrane Conductance Regulator−/− Mice. Am J Respir Cell Mol Biol 40: 295–304.
34. Verhoef PA, Kertesy SB, Lundberg K, Kahlenberg JM, Dubyak GR (2005) Inhibitory Effects of Chloride on the Activation of Caspase-1, IL-1β Secretion, and Cytolysis by the P2X7 Receptor. The Journal of Immunology 175: 7623–7634.
35. Miggin SM, Palsson-McDermott E, Dunne A, Jefferies C, Pinteaux E, et al. (2007) NF-kappaB activation by the Toll-IL-1 receptor domain protein MyD88 adapter-like is regulated by caspase-1. Proc Natl Acad Sci U S A 104: 3372–3377.
36. Vij N, Mazur S, Zeitlin PL (2009) CFTR is a negative regulator of NFkappaB mediated innate immune response. PLoS One 4: e4664.
37. Hunter MJ, Treharne KJ, Winter AK, Cassidy DM, Land S, et al. (2010) Expression of Wild-Type CFTR Suppresses NF-κB-Driven Inflammatory Signalling. PLoS ONE 5: e11598.
38. Juliana C, Fernandes-Alnemri T, Wu J, Datta P, Solorzano L, et al. (2010) Anti-inflammatory compounds parthenolide and Bay 11-7082 are direct inhibitors of the inflammasome. J Biol Chem 285: 9792–9802.
39. Di A, Brown ME, Deriy LV, Li C, Szeto FL, et al. (2006) CFTR regulates phagosome acidification in macrophages and alters bactericidal activity. Nat Cell Biol 8: 933–944.
40. Averna M, Stifanese R, Grosso R, Pedrazzi M, De Tullio R, et al. (2011) Calpain digestion and HSP90-based chaperone protection modulate the level of plasma membrane F508del-CFTR. Biochimica et Biophysica Acta (BBA) - Molecular Cell Research 1813: 50–59.
41. Rzemieniak SE, Hirschfeld AF, Victor RE, Chilvers MA, Zheng D, et al. Acidification-dependent activation of CD1d-restricted natural killer T cells is intact in cystic fibrosis. Immunology 130: 288–295.
42. LeibundGut-Landmann S, Weidner K, Hilbi H, Oxenius A (2011) Nonhematopoietic Cells Are Key Players in Innate Control of Bacterial Airway Infection. The Journal of Immunology 186: 3130–3137.

43. Reiniger N, Lee MM, Coleman FT, Ray C, Golan DE, et al. (2007) Resistance to Pseudomonas aeruginosa Chronic Lung Infection Requires Cystic Fibrosis Transmembrane Conductance Regulator-Modulated Interleukin-1 (IL-1) Release and Signaling through the IL-1 Receptor. Infect Immun 75: 1598–1608.
44. Gasse P, Mary C, Guenon I, Noulin N, Charron S, et al. (2007) IL-1R1/MyD88 signaling and the inflammasome are essential in pulmonary inflammation and fibrosis in mice. The Journal of Clinical Investigation 117: 3786–3799.
45. Churg A, Zhou S, Wang X, Wang R, Wright JL (2009) The role of interleukin-1beta in murine cigarette smoke-induced emphysema and small airway remodeling. Am J Respir Cell Mol Biol 40: 482–490.
46. Blohmke CJ, Victor RE, Hirschfeld AF, Elias IM, Hancock DG, et al. (2008) Innate immunity mediated by TLR5 as a novel antiinflammatory target for cystic fibrosis lung disease. J Immunol 180: 7764–7773.
47. Ward JR, West PW, Ariaans MP, Parker LC, Francis SE, et al. (2010) Temporal interleukin-1beta secretion from primary human peripheral blood monocytes by P2X7-independent and P2X7-dependent mechanisms. J Biol Chem 285: 23147–23158.
48. Netea MG, Nold-Petry CA, Nold MF, Joosten LA, Opitz B, et al. (2009) Differential requirement for the activation of the inflammasome for processing and release of IL-1beta in monocytes and macrophages. Blood 113: 2324–2335.
49. Piccini A, Carta S, Tassi S, Lasiglié D, Fossati G, et al. (2008) ATP is released by monocytes stimulated with pathogen-sensing receptor ligands and induces IL-1β and IL-18 secretion in an autocrine way. Proceedings of the National Academy of Sciences 105: 8067–8072.
50. Del Porto P, Cifani N, Guarnieri S, Di Domenico EG, Mariggio MA, et al. (2011) Dysfunctional CFTR alters the bactericidal activity of human macrophages against Pseudomonas aeruginosa. PLoS ONE 6: e19970.
51. Sorio C, Buffelli M, Angiari C, Ettorre M, Johansson J, et al. (2011) Defective CFTR expression and function are detectable in blood monocytes: development of a new blood test for cystic fibrosis. PLoS ONE 6: e22212.
52. Konstan MW, Hilliard KA, Norvell TM, Berger M (1994) Bronchoalveolar lavage findings in cystic fibrosis patients with stable, clinically mild lung disease suggest ongoing infection and inflammation. Am J Respir Crit Care Med 150: 448–454.
53. Hilliard TN, Regamey N, Shute JK, Nicholson AG, Alton EW, et al. (2007) Airway remodelling in children with cystic fibrosis. Thorax 62: 1074–1080.
54. Khan TZ, Wagener JS, Bost T, Martinez J, Accurso FJ, et al. (1995) Early pulmonary inflammation in infants with cystic fibrosis. Am J Respir Crit Care Med 151: 1075–1082.
55. van de Veerdonk FL, Netea MG, Dinarello CA, Joosten LA. Inflammasome activation and IL-1beta and IL-18 processing during infection. Trends Immunol 32: 110–116.
56. Greten FR, Arkan MC, Bollrath J, Hsu L-C, Goode J, et al. (2007) NF-κB Is a Negative Regulator of IL-1β Secretion as Revealed by Genetic and Pharmacological Inhibition of IKKβ. Cell 130: 918–931.
57. Zheng Y, Lilo S, Brodsky IE, Zhang Y, Medzhitov R, et al. (2011) A Yersinia effector with enhanced inhibitory activity on the NF-kappaB pathway activates the NLRP3/ASC/caspase-1 inflammasome in macrophages. PLoS Pathog 7: e1002026.
58. Kunsch C, Rosen CA (1993) NF-kappa B subunit-specific regulation of the interleukin-8 promoter. Mol Cell Biol 13: 6137–6146.
59. Sander LE, Davis MJ, Boekschoten MV, Amsen D, Dascher CC, et al. (2011) Detection of prokaryotic mRNA signifies microbial viability and promotes immunity. Nature 474: 385–389.
60. Smith EE, Buckley DG, Wu Z, Saenphimmachak C, Hoffman LR, et al. (2006) Genetic adaptation by Pseudomonas aeruginosa to the airways of cystic fibrosis patients. Proc Natl Acad Sci U S A 103: 8487–8492.
61. Roy-Burman A, Savel RH, Racine S, Swanson BL, Revadigar NS, et al. (2001) Type III Protein Secretion Is Associated with Death in Lower Respiratory and Systemic Pseudomonas aeruginosa Infections. Journal of Infectious Diseases 183: 1767–1774.
62. Blohmke CJ, Park J, Hirschfeld AF, Victor RE, Schneiderman J, et al. (2010) TLR5 as an Anti-Inflammatory Target and Modifier Gene in Cystic Fibrosis. The Journal of Immunology 185: 7731–7738.
63. Hirschfeld AF, Bettinger JA, Victor RE, Davidson DJ, Currie AJ, et al. (2007) Prevalence of Toll-like receptor signalling defects in apparently healthy children who developed invasive pneumococcal infection. Clin Immunol 122: 271–278.

12

Plasma sCD14 as a Biomarker to Predict Pulmonary Exacerbations in Cystic Fibrosis

Bradley S. Quon[1,2*], David A. Ngan[1], Pearce G. Wilcox[1,2], S. F. Paul Man[1,2], Don D. Sin[1,2]

1 Centre for Heart Lung Innovation, St. Paul's Hospital, University of British Columbia, Vancouver, British Columbia, Canada, **2** Division of Respiratory Medicine, St. Paul's Hospital, University of British Columbia, Vancouver, British Columbia, Canada

Abstract

Background: One in four cystic fibrosis (CF) patients diagnosed with a pulmonary exacerbation will not recover their baseline lung function despite standard treatment. This highlights the importance of preventing such events. Clinical decision-making can be improved through a simple blood test that predicts individuals at elevated short-term risk of an exacerbation.

Methods: We obtained plasma samples from 30 stable CF patients from the St. Paul's Hospital Adult CF Clinic (Vancouver, Canada). For 15 patients, an additional plasma sample was obtained during an exacerbation. Soluble CD14 (sCD14) and C-reactive protein (CRP) were quantified using ELISA kits. Myeloperoxidase (MPO), interleukin(IL)-6, IL-1β, monocyte chemoattractant protein-1 (MCP-1), vascular endothelial growth factor (VEGF), and granulocyte colony-stimulating factor (G-CSF) were quantified using Luminex™ immunoassays. Stable state biomarker levels were examined in their ability to predict individuals that would experience a pulmonary exacerbation requiring intravenous (IV) antibiotics within 4 months. Paired stable and exacerbation plasma biomarker levels were also compared.

Results: sCD14 levels were significantly higher in patients that experienced a pulmonary exacerbation requiring IV antibiotics within 4 months ($p = 0.001$). sCD14 cut-off value of 1450 ng/mL was associated with an area under the curve of 0.91 (95% CI 0.83–0.99) for predicting an exacerbation within 4 months of a stable visit, with a sensitivity of 100% and specificity of 82%. Plasma sCD14 levels were significantly higher during exacerbations than during periods of clinical stability ($p = 0.03$).

Conclusions: Plasma sCD14 is a promising biomarker for identifying CF patients who will exacerbate within 4 months of a stable visit but requires further study in larger, independent cohorts.

Editor: Dominik Hartl, University of Tübingen, Germany

Funding: This study was supported by a British Columbia Lung Association Grant-in-Aid (http://www.bc.lung.ca/association_and_services/research.html). The funders had no role in study design, data collection and analysis, decision to publish, or preparation of the manuscript.

Competing Interests: The authors have declared that no competing interests exist.

* E-mail: bradley.quon@hli.ubc.ca

Introduction

Cystic fibrosis (CF) pulmonary exacerbations are clinically important events for CF patients. They are associated with reduced quality of life and survival [1,2,3,4]. Despite aggressive treatment with intravenous (IV) antibiotics targeting airway infection, one in four CF patients diagnosed with an exacerbation will fail to regain their prior baseline lung function post-treatment [5]. This suggests exacerbations may lead to irreversible lung damage, thus highlighting the importance of exacerbation prevention and early diagnosis.

Although CF pulmonary exacerbation definitions vary, they are characterized by a combination of changes in symptoms and lung function (e.g. FEV1% predicted) necessitating an augmentation in treatment [6]. However, because these changes occur downstream from the underlying pathogenic processes, there is invariably a delay of several days (if not weeks) between onset of the exacerbation and diagnosis and treatment of these events. This delay contributes to incomplete recovery of patients' health status and lung function. To prevent these delays, however, clinicians would require a highly sensitive and specific (and inexpensive) test that can accurately risk-stratify these patients for imminent exacerbation even when their symptoms and lung function are stable. Exacerbation outcomes can potentially be improved by identifying patients that are at elevated short-term risk of developing an exacerbation. Such individuals can be selectively targeted for initiation or intensification of maintenance therapies to prevent exacerbations. Exacerbations can potentially be prevented with medications such as mucolytic agents and inhaled antibiotics [7]. These individuals can also be monitored more closely, which may lead to earlier exacerbation detection and treatment. Biomarkers reflective of systemic inflammation have demonstrated promise in monitoring CF lung disease activity, even when patient symptoms are stable [8]. Systemic inflammatory changes likely occur upstream from changes in clinical parameters and thus may enhance exacerbation risk-stratification.

The objectives of this study were to identify systemic inflammatory biomarkers that can be used to: 1) predict CF individuals that are at elevated risk of developing an exacerbation within 4 months of a stable visit; and 2) discriminate between CF individuals that are clinically stable vs. those experiencing an exacerbation.

Methods

Study Population

We enrolled 64 adult patients from the Adult Cystic Fibrosis (CF) Clinic at St. Paul's Hospital (Vancouver, British Columbia, Canada) between April 2009 and June 2010 who were clinically stable at the time of baseline assessment. We included patients with two disease-causing CF transmembrane conductance regulator (CFTR) mutations and at least two sweat chloride measurements of greater than 60 mmol/L. Patients who had experienced an exacerbation within 4 weeks of the initial stable visit or had previously undergone a solid organ transplant were excluded. Patients were not required to have a prior history of exacerbations. Written informed consent was obtained from the research subjects and the University of British Columbia – Providence Health Care Research Ethics Board (UBC-PHC REB) approved the study protocol and consent procedure.

Blood Collection

Venous blood samples were collected in clinic, processed for plasma, and stored at −80°C until thawing for batched analysis. Blood was collected during the initial stable assessment and longitudinally during subsequent stable or exacerbation clinic visits up to August 2010. If an enrolled patient missed a clinic appointment, they were not approached outside of clinic to obtain blood samples. Blood samples were classified as being from a stable clinic visit if the subject did not have a significant change in symptoms warranting escalation in therapy within 4 weeks of the blood draw. Blood samples were classified as being from an exacerbation clinic visit if the subject had the need for additional antibiotic treatment (oral or intravenous) as indicated by a recent change in at least two of the following: change in sputum volume or colour, increased cough, increased malaise, fatigue or lethargy, anorexia or weight loss, increased dyspnea, decrease in pulmonary function by 10% or more, radiographic changes [6,9]. Blood was not collected if the patient was already started on antibiotics prior to the exacerbation clinic visit. CF physicians were not blinded to study participation but were blinded to the blood biomarker results, which were performed several months following the clinic visit.

Clinical Information

Spirometric data were obtained using standard techniques, in accordance with guidelines from the American Thoracic Society [10]. Demographic and other clinical data were extracted through chart review. Exacerbations during the follow-up period were ascertained through chart review (up to 2 years following enrollment) by study personnel blinded to the biomarker results. Because follow-up exacerbations were based on chart review, we could not reliably separate out the use of oral antibiotics for prophylaxis, or extra-pulmonary indications (e.g. sinusitis) versus those used for acute exacerbations. Thus, follow-up exacerbations were defined based on the need for intravenous antibiotic treatment as indicated by a recent change in at least two of the following: change in sputum volume or colour, increased cough, increased malaise, fatigue or lethargy, anorexia or weight loss, increased dyspnea, decrease in pulmonary function by 10% or more, radiographic changes [6,9]. Infection status was defined based on the sputum culture results reported at the time of the CF clinic encounter.

Samples Analyzed

A priori, we decided to analyze plasma samples from 30 out of 64 patients in this pilot study. We selected all 15 (out of 64) patients who had a paired sample collected during clinical stability followed by an exacerbation visit. We then randomly selected an additional 15 patients from the remaining 49 patients. All 15 patients had at least one initial stable sample and 10 of the 15 patients had 2 subsequent stable samples to allow for the analysis of variability in measurements over 3 consecutive stable clinic visits (**Figure 1**).

Biomarker Assays

Circulating proteins from the following inflammatory pathways were selected based on review of the literature and the availability of reliable commercial immunoassays: 1) acute phase proteins; 2) pro-inflammatory cytokines; 3) markers of neutrophilic inflammation; and 4) markers of tissue injury/hypoxia. Acute phase proteins included C-reactive protein (CRP) and soluble cluster of differentiation 14 (sCD14), which were measured using enzyme-linked immunosorbent assay (ELISA) kits (R&D Systems, Minneapolis, MN) with a coefficient of variation of 2.8% and 3.1%, respectively. Cytokines involved in the early phase inflammatory response included interleukin-6 (IL-6), IL-1β, and monocyte chemoattractant protein-1 (MCP-1), which were quantified using high-sensitivity Luminex® bead-based multiplex assays (R&D Systems, Minneapolis, MN) with a coefficient of variation of 3.5%, 6.9%, and 3.3%, respectively. Markers of neutrophilic inflammation included granulocyte colony-stimulating factor (G-CSF) and myeloperoxidase (MPO), and a marker of tissue injury/hypoxia included vascular endothelial growth factor (VEGF). These markers were also quantified using high-sensitivity Luminex® bead-based multiplex assays (R&D Systems, Minneapolis, MN) with a coefficient of variation of 5.3%, 3.9%, and 5.7% respectively. All samples were measured in duplicate and by study personnel who were blinded to patient characteristics and to the study visit number. To mitigate batch effect, baseline and exacerbation paired samples were assayed on the same plates.

Statistical Analysis

Descriptive statistics were presented as medians/interquartile ranges or numbers/proportions. The relationship between stable visit biomarker level and FEV1% predicted was examined using Spearman's rank correlation coefficient. Variability in biomarker measurement, including FEV1% predicted, over three consecutive stable clinic visits was examined using a coefficient of variation (calculated as standard deviation divided by the mean).

Following log transformation to normalize the data, we used the two-group t-test to compare stable visit biomarker levels in patients who did vs. did not develop a pulmonary exacerbation requiring IV antibiotics within 4 months. For biomarkers that were significantly different between the two groups, we performed an area under receiver operating characteristic (ROC) curve analysis to evaluate various biomarker cut-off values to predict exacerbations requiring IV antibiotics within 4 months of the stable visit. We also conducted a post-hoc sub-group analysis to examine area under ROC curve stratified by *Pseudomonas* infection status (positive vs. negative) and median baseline lung function (below median FEV1% predicted vs. equal to or above median FEV1% predicted).

Lastly, biomarker levels when a patient was clinically stable vs. experiencing a pulmonary exacerbation were compared using a paired t-test, following log transformation to normalize the data if

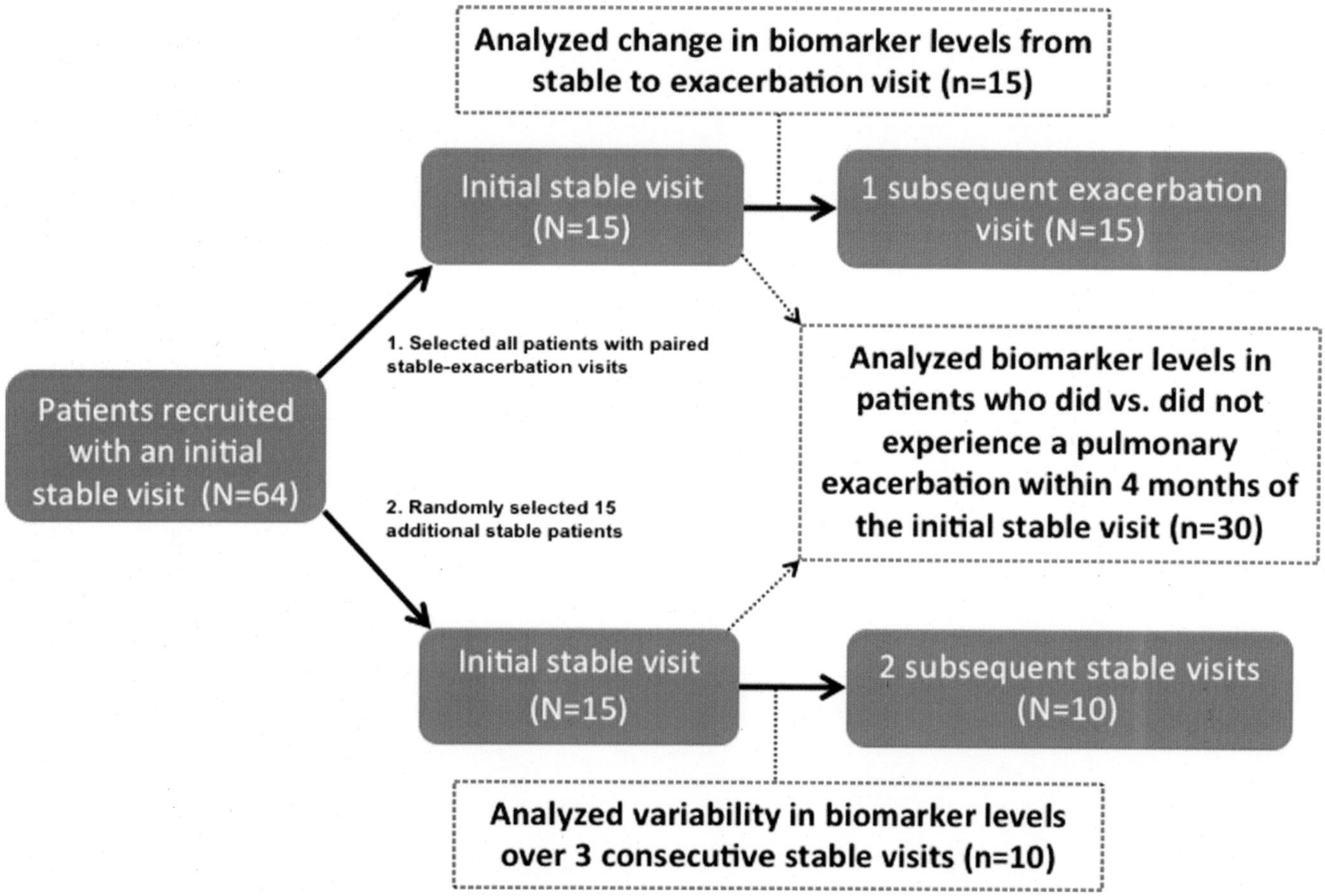

Figure 1. Blood collection schedule and analysis plan.

the paired differences were not normally distributed. P-values of less than 0.05 were considered statistically significant (two-tailed test). All analyses were conducted using STATA 12.1 (College Station, TX) and figures were created using GraphPad PRISM 6 (LaJolla, CA).

Results

Patient Demographics

The study population was generally representative of patients typically followed at an adult CF clinic with a few notable exceptions (**Table 1**). There was a slight over-representation of males and the prevalence of CF-related diabetes was lower than reported in the literature, as it was stringently defined based on the need for insulin therapy. Seven of 30 (23%) patients were diagnosed with an exacerbation requiring IV antibiotics in the year prior to enrolment.

Blood Biomarker Levels and Stable Lung Function

CRP and G-CSF levels inversely correlated with FEV1% predicted at the time of initial assessment, when the patients were deemed clinically stable (**Table 2**). There was also an inverse relationship between MPO level and FEV1% predicted, but did not reach statistical significance ($p = 0.09$). sCD14, IL-6, IL-1β, MCP-1, and VEGF levels were not related with lung function measurements during clinical stability.

Stable Visit Variability in Blood Biomarker Levels

Based on three consecutive stable visit measurements from 10 patients collected longitudinally over a median period of 9.2 (7.1 to 12.4) months, there was wide variability in levels (based on coefficient of variation) of most biomarkers except FEV1% predicted and sCD14 (**Table 3**).

Stable Visit Blood Biomarker Levels in Patients who did vs. did not have an Exacerbation Requiring IV Antibiotics within 4 Months

Eight out of 30 (27%) patients were diagnosed with a pulmonary exacerbation requiring IV antibiotics within 4 months of the stable visit. sCD14 levels measured at the time of stable assessment were significantly higher in patients who went on to develop a pulmonary exacerbation in 4 months, compared to those who did not ($p = 0.001$) (Figure 2). No other biomarker levels were significantly different in patients who did vs. did not exacerbate within 4 months of a stable blood draw (Table 4).

sCD14 Level and the Short-term Risk of Exacerbation Requiring IV Antibiotics

Various sCD14 cut-off values were examined and a cut-off value of 1450 ng/mL resulted in a maximum area under the ROC curve of 0.91 (95% CI 0.83–0.99) (**Figure 3**). This cut-off corresponded to a sensitivity of 100% (8 of 8 patients) and specificity of 82% (18 of 22 patients). In a post-hoc sub-group analysis comparing ROC curves according to baseline *Pseudomonas*

Table 1. Baseline patient characteristics.

Baseline Characteristic*	All Participants (N = 30)	Participants with paired stable-exacerbation visits (N = 15)	Participants with three consecutive stable visits (N = 10)
Age (years)	28 (20–37)	27 (21–33)	27 (22–34)
Male	19 (63%)	11 (73%)	5 (50%)
FEV1% predicted	68 (39–96)	66 (35–92)	78 (59–92)
BMI (kg/m^2)	22 (20–26)	22 (21–23)	23 (22–24)
***Pseudomonas* culture (+)**	16 (53%)	10 (67%)	3 (30%)
CF-related diabetes (on insulin)	5 (17%)	1 (7%)	2 (20%)
Use of IV antibiotics in the prior year	7 (23%)	5 (33%)	2 (20%)
Number of exacerbations requiring IV antibiotics in the prior year	0 (0–0)	0 (0–1)	0 (0–0)

*Median (interquartile range) or Number (proportion).
Abbreviations: BMI = body mass index; FEV1 = forced expiratory volume in 1 second; IV = intravenous.

infection status (positive vs. negative) and lung disease severity (below vs. equal to or above median value of 75% predicted), the area under ROC curves were similar across all sub-groups (data not presented).

Paired Stable and Exacerbation Biomarker Measurements

Fifteen out of 30 (50%) patients had paired stable-exacerbation blood samples collected during consecutive CF clinic visits. The median time between paired samples was 3.0 (2.1 to 4.9) months. There was a significant decrease in the geometric mean FEV1% predicted from stable to exacerbation measurement (**Table 5**). Six out of fifteen (40%) exacerbations required treatment with IV antibiotics and the remainder were treated with oral antibiotics. Six out of fifteen (40%) patients had a new bacterium isolated from their exacerbation sputum culture relative to their stable sputum culture (3 *Haemophilus influenza*, 1 *Burkholderia cepacia complex* – genomovar multivorans, 1 *Streptococcus pneumonia*, and 1 *Acinetobacter baumanni*). sCD14 was the only biomarker that changed significantly from paired stable to exacerbation measurements ($p = 0.03$) (**Table 5**). There was a trend toward a significant increase of CRP, MCP-1, and MPO levels from stable to exacerbation measurements (all $p<0.10$). Subgroup analyses based on potential predictors of more severe systemic inflammation at the time of exacerbation, such as the need for IV antibiotics and growth of new bacteria on sputum culture, did not significantly modify any of the results (data not presented).

Discussion

New biomarkers of CF lung disease activity are urgently required to enhance clinical decision-making and improve exacerbation outcomes. Given the adverse impact that exacerbation events have on CF patients, it is a priority to prevent them. A biomarker to identify individuals that are at elevated short-term risk of developing an exacerbation will allow for more selective targeting of preventive therapies (such as mucolytics and inhaled antibiotics) in those most likely to benefit. Discovery of a biomarker that reliably increases early in the course of an exacerbation is also desirable as it may lead to earlier detection

Table 2. Correlation between blood biomarker levels and stable (baseline) lung function.

Biomarker	N	Rho (ρ)	P-value†
sCD14	30	−0.15	0.4
CRP	30	−0.42	0.02
IL-6	29*	0.16	0.4
IL-1β	23*	−0.27	0.2
MCP-1	30	0.11	0.6
G-CSF	30	−0.49	0.01
MPO	30	−0.31	0.09
VEGF	26*	0.26	0.2

*Missing individuals had undetectable levels.
†Spearman's rank correlation.
Abbreviations: sCD14 = soluble cluster of differentiation 14; CRP = C-reactive protein; IL = interleukin; MCP-1 = monocyte chemotattractant protein-1; G-CSF = granulocyte colony-stimulating factor; MPO = myeloperoxidase; VEGF = vascular endothelial growth factor.

Table 3. Coefficient of variation for blood biomarker levels over 3 consecutive stable visits.

Biomarker	N	Coefficient of Variation†
FEV1 % Predicted	10	4
sCD14	10	7
CRP	10	44
IL-6	7*	43
IL-1β	4*	55
MCP-1	10	25
G-CSF	6*	27
MPO	10	26
VEGF	10	52

*Missing individuals had less than 3 measurements due to undetectable levels
†Standard deviation divided by mean
Abbreviations: sCD14 = soluble cluster of differentiation 14; CRP = C-reactive protein; IL = interleukin; MCP-1 = monocyte chemoattractant protein-1; G-CSF = granulocyte colony-stimulating factor; MPO = myeloperoxidase; VEGF = vascular endothelial growth factor

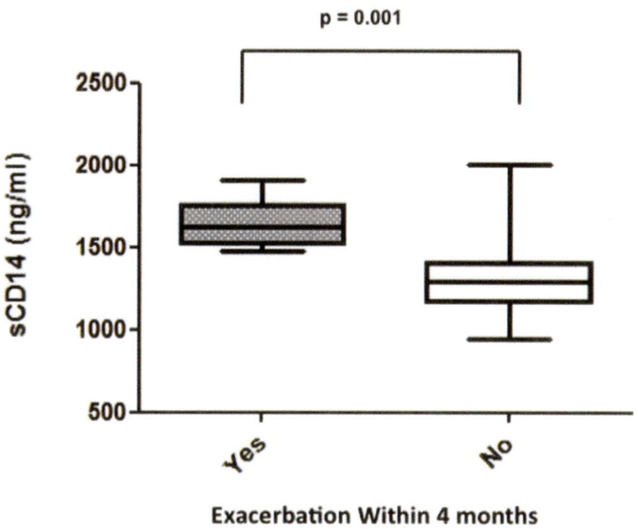

Figure 2. Boxplot of sCD14 levels in patients who did vs. did not experience a pulmonary exacerbation within 4 months.

Table 4. Comparison of blood biomarker levels in patients who did vs. did not experience a pulmonary exacerbation requiring IV antibiotics within 4 months of a stable blood collection.

	Exacerbation within 4 months*		
Biomarker	**Yes (n = 8)**	**No (n = 22)**	**P-value**†
sCD14 (ng/mL)	1645.7 (1.1)	1297.4 (1.2)	0.001
CRP (mg/L)	4.1 (5.3)	2.1 (3.5)	0.2
IL-6 (pg/mL)	2.1 (2.2)	2.8 (3.4)	0.5
IL-1β (pg/mL)	0.5 (2.0)	0.5 (1.8)	0.9
MCP-1 (pg/mL)	95.4 (1.2)	102.3 (1.5)	0.7
G-CSF (pg/mL)	53.0 (3.4)	22.1 (2.8)	0.1
MPO (ng/mL)	454.8 (1.6)	319.6 (1.8)	0.1
VEGF (pg/mL)	53.0 (3.4)	22.1 (2.3)	0.8

*Geometric mean (standard deviation)
†Two-group t-test
Abbreviations: sCD14 = soluble cluster of differentiation 14; CRP = C-reactive protein; IL = interleukin; MCP-1 = monocyte chemoattractant protein-1; G-CSF = granulocyte colony-stimulating factor; MPO = myeloperoxidase; VEGF = vascular endothelial growth factor

and treatment, prior to the establishment of irreversible lung damage.

In this study, we examined several biologically plausible biomarkers of disease activity that could be measured in the systemic circulation. Blood is an attractive biological compartment for biomarker measurement in CF as it can be obtained non-invasively in most clinical laboratories and has the potential for clinical application in patients of all ages and with all stages of lung disease severity. First, we examined whether stable visit biomarker levels were different in patients who were prone to experiencing an exacerbation requiring IV antibiotics within 4 months, compared to those who did not. sCD14 levels were significantly higher in patients who experienced an exacerbation in short-term follow-up. In identifying patients who do vs. do not exacerbate within 4 months of a stable clinic visit, test performance accuracy was optimized using a sCD14 cut-off value of 1450 ng/mL, with an area under ROC curve of 0.91 (95% CI 0.83–0.99). sCD14 possesses other desirable characteristics as a disease activity biomarker as it does not relate to underlying lung disease severity (i.e. FEV1% predicted) and exhibits minimal measurement variability over time when a patient is deemed clinically stable. sCD14 is biologically plausible as a biomarker of disease activity as it is involved in the innate immune response to infection and can mediate phagocytosis by binding to bacterial ligands, such as lipopolyassacharide (LPS), on the surface of gram-negative bacteria [11,12]. It is secreted in a protease-independent manner by monocytes and is cleaved from membrane-bound forms of CD14 on the surface of monocytes and macrophages by proteases such as neutrophil elastase [13]. It is also released as class 2 acute phase proteins from the liver (in response to IL-6), possibly bridging the gap between innate and adaptive immunity [14]. sCD14 has showed promise as a biomarker of pneumonia in children and sepsis in adults [13,15,16].

In our comparison of biomarker levels when a patient was clinically stable vs. experiencing a pulmonary exacerbation, the only biomarker (other than FEV1% predicted) that demonstrated significant change in paired analysis was sCD14. There was also a trend toward a significant increase in CRP, MCP-1, and MPO. For each biomarker, there was substantial overlap observed in stable and exacerbation biomarker levels between patients, which makes the establishment of an absolute cut-off for normal vs. abnormal highly unlikely, which may limit clinical application (**Figure 3**). Moreover, while most patients had an increase in sCD14, CRP, MCP-1 and MPO levels when transitioning from a stable to exacerbation health state, some individual patients had no change or even a slight decrease in biomarker levels (**Figure 4**).

There are several potential limitations to our study. First, this was a pilot study so we selected all 15 patients with paired stable-exacerbation visits and an additional 15 patients of those remaining at random. This aspect of our study design potentially limits the generalizability of our findings but unlikely introduced any systematic bias as this was defined *a priori*. For prediction of exacerbations within 4 months, such events were defined based on IV antibiotic requirement, which allowed for more reliable

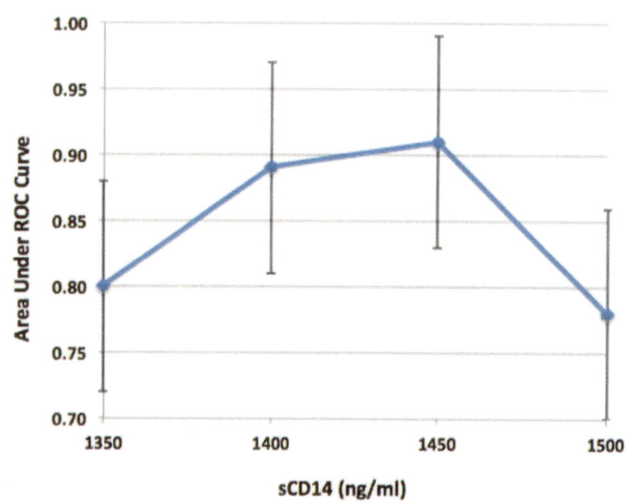

Figure 3. Defining an optimal sCD14 threshold value to predict pulmonary exacerbations requiring IV antibiotics within 4 months.

Table 5. Comparison of paired stable-exacerbation biomarker levels.

Biomarker	N	Stable*	Exacerbation*	P-value†
FEV1 % Predicted	15	64.3 (1.4)	54.6 (1.5)	0.0002
sCD14 (ng/mL)	15	1357.3 (1.2)	1475.0 (1.2)	0.03
CRP (mg/L)	15	4.1 (3.6)	6.7 (3.0)	0.09
IL-6 (pg/mL)	14**	2.2 (2.6)	3.7 (2.3)	0.2
IL-1β (pg/mL)	9**	0.7 (1.8)	0.9 (1.6)	0.8
MCP-1 (pg/mL)	15	95.8 (1.2)	111.7 (1.4)	0.06
G-CSF (pg/mL)	15	46.1 (2.9)	58.4 (3.1)	0.4
MPO (ng/mL)	15	383.2 (1.9)	478.9 (1.8)	0.08
VEGF (pg/mL)	15	10.2 (1.8)	10.0 (1.6)	0.8

*Geometric mean (standard deviation)
**Missing individuals had undetectable levels
†Paired t-test
Abbreviations: sCD14 = soluble cluster of differentiation 14; CRP = C-reactive protein; IL = interleukin; MCP-1 = monocyte chemoattractant protein-1; G-CSF = granulocyte colony-stimulating factor; MPO = myeloperoxidase; VEGF = vascular endothelial growth factor

identification of these events through chart review, as exacerbations requiring oral antibiotics are inconsistently documented in our clinic and are confounded by the fact that almost all patients in the clinic are prophylactically treated with oral macrolides (or a similar antibiotic for those intolerant to macrolides) for exacerbation prevention. This definition resulted in the selection of more severe exacerbations with the likely omission of milder events. Another potential limitation of this definition is that the decision to treat an exacerbation with IV (vs. oral) antibiotics may extend beyond severity of the attack and may relate to the discretion of the treating physician or the preference of the patient. Notwithstanding, it is clinically relevant to focus on the prediction of exacerbations requiring IV antibiotics as they have the greatest impact on patient quality of life and survival and thus should be prioritized for prevention [17,18].

In contrast to the prediction analysis, which exclusively relied on chart review for determining exacerbations, we prospectively collected exacerbation information for the paired analysis. Thus, we could reliably ascertain both mild exacerbations, requiring only oral antibiotics as well as more severe exacerbations requiring IV antibiotic therapy. Indeed, most of the exacerbations determined prospectively were mild events. The enrichment of mild events in the paired analysis may explain the lack of significant change observed in CRP and MPO levels from stable to exacerbation state, both of which have been shown to increase during

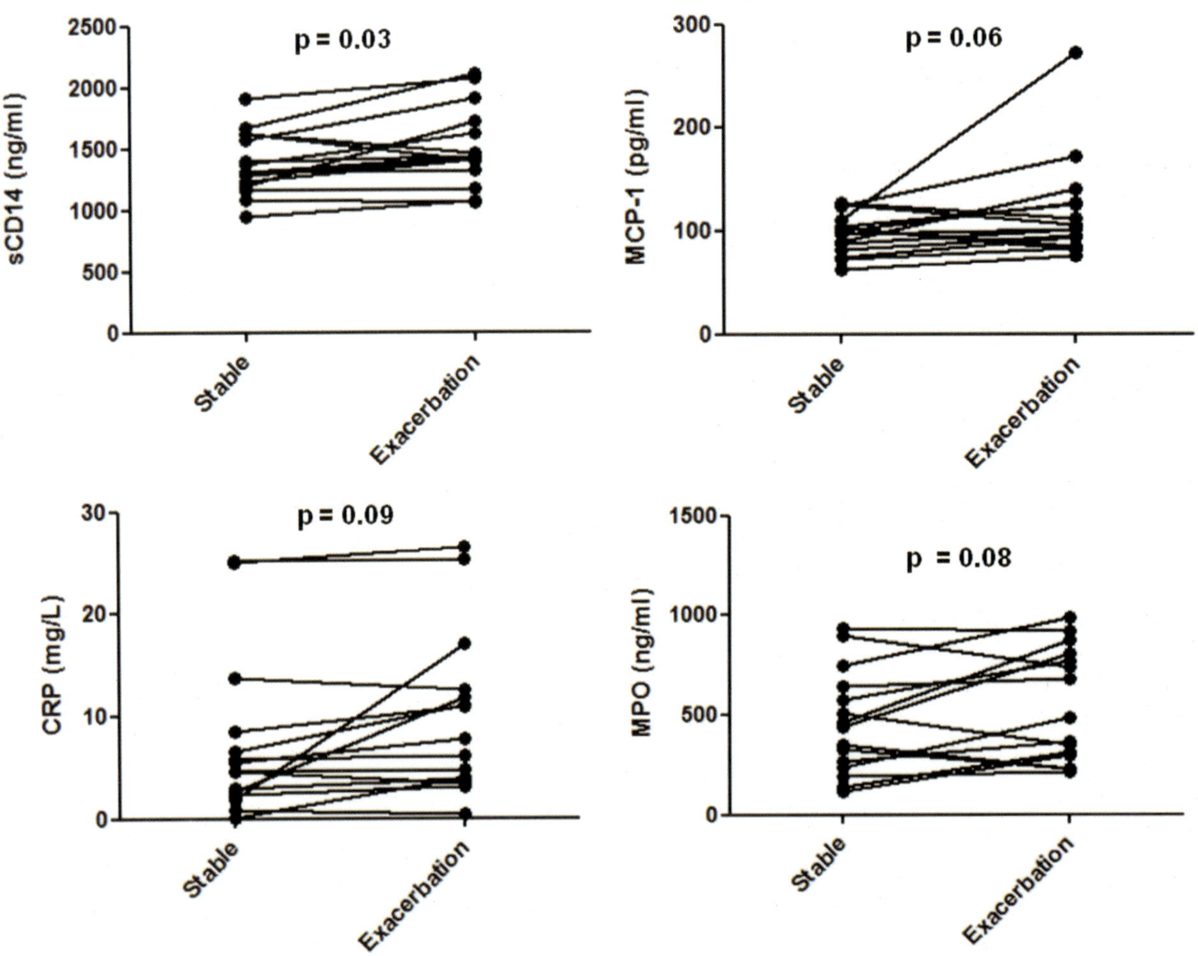

Figure 4. Paired stable-exacerbation biomarker levels for biomarkers with statistically significant (<0.05) or borderline significant change (p<0.10).

exacerbations in prior studies [8,19,20,21,22,23]. We chose four months as the exacerbation prediction interval of interest as most patients are followed-up routinely in the CF clinic every 3 to 4 months and therefore prediction of an event prior to the next clinic visit has the most clinical utility. In a sensitivity analysis, we did not observe a significant difference in the prediction accuracy of sCD14 if the prediction interval was changed to 3 or 6 months (data not presented). Due to our small sample size, we were limited in our ability to combine clinical variables and biomarkers into a multivariate prediction model. However, the high performance accuracy observed for sCD14 alone makes it unlikely that clinical variables would have further improved prognostic accuracy. The small sample size also precluded our ability to identify a high-risk subgroup that is more likely to benefit from blood biomarker analysis.

In conclusion, plasma sCD14 holds promise as a biomarker to identify individuals at elevated short-term risk of a pulmonary exacerbation requiring IV antibiotics but these results must be confirmed in a larger, independent cohort. No plasma biomarkers demonstrated sufficient discriminatory power for the detection of pulmonary exacerbations and therefore new biomarkers of disease activity must be discovered to enhance the early detection of exacerbations.

Author Contributions

Conceived and designed the experiments: BSQ SFPM DDS. Performed the experiments: BSQ DAN. Analyzed the data: BSQ DAN. Contributed reagents/materials/analysis tools: DDS. Wrote the paper: BSQ DAN PGW SFPM DDS.

References

1. Liou TG, Adler FR, Fitzsimmons SC, Cahill BC, Hibbs JR, et al. (2001) Predictive 5-year survivorship model of cystic fibrosis. American journal of epidemiology 153: 345–352.
2. Britto MT, Kotagal UR, Hornung RW, Atherton HD, Tsevat J, et al. (2002) Impact of recent pulmonary exacerbations on quality of life in patients with cystic fibrosis. Chest 121: 64–72.
3. Mayer-Hamblett N, Rosenfeld M, Emerson J, Goss CH, Aitken ML (2002) Developing cystic fibrosis lung transplant referral criteria using predictors of 2-year mortality. American journal of respiratory and critical care medicine 166: 1550–1555.
4. Yi MS, Tsevat J, Wilmott RW, Kotagal UR, Britto MT (2004) The impact of treatment of pulmonary exacerbations on the health-related quality of life of patients with cystic fibrosis: does hospitalization make a difference? The Journal of pediatrics 144: 711–718.
5. Sanders DB, Bittner RC, Rosenfeld M, Hoffman LR, Redding GJ, et al. (2010) Failure to recover to baseline pulmonary function after cystic fibrosis pulmonary exacerbation. American journal of respiratory and critical care medicine 182: 627–632.
6. Bilton D, Canny G, Conway S, Dumcius S, Hjelte L, et al. (2011) Pulmonary exacerbation: towards a definition for use in clinical trials. Report from the EuroCareCF Working Group on outcome parameters in clinical trials. Journal of cystic fibrosis: official journal of the European Cystic Fibrosis Society 10 Suppl 2: S79–81.
7. Flume PA, O'Sullivan BP, Robinson KA, Goss CH, Mogayzel PJ, Jr., et al. (2007) Cystic fibrosis pulmonary guidelines: chronic medications for maintenance of lung health. American journal of respiratory and critical care medicine 176: 957–969.
8. Hakimi Shoki A, Mayer-Hamblett N, Wilcox PG, Sin DD, Quon BS (2013) Systematic Review of Blood Biomarkers in Cystic Fibrosis Pulmonary Exacerbations. Chest.
9. Fuchs HJ, Borowitz DS, Christiansen DH, Morris EM, Nash ML, et al. (1994) Effect of aerosolized recombinant human DNase on exacerbations of respiratory symptoms and on pulmonary function in patients with cystic fibrosis. The Pulmozyme Study Group. The New England journal of medicine 331: 637–642.
10. (1987) Standardization of spirometry–1987 update. Statement of the American Thoracic Society. The American review of respiratory disease 136: 1285–1298.
11. Wright SD (1995) CD14 and innate recognition of bacteria. Journal of immunology 155: 6–8.
12. Wright SD, Ramos RA, Tobias PS, Ulevitch RJ, Mathison JC (1990) CD14, a receptor for complexes of lipopolysaccharide (LPS) and LPS binding protein. Science 249: 1431–1433.
13. Marcos V, Latzin P, Hector A, Sonanini S, Hoffmann F, et al. (2010) Expression, regulation and clinical significance of soluble and membrane CD14 receptors in pediatric inflammatory lung diseases. Respiratory research 11: 32.
14. Bas S, Gauthier BR, Spenato U, Stingelin S, Gabay C (2004) CD14 is an acute-phase protein. Journal of immunology 172: 4470–4479.
15. Landmann R, Zimmerli W, Sansano S, Link S, Hahn A, et al. (1995) Increased circulating soluble CD14 is associated with high mortality in gram-negative septic shock. The Journal of infectious diseases 171: 639–644.
16. Burgmann H, Winkler S, Locker GJ, Presterl E, Laczika K, et al. (1996) Increased serum concentration of soluble CD14 is a prognostic marker in gram-positive sepsis. Clinical immunology and immunopathology 80: 307–310.
17. Hegarty M, Macdonald J, Watter P, Wilson C (2009) Quality of life in young people with cystic fibrosis: effects of hospitalization, age and gender, and differences in parent/child perceptions. Child: care, health and development 35: 462–468.
18. Ellaffi M, Vinsonneau C, Coste J, Hubert D, Burgel PR, et al. (2005) One-year outcome after severe pulmonary exacerbation in adults with cystic fibrosis. American journal of respiratory and critical care medicine 171: 158–164.
19. Eichler I, Nilsson M, Rath R, Enander I, Venge P, et al. (1999) Human neutrophil lipocalin, a highly specific marker for acute exacerbation in cystic fibrosis. The European respiratory journal: official journal of the European Society for Clinical Respiratory Physiology 14: 1145–1149.
20. Rayner RJ, Wiseman MS, Cordon SM, Norman D, Hiller EJ, et al. (1991) Inflammatory markers in cystic fibrosis. Respiratory medicine 85: 139–145.
21. Hendry J, Elborn JS, Nixon L, Shale DJ, Webb AK (1999) Cystic fibrosis: inflammatory response to infection with Burkholderia cepacia and Pseudomonas aeruginosa. The European respiratory journal: official journal of the European Society for Clinical Respiratory Physiology 14: 435–438.
22. Roderfeld M, Rath T, Schulz R, Seeger W, Tschuschner A, et al. (2009) Serum matrix metalloproteinases in adult CF patients: Relation to pulmonary exacerbation. Journal of cystic fibrosis: official journal of the European Cystic Fibrosis Society 8: 338–347.
23. Davidson SJ, Paramothayan S, Hodson ME (2009) Adult cystic fibrosis patients with and without infective exacerbations and their factor XII levels. Blood coagulation & fibrinolysis: an international journal in haemostasis and thrombosis 20: 400–402.

13

Phenotypic Heterogeneity of *Pseudomonas aeruginosa* Populations in a Cystic Fibrosis Patient

Matthew L. Workentine[1,2], Christopher D. Sibley[4], Bryan Glezerson[4], Swathi Purighalla[4], Jens C. Norgaard-Gron[4], Michael D. Parkins[4,5,6], Harvey R. Rabin[4,5,6], Michael G. Surette[1,2,3,4]*

1 Farncombe Family Digestive Health Research Institute, McMaster University, Hamilton, Ontario, Canada, **2** Department of Medicine, McMaster University, Hamilton, Ontario, Canada, **3** Department of Biochemistry and Biomedical Sciences, McMaster University, Hamilton, Ontario, Canada, **4** Department of Microbiology, Immunology and Infectious Diseases, University of Calgary, Calgary, Alberta, Canada, **5** Department of Medicine, University of Calgary, Calgary, Alberta, Canada, **6** Adult Cystic Fibrosis Clinic, University of Calgary, Calgary, Alberta, Canada

Abstract

The opportunistic pathogen *Pseudomonas aeruginosa* chronically infects the lower airways of patients with cystic fibrosis. Throughout the course of infection this organism undergoes adaptations that contribute to its long-term persistence in the airways. While *P. aeruginosa* diversity has been documented, it is less clear to what extent within-patient diversity contributes to the overall population structure as most studies have been limited to the analysis of only a few isolates per patient per time point. To examine *P. aeruginosa* population structure in more detail we collected multiple isolates from individual sputum samples of a patient chronically colonized with *P. aeruginosa*. This strain collection, comprised of 169 clonal isolates and representing three pulmonary exacerbations as well as clinically stable periods, was assayed for a wide selection of phenotypes. These phenotypes included colony morphology, motility, quorum sensing, protease activity, auxotrophy, siderophore levels, antibiotic resistance, and growth profiles. Each phenotype displayed significant variation even within isolates of the same colony morphotype from the same sample. Isolates demonstrated a large degree of individuality across phenotypes, despite being part of a single clonal lineage, suggesting that the *P. aeruginosa* population in the cystic fibrosis airways is being significantly under-sampled.

Editor: John R. Battista, Louisiana State University and A & M College, United States of America

Funding: This work was supported by grants from Cystic Fibrosis Canada to M.G.S and to M.D.P. and a postdoctoral fellowship to M.L.W. M.G.S. is also supported as a Canada Research Chair in Interdisciplinary Microbiome Research. C.D.S. was supported by a Canada Graduate Scholarship from the Canadian Institutes of Health Research. The funders had no role in study design, data collection and analysis, decision to publish, or preparation of the manuscript.

Competing Interests: The authors have declared that no competing interests exist.

* E-mail: surette@mcmaster.ca

Introduction

Cystic fibrosis (CF) is an autosomal recessive disorder where mutations in the CF transmembrane conductance regulator lead to altered ion flux and the reduction of fluid covering the surface of airway epithelial cells [1–3]. Compromised innate immunity including reduced mucociliary clearance in patients with CF, gives a variety of species the opportunity to colonize the lower airways, ultimately generating long-term complex bacterial infections [2,4–6]. The microbial community in the CF lung is known to be complex[7–15] and its changing dynamics can influence severity of disease [10,16]. However, *Pseudomonas aeruginosa* infection is traditionally considered to be the most common agent contributing to lung function decline and ultimate mortality in CF patients [17–19]. *P. aeruginosa* infections in the lower airways can be maintained for decades. Throughout this time *P. aeruginosa* exhibits genetic and phenotypic diversity thought to occur as the organism adapts to the lower airway environment [20,21]. Some factors considered to be the hallmarks of *P. aeruginosa* adaption to the CF airways include a switch to the mucoid phenotype [22] and loss of motility [23]. Diverse colony morphologies from clonal populations of *P. aeruginosa* are also routinely observed in clinical laboratories and some have been linked to increased antibiotic resistance and enhanced cytotoxicity [24–26]. It has been suggested that these colony variants have adaptations specific for persistence in the lower airways [27].

Although such genetic and phenotypic changes have been documented, cross-sectional studies are often limited to a small number time points from a large number of patients [28] and longitudinal studies by a large number of time points from a small number of patients [20] thus the full extent of micro-evolutionary dynamics that might be present throughout the course of infection is not yet well defined. Furthermore, most studies have analyzed a limited number of isolates per sample. Recent evidence suggests that this leads to an underestimation of the true diversity present in a sample. For example, Wilder and colleagues examined quorum-sensing phenotypes in clinical *P. aeruginosa* isolates and found very high within-patient diversity [29]. In addition, large variation in antibiotic resistance profiles was found for *P. aeruginosa* isolates with the same morphotype [30,31]. By way of screening multiple phenotypes Mowat *et al.* have demonstrated high intraspecific diversity in the *P. aeruginosa* Liverpool Epidemic Strain (LES) that is responsible for a significant burden of infection in both Europe and North America [32]. One implication of high intraspecific diversity in the CF airways is that analysis of only a few isolates may lead to a misrepresentation of the *P. aeruginosa* phenotype, such as oversimplified antibiotic resistance profiles. Therefore a clear understanding of *P. aeruginosa* evolutionary dynamics in the CF airways that includes intraspecific diversity is necessary.

In the present study we examined the population dynamics of a newly described transmissible strain of *P. aeruginosa* [33] in a single patient over the course of one year. A number of phenotypes linked to survival and persistence in the CF airways were measured including colony morphology, motility, quorum sensing, proteases, auxotrophy, siderophores, growth profiles and antibiotic resistance. This represents more phenotypes than have been previously examined in single studies of *P. aeruginosa* intraspecific diversity. We observed very high diversity across all phenotypes even within isolates of a single colony morphotype recovered from a single sputum sample, which has been noted previously in LES epidemic *P. aeruginosa* strain [32]. However, we find that each phenotype is highly variable between isolates and not accurately characterized as simply the presence or absence of a phenotype. No obvious patterns in phenotype prevalence or activity was strongly correlated with early exacerbation samples or periods of clinical stability. This suggests that *P. aeruginosa* contribution to acute exacerbation may arise in part through complex population interactions rather than fluctuations in specific virulent strains within the population.

Results

The source patient was a 31 year old male (genotype F508del/F508del) with advanced CF airways disease, whom had been chronically infected with *P. aeruginosa* for 20 years. Thirty-four expectorated sputum samples were collected from the patient over one year, and comprised 16 samples collected during periods of clinical stability and 18 samples collected through three acute pulmonary exacerbations during which the patient was hospitalized and treated with parenteral anti-pseudomonal therapies (Table S1). Multiple *P. aeruginosa* isolates were collected from each sample as well as multiple isolates with identical colony morphologies (representative plate image shown in Figure S1). To ensure that slow growing colonies were not overlooked the plates were allowed to incubate for 72 h, which is longer than usual for a clinical lab. Fourteen unique colony morphologies were identified in a total of 169 isolates and were comprised of equal numbers of mucoid and non-mucoid isolates (Figure 1A). The cell counts for each colony type varied greatly throughout the exacerbation periods and no associations between exacerbation and a particular colony type were observed (Figure 1B). We also noted for all three exacerbations that the total levels of *P. aeruginosa* did not show any decrease, despite antibiotic therapy and resolution of symptoms.

The genetic variability of this population was monitored using pulse field gel electrophoresis (PFGE). The pulse-field patterns reveal that all isolates belong to a single clonal group with only 2–3 band differences between them (Figure 2 and Figure S2), which is indicated by a Dice coefficient of greater than 80% for all the pairwise combinations of isolates. The PFGE patterns of the isolates matched the pattern of a recently identified epidemic strain (highlighted in yellow in Figure 2 and indicated in Figure S2), the Prairie Epidemic Strain (PES), which is known to be present in ~30% of the patients in the clinic that the source patient was attending [33].

To assemble phenotype profiles we measured 21 different phenotypes related to virulence, including swimming, swarming and twitching motility, activity of several proteases, quorum sensing signal molecule production, siderophore levels, antibiotic resistance to five antibiotics, and growth profiles in different media types, including nutrient rich medium, minimal medium, synthetic CF medium and medium lacking amino acids to measure the prevalence of auxotrophy. The most prominent feature that emerged from this analysis (summarized in Figure 3) is the large amount of variance within each phenotype. Each isolate demonstrated a high degree of individuality from the other isolates (i.e. no two isolates were the same) and we observed a large range in values for every phenotype measured beyond the normal variation inherent to the assays (Figure S3). We also noted that although some phenotypes, such as gelatinase and protease activity were highly correlated, for the most part, phenotypes behaved independently (Figure S4). Moreover, there were no significant changes in mean phenotype values over time (Figure S5). It is also interesting to note that there were approximately equal numbers of motile and non-motile organisms. In the swimming assay 51% of all the isolates were motile and in the swarming assay 56% were motile. There was also an approximately equal number of mucoid and non-mucoid colony types in both the motile and non-motile isolates (data not shown). That is to say, loss of motility was not correlated to mucoidy.

Disk diffusion assays were used to assess antibiotic susceptibility, which also showed a high level of variation (Figure 4). Many of the morphotypes had both sensitive and resistant isolates but even among the sensitive isolates there was large variability in the zone of clearing (colistin is a good example of this). Although all isolates were susceptible to colistin there was a range of zone sizes observed, with some approaching resistant. Importantly, this patient was exposed to colistin for only a few weeks during a clinically stable period and had no colistin exposure during exacerbation periods that samples were collected from (Table S1). In this set of isolates there was no association with acute antibiotic exposure during exacerbation and the abundance of resistant isolates in the population (Figure S6). We also noted that neither morphotype nor mucoidy were associated with any particular antibiotic resistance profile (Figure 4).

A clustering analysis of all the phenotypes measured (Figure 5) reveals a high level of individuality present in these isolates. What is noteworthy from the clustering is that the isolates do not cluster by morphotype or mucoidy or any of the other metadata variables, including date of isolation (not shown). Rather, the isolates clustered into 3 main phenotypic groups, which can also be seen in the principle components analysis (PCA) (Figure S7). To determine if there was any correlation between the genetic (PFGE profile) and phenotypic measures each isolate in the UPGMA tree was coloured according to the phenotypic groups it fell into (Figure 2). In general there was not good agreement between the genetic and phenotypic clustering with the exception of one group of isolates. The group is highlighted in purple in both the genetic (Figure 2) and phenotypic (Figure 5) data. The functional importance of any groups remains to be explored, however, these findings do highlight the depth of diversity even within a single morphotype.

The diversity present within a single sample was analyzed more in depth by selecting 44 individual isolates from each of two different morphotypes (4 and 5) from one sputum sample that was collected at later date. For these additional 88 isolates we measured a subset of phenotypes; antibiotic sensitivity, protease production and swimming motility. As shown in Figure 6 there was a large degree of phenotypic variation even within isolates from a single sample and of a single colony morphotype. Both morphotypes had motile and non-motile isolates and morphotype 5 had both protease positive and negative isolates. Both morphotypes also had a large distribution of antibiotic sensitive isolates and with the exception of colistin, a good number of resistant isolates. The large phenotypic variation observed in

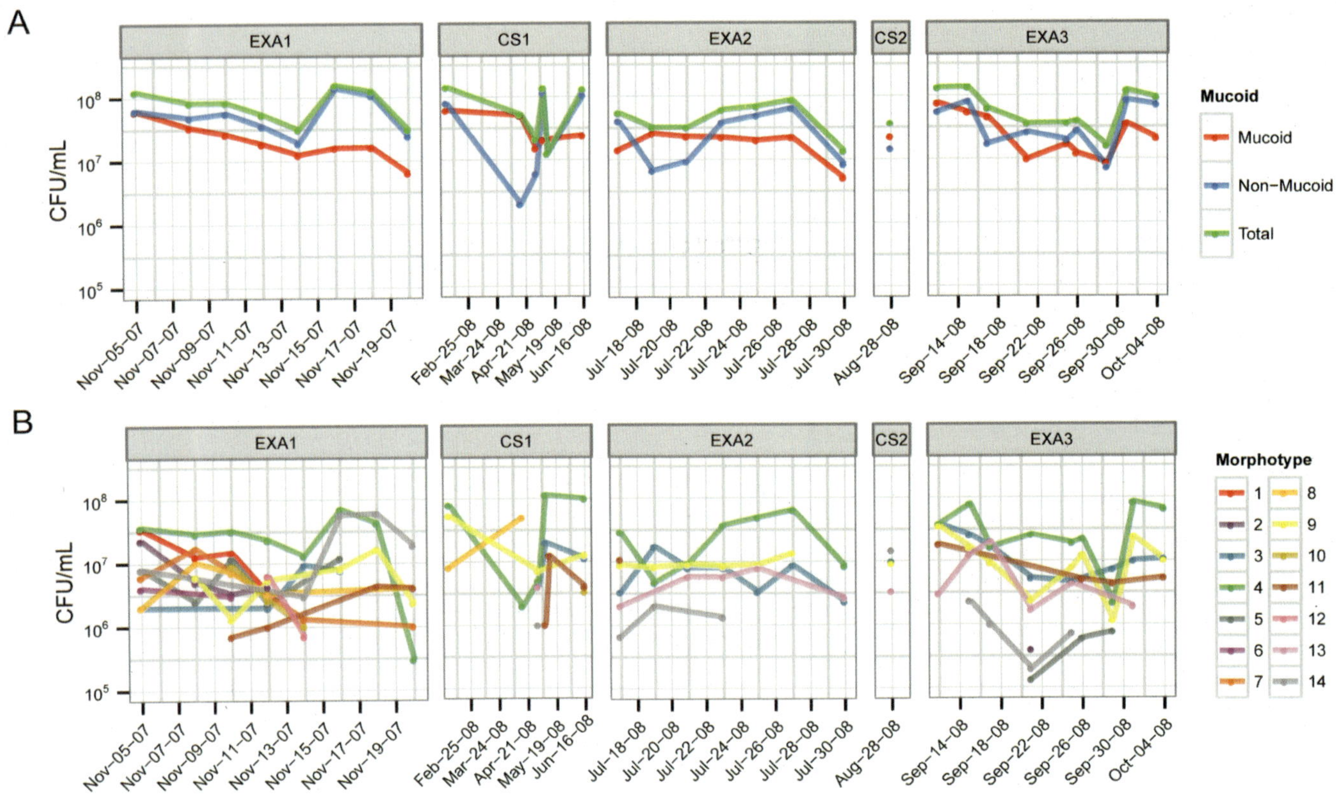

Figure 1. Levels of *P. aeruginosa* during three pulmonary exacerbation periods over the course of one year. A, Total levels, expressed as colony forming units (CFU) per mL of sputum are shown in green and the numbers of mucoid and non-mucoid isolates are indicated in red and blue, respectively. B, The CFU per ml for each of the 14 colony types are shown.

similar morphotypes was still present at a higher sampling depth, indicating that even with this number of isolates under-sampling is still occurring.

To verify that such high diversity is not limited to a single patient, samples were collected from an additional 3 patients during a single pulmonary exacerbation. We found high phenotypic diversity among the *P. aeruginosa* isolates from all patients

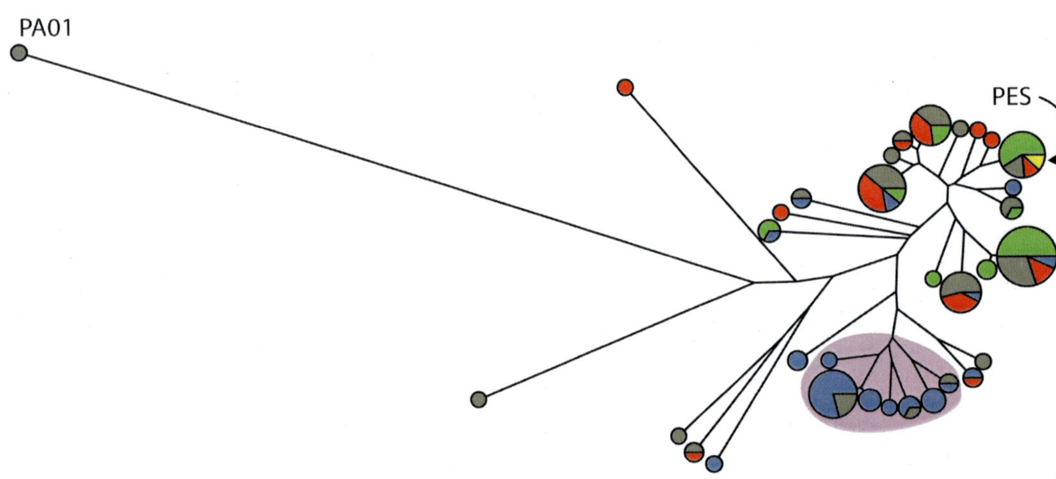

Figure 2. Genetic diversity present in collected *P. aeruginosa* isolates from a single patient. The Dice coefficient from pulse field gel electrophoresis patterns of each isolate was used to construct a UPGMA tree (unrooted). Isolates from this study were no more than 20% different from each other but were more than 40% different from PA01. Isolates with identical PFGE patterns are grouped into a single node where the size of that node represents the number of isolates. Colouring represents the phenotypic group that the isolate falls into and the colours match the colouring in Figure 5. Two PES strains were included in the analysis and are coloured in yellow. The cluster highlighted by purple is a cluster where the phenotypic and genetic groups are similar.

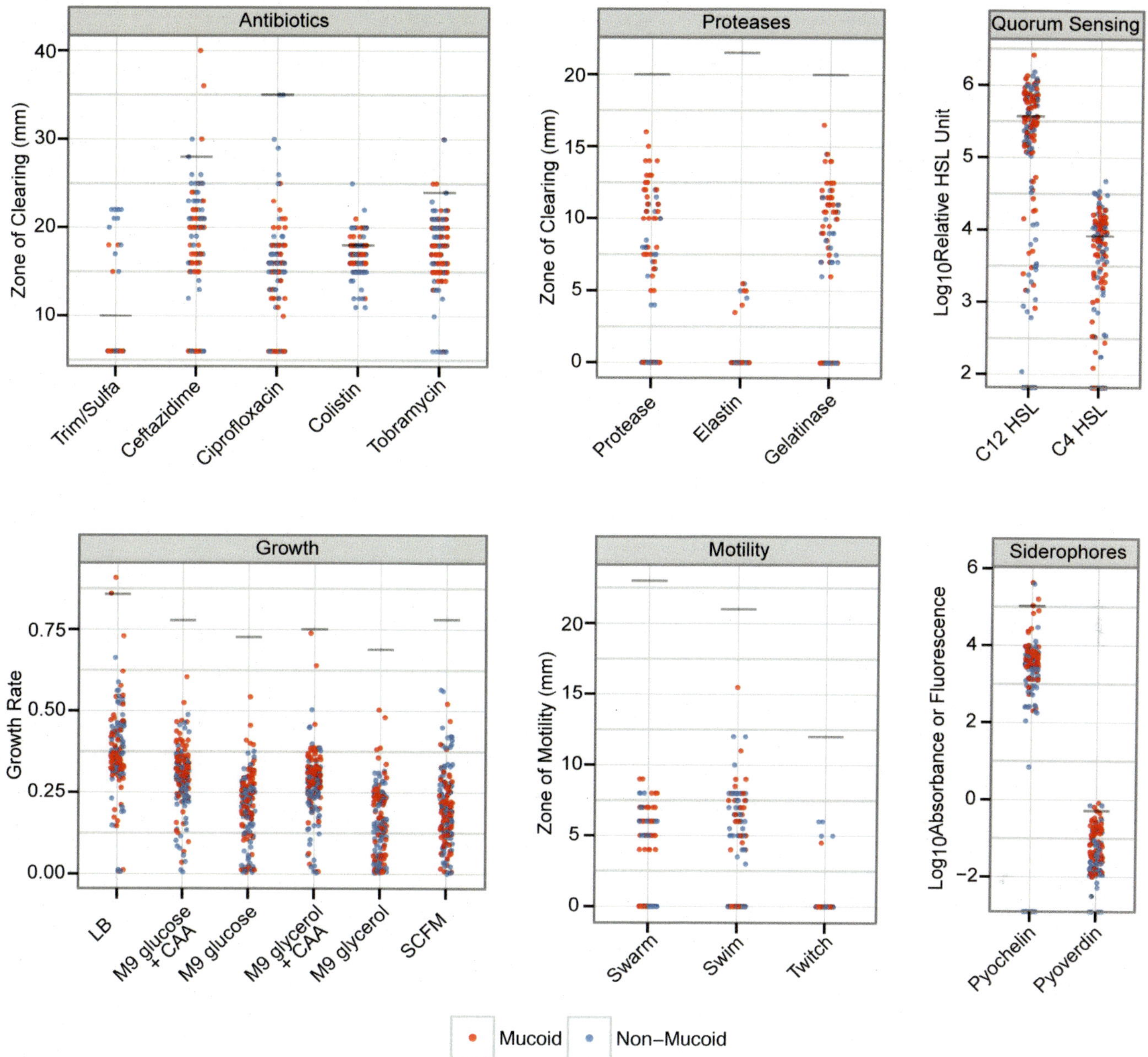

Figure 3. Phenotypic diversity present in collected *P. aeruginosa* isolates from a single patient. The data points are coloured according to whether the isolate was classified as mucoid or not. Grey lines indicate the phenotype value measured for the common lab strain, PA01.

examined, which were comprised of both PES and non-PES strains (Figure S8). Levels of *P. aeruginosa* were monitored throughout the course of the exacerbation and we found that in one of the three patients *P. aeruginosa* levels did not decrease (Figure S9C), as we observed for the main patient (Figure 1A and Figure S9D). However, in two of the patients there was a noticeable drop in *P. aeruginosa* levels near the end of the exacerbation period (Figure S9 A and B). For all patients examined we found that levels of mucoid and non-mucoid isolates were approximately the same and this did not change during exacerbation periods (Figure S9). Furthermore in the patients where the levels of *P. aeruginosa* dropped during the exacerbation we did not observe any corresponding decrease in measured antibiotic resistance (data not shown), however, deeper sampling will be required to fully resolve this.

Discussion

The phenotypic variability in *P. aeruginosa* isolates from chronic CF patients is documented in the literature. *P. aeruginosa* isolates, even clonal isolates from the same sample, have been shown to have large variations in motility [34,35], quorum sensing [29,34], virulence factor production [34–36], antibiotic susceptibility [30,31,36] and biofilm formation [34]. A recent study examined phenotypic and genetic variability in the *P. aeruginosa* Liverpool Epidemic Strain (LES) from 10 adult CF patients and found large diversity in virulence factors, auxotrophy, hypermutability, antibiotic resistance, presence of prophage, and colony morphotype [32]. Here we expand the range of phenotypes examined and identify high phenotypic diversity within a novel epidemic strain, PES. There are several key similarities between the LES and PES

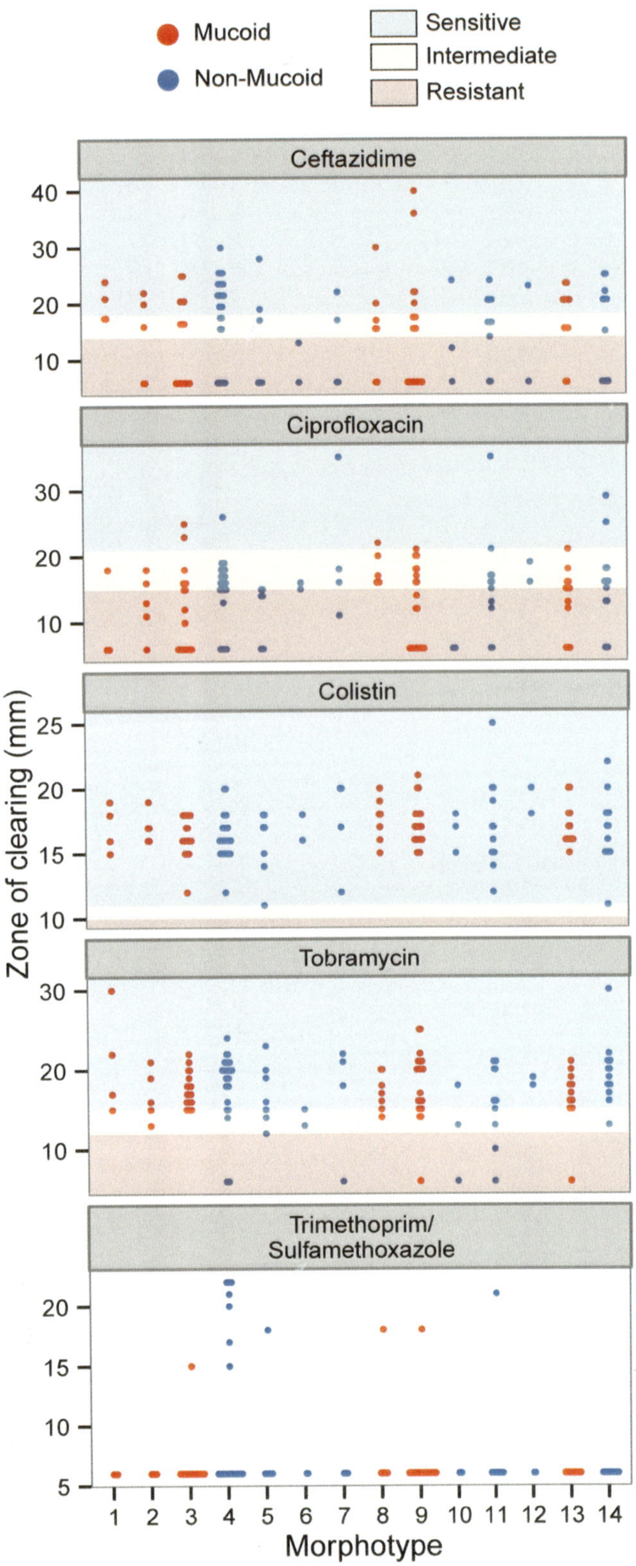

Figure 4. Distribution of antibiotic resistance among the analyzed isolates. Shown are zones of clearing from disc diffusion assays for five commonly used antibiotics in CF clinics and the resistance cutoffs for each antibiotic are given by the dashed lines. Resistance profiles for each colony morphotype are shown individually and coloured according to whether that colony type was initially identified as mucoid or not. Cutoff values for resistant, intermediate and sensitive are indicated by the colour of the background; red, yellow and blue, respectively. Cutoff values for trimethoprim/sulfamethoxazole are not published for *P. aeruginosa* by the CLSI.

isolate collections. First, both demonstrate a high degree of variability within isolates from a single sample, indicating the need for deeper sampling. In addition, the heterogeneity in antibiotic resistant profiles of both sets of isolates remained consistent during and after antibiotic treatment, indicating a lack of positive selection for resistance or negative selection for sensitivity. An important observation from our analysis of the PES isolates is that

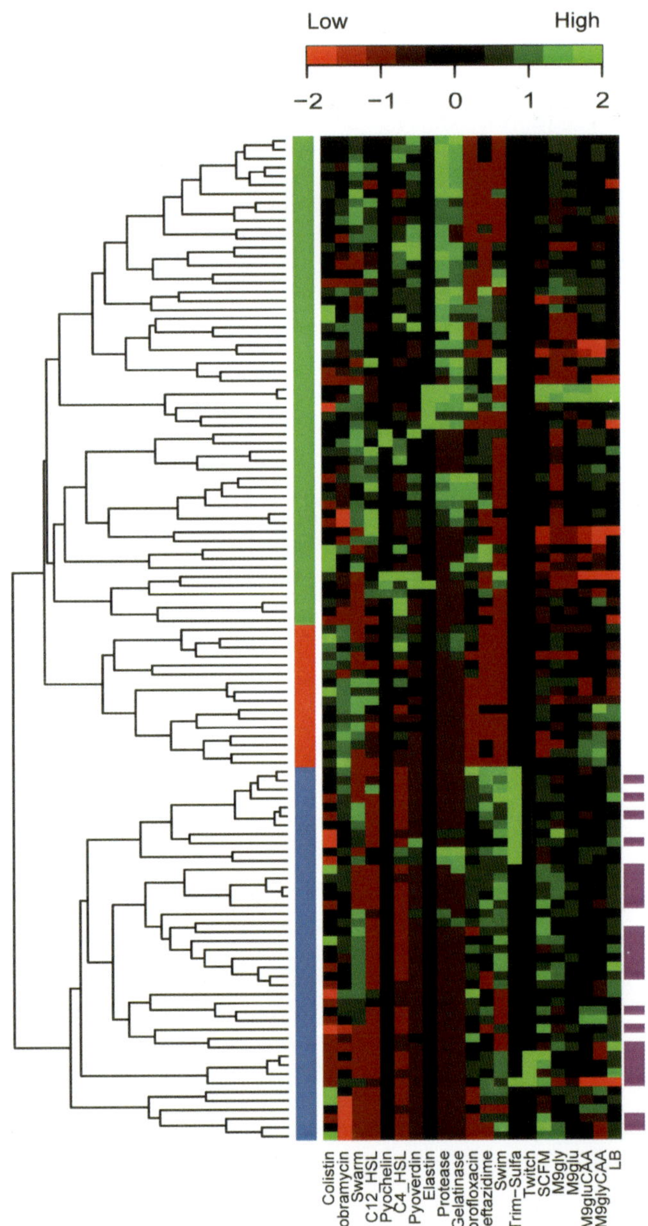

Figure 5. Hierarchical cluster analysis of the phenotype profiles. Green indicates a value above the mean and red indicates a value below the mean. The three colours on the left side indicate the three main cluster groups. Purple bars on the right side indicate the isolates that group closely in both the phenotypic and genetic analysis. Missing values were removed prior to analysis.

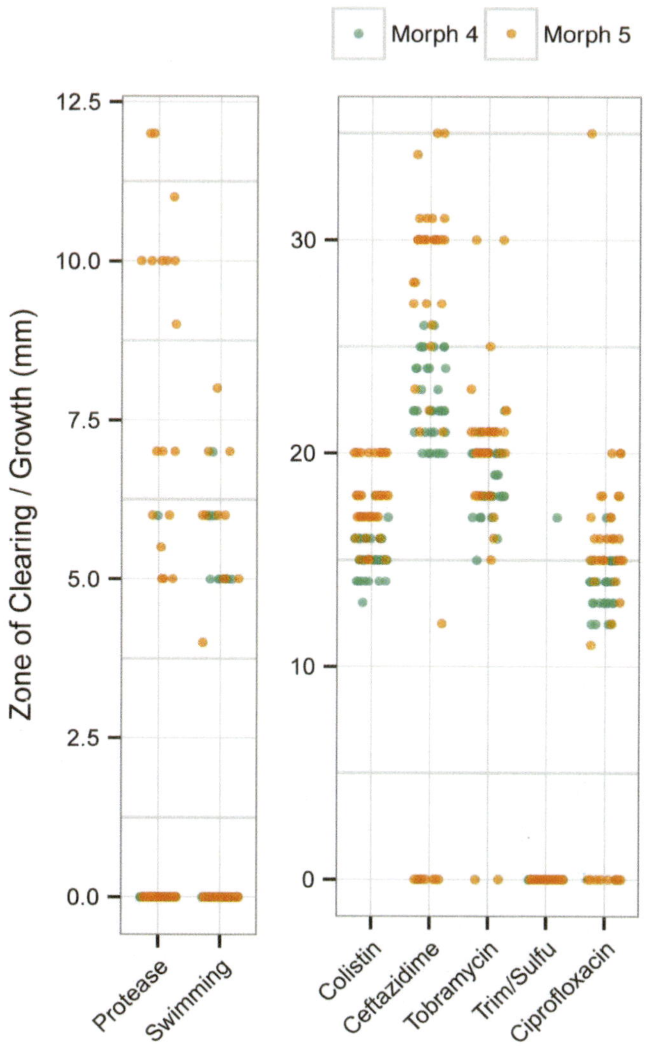

Figure 6. Phenotypic diversity of *P. aeruginosa* isolates from a single sample. Phenotype profiles were obtained from a total of 88 isolates and were comprised of two different colony morphologies, which are shown as orange and green on the plot.

binning a phenotype into categories such as 'high' or 'low' will lead to the underestimation of the true diversity in a sample. For example even though many of our isolates would be classified as sensitive to a number of antibiotics there was still variability within the measured zones of clearing. As such, if isolates are to be clustered for further analysis, as done by Mowat *et al.*, [32], binning the phenotypes will underestimate the diversity and may not represent an accurate population structure. What is clear however, from the current study and others [29,30,32,36] is that the *P. aeruginosa* population is being under-sampled based on morphotype assessment alone. How many isolates per sample are required to accurately describe the population structure and how best to measure diversity are significant challenges.

Many studies have also documented the genetic variability inherent to *P. aeruginosa* during chronic lower airway infections. Mutational targets often identified are *mexZ*, *lasR*, and *mucA*, a regulator of alginate biosynthesis [20,28,37–39]. For some time many *P. aeruginosa* adaptations have been associated with adaptation to and chronic persistence of the bacterium in the lower airways. Examples of this include loss of motility, thought to be associated with decreased immunogenicity [23,40], and conversion to the mucoid phenotype, a key indicator of poor prognosis [22,41,42]. Evidence presented in the current study suggests that non-mucoid isolates are just as prevalent as mucoid isolates. Similarly, we found both motile and non-motile isolates in relatively equal abundance, which has been observed previously [32,35,36]. The implication of this is that rather than a single phenotype dominating the lung environment, a number of phenotypes can evolve, including but not restricted to, mucoid phenotypes. Given that environmental heterogeneity is very good explanation for the maintenance of diversity [43], the rapid emergence of large diversity in the *Pseudomonas* population is suggestive of many diverse niches within the lower airways leading to a number of sub-populations [29]. It is also important to note that expectorated sputum by its very nature is not necessarily representative of the entire lung and we do not know whether it represents a sample from one lobe or a mixture (and will vary between samples). However, most of our samples were collected during physiotherapy and therefore may be more representative than single spontaneous sputum samples.

Adaptive radiation, the evolution of multiple lineages to fill available niches [44,45], is perhaps the most attractive theory to account for the emergence of such diversity in lower airway *Pseudomonas* populations. Lee *et al.*, observed large diversification of *E. coli* populations in monoassociated mice over a period of 1000 days, which corresponded to approximately 20,000 *E. coli* generations [46]. In a very reproducible manner, *P. fluorescens* rapidly diversifies into multiple niche specialists within a matter of days [47]. In *Salmonella*, laboratory passage leads to rapid loss of a spatial phenotype and accumulation of *rpoS* mutations [48]. The evolved populations exhibited a complex distribution of *rpoS* activity indicating that many different types of mutations were being generated even in the absence of spatial heterogeneity [48]. These examples highlight how spatial heterogeneity and niche partitioning can drive diversification, both of which are relevant in the complex and dynamic CF airways. It is important to note as well, that it is not clear if underlying cause of the phenotypic diversity is exclusively genetic in origin or partly a result of phenotypic plasticity. Although there were certainly genetic differences between the isolates, PFGE was not able to distinguish all the individual isolates due to inherent lack of resolution.

In conclusion, the high intraspecific diversity of *P. aeruginosa* populations demonstrated here and in other studies, indicates that caution is in order when making conclusions based on the analysis of a small number of samples. Assuming that one (or a few) isolates is representative of the entire population can lead to under-estimations of the true diversity present. This may also lead to inaccurate descriptions of *P. aeruginosa* phenotypes such as antibiotic resistance, which would have significant implications for antibiotic therapy [31]. There are also implications for detailed genetic and physiological studies that usually focus on a single isolate [27]. Such studies can provide useful information, however, to extend these conclusions to the whole population may not be accurate. Furthermore, from an ecological standpoint, under-estimating the diversity can also hinder attempts to fully understand the population structure and persistence of this organism in the lower airways. Given the polymicrobial nature of the CF lower airway infection it will be paramount to understand how *P. aeruginosa* diversity can influence the population structure of the whole polymicrobial community and vice versa. *P. aeruginosa* contribution to disease progression in CF may require an understanding of the interaction of a complex population of *P. aeruginosa* as a whole with the host and other microbes. Variants within the *P. aeruginosa* population may contribute to different aspects of disease progression such as the transition to a pulmonary exacerbation. Furthermore we know that other organisms in the lower airway community can modulate *P. aeruginosa* virulence [49,50] and it may be that the key to understanding these infections lies in the interplay between the various community members, including diverse *P. aeruginosa* sub-populations.

Materials and Methods

Ethics Statement

The research performed in this study including sample collection and subject consent procedures has been approved by the Conjoint Health Research Ethics Board of the Faculties of Medicine, Nursing and Kinesiology, University of Calgary (CHREB), approval number E-23087: Collection, Storage and Banking of Tissue Samples (Blood and Sputum) and Sputum Microbial Isolates of Patients Attending the Adult Cystic Fibrosis Clinic, University of Calgary Medical Clinic of the Foothills Medical Center for the purposes of CF research. Subject consent was provided in written format through an informed consent form approved by the CHREB.

Sample collection and bacterial isolation

Starting in the fall of 2007 serial sputum samples were collected from an adult CF patient from the Southern Alberta Adult CF clinic. After physical therapy targeting the four quadrants of the lungs, sputum was ptyalized four times and pooled into sterile containers. Within a period of two hours after collection, sputum samples were sheared by passage through a 1-cc needleless syringe to help emulsify the sample and then serially diluted in nutrient rich brain heart infusion (BHI) broth (BD). The 10^{-3}, 10^{-4} and 10^{-5} dilutions were first rigorously vortexed and 300 µL was plated on large (150 mm diameter, VWR) MacConkey (BD) (MAC) agar plates. After incubation for a minimum of 72 h and up to 96 h at 37°C, plates were visually inspected for growth of *P. aeruginosa* and morphotypes were identified based on colony size, pigment production, texture and mucoidy. A representative colony of each morphotype was purified three times on MAC plates and on Pseudomonas Isolation Agar (BD) (PIA) to confirm that the isolated colony was *P. aeruginosa.* Upon purification, colony morphology was compared to the morphology found on the initial sample plate. Morphotype stability of each isolate was checked by plating isolates on MAC plates and inspecting for changes in colony morphology after 48 hours of incubation at 37°C. Isolates were frozen at −80°C in 10% (w/v) skim milk powder (BD). One hundred sixty-nine *P. aeruginosa* isolates were collected through three exacerbations and 7 separate samples collected from routine visits to the CF clinic. An additional 88 isolates, comprised from two colony types, were collected at a later date from a single sputum sample.

For storage and routine assays the isolates were arrayed in multi-well plates containing TSB broth with 20% (w/v) glycerol and frozen at −80°C. For phenotyping, multi-well plates containing TSB or BHI were inoculated from the frozen storage plates using a pin replicator. Plates were then sealed with sealing tape and incubated for 24 or 48 hours with shaking at 37°C. After incubation, cultures were diluted (1/10) into 100 µl of fresh media and incubated for a further 4 hours at 37°C before being used as inoculants for phenotype assays. All isolates exhibited reproducible phenotypes when assayed as described. Many of the assays (e.g. motility) show day-to-day variability due to subtle differences in conditions but the relative phenotype measurements compared to control strains were consistent.

Phenotype Assays

Phenotype assays were performed according standard protocols previously described in the literature and summarized below. Full method details can be found in the supplementary information. Protease production was measured using dialyzed brain heart infusion (D-BHI) milk media [51]. Gelatinase and elastin activity were assayed using previously described assays [52,53]. Swimming motility of *P. aeruginosa* was investigated by using 0.3% (w/v) agar LB plates and swarming was assayed using nutrient glucose media solidified with 0.5% (w/v) agar [54]. Twitching was measured using thin LB media without salt (LBNS) [55]. *P. aeruginosa* was tested for resistance to commonly used anti-pseudomomal drugs using a modified Kirby Bauer disk diffusion method. Five common anti-pseudomonal antibiotics at clinically relevant concentrations were tested, ceftazidime 30 µg (CAZ, Sigma, Aldrich); ciprofloxacin 5 µg (CIP, Sigma, Aldrich), tobramycin 10 µg (NN, Sigma, Aldrich), trimethoprim/sulfamethoxazole 1.25 µg/23.75 µg (SXT, Sigma, Aldrich), colistin 10 µg (CL, Sigma, Aldrich). Zone diameters of clearing were measured and isolates were classified as described by the Clinical Laboratory Standards Institute, (formerly National Committee on Clinical Laboratory Standards) guidelines as resistant, intermediate or susceptible to the antibiotic [56]. Both 3-oxo-C12 HSL and C4 HSL autoinducer production of *P. aeruginosa* isolates were measured using previously described assays [57]. Growth in auxotrophic conditions was tested with M9 minimal media supplemented with either 0.5% (w/v) dextrose or glycerol, with and without 0.2% (w/v) casamino acids (CAA). Growth in high nutrient media was measured using LB media and growth was also measured in synthetic CF medium [58]. Siderophores were directly measured from spent media of cultures that were grown in M9 minimal media supplemented with glucose and CAA as described [59]. The presence of pyoverdin was assayed by measuring absorbance at 405 nm and pyochelin was assayed by measuring fluorescence with an excitation of 355 nm and emission at 460 nm. Raw data for the phenotype measurements is available upon request.

Data analysis

For comparison across different phenotypes mean measurements were normalized by unit variance scaling (dividing each value by the standard deviation of that phenotype) and then by mean centering. Principal component analysis and clustering using the Pearson correlation and un-weighted pair group average (UPGMA) was done in R [60]. Growth curves were fit using a spline method and growth parameters estimated from the fits [61]. Maximum growth rates were used for further analysis.

Pulse-field gel electrophoresis

Strains were inoculated from frozen stocks onto BHI agar and cultured at 37°C for 48 hours. A cell suspension equivalent to a 1.5 MacFarland standard was prepared in suspension buffer (1 M NaCl, 10 mM Tris-HCL, pH 7.6) and mixed with an equal volume of molton 1% (w/v) SeaKem Gold Agarose in TE_1 buffer (10 mM Tris-HCL, 1 mM EDTA, pH 7.6). This mixture was added immediately to a prepared PFGE plug mold (BioRad). Once the plugs were solidified the embedded cells were lysed for 4 h at 37°C in lysis solution (1 M NaCl, 100 mM EDTA, 0.5% Brij-58, 0.5% sarcosyl, 0.2% deoxycholate, 6 mM Tris-HCl [pH 7.6], 1 mg/mL lysozyme, 20 µg/mL RNase). This was followed by an overnight incubation at 50°C in ESP solution (0.5 M EDTA [pH 9], 1% sarcosyl, 70 µg/mL proteinase K) to digest proteins. Lysed plugs were washed 5 times in $TE_{0.1}$ (T10 mM Tris-HCL, 0.1 mM EDTA, pH 7.6) to remove all traces of lysis and ESP solutions. Plugs were stored temporarily at 4°C in

$TE_{0.1}$. Prior to restriction digest the plugs were incubated with 1X reaction buffer (NEBuffer 4) for 15 min at room temperature to allow the buffer to fully penetrate the plug. Each plug was digested with 20U *SpeI* (New England Biolabs) for 4 h at 37°C in 1X reaction buffer with agitation every hour to ensure complete restriction.

Electrophoresis was performed using the BioRad CHEF Mapper PFGE system according to manufacturers instructions. 1% agarorse gels were prepared with SeaKem Gold agarose in 0.5X TBE. Plugs were loaded along with the lambda ladder (New England Biolabs) and overlayed with more agarose. Running conditions were as follows: running buffer: 0.5X TBE, temperature: 10°C, initial switch time: 5 sec, final switch time: 45 sec, included angle: 120°, cell voltage: 6 V/cm, run time: 20 hours. Gels were stained for 60 min with 0.5X GelRed fluorescent nucleic acid stain (Biotium), rinsed 3X in distilled water and imaged on a UV transilluminator.

Gel images were inverted and the contrast and brightness optimized in Adobe Photoshop using the 'Curves' tool. Optimized images were analyzed with BioNumerics (Applied Maths). After gel normalization bands were assigned manually. Sample lanes were compared using the Dice coefficient, allowing for a 1% tolerance in band matching. Hierarchical clustering was performed using the un-weighted pair group average (UPGMA) linkage and selecting the highest scoring tree from 200 permutations.

Supporting Information

Figure S1 Representative plate showing the diversity of colony morphologies of *P. aeruginosa* isolates from a single sputum sample.

Figure S2 Pulse-field gel electrophoresis. A UPGMA tree based on PFGE patterns across all the isolates compared using the Dice coefficient. The tree is identical to the one shown in Figure 2, but has been rooted to allow for display of the gel images.

Figure S3 Variation in growth measures. Growth rates for each isolate under different media types are shown with error bars (standard deviation). Isolates were sorted according to their growth in M9 minimal media with glucose and case amino acids.

Figure S4 Correlation matrix of the measured phenotypes. The Pearson correlation coefficient was calculated for each phenotype pair where the yellow represents a high correlation (close to 1) and blue represents no correlation (close to 0).

Figure S5 Changes in mean phenotype values over time. The mean of each phenotype was calculated for each sputum sample. The point are coloured according to the clinical status. A local smoothing function, shown with a blue line (shaded area represents 95% confidence intervals) was added to identify any trends present in the data.

Figure S6 Antibiotic susceptibility profiles of the collected isolates during the three pulmonary exacerbations. Isolates were classified based on zone sizes from disk diffusion assays. For each sputum sample the relative proportion of resistant (red), intermediate (blue), and sensitive (green) isolates is shown for the four antibiotics where standardized cutoff values for *P. aeruginosa* are available.

Figure S7 PCA analysis of the measured phenotype profiles. The first two components are shown and the data points are coloured according to the cluster pattern observed in the hierarchical cluster analysis. The amount of variation (in percent) explained by each principle component is shown on the axis.

Figure S8 Phenotypic diversity of *P. aeruginosa* isolates from multiple CF patients. Isolates were collected from an additional 3 CF patients to determine the extent of phenotypic diversity. Samples were collected during a single exacerbation period and processed as before. Multiple isolates were collected from each sample, which often contained both mucoid (red) and non-mucoid (blue) isolates. Patient 1 was colonized with a non-PES strain while both patients 2 and 3 were colonized with PES.

Figure S9 Responders versus non-responders. Cell counts for mucoid (red), non-mucoid (blue), and total (green) *P. aeruginosa* in 4 CF patients throughout the course of a pulmonary exacerbation. Patient 4 is the patient from which the isolates in the current study were collected. Patients 2, 3 and 4 were colonized with the PES strain while the Patient 1 had a non-PES strain. Patients 1 and 2 showed a decline in total *P. aeruginosa* levels and are defined as 'responders', i.e. the drop in cell count corresponded with administration of antibiotic therapy. Patients 3 and 4 did not show any drop in *P. aeruginosa* levels despite resolution of exacerbation symptoms and can defined as 'non-responders'.

Table S1 Sample Details.

Acknowledgments

We acknowledge the Southern Alberta CF Clinic for their contribution, in particular Julie Wilson, for efforts to coordinate specimen processing. We would also like to thank the patient for his participation in this study.

Author Contributions

Conceived and designed the experiments: MLW CDS HRR MGS. Performed the experiments: MLW CDS BG SP JCN. Analyzed the data: MLW CDS MDP MGS. Wrote the paper: MLW MDP MGS.

References

1. Matsui H, Grubb BR, Tarran R, Randell SH, Gatzy JT, et al. (1998) Evidence for periciliary liquid layer depletion, not abnormal ion composition, in the pathogenesis of cystic fibrosis airways disease. Cell 95: 1005–1015.
2. Lipuma JJ (2010) The changing microbial epidemiology in cystic fibrosis. Clinical Microbiology Reviews 23: 299–323. doi:10.1128/CMR.00068-09.
3. Davis PB, Drumm M, Konstan MW (1996) Cystic fibrosis. Am J Respir Crit Care Med 154: 1229–1256.
4. Lyczak JB, Cannon CL, Pier GB (2002) Lung infections associated with cystic fibrosis. Clinical Microbiology Reviews 15: 194–222.
5. Hauser AR, Jain M, Bar-Meir M, McColley SA (2011) Clinical significance of microbial infection and adaptation in cystic fibrosis. Clinical Microbiology Reviews 24: 29–70. doi:10.1128/CMR.00036-10.
6. Sibley CD, Surette MG (2011) The polymicrobial nature of airway infections in cystic fibrosis: Cangene Gold Medal Lecture. Can J Microbiol 57: 69–77. doi:10.1139/w10-105.
7. Stressmann FA, Rogers GB, van der Gast CJ, Marsh P, Vermeer LS, et al. (2012) Long-term cultivation-independent microbial diversity analysis demonstrates that bacterial communities infecting the adult cystic fibrosis lung show stability and resilience. Thorax. doi:10.1136/thoraxjnl-2011-200932.

8. Zhao J, Schloss PD, Kalikin LM, Carmody LA, Foster BK, et al. (2012) Decade-long bacterial community dynamics in cystic fibrosis airways. P Natl Acad Sci Usa 109: 5809–5814. doi:10.1073/pnas.1120577109.
9. Tunney MM, Klem ER, Fodor AA, Gilpin DF, Moriarty TF, et al. (2011) Use of culture and molecular analysis to determine the effect of antibiotic treatment on microbial community diversity and abundance during exacerbation in patients with cystic fibrosis. Thorax. doi:10.1136/thx.2010.137281.
10. Sibley CD, Parkins MD, Rabin HR, Duan K, Norgaard JC, et al. (2008) A polymicrobial perspective of pulmonary infections exposes an enigmatic pathogen in cystic fibrosis patients. P Natl Acad Sci Usa 105: 15070–15075. doi:10.1073/pnas.0804326105.
11. Sibley CD, Grinwis ME, Field TR, Eshaghurshan CS, Faria MM, et al. (2011) Culture enriched molecular profiling of the cystic fibrosis airway microbiome. PLoS ONE 6: e22702. doi:10.1371/journal.pone.0022702.
12. Parkins MD, Sibley CD, Surette MG, Rabin HR (2008) The Streptococcus milleri group–an unrecognized cause of disease in cystic fibrosis: a case series and literature review. Pediatr Pulmonol 43: 490–497. doi:10.1002/ppul.20809.
13. Rogers GB, Carroll MP, Serisier DJ, Hockey PM, Jones G, et al. (2004) Characterization of bacterial community diversity in cystic fibrosis lung infections by use of 16 s ribosomal DNA terminal restriction fragment length polymorphism profiling. Journal of Clinical Microbiology 42: 5176–5183. doi:10.1128/JCM.42.11.5176–5183.2004.
14. Stressmann FA, Rogers GB, Klem ER, Lilley AK, Donaldson SH, et al. (2011) Analysis of the bacterial communities present in lungs of patients with cystic fibrosis from American and British centers. Journal of Clinical Microbiology 49: 281–291. doi:10.1128/JCM.01650–10.
15. van der Gast CJ, Walker AW, Stressmann FA, Rogers GB, Scott P, et al. (2010) Partitioning core and satellite taxa from within cystic fibrosis lung bacterial communities. ISME J. doi:10.1038/ismej.2010.175.
16. Sibley CD, Parkins MD, Rabin HR, Surette MG (2009) The relevance of the polymicrobial nature of airway infection in the acute and chronic management of patients with cystic fibrosis. Curr Opin Investig Drugs 10: 787–794.
17. Emerson J, Rosenfeld M, McNamara S, Ramsey B, Gibson RL (2002) Pseudomonas aeruginosa and other predictors of mortality and morbidity in young children with cystic fibrosis. Pediatr Pulmonol 34: 91–100. doi:10.1002/ppul.10127.
18. Kerem E, Corey M, Gold R, Levison H (1990) Pulmonary function and clinical course in patients with cystic fibrosis after pulmonary colonization with Pseudomonas aeruginosa. J Pediatr 116: 714–719. doi:10.1016/S0022-3476(05)82653–8.
19. Kosorok MR, Zeng L, West SE, Rock MJ, Splaingard ML, et al. (2001) Acceleration of lung disease in children with cystic fibrosis after Pseudomonas aeruginosa acquisition. Pediatr Pulmonol 32: 277–287.
20. Smith EE, Buckley DG, Wu Z, Saenphimmachak C, Hoffman LR, et al. (2006) Genetic adaptation by Pseudomonas aeruginosa to the airways of cystic fibrosis patients. P Natl Acad Sci Usa 103: 8487–8492. doi:10.1073/pnas.0602138103.
21. Hogardt M, Heesemann J (2010) Adaptation of Pseudomonas aeruginosa during persistence in the cystic fibrosis lung. Int J Med Microbiol. doi:10.1016/j.ijmm.2010.08.008.
22. Govan JR, Deretic V (1996) Microbial pathogenesis in cystic fibrosis: mucoid Pseudomonas aeruginosa and Burkholderia cepacia. Microbiol Rev 60: 539–574.
23. Mahenthiralingam E, Campbell ME, Speert DP (1994) Nonmotility and phagocytic resistance of Pseudomonas aeruginosa isolates from chronically colonized patients with cystic fibrosis. Infection and Immunity 62: 596–605.
24. Drenkard E, Ausubel FM (2002) Pseudomonas biofilm formation and antibiotic resistance are linked to phenotypic variation. Nature 416: 740–743. doi:10.1038/416740a.
25. Götz von F, Häussler S, Jordan D, Saravanamuthu SS, Wehmhöner D, et al. (2004) Expression analysis of a highly adherent and cytotoxic small colony variant of Pseudomonas aeruginosa isolated from a lung of a patient with cystic fibrosis. J Bacteriol 186: 3837–3847. doi:10.1128/JB.186.12.3837–3847.2004.
26. Häussler S, Ziegler I, Löttel A, Götz von F, Rohde M, et al. (2003) Highly adherent small-colony variants of Pseudomonas aeruginosa in cystic fibrosis lung infection. J Med Microbiol 52: 295–301.
27. Starkey M, Hickman JH, Ma L, Zhang N, de Long S, et al. (2009) Pseudomonas aeruginosa rugose small-colony variants have adaptations that likely promote persistence in the cystic fibrosis lung. J Bacteriol 191: 3492–3503. doi:10.1128/JB.00119–09.
28. Feliziani S, Luján AM, Moyano AJ, Sola C, Bocco JL, et al. (2010) Mucoidy, Quorum Sensing, Mismatch Repair and Antibiotic Resistance in Pseudomonas aeruginosa from Cystic Fibrosis Chronic Airways Infections. PLoS ONE 5. doi:10.1371/journal.pone.0012669.
29. Wilder CN, Allada G, Schuster M (2009) Instantaneous within-patient diversity of Pseudomonas aeruginosa quorum-sensing populations from cystic fibrosis lung infections. Infection and Immunity 77: 5631–5639. doi:10.1128/IAI.00755–09.
30. Foweraker JE, Laughton CR, Brown DFJ, Bilton D (2005) Phenotypic variability of Pseudomonas aeruginosa in sputa from patients with acute infective exacerbation of cystic fibrosis and its impact on the validity of antimicrobial susceptibility testing. J Antimicrob Chemother 55: 921–927. doi:10.1093/jac/dki146.
31. Foweraker JE, Laughton CR, Brown DF, Bilton D (2009) Comparison of methods to test antibiotic combinations against heterogeneous populations of multiresistant Pseudomonas aeruginosa from patients with acute infective exacerbations in cystic fibrosis. Antimicrob Agents Chemother 53: 4809–4815. doi:10.1128/AAC.00269–09.
32. Mowat E, Paterson S, Fothergill JL, Wright EA, Ledson MJ, et al. (2011) Pseudomonas Aeruginosa Population Diversity and Turnover in Cystic Fibrosis Chronic Infections. Am J Respir Crit Care Med: 201009–1430OCv1. doi:10.1164/rccm.201009–1430OC.
33. Glezerson BA, Sibley CD, Sibley KE, Surette MG, Rabin HR, et al. (2012) A twenty-five year outbreak of Pseudomonas aeruginosa: identification of the Prairie Epidemic Strain (PES). Journal of Cystic Fibrosis 11(S1) :S41.
34. Lee B, Haagensen JAJ, Ciofu O, Andersen JB, Høiby N, et al. (2005) Heterogeneity of biofilms formed by nonmucoid Pseudomonas aeruginosa isolates from patients with cystic fibrosis. Journal of Clinical Microbiology 43: 5247–5255. doi:10.1128/JCM.43.10.5247–5255.2005.
35. Leone I, Chirillo MG, Raso T, Zucca M, Savoia D (2008) Phenotypic and genotypic characterization of Pseudomonas aeruginosa from cystic fibrosis patients. Eur J Clin Microbiol Infect Dis 27: 1093–1099. doi:10.1007/s10096-008–0551–1.
36. Fothergill JL, Mowat E, Ledson MJ, Walshaw MJ, Winstanley C (2010) Fluctuations in phenotypes and genotypes within populations of Pseudomonas aeruginosa in the cystic fibrosis lung during pulmonary exacerbations. J Med Microbiol 59: 472–481. doi:10.1099/jmm.0.015875–0.
37. D'Argenio DA, Wu M, Hoffman LR, Kulasekara HD, Déziel E, et al. (2007) Growth phenotypes of Pseudomonas aeruginosa lasR mutants adapted to the airways of cystic fibrosis patients. Mol Microbiol 64: 512–533. doi:10.1111/j.1365–2958.2007.05678.x
38. Mena A, Smith EE, Burns JL, Speert DP, Moskowitz SM, et al. (2008) Genetic adaptation of Pseudomonas aeruginosa to the airways of cystic fibrosis patients is catalyzed by hypermutation. J Bacteriol 190: 7910–7917. doi:10.1128/JB.01147–08.
39. Ciofu O, Mandsberg LF, Bjarnsholt T, Wassermann T, Høiby N (2010) Genetic adaptation of Pseudomonas aeruginosa during chronic lung infection of patients with cystic fibrosis: strong and weak mutators with heterogeneous genetic backgrounds emerge in mucA and/or lasR mutants. Microbiology (Reading, Engl) 156: 1108–1119. doi:10.1099/mic.0.033993–0.
40. Amiel E, Lovewell RR, O'Toole GA, Hogan DA, Berwin B (2010) Pseudomonas aeruginosa evasion of phagocytosis is mediated by loss of swimming motility and is independent of flagellum expression. Infection and Immunity 78: 2937–2945. doi:10.1128/IAI.00144–10.
41. Henry RL, Mellis CM, Petrovic L (1992) Mucoid Pseudomonas aeruginosa is a marker of poor survival in cystic fibrosis. Pediatr Pulmonol 12: 158–161.
42. Li Z, Kosorok MR, Farrell PM, Laxova A, West SEH, et al. (2005) Longitudinal development of mucoid Pseudomonas aeruginosa infection and lung disease progression in children with cystic fibrosis. JAMA 293: 581–588. doi:10.1001/jama.293.5.581.
43. Kassen R (2002) The experimental evolution of specialists, generalists, and the maintenance of diversity. J Evolution Biol 15: 173–190.
44. Schluter D (2000) The Ecology of Adaptive Radiation. Oxford Univ Press.
45. Kassen R (2009) Toward a general theory of adaptive radiation: insights from microbial experimental evolution. Annals of the New York Academy of Sciences 1168: 3–22. doi:10.1111/j.1749–6632.2009.04574.x.
46. Lee SM, Wyse A, Lesher A, Everett ML, Lou L, et al. (2010) Adaptation in a mouse colony monoassociated with Escherichia coli K-12 for more than 1,000 days. Appl Environ Microbiol 76: 4655–4663. doi:10.1128/AEM.00358–10.
47. Rainey PB, Travisano M (1998) Adaptive radiation in a heterogeneous environment. Nature 394: 69–72.
48. Davidson CJ, White AP, Surette MG (2008) Evolutionary loss of the rdar morphotype in Salmonella as a result of high mutation rates during laboratory passage. ISME J 2: 293–307. doi:10.1038/ismej.2008.4.
49. Duan K, Dammel C, Stein J, Rabin H, Surette MG (2003) Modulation of Pseudomonas aeruginosa gene expression by host microflora through interspecies communication. Mol Microbiol 50: 1477–1491.
50. Sibley CD, Duan K, Fischer C, Parkins MD, Storey DG, et al. (2008) Discerning the Complexity of Community Interactions Using a Drosophila Model of Polymicrobial Infections. PLoS Pathog 4: e1000184. doi:10.1371/journal.ppat.1000184.
51. Sokol PA, Ohman DE, Iglewski BH (1979) A more sensitive plate assay for detection of protease production by Pseudomanas aeruginosa. Journal of Clinical Microbiology 9: 538–540.
52. Smith HL, Goodner K (1958) Detection of bacterial gelatinases by gelatin-agar plate methods. J Bacteriol 76: 662–665.
53. Sokol PA, Cox CD, Iglewski BH (1982) Pseudomonas aeruginosa mutants altered in their sensitivity to the effect of iron on toxin A or elastase yields. J Bacteriol 151: 783–787.
54. Rashid MH, Kornberg A (2000) Inorganic polyphosphate is needed for swimming, swarming, and twitching motilities of Pseudomonas aeruginosa. P Natl Acad Sci Usa 97: 4885–4890. doi:10.1073/pnas.060030097.
55. Baynham PJ, Ramsey DM, Gvozdyev BV, Cordonnier EM, Wozniak DJ (2006) The Pseudomonas aeruginosa ribbon-helix-helix DNA-binding protein AlgZ (AmrZ) controls twitching motility and biogenesis of type IV pili. J Bacteriol 188: 132–140. doi:10.1128/JB.188.1.132–140.2006
56. CLSI (2009) Performance Standards for Antimicrobial Susceptibility Testing; Nineteenth Informational Supplement. Wayne, PA: Clinical and Laboratory Standards Institute.

57. Duan K, Surette MG (2007) Environmental regulation of Pseudomonas aeruginosa PAO1 Las and Rhl quorum-sensing systems. J Bacteriol 189: 4827–4836. doi:10.1128/JB.00043-07
58. Palmer KL, Aye LM, Whiteley M (2007) Nutritional cues control Pseudomonas aeruginosa multicellular behavior in cystic fibrosis sputum. J Bacteriol 189: 8079–8087. doi:10.1128/JB.01138-07
59. Wagner T, Soong G, Sokol S, Saiman L, Prince A (2005) Effects of azithromycin on clinical isolates of Pseudomonas aeruginosa from cystic fibrosis patients. Chest 128: 912–919. doi:10.1378/chest.128.2.912
60. Core R Team (2012) R: A Language and Environment for Statistical Computing. R Foundation for Statistical Computing. Available: http://www.R-project.org/
61. Kahm M, Hasenbrink G, Lichtenberg-Fraté H, Ludwig J, Kschischo M (2010) grofit: fitting biological growth curves with R. Journal of Statistical Software 33: 1–21.

Non-Apoptotic Toxicity of *Pseudomonas aeruginosa* toward Murine Cells

Sanhita Roy[1], Tracey Bonfield[2], Alan M. Tartakoff[3]*

1 Department of Ophthalmology and Visual Sciences, Case Western Reserve University, Cleveland, Ohio, United States of America, **2** Department of Pediatrics, Case Western Reserve University, Cleveland, Ohio, United States of America, **3** Pathology Department and Cell Biology Program, Case Western Reserve University, Cleveland, Ohio, United States of America

Abstract

Although *P. aeruginosa* is especially dangerous in cystic fibrosis (CF), there is no consensus as to how it kills representative cell types that are of key importance in the lung. This study concerns the acute toxicity of the sequenced strain, PAO1, toward a murine macrophage cell line (RAW 264.7). Toxicity requires brief contact with the target cell, but is then delayed for more than 12 h. None of the classical toxic effectors of this organism is required and cell death occurs without phagocytosis or acute perturbation of the actin cytoskeleton. Apoptosis is not required for toxicity toward either RAW 264.7 cells or for alveolar macrophages. Transcriptional profiling shows that encounter between PAO1 and RAW 264.7 cells elicits an early inflammatory response, followed by growth arrest. As an independent strategy to understand the mechanism of toxicity, we selected variant RAW 264.7 cells that resist PAO1. Upon exposure to *P. aeruginosa*, they are hyper-responsive with regard to classical inflammatory cytokine production and show transient downregulation of transcripts that are required for cell growth. They do not show obvious morphologic changes. Although they do not increase interferon transcripts, when exposed to PAO1 they dramatically upregulate a subset of the responses that are characteristic of exposure to g-interferon, including several guanylate-binding proteins. The present observations provide a novel foundation for learning how to equip cells with resistance to a complex challenge.

Editor: Gunnar F. Kaufmann, The Scripps Research Institute and Sorrento Therapeutics, Inc., United States of America

Funding: This work was supported through a grant from the Cystic Fibrosis Foundation (www.cff.org/mobile/index.cfm?menu = 1&)(R447-CR07) and from the Case Western Reserve University/Cleveland Clinic CTSA Grant (no. UL1 RR024989) from the National Center for Research Resources (NCRR), a component of the National Institutes of Health (NIH) and NIH roadmap for Medical Research. The funders had no role in study design, data collection and analysis, decision to publish, or preparation of the manuscript.

Competing Interests: The authors have declared that no competing interests exist.

* E-mail: amt10@case.edu

Introduction

Although many microorganisms kill target cells by specific well-characterized mechanisms, for others the causes of toxicity are unknown. A case of particular interest is that of *P. aeruginosa*. This organism is acutely dangerous for individuals with cystic fibrosis (CF). Its large genome encodes multiple potentially toxic secretion systems [1,2]. Moreover, it triggers multiple responses in host cells, e.g. [3,4]. Adding to the complexity of the pathogen-host encounter are the changes of phenotype of the organism during infection, e.g. as a result of quorum sensing, differentiation into a mucoid state characterized by alginate production, establishment of biofilms, etc. [5–7].

Much attention has focused on the possible contribution to pathogenicity of protein secretion. Thus, the type III secretion apparatus injects bacterial enzymes into the target cell cytoplasm [8,9] and the type II pathway releases multiple hydrolytic enzymes to the medium [10,11]. Furthermore, *P. aeruginosa* lipopeptides and lipopolysaccharide (LPS) stimulate target cell Toll-like receptors, TLR2 and TLR4, respectively [12]. TLR4 signaling is proinflammatory, leading to nuclear translocation of NF-kB and activation of MAPK, while TLR2 signaling appears to oppose TLR4, e.g. [13–15]. Nevertheless, studies of knockout mice argue against a central role for TLR4 (or TLR2) in the acute pathogenesis that is characteristic of CF [16,17].

Binding of *P. aeruginosa* to cell surfaces has been suggested to be mediated by the ganglioside GM1, fibronectin, integrins, and by the cystic fibrosis transmembrane regulator (CFTR). Internalization requires the kinases, PI3K and Akt, and the actin cytoskeleton [18,19]. *P. aeruginosa* also produces two potentially toxic lectins [20].

To investigate the causes of toxicity by *P. aeruginosa*, we developed a highly sensitive assay using RAW 264.7 murine macrophage-monocytes as the target. Although human macrophages express surface CFTR, RAW 264.7 cells (and murine macrophages) do not [21,22]. Reduced expression of CFTR is also characteristic of many cell type in cystic fibrosis [12,23].

Among the issues of broader significance raised by the present observations is the question of what distinguishes inflammatory responses that are protective from those that damage target cells. We have generated variant cells that resist the toxicity of *P. aeruginosa*. Their transcriptional profiles, when compared to wildtype, show that many pro-inflammatory changes need not culminate in toxicity.

Results

1. Characterization of Toxicity

A minimal toxicity assay for P. aeruginosa. Resting murine RAW 264.7 cells were exposed to the sequenced strain of *P. aeruginosa*, PAO1 - that is proficient in secretion of potentially toxic proteins [24] - for 1 h at low multiplicity of infection (MOI = 10). Cells were then washed and returned to culture in the presence of gentamicin and streptomycin, to eliminate extracellular *P. aeruginosa*. After 12 h, viability was still excellent, judging from MTT (3-[4,5-Dimethylthiazol-2-yl]-2,5-diphenyltetrazolium bromide) assays and the lack of release of cytoplasmic green fluorescent protein, GFP (when GFP-expressing target cells were used). Moreover, most cells had elongated and increased in size – as in many examples of macrophage activation (Figure 1A), and up to 25% of the cells had become binucleate [25] (Figure 1B). Nevertheless, the actin cytoskeleton still extended into filipodia (Figure 1B), distinguishing this response from that of cells that were exposed to higher multiplicities of *P. aeruginosa* or to other microorganisms, e.g. [9,26,27]. By 24 h, it was obvious that cell number and total MTT activity had not increased (Figure 1C). Moreover, in experiments with cells that expressed cytosolic GFP - ~70% of the target cells were no longer fluorescent. Within 2–3 days the small number of remaining cells was severely vacuolated (not shown).

Contact is required for toxicity, but phagocytosis is not required. To learn whether contact between the bacteria and the host cell is required for toxicity, we ultracentrifuged bacterial cultures and passed the supernatant through a Millipore filter before diluting samples into media that were added to cell cultures for 1 h. Even at concentrations corresponding to MOI = 50, MTT assays and visual inspection showed no toxicity during the following days (not shown).

By using PAO1 that expresses GFP in standard 1 h exposure toxicity protocols, we observed that only a small number of bacteria remained adherent to the filipodia after washing (Figure 2A). Upon reincubation for several hours, they then progressively deteriorated. We saw no visual evidence for internalization. The amount of internalization was also quantitated by washing the target cells after exposure to *P. aeruginosa*, preparing cell lysates under conditions that do not to kill the organism [28], plating the extracts on LB agar plates and incubating overnight. These experiments show that fewer than 1/20 of the target cells harbor a bacterium (not shown).

2. Requirements for toxicity

Toxicity is not due to factors released from RAW 264.7 cells exposed to PAO1. To learn whether soluble factors released from target cells cause toxicity, bacteria were incubated at MOI = 10 for 1–3 h with RAW 264.7 cells prior to collecting the medium, centrifuging it to remove bacteria, and Millipore filtration. The filtrates were then added to naïve cultures of RAW 264.7 cells for 1 h. Again, no toxicity was seen over the following days (not shown).

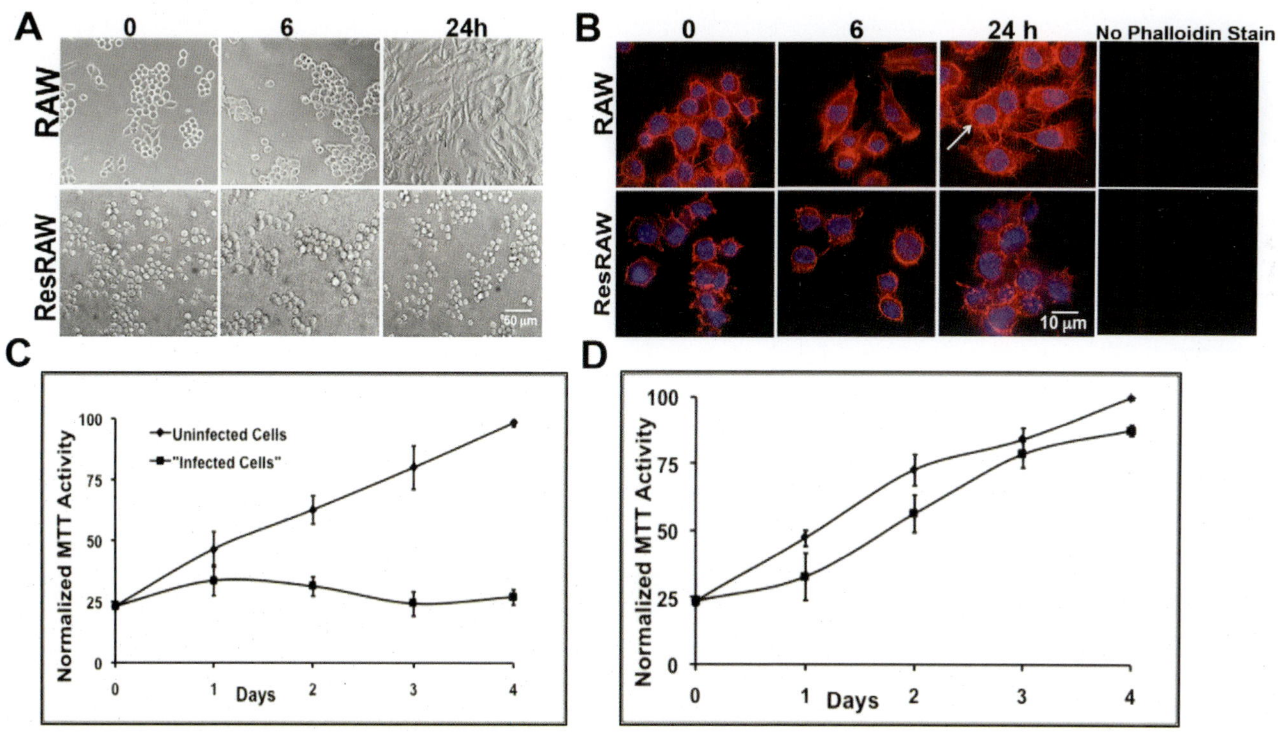

Figure 1. Impact of *P. aeruginosa* on viability on RAW 264.7 cells. A) Phase overview of cell morphology, uninfected cells (RAW) and resistant cells (ResRAW - see text) were exposed to *P. aeruginosa* (MOI 10) and returned to culture for 6 or 24 h. Note the major change in cell shape and size of the wt cells upon exposure to *P. aeruginosa*. The resistant cells appear unaffected over the same time period. **B**) Actin cytoskeleton, stained with rhodamine-phalloidin after fixation. Uninfected cells compared to resistant cells after exposure to *P. aeruginosa* (MOI 10) and reculture for 6 or 24 h. Note the enlargement of wt cells and appearance of a subset of cells with double nuclei (shown by an arrow). The nuclei were stained blue with DAPI. For the panels at the right, phalloidin staining was omitted and the images were viewed with the red filter. **C** and **D**: MTT assays to quantitate cell number. Uninfected cells compared to cells exposed to *P. aeruginosa* and then recultured over 4 days for both naïve RAW 264.7 (**C**) and resistant cells (**D**). In both cases, cells were exposed to *P. aeruginosa* for 1 h before washing and return to culture. Activity measurements (per culture) were normalized to values for cells cultured without PAO1 over four days.

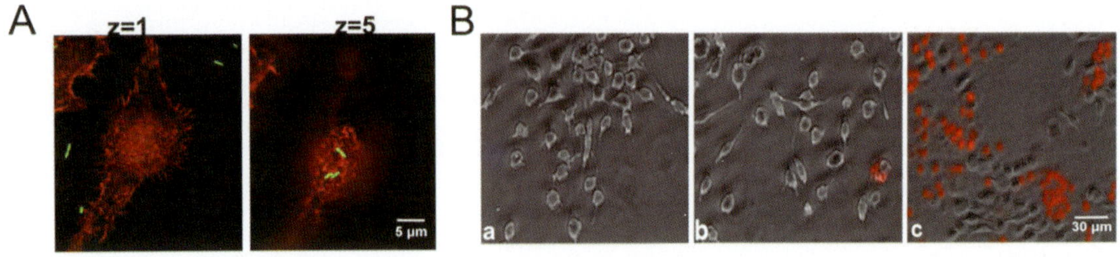

Figure 2. Morphological changes of naïve RAW 264.7 cells in response to PAO1. A) Fluorescent microscope images of RAW 264.7 cells exposed to PAO1 expressing GFP at MOI 10 for 1 h. After washing, cells were fixed and stained with phalloidin. Two different z planes are shown. **B**) Killing of RAW 264.7 cells exposed to PAO1 as indicated by appearance of propidium iodide stained cells after 48 h. a) Uninfected cells, b) Cells cocultured with cells exposed to PAO1, c) Cells directly exposed to PAO1.

In parallel experiments, we performed cocultures in which a coverslip of cells was exposed to PAO1, washed, and then placed in a Petri dish that already contained a coverslip of naïve RAW 264.7 cells. After two days of culture with antibiotics, both coverslips were stained with propidium iodide: only the former showed evidence of toxicity (Figure 2B, panel c). The cells that never received bacteria but were cocultured with cells that had been exposed to bacteria (panel b) could not be distinguished from cells that were neither cocultured nor received any bacteria (panel a). Thus, contact between bacterium and target is required for toxicity and toxicity is cell-autonomous.

Type II and III Secretion. PAO1 produces several toxins. Some are secreted by its Type II secretion system, while the Type III system delivers others directly into the cytoplasm of target cells. To learn whether toxicity toward RAW 264.7 involves these systems, we tested the impact of two PAO1 mutants. The first lacks the type II secretion system (*xcp*), while the second lacks the type III secretion system (*pscC*) [29,30]. Both mutants are as toxic as wildtype in our standard protocol (Figure 3A). A double mutant that lacks both systems is also obviously toxic (not shown).

Importance of bacterial metabolism. Toxicity appears to be due to components that are present at the time of addition of bacteria to the target cells. Neither inclusion of inhibitors of translation or transcription (Figure 3B) nor heat treatment (85°C, 60 min), has a major effect on toxicity. Taken together, we conclude that the bacteria do not need to be metabolically active to cause toxicity. We therefore investigated the importance of surface components of *P. aeruginosa*.

Surface components, lectins, muramyldipeptide, DNA. To learn whether appendages contribute to toxicity, we tested the impact of PAO1 mutants that lack flagella (*ΔfliC*, *ΔfliQ*) or pili (*ΔpilA*). The known pro-inflammatory impact of flagellin is mediated by TLR5, that binds bacterial flagellin [31], that is not expressed on RAW 264.7 [17,32]. All three mutants were clearly toxic (Figure 3C).

Lectins of *P. aeruginosa* bind preferentially to galactose and fucose and could contribute to toxicity. We therefore conducted standard assays in the absence or presence of fucose (50 mM), galactose (50 mM), p-nitro-phenyl-fucoside (25 mM) and IPTG (0.5 mM),

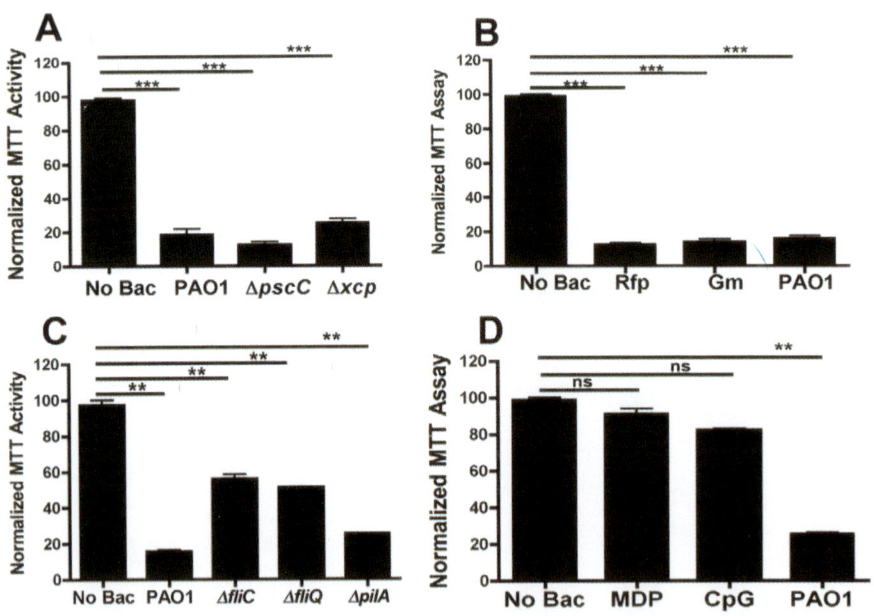

Figure 3. MTT assay to determine the viability of RAW 264.7 cells. RAW 264.7 cells were (**A**) exposed to Type II and Type III mutants of PAO1 for 1 h, or (**B**) to PAO1 in the presence of rifampicin (Rfp, 40 μg/ml), or gentamicin (Gm, 200 μg/ml). In (**C**), cells were exposed to different mutant strains of PAO1 containing mutations in pili and flagella. In (**D**), cells were exposed to muramyldipeptide (MDP, 25 μg/ml) or CpG DNA (5 μg/ml). In all cases cell viability was estimated by measuring MTT activity after 24–48 h as mentioned in text. (***) designates $p<0.0003$. ns: not-significant.

both singly and in combination with each other. No reduction in toxicity was detected (not shown).

Muramyldipeptide (MDP), a minimal structural unit of peptidoglycan, is present in the outer wall of Gram-positive bacteria and Gram-negative bacteria and is known to stimulate the immune system [33]. When RAW 264.7 cells were treated with high doses of MDP for 2 days there was no evidence of cell death (Figure 3D).

Proinflammatory stimulation by bacterial DNA is mediated by TLR9, that resides in endocytic compartments, e.g. [34]. The TLR9 ligand, CpG DNA, was therefore tested for toxicity; however, a high dose of B type CpG DNA caused only modest toxicity over 2 days (Figure 3D).

Lipopolysaccharide. The major *P. aeruginosa* surface-associated virulence factor, lipopolysaccharide (LPS), plays an important immunogenic and structural role, mediates interactions between the bacterial cell surface and the external environment, and binds TLR4 [35]. To evaluate the contribution of LPS to toxicity, we challenged cells with graded doses of soluble LPS purified from *P. aeruginosa*, serotype 10**.** Continuous exposure for 5 days is toxic; however, the LD_{50} for such preparations is at least 100× higher than the amount of LPS that we calculate is present on bacteria at MOI = 10 (Table 1). This could reflect the increased impact of clustering of binding sites on the target cell.

The toxicity of LPS is generally thought to be due to its lipid A moiety [35]. Consistent with this information, we observe that *P. aeruginosa* expressing LPS with truncated glycans is also potent (Figures S1A and S1B).

As a further test of the contribution of LPS to toxicity, we evaluated the possible protective effect of polymyxin B, an agent that sequesters LPS in a stoichiometric complex [36]. We find that polymyxin B is an effective inhibitor of the toxicity of soluble LPS; however, it provides only minimal protection against PAO1 (Figure S1C).

3. Response to *P. aeruginosa*

NF-kB Activation. Nuclear factor-kB (NF-kB) is a critical participant in the immediate early pathogen response, regulating inflammation, cell proliferation and survival. In resting cells, NF-kB is bound to cytoplasmic inhibitors (IkBs), while it translocates to the nucleus in response to various stimuli, e.g. [37]. As expected, we observe that the p65 subunit of NF-kB enters the nucleus within one hour of exposure to bacteria (Figure 4A, 4B). It is excluded from the nucleolus and from the most chromatin-rich regions of the nucleoplasm, judging from preparations stained with DAPI. Treatment of cells with soluble LPS also causes nuclear translocation of p65 (Figure 4A). As shown in Figure 4B, total IkB decreases in RAW cells upon 1 h exposure to PAO1. Parallel assessment of phosphorylation of IkB shows a variable increase (not shown).

Cytokine Profiles. Supernatants harvested at 1, 6 and 24 h of exposure to PAO-1 were assayed for IL-6, MIP-2, and TNFα, secretion. Figure 5 shows that MIP-2 and TNFα were significantly elevated as early as 1 h, consistent with the rapid activation of NF-kB. IL-6 secretion became obvious by 6 h (Figure 5).

Transcriptional changes [Note: For references pertaining to specific proteins see Table S3.]. We recovered RNA for microarray analysis from cells before exposure to PAO1, after 1 h exposure, and after exposure for 1 h followed by washing and 8 h reculture with antibiotics ("1+8 h"). *P. aeruginosa* is known to elicit major transcriptional changes in other target cells, e.g. [38–40]. Table 1 (and Table S2) provide an overview of these data. Both Tables are based on the gene ontology analysis.

Table 1. Overview of Transcript Changes.

Condition	Increases		Decreases	
	Categories		Categories	
Wt cells+P.a. 1 h	apoptosis, inflammatory response, immune response, positive regulation of the I-kB kinase-NF-kB cascade	$p<10^{-11}$	modest	marginal
Wt cells+P.a. 1+8 h	apoptosis, inflammatory response, immune response, positive regulation of the I-kB kinase-NF-kB cascade, positive regulation of cell proliferation, chemotaxis, anti-apoptosis, neutrophil chemotaxis, regulation of apoptosis, response to LPS, PDGF receptor signaling pathway	$p<10^{-10}$	cell cycle progression, cell division, mitosis, cell cycle regulation, nucleosome assembly	$p<10^{-13}$
mutant cells vs wt	signal transduction, prostaglandin biology	$10^{-6}<p<10^{-3}$	immune and inflammatory responses	$10^{-7}<p<10^{-3}$
Mutant+P.a. 1 h	apoptosis, immune response, inflammatory response, positive regulation of I-kB kinase-NF-kB cascade, anti-apoptosis	$10^{-16}<p<10^{-6}$	various	$10^{-16}<p<10^{-6}$
Mutant+P.a. 1+8 h	apoptosis, immune response, inflammatory response, positive regulation of I-kB kinase-NF-kB cascade, anti-apoptosis		cell cycle progression, cell division, mitosis, cell cycle regulation, nucleosome assembly	$10^{-22}<p<10^{-14}$
Wt: 1+8 h vs 1 h	Ccl2, Cd274, Edn1, Gbp1, Il1f6, Isg15, Rsad2, and Serpinb9		Little change	
Mutant: 1+8 h vs 1 h	Many g-interferon targets, Rsad2, Gbp1, Isg15, Gbp3, Gbp5, Gbp6, Ifi202b, tenascin		Little change	

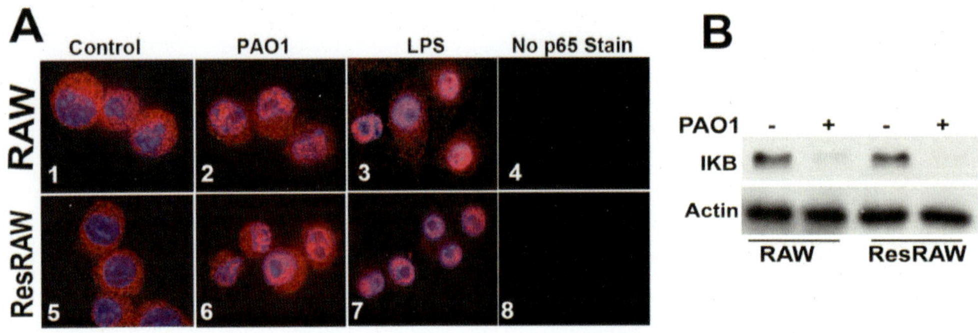

Figure 4. NF-kB activation in naïve and resistant RAW 264.7 cells. A) Naïve and resistant RAW 264.7 cells (ResRAW) were exposed to PAO1 (MOI 10) or to LPS (100 ng/ml) for 1 h. Note the translocation of the p65 subunit of NF-kB to the nucleus in both cell types. For the right-hand most images, preparations that received no primary antibody were viewed in the red channel. **B**) To quantitate the inhibitor of NF-kB (IKB), cells were exposed to PAO1 for 1 h, harvested and processed for Western blot analysis to detect IkB and b-actin. Note the major reduction in total IKB.

After 1 h exposure, changes by comparison to t 0 are summarized in Table S5A. In Table S6A the data have been trimmed to remove unannotated genes and changes of lesser statistical significance. Table S7(1d) and S7(1i) group the entries in Table S6A according to gene ontology/pathway criteria, where the suffixes (i) and (d) designate tabulations of the increases *vs* decreases.

Categories that show major increase after 1 h exposure (Table S7(1i)) include ($p<10^{-11}$): apoptosis, inflammatory response, immune response, and positive regulation of the I-kB kinase-NF-kB cascade. Specific transcripts encode cytokines that we have measured (MIP-2 and TNFα), as well as many others (CCL2, CCL4, CCL5, CCL7, Csf3, CXCL3, CXCL10, Edn1, IL1a, IL1b, Il1f6 and Lif). Most of these increases are also seen at 1+8 h (Table S7(2), S6C/D). Those that appear only at +1 h are the transcription factor, Bhlhb2, Irf4 (that negatively regulates NF-kB signaling), and the TNF family member, Tnfsf9. Decreases seen only at +1 h are for two little-characterized g-interferon-responsive proteins, Ifi27 and Ifi44. None of the decreases have p-values that are nearly comparable to those of the increases.

Categories that increase after 1+8 h ($p<10^{-10}$) (S7(2i)) include those noted after 1 h, with addition of: positive regulation of cell proliferation, chemotaxis, anti-apoptosis, neutrophil chemotaxis, regulation of apoptosis, response to LPS, and PDGF receptor signaling pathway.

The group that increases >10x includes selected cytokines (Ccl2, Il1f6) and, interestingly, some responses that can be triggered by g-interferon (CD274, endothelin-1, Gbp1, Isg15, Rsad2/viperin, Serpinb9). Since there is no increase in g-interferon transcripts, these latter changes are likely to reflect cross-talk between pathways.

Categories that decrease after 1+8 h show greater statistical significance ($p<10^{-13}$) than increases (Tables S7(2i/d)). Thus, many decreases reflect strong inhibition of cell proliferation: cell cycle progression, cell division, mitosis, cell cycle regulation and nucleosome assembly. The group of strongest decreases encodes many histones, ribosomal proteins, subunits of the mitochondrial Fo-ATPase, and the actin-binding protein, anillin

Transcripts that are most strongly downregulated at 1+8 h by comparison to 1 h, as is evident in the categories, include many that are required for cell growth (Table S7(2)). Table S6C lists transcripts that are changed at 1+8 h but not more than 2x at 1 h.

Among entries that decrease selectively at 1 h compared to 1+8 h (Table S6D), none show changes of >10x.

4. Mechanism of Toxicity

What signaling pathway mediates toxicity?. To examine the role of signaling pathways in cell death, we monitored the possible protective effect of adding kinase inhibitors 3 h before PAO1 treatment. SP600125, that inhibits the phosphorylation of c-Jun and expression of inflammatory genes, reduced cell death by almost 50% at 10 μg/ml (Figure 6A). Other inhibitors, U0126 (for MEK) and BMS345541 (for IKK), had little effect.

A Role for Apoptosis?. Many host-pathogen interactions are linked to activation of cascades that converge on caspase 3, stimulating both extrinsic and intrinsic pathways, e.g. [41,42]. We

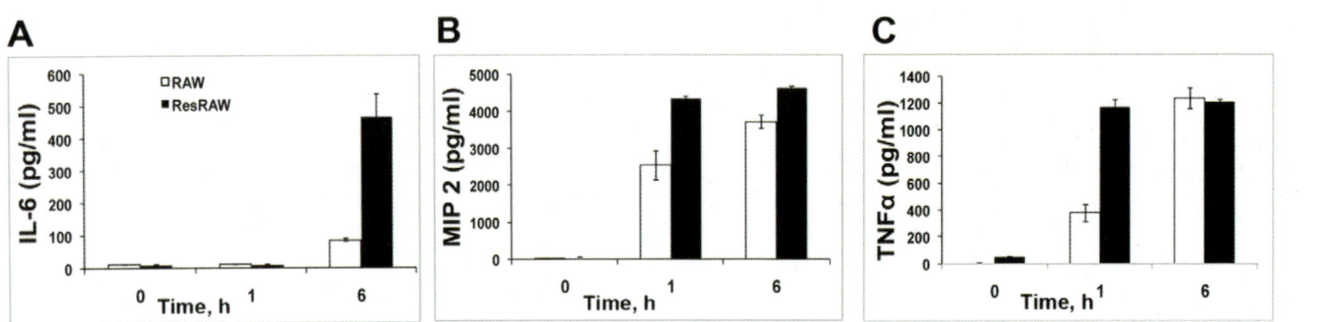

Figure 5. Cytokine production in response to PAO1. IL6 (**A**), MIP2 (**B**) and TNFα (**C**) secretion by naïve (solid line) and resistant (dotted line) RAW 264.7 cells were quantitated by ELISA, as described in Methods. Cells were exposed to PAO1 at MOI 10 for 1 h and recultured. Supernatants were collected at 0, 1 and 6 h. Cytokine production of mean +/− SD of three wells for each condition.

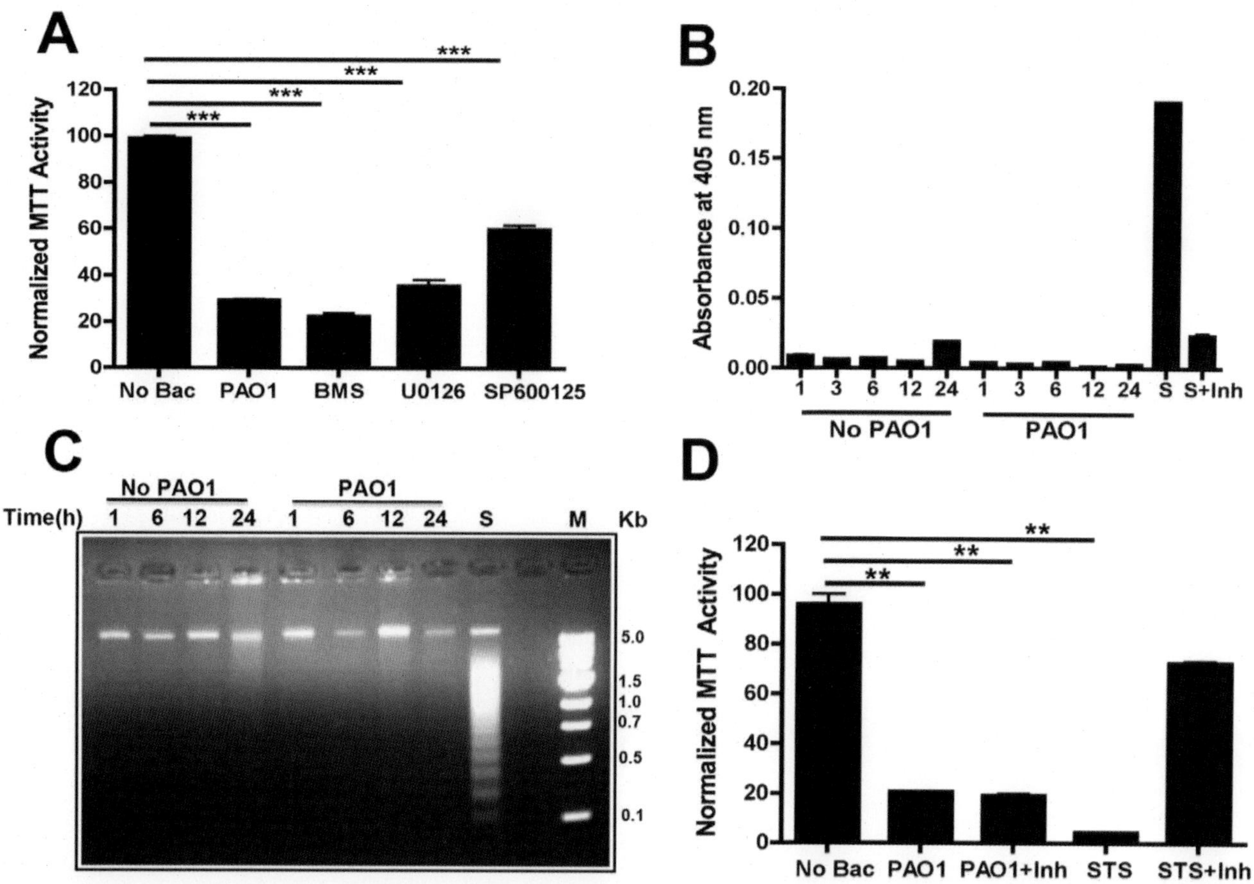

Figure 6. Toxicity of PAO1 toward RAW 264.7 cells. A) RAW 264.7 cells were exposed to PAO1 in the presence of different kinase inhibitors: SP600125 (for JNK, 10 mg/ml), U0126 (for MEK, 10 mg/ml) and BMS345541 (for IKK, 10 mg/ml). MTT assays quantitated cell viability after 1 day. **B**) RAW 264.7 cells were treated with PAO1 (MOI 10, 1 h) and washed. Caspase-3 activity was measured by colorimetric assays after 1–24 h. Control cells not exposed to bacteria were collected at the same time points. Sample treated with staurosporine (STS, 1 µg/ml) with or without caspase-3 inhibitor (Inh) for 3 h were used as a positive control. **C**) RAW 264.7 cells were exposed to PAO1 (MOI 10) for 1 h. DNA was isolated from cells at the indicated time points and analyzed by agarose gel electrophoresis. Control cells were not exposed to PAO1. Cells incubated with staurosporine (S) for 3 h were used as a positive control. M denotes the DNA ladder. **D**) RAW 264.7 cells were exposed to PAO1 +/− prior incubation with caspase 3 inhibitor (Inh). The viability of the cells was measured by MTT assay after 2 days. Cells treated with staurosporine were used as a positive control. Data are indicative of three repeat experiments with similar results and error bars represent standard deviations. (***) designates $p<0.0003$.

therefore evaluated caspase 3 activity after exposure to PAO1. Negative controls (unstimulated cells) and a positive control consisting of cells treated with staurosporine, were analyzed in parallel. As expected, staurosporine strongly increased activity, but no increase was detected even after 24 h in cells exposed to PAO1 (Figure 6B). Consistent with this apparent lack of involvement of apoptosis, in protocols that show obvious DNA laddering after treatment with staurosporine we do not see laddering for cells treated with PAO1, even after 24 h (Figure 6C).

To learn whether toxicity nevertheless could be due to apoptosis, we added the cell-permeable caspase-3 inhibitor, Ac-DEVD-CHO, 4 h prior to addition of bacteria and also included it during the subsequent 1–2 day incubation. As illustrated in Figure 6D, this inhibitor blocked killing by staurosporine but had no effect on the toxicity of *P. aeruginosa*. Parallel experiments show that murine alveolar macrophages are also killed by *P. aeruginosa* and that that apoptosis is not involved (Figure S2). Possibly, although DNA cleavage and internalization of *Pseudomonas* do not appear to be involved, *Pseudomonas* toxicity is mechanistically related to necrosis or pyroptosis [43–46].

5. Selection of resistant cells

To further explore the mechanism of toxicity, we recovered RAW 264.7 mutants that resist *P. aeruginosa*. Thus, unmutagenized cells were exposed to wild type bacteria for 1 h at MOI = 10, washed, and then recultured for 4 days, at which point the majority of the cells had died. The survivors were allowed to recover, and were again exposed to *P. aeruginosa* for 1 h. After ten iterations of this protocol the survivors tolerated exposure to *P. aeruginosa* to a much greater extent than naïve cells (Figure 1D). Their resistance is thus a stable characteristic. Although we have not proven that these cells carry chromosomal mutations, we refer to them as "mutants." They also are much more resistant than naïve cells when exposed to *P. aeruginosa* for as long as 5 h at MOI 50 (not shown).

We recovered five clones of resistant cells by limiting dilution. Since they all originated from a single pool of cells, they could be identical to each other. We do not think that they preexisted among the naïve cells, since exposure of naïve cells to doses of *P. aeruginosa* that are tolerated by the mutants totally eradicates the naïve population. In the following studies we focus on one clone (#2).

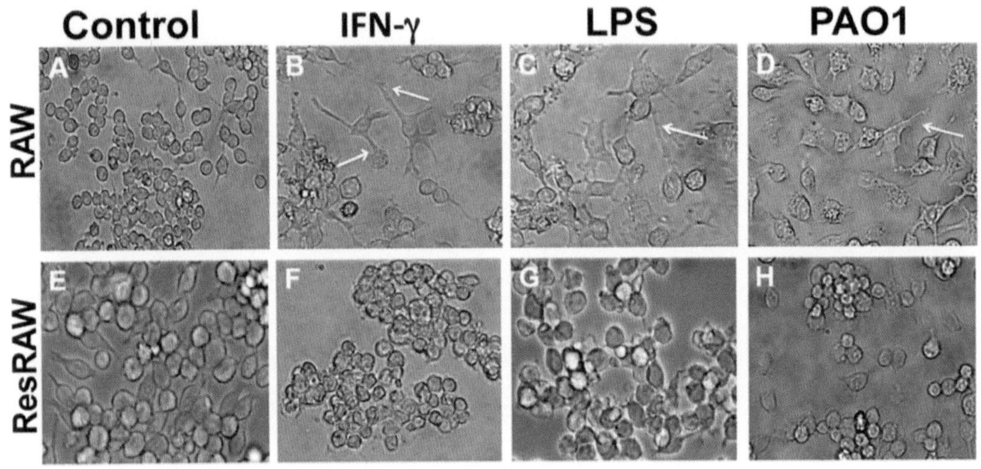

Figure 7. Morphological changes of naïve and resistant RAW 264.7 cells. Both naïve and resistant cells were exposed to g-interferon (25 ng/ml), soluble LPS (2 mg/ml) and PAO1 (MOI 10). After 1 h they were returned to culture for 48 h. The large differences of responsiveness of between the naïve and resistant cells are indicated by arrows. The naïve cells upon exposure to g-interferon, LPS, and PAO1 have extended processes and appear vacuolated, whereas the appearance of the resistant cells upon treatment does not differ from that of untreated control cells.

6. Characterization of Mutants

Morphology, cross-resistance. Upon treatment with PAO1, soluble LPS of *P. aeruginosa*, or mouse g-interferon for 24 h, wild type cells spread and (especially with g-interferon), extend processes (Figure 7B), and ultimately become highly vacuolated (Figure 7C and 7D). By contrast, the mutant cells do not change shape or size or generate binucleated cells upon exposure to *P. aeruginosa* (Figure 1A). They also do not spread in response to soluble LPS or to g-interferon (Figure 7F and 7G). The mutant is also significantly more resistant to *E. coli* than wild type (not shown).

Since a MDCK mutant selected for resistance to Concanavalin A is coincidentally resistant to ricin and to *P. aeruginosa* [47], we asked the inverse question of whether the RAW 264.7 mutant resists these lectins. When grown continuously in their presence, the mutant is at least 2x more resistant to both ConA and RCA I than wildtype (Table 2).

Signaling. Since the mutant cells resist exposure to PAO1, they could have lesions at the level of TLR4 or downstream lesions along a signaling pathway. Nevertheless, as for wildtype cells, the p65 subunit of NF-kB relocates massively to the nucleus of the mutant cells within 1 h of exposure to PAO1 at MOI 10 (Figure 4A – panel 6). Relocation of p65 is also observed with soluble LPS (Figure 4A – panel 7). Consistent with the, Western blotting shows that the level of IkBα in the mutant decreases after exposure to PAO1 (Figure 4B).

Table 2. Comparative Sensitivity of the Mutant and Wildtype Cells.

Clones	LD_{50} (μg/ml)		
	ConA	RCA	LPS
RAW	~20	~0.1	~0.1
ResRAW	~70	~0.5	~5

Sensitivity was evaluated by exposing cells to the lectins or to LPS continuously for 2–3 days.

Furthermore, exposure of the mutant to PAO1 strongly stimulates the release of several cytokines (Figure 5). In fact, the levels of secreted IL-6, MIP2 and TNF-α increase more rapidly than for wildtype. Thus, judging from both the relocation of p65 and from cytokine release, TLR4 signaling occurs in the mutant cells.

Transcriptional Profiles. The ability of the mutant cells to tolerate *P. aeruginosa* could reflect their steady-state phenotype or their differential hyper- or hypo-responsiveness when exposed to *P. aeruginosa*. We therefore compared the transcriptional profiles of these cells to wildtype, both before and after exposure. The following paragraphs summarize these observations.

Steady-state profiles (Tables S5C, S6I; S7(9i), S7(9d)). Before exposure to PAO1, the mutant has a transcriptional profile that differs from wildtype. Resistant cells show relative upregulation ($10^{-6}<p<10^{-3}$) of categories that are most enriched in signal transduction and prostaglandin biology. Specific transcripts encode

- The TGFb receptor,
- G-protein-coupled receptors for two bioactive lipids (platelet-activating factor, sphingosine phosphate),
- The receptor for programmed cell death ligand 1, and two semaphorin receptors (plexins). The semaphorins and corresponding receptors are best-characterized regarding neuronal migration and outgrowth of neuronal processes; however, they have also been implicated in inflammatory responses in conjunction with TGFb [48].
- Curiously, a GTPase-activating protein (Rgs1) that inhibits GPCR signaling is also upregulated.

The most strongly downregulated categories ($10^{-7}<p<10^{-3}$) before exposure to PAO1 are immune and inflammatory responses. They include transcripts that encode one of the subunits that functions in conjunction with Tlr4 (CD14), as well as Tlr8.

Transcripts related to prostaglandin biology are either upregulated (Cox-1, Ptgds-2) or downregulated (Cox-2, protaglandin E4 receptor). A similar lack of uniformity is seen for proteins important for anti-viral responses (RNase L *vs* Ifitm3, Ifih1, Oas2).

Responses of resistant cells (1 h exposure: Tables S5D, S6E, S7(5i/d); 1+8 h exposure: Tables S5E, S6F, S7(6i/d)). When the mutant cells are exposed to *P. aeruginosa* for 1 h or for 1 h followed by 8 h, major transcriptional changes occur. As for wildtype, the following categories are most strongly upregulated ($10^{-16}<p<10^{-6}$) at both time points: apoptosis, immune response, inflammatory response, positive regulation of I-kB kinase-NF-kB cascade, anti-apoptosis.

At the 1 h time point, the most strongly downregulated categories ($10^{-16}<p<10^{-6}$) seem not to fall into coherent groupings. At 1+8 h, the categories that show strongest downregulation ($10^{-22}<p<10^{-14}$) are indicative of cell cycle arrest, as for wildtype. This similarity is notable since the resistant cells are destined to survive.

The progression of these responses through time is indicated in Tables S6C and S6D (wildtype) and S6G/H (mutant). To make this assessment, we have focused on transcripts whose levels do not change more than 2x in the 1 h *vs* 0 h tabulation. We then enumerate the intensity levels of the same group of transcripts in the tabulation of 1+8 h *vs* 0 h data for the same cell type.

For wildtype cells, transcripts that show >10x induction at 1+8 h (but not at 1 h) are Ccl2, Cd274, Edn1, Gbp1, Il1f6, Isg15, Rsad2, and Serpinb9. For the mutant, some responses are shared (Rsad2, Gbp1, Isg15); however, a distinctive new signature group of increases emerges. In this group, the recurrence of guanylate-binding proteins (Gbp3, Gbp5, Gbp6, as well as Gbp1) is striking. These proteins are also strongly induced by g-interferon, but their biological significance remains incompletely characterized [49]. Their induction by LPS is an order of magnitude less than induction by g-interferon and appears to be only transient [50]. Other proteins of possible importance for survival are Ifi202b, that promotes NF-kB signaling, and tenascin, that promotes cell rounding. No transcripts show strong downregulation when the 1+8 h data for resistant cells are compared to 1 h (Table S6H).

Wildtype vs resistant cell comparisons: (1 h exposure: (Tables S6J/J′; 1+8 h exposure: Tables S6K/K′). The distinctive characteristics of a sensitive cell could be either positive or negative by comparison to a resistant cell. The top-to-bottom order of entries in Table S3 displays a) increases seen in the resistant cells after 1+8 h, that do not occur after 1+8 h in wildtype, b) increases seen in the wt after 1+8 h, that do not occur after 1+8 h in resistant cells, c) base-line comparison of mutant cells to wildtype, and d) transcripts thought to be relevant to survival (<0.5x or >2.0x).

In the 1+8 h samples for the mutant, points of particular interest are summarized in Table S4. It includes

- Transcripts that are expected to promote TLR signaling, including CD14, If202b, Nfkb1 and Traf5, that increase, and Nfkbie and Gpr109a, that decrease. TLR signaling could also be reduced by the increase in Tnip and the decrease in Tlr4 and Tlr13.
- Transcripts that are expected to promote JAK/STAT signaling, including Grap and Nfam, that increase, and Socs3 that decreases. JAK/STAT signaling could also be reduced by the decrease of JAK2 and the spingosine-phosphate receptor, S1pr1, that sustains SOX3 signaling.
- Transcripts that are expected to promote GPCR signaling, including E2f8, that increases, and Rgs1 and Trem2, that decrease.
- Transcripts that are expected to promote growth, including Gbp3, Gbp5, Gbp6, Myc, Plk2, Pkrir and Rasgrp3, that increase, and the decrease of CD274 (the receptor for the programmed cell death ligand), Fas, Phlda1 and Serpin b9. Growth could be opposed by the relative increase of Wee1.

Although the mutant cells survive, they show many of the initial changes that are also characteristic of the wildtype, e.g. major downregulation of histone transcripts. One might expect that resistance results from dampening of the initial changes. Nevertheless, only very few transcripts that are upregulated in wildtype at both +1 h and 1+8 h are upregulated in the mutant only at the initial time point. These are the transcription factor, Bhlbhb2, and Ifrd1.

Discussion

The encounter between *P. aeruginosa* and host cells in the lung is seldom catastrophic unless the host is compromised. The case of cystic fibrosis (CF) is striking, in that *P. aeruginosa* infections account for a large fraction of CF deaths [6]. Several hypotheses can account for the exaggerated inflammatory responses of cells of CF patients: 1) that binding of bacterial LPS to cell surface CFTR normally elicits protective responses, e.g. phagocytosis and rapid initiation of signaling mediated by IL-1 [12,23], 2) that alterations of glycosylation that are characteristic of the surfaces of CF cells sensitize them to *P. aeruginosa*, e.g. [6], or 3) that alteration of the composition of airway surface liquid by CFTR activity affects bacterial clearance. Given this lack of unanimity, additional approaches will be needed to learn how to make cells resistant to *P. aeruginosa*.

This study aims to identify especially sensitive features of the target cell, rather than describing all possible means by which the bacterium could kill this target. For this reason, we have abbreviated the time of exposure to pathogen and used a low multiplicity of infection. As for many cell types in CF, the target cells that we have chosen (RAW 264.7 monocyte/macrophages) do not express the cystic fibrosis transmembrane regulator. We surprisingly observe that several classical mechanisms of toxicity are irrelevant: Neither type II and type III secretion, pili nor flagella are required. Although cell contact is required, the only way to implicate LPS in toxicity is with the proviso that it must be in concentrated form, i.e. soluble LPS is toxic but on a molar basis it is orders of magnitude less toxic than intact *P. aeruginosa*.

Since *P. aeruginosa* seems not to be phagocytosed under the conditions used, a powerful signaling cascade(s) is presumably initiated upon contact with the cell surface. This same pathway could be responsible for initiating translocation of the p65 subunit of NF-kB into the nucleus and eliciting cytokine secretion. Intriguingly, toxicity is not accompanied by caspase 3 activation and inhibition of this enzyme does not block toxicity, although apoptosis can result from the interaction of *P. aeruginosa* with other cell targets [51,52]. Thus, in agreement with observations of some other host-pathogen interactions, death does not require apoptosis [53–55]. Judging from the impact of a JNK inhibitor, this kinase may be central to the toxicity of PAO1 [56,57].

To identify functionally significant intermediates, we generated cells that resist the toxicity of *P. aeruginosa*. As summarized in Figure 8, they show some but not all of the responses that are characteristic of wildtype cells. Strikingly, these cells do not show morphological signs of activation (spreading); however, they do respond strongly to PAO1. In fact, they are hyper-responsive in the sense that PAO1 elicits cytokine secretion and selected transcriptional changes even more dramatically than for wildtype. Over-reaction could be part of a protective response due either to induction of protective factors or to repression of factors that normally oppose activation. Analysis of the possible mechanism(s) of toxicity is simplified by the demonstration that factors released

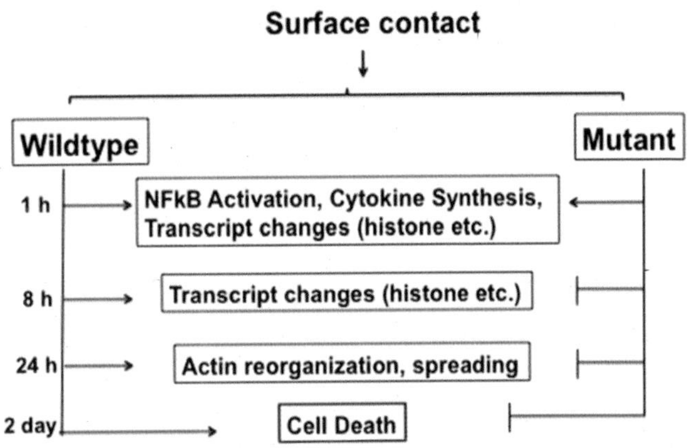

Figure 8. Overeview of the responses of wildtype and mutant cells. As is detailed in the text, the present observations show that both cell types exhibit comparable initial changes, including NF-kB activation, cytokine secretion, and downregulation of transcripts that are essential for continued growth. Nevertheless, only the wildtype cells are ultimately killed. The mutant cells show distinct upregulation of transcripts that are associated with responses to g-interferon. These changes could be of central importance for survival.

from wildtype target cells and bacterial supernatants are not themselves toxic. Moreover, supernatants from stimulated mutant cells do not protect naïve wildtype cells. We conclude that, although corresponding autocrine loops surely exist, they are not key to toxicity.

Although cells resistant to *E. coli* LPS have been studied previously, we are not aware of studies that have used live *P. aeruginosa* for selection. Among LPS-resistant cells are

- Cells that cannot signal through TLR4: A J774.1 macrophage mutant [58], and a CHO cell mutant that has a defect in the LPS co-receptor, MD-2 [59].
- Cells that bind LPS: A WEHI-3 macrophage-derived mutant [60], and a CHO cell mutant that shows normal translocation of NF-kB upon LPS treatment [61]. Like the CHO cell mutant, the new mutants are still responsive to PAO1.

Our transcription profile data provide a point of reference for understanding the sensitivity/resistance of both the normal RAW 264.7 cell and the mutant. These stable phenotypic differences could result from multiple ramifications of a single genetic change, from a widespread epigenetic change, or from chromosomal rearrangements.

The differences of steady state profiles of mutant *vs* wildtype before stimulation suggest that the mutant is well-prepared to participate in several types of signaling: multiple receptors are upregulated (for TGF, lipid mediators, semaphorins). Moreover, although they do respond to *P. aeruginosa*, the titer of two Tlr receptors (CD14, Tlr8) is reduced. They also exhibit a reduced level of at least one pro-apoptotic protein (Ifi27).

When wildtype cells are stimulated for 1 h, they already show strong proinflammatory responses that persist through time, along with dramatic down-regulation of housekeeping genes (encoding histones, ribosomal proteins, etc.) and selected receptors. These changes provide a molecular signature of the non-apoptotic form of toxicity that is triggered in this situation. Very comparable changes occur in the mutant, but by the 1+8 h time point, several novel increases occur. The strongest of these encode several of the "guanylate-binding proteins," tenascin, that promotes spreading, and Ifi202b, that promotes NF-kB signaling. Also striking is the upregulation of several growth-promoting transcripts (Myc, Rasgpr3, Plk2, Pkrir) along with downregulation of several that could oppose survival (CD274, Fas, Phlda1, Serpin b9). Taken together, these observations suggest the value of preliminary expression of multiple receptors, and induction of a cluster of powerful growth-promoting factors (Figure 8).

Interestingly, there is a very striking enrichment of a repertoire of g-interferon-inducible transcripts among the responses that are stronger in the mutant than in wildtype – Table S3. As g-interferon transcripts do not increase, these observations could signify that the mutant allows extensive input into g-interferon signaling pathways. Nevertheless, we do not observe upregulation of transcription factors (e.g. DRAF, VAF, VIF) that mediate the induction of subsets of g-interferon targets, either by g-interferon itself or by dsRNA [62]. Perhaps the induced repertoire results from "cross-talk" between signaling pathways. "Cross-talk" has been detected under other circumstances, with emphasis on g-interferon's non-classical stimulation of pathways other than those normally under control of STAT1 [63,64].

Few transcription factors appear to be up- or down-regulated in the mutant and those that are affected are not obviously linked to g-interferon. Thus, the widely-expressed factor, bhlbh2, is increased in the mutant before exposure to *P. aeruginosa*, while bhlbh3 [65] is selectively reduced in the mutant after stimulation. E2f8 is selectively reduced after stimulation only in wildtype. Other possible contributors are kinases that impact STAT proteins or their regulators, e.g. Socs proteins.

g-interferon signals principally through JAK1, JAK2 and STAT1. Nevertheless, g-interferon signaling can also lead to STAT-independent activation of ERK1/2 and PI3-kinase, e.g. [63].

There has been no agreement as to whether g-interferon can protect cells against *P. aeruginosa* [66,67] perhaps because one of the secretory proteases of this organism can degrade g-interferon [68]. The present observations reopen this issue and forcefully raise the question of whether a subset of g-interferon-responsive proteins effectively opposes *P. aeruginosa* [69].

The ease with which resistant cells can be obtained suggests that comparable shifts of transcriptional specificity could normally enable wildtype cells in the host organism to resist *P. aeruginosa*. Identification of factors that mediate these shifts could therefore help identify molecular targets of therapeutic value.

g-interferon-induced proteins are often critical for responses to intracellular pathogens; however, evidence for the importance of Gbp's in defense against viral and bacterial infections remains fragmentary. Moreover, although *Listeria monocytogenes* and *Toxoplasma gondii* upregulate multiple GBPs *in vivo*, the toxicity of *Salmonella* (toward RAW 264.7 cells) is actually potentiated by GBP-5 [44,70]. Other studies have shown that increased Gbp expression can inhibit cell growth and spreading, metalloprotease production and angiogenesis [71–74]. The present data set therefore presents a challenge for interpretation. One or more of the Gbp's - or other g-interferon-responsive proteins - could account for the resistance of the mutant cells.

Materials and Methods

Source of reagents

Except where indicated otherwise, all chemicals were from Sigma-Aldrich Chemical Co.

Bacterial Strains and Growth Conditions

Strains and plasmids used are listed in Table S1. The strain of PAO1 is proficient in Type I, II and III secretion (Dr. A. Rietsch, personal communication). Bacteria were routinely grown overnight with shaking at 37°C in Luria-Bertani medium. The concentration of bacteria was determined by spectrophotometry (OD_{600} of 0.1 was equivalent to 1×10^8 cfu/ml). The growth of the bacteria could be completely inhibited with a mixture of 200 µg/ml of gentamicin (Sigma-Aldrich, G-1914) and 200 µg/ml streptomycin (Sigma-Aldrich, S-6501).

Cell Culture

RAW 264.7 (ATCC T1B-71), a mouse monocyte-derived cell line, was grown in DMEM (Invitrogen, Carlsbad, CA), supplemented with 10% heat inactivated fetal bovine serum (Invitrogen), 5% CO_2 at 37°C. Cells were seeded at 1×10^4 cells/500 µl on coverslips (for microscopy) or 1×10^5 cells/well in 12 well plates (for MTT assays) or 2×10^5 cells/well in 6 well plates (for other assays). For selected experiments, 1×10^6 cells were transduced with a hrGFP retroviral supernatant (Stratagene) and cells expressing green fluorescent protein (GFP) were cloned by limiting dilution.

Exposure to *P. aeruginosa*

P. aeruginosa were grown overnight, diluted and regrown for another 2 h to an OD_{600} of 0.1 so that they were in exponential growth phase. Cultures were centrifuged at 10,000 rpm for 10 min and were resuspended in tissue culture medium. *P. aeruginosa* was added to RAW 264.7 cells in their serum-containing growth medium at a MOI of 10:1 (if not mentioned otherwise). After 1 h, the cells were washed 3× with PBS and fresh medium containing gentamicin (200 µg/ml) and streptomycin (200 µg/ml) was added to kill extracellular bacteria during continued culture. To estimate the titer of internalized bacteria, we prepared cell lysates according to [28] and plated them on LB plates for quantitation.

Mutant Selection

5×10^5 RAW 264.7 cells were exposed to PAO1 at MOI = 5 for 1 h in medium without antibiotics at 37°C. Cells were washed with PBS and received fresh medium supplemented with 200 µg/ml gentamicin and 200 µg/ml streptomycin. The surviving cells (viability 5–10%) were allowed to grow for 3–5 days until viability was again excellent. The cells were then split and again exposed to *P. aeruginosa*. This process was iterated 10×. Both naïve and cycled RAW 264.7 cells were cloned by limiting dilution.

Cytotoxicity Assays

Cytotoxicity was determined quantitatively using a 3-[4,5-Dimethylthiazol-2-yl]-2,5-diphenyltetrazolium bromide (MTT) (Invitrogen, M-6494) cleavage assay (Mosmann, 1983). For this assay, 1×10^5 cells were plated onto 12-well plates 1 day prior to the experiment and exposed to bacteria as above. After removal of the supernatant the cells were rinsed with PBS. At this point, 100 µl of 5 mg/ml MTT in PBS was added per ml of culture media and incubated for 1 h at 37°C. The supernatant was discarded and 1 ml of stop solution (20% SDS, 50% dimethylformamide) was added to each well to dissolve the formazone crystals. Absorbance was recorded at 570 nm. Readings taken for uninfected control cells were used for normalization. The percent viability was calculated by the formula $(A_{570\ nm})_{sample}/(A_{570\ nm})_{control}\times100$. The controls were not exposed to bacteria. For these and all other quantitative assays, standard deviations were calculated and illustrated as error bars.

Statistical analysis

Statistical analysis was performed using an unpaired t test (Prism; GraphPad Software). p values less than 0.05 were considered significant.

Preparation of culture supernatants

To ascertain whether toxicity was due to soluble factors released by bacteria or RAW 264.7 cells, several experiments were performed. To investigate the toxicity of bacterial supernatants, two procedures were used: 1) graded amount of bacterial culture were centrifuged for 5 min at 10,000 rpm. The pellets were discarded and the supernatants were passed through 0.22 µm filters (Millipore), mixed 1:10 with growth medium and added to RAW 264.7 cultures (2.5×10^5 cells/well) for 1 h. Control plates received the same volume of LB medium. 2) PAO1 was added at MOI = 10 and 50 to culture wells either with or lacking RAW cells. After 1 h, the resulting supernatants were recovered, centrifuged for 5 min at 10,000 rpm and filtered through 0.22 µm filters. They were then added (without dilution) to naïve RAW 264.7 cultures. After incubation for 1 h at 37°C, they were transferred to fresh medium for two days for examination and MTT assay.

Microscopy

RAW 264.7 cells (5×10^3) were grown overnight on 12 mm glass coverslips and exposed to bacteria at MOI = 10 and 50 at 37°C. After 1 h, the cells were washed with PBS and fixed with 4% paraformaldehyde in PBS for 15 min at room temperature, washed with PBS, incubated with 0.1 M glycine in PBS for 5 min followed by 0.1% (v/v) Triton X-100 in PBS for 1 min at room temperature. They were then stained with 0.15 µM phalloidin in PBS (Sigma, P-1951) for 15 min at room temperature in the dark and washed with PBS. The coverslips were then stained with 0.015 µM 4,6-diamidino-2-phenylindole (DAPI) (Sigma-Aldrich, D-9542) in PBS for 2 min in the dark, washed with PBS, and mounted on glass slides using gel mount antifade reagent (Biomeda Corp.). The slides were viewed at 100× magnification under oil immersion in an epifluorescence microscope and by Deltavision microscopy.

p65 Translocation Assays

For indirect immunofluorescence analysis, 5×10^3 cells were grown on 18 mm glass coverslips and exposed to either PAO1, MOI = 10 or to 100 µg/ml LPS of *P. aeruginosa*, serotype 10 (Sigma-Aldrich L-9143), for 1 h, washed, and recultured as required. Cells were fixed with 4% paraformaldehyde in PBS for 15 min at room temperature, permeabilized with 0.1% Triton X-100 in PBS for 1 min at room temperature and stained with rabbit anti-p65 (1:100; eBioscience Ltd) in PBS containing 10% goat serum for 30 min at room temperature. Cells were incubated with Lissamine-Rhodamine conjugated goat anti-rabbit IgG (Jackson ImmunoResearch Laboratories) in PBS at room temperature for 30 min and washed 3× with PBS. Nuclei were stained using DAPI as above, washed, mounted and examined. For detecting activation of the cells, the cells were treated with LPS or PAO1 as described, fixed and viewed at 40× in phase contrast microscope.

Apoptosis Assays

DNA Fragmentation. RAW 264.7 cells were plated in six well plates (1×10^6 cells/well) and were exposed to PAO1, MOI = 10 for 1 h. The cells were then washed 3× in PBS and recultured. After 1–24 h the cells were collected by centrifugation and lysed with 200 µl of lysis buffer (10 mM Tris-Cl, pH 8.0, 10 mM EDTA and 0.05% Triton X-100) [75]. Lysates were incubated with 1 µg/ml of RNaseA, followed by 0.5 µg/ml of Proteinase K for 1 h at 37°C and 50°C respectively. DNA was extracted using Tris-saturated phenol, pH 7.4, chloroform and isoamyl alcohol (25:24:1) and precipitated with isopropyl alcohol at −20°C. The precipitate was centrifuged at 12,000×g for 15 min and the pellet was air dried and suspended in 10 mM Tris-Cl, pH 8.0. Samples of DNA (2.5 µg) were electrophoresed in 1.2% agarose gels in TAE, and stained with ethidium bromide. As a positive control, cells were also treated with staurosporine (1 µg/ml for 2 h), a kinase inhibitor that induces apoptosis [76], and DNA samples were processed exactly as above.

Caspase-3 Assay

Cells in six well plates (1×10^6 cells/well) were exposed to PAO1 and samples were collected at different time points by centrifugation at 1,000×g for 15 min. The pelleted cells were lysed in 100 µl lysis buffer (250 mM HEPES, pH 7.4; 25 mM CHAPS and 25 mM DTT), incubated on ice for 30 min and then centrifuged at 12,000×g for 15 min. Supernatants were incubated with the caspase-3 substrate, 0.2 mM Ac-DEVD-pNA (Sigma-Aldrich) overnight at 37°C. Product formation was measured spectrophotometricaly at 405 nm. As controls, the cells were pretreated for 4 h with 0.02 mM cell-permeable inhibitor of caspase-3 (Ac-DEVD-CHO) prior to exposure to bacteria. The inhibitors were also present after the cells were washed free of bacteria.

Western Blot Analysis

Both wildtype and mutant cells were exposed (or not) to PAO1 as mentioned above. The cells were washed 3× in PBS, and lysed using cold 1× lysis buffer (Cell Signaling Technology, Beverly, MA). Total protein was quantified using standard BCA assay, and 10 µg of protein were separated by 12% SDS-polyacrylamide gel, transferred to nitrocellulose membrane, and probed for total IkB and ß-actin (Cell Signaling Technology). Proteins were detected using HRP-conjugated secondary antibodies and developed with Supersignal West Femto Maximum Sensitivity Substrate (Pierce).

Cytokine Measurements

To quantify cytokine secretion, cells were grown overnight in a 12 well plate (1×10^5 cells/well) and exposed to PAO1 at MOI = 10 for 1 h. The cells were then recultured. Supernatants were collected after 0, 1, 6 and 24 h to measure released cytokines. The Mouse Cytokine FMAP BASE kit (R&D Bioscience) was used to quantitate interleukins IL-6, MIP-2 and TNF-α. For this purpose, 100 µl of the supernatants were added to 96 well microtiter plates containing antibody-coated bead complexes. Plates were analyzed using the Luminex 100 analyzer, version 7.1 (Luminex Corp., Austin, TX). A minimum of 100 events (beads) was collected for each cytokine/sample and median fluorescence intensities were obtained. Cytokine concentrations were calculated based on standard curve data using STATLIA from Brendan version 3.2.

Microarray Analysis

Triplicate cultures of RAW 264.7 cells and mutants were harvested 0, 1 and 8 h after 1 h exposure to PAO1, MOI = 10 for 1 h; control samples (0 h time point) were not exposed to bacteria. In each case cells were washed 3× with cold PBS and total RNA was isolated using RNeasy kit (QIAGEN) and then further processed by the Gene Expression and Genotyping Facility of the Case Comprehensive Cancer Center. Affymetrix analysis of ~1 µg of RNA used mouse whole transcriptome arrays (Mouse GeneChip 1.0 ST chip) and Affymetrix software. Hybridization was conducted overnight at 45°C with agitation. Post-hybridization, washing and staining were performed in a Fluidics Station 450 (Affymetrix). Hybridization signal was measured using a GeneChip scanner (Affymetrix GC3000) to detect the fluorescence at each probe loci. Signal values were generated using Expression Console 1.1 (EC, Affymetrix). Signals were normalized using the RMA (Robust multichip Analysis) feature of EC. Fold changes in expression were filtered by means of a 1.5 fold change in a binary comparison ratio data between group means.

BAMarray analysis (incorporating Bayesian Analysis of Microarray data) was also used to analyze our data set. This software is a statistical tool which is capable of conferring significance upon observed differences between the means of individual gene expression signals of groups of samples. False detection rates get smaller with increasing numbers of replicates per group. The software is freely available to academic users. Data were exported as space-delimited text files which were imported into MS excel. Probset identifiers are accompanied by the following significance indices: "1" (significantly increased over the base line group); "0" (not significantly different from the baseline group) and "−1" (significantly decreased compared to the baseline group). BAM analysis deals only with statistical significance and does not comment on the magnitude of the fold change. We cross-referenced our gene change results from BAMarray with the 1.5 fold changes between group means describe above. This produced a keeper data set which we subsequently took into other software for pattern and pathway mining analyses.

Functional gene classifications were derived from Gene Ontology information found in National Center for Biotechnology Information (NCBI) database and from independent literature searches.

There are three sets of supplementary Tables (Tables S5, S6, S7), as inventoried end of the list of supplementary tables:

Tables S5A–S5B, S5D–S5E "Full Data Sets: Comparisons to t 0" provide the basic data sets in which the values for each condition (e.g. after 1 h exposure to *P. aeruginosa*) is compared to that of resting cells (t 0) of the same type. Table S5C compares the transcript levels for the resistant cells to wildtype cells.

In Tables S6A–K "Homotypic and Heterotypic Comparisons for Annotated Genes," the data sets have been simplified by including only annotated genes, e.g. Table S6A is a simplified version of Table S5A. Tables S6A, S6B, S6E, S6F include comparative information, listing genes that change in one time interval but not more than 1.5× in another (e.g. in the wildtype t1+8 h vs t 0 comparison but not more than 1.5× in the wildtype t1 h vs t 0 comparison). Tables S6C and S6D (for wt cells, like S6G and S6H for the resistant cells) lists entries for which changes are seen at one time point (e.g. 1+8 h vs t0) but not at another (e.g. 1 h vs t 0). Table S6I (as well as S7(9i)/7(9d)) compares the transcriptome of resting wildtype cells with that of resting resistant cells. Tables S6J and S6K make comparisons between the wildtype and resistant cells. The comparisons designated (') are inverse to those lacking this designation, e.g. Table S6J is "changed in wildtype 1 h vs t 0 but not more than 1.5× in resistant cells 1 h vs t

0", while Table S6J′ is "changed in resistant 1 h vs t 0 but not in wildtype 1 h vs t 0". In the comparative tables, changes must be >1.5 x to be included.

Tables S7(1,2,5,6,9) - "Gene Ontology Groups" summarize gene ontology classifications and therefore include only annotated genes. An overview summary of these data is given in Tables 1 and S2. We have eliminated categories for which there was only a single entry. The suffixes (i) or (d) indicate whether increases or decreases are observed.

In these Tables, the columns specify probe set IDs, average values for one condition, average values for the second condition, the quotient of the two, the "posterior call" [that indicates whether, according to Bam analysis, the change is significant and is an increase (+1) or decrease (−1)], the gene symbol (if known) and gene description (if known). The columns specify the functional category, its type, the total number of genes within that category in the spread sheet, the expanded number of such genes, the number of genes in this analysis that are included in the category, the number expressed as a percent of genes in the category, the specific genes in question, the p-value for having this overlap, the data source for annotations, and the rank order of each entry. The successive spread sheets are either total, or successively trimmed by p-value, or trimmed to eliminate entries where there is only a single entry.

Supporting Information

Figure S1 Investigations of the importance of LPS. A) A schematic of LPS structure, indicating the portions of the glycan that are absent in selected mutants. **B**) A two-day assay of the toxicity of *Pseudomonas* expressing truncated forms of LPS, by comparison to wt PAO1. **C**) Standard two-day assays show that polymyxin B blocks the toxicity of soluble LPS, but not intact PAO1.

Figure S2 Studies of Murine Alveolar Macrophages. A) MTT assays to quantitate cell number. Uninfected cells compared to cells exposed to *P. aeruginosa* and then recultured over 4 days. **B**) Annexin V binding evaluated by flow cytometry: Black: non-specific signal detected with an isotype-matched control antibody. Red: Cells not exposed to bacteria or to staurosporin. Blue: Cells exposed to bacteria or to staurosporin, as indicated. **C**) Caspase involvement, as in Figure 6B. Cells were exposed to PAO1 (MOI 10, 1 h) washed, and returned to culture. Caspase-3 activity was measured after 1–24 h (P1, P3 etc). Control cells not exposed to bacteria were collected at the same time points (C1, C3 etc.). Sample treated with staurosporine (STS, 1 μg/ml) with or without caspase-3 inhibitor (Inh) for 3 h were used as a positive control.

Methods S1 Supplementary Methods.

Table S1 Bacterial strains and plasmids used in this study are listed in Table S1.

Table S2 Summary of Gene Ontology Information.

Table S3 Comparison of wildtype and resistant cell responses.

Table S4 Summary of Relative Changes After 1+8 h Exposure to *Pseudomonas aeruginosa*.

Table S5 Full Data Sets: Comparisons to t0 - Tables S5A–S5E. Table S5A: WT t1 hr vs WT t0. Table S5B: WT t1+8 h vs WT t0. Table S5C: Resistant t0 vs WT t0. Table S5D: Resistant t1 hr vs t0. Table S5E: Resistant t1+8 hr vs t0.

Table S6 Homotypic and Heterotypic Comparisons for Annotated Genes - Tables S6A–S6K. Table S6A: Changes in WT t1 vs WT t0. Table S6B: Changes in WT t1+8 vs WT t0. Table S6C: Changes in WT t1+8 vs WT t0, not in WT t1 vs t0. Table S6D: Changes in WT t1 vs WT t0, not in WT t1+8 vs t0. Table S6E: Changes in resistant t1 vs t0. Table S6F: Changes in resistant t1+8 vs t0. Table S6G: Changes in resistant t1+8 vs t0, not in resistant t1 vs t0. Table S6H: Changes in resistant t1 vs t0, not in resistant t1+8 vs t0. Table S6I: Changes in resistant t0 vs WT t0. Table S6J: Changes in WT t1 vs WT t0, not in resistant t1 vs t0. Table S6J′: Changes in resistant t1 vs t0, not in WT t1 vs t0. Table S6K: Changes in WT t1+8 vs WT t0, not in resistant t1+8 vs t0. Table S6K′: Changes in resistant t1+8 vs t0, not in WT t1+8 vs t0.

Table S7 Gene Ontology Groups – S7(1)–S7(9). Table S7(1d): Groups associated with WT t1 vs WT t0 decreases. Table S7(1i): Groups associated with WT t1 vs WT t0 increases. Table S7(2d): Groups associated with WT t1+8 vs WT t0 decreases. Table S7(2i): Groups associated with WT t1+8 vs WT t0 increases. Table S7(5d): Groups associated with resistant t1 vs resistant t0 decreases. Table S7(5i): Groups associated with resistant t1 vs resistant t0 increases. Table S7(6d): Groups associated with resistant t1+8 vs resistant t0 decreases. Table S7(6i): Groups associated with resistant t1+8 vs resistant t0 increases. Table S7(9d): Groups associated with resistant t0 vs WT t0 decreases. Table S7(9i): Groups associated with resistant t0 vs WT t0 increases.

Acknowledgments

We thank the following for help in selected experiments: C. Hollegian, P. Jaiswal, J. Saks. Thanks to the following for bacterial strains and advice: D. Abbott, J. Lam, V. Lee, G. Pier, A. Rietsch, and G. Toole.

Author Contributions

Conceived and designed the experiments: SR TB AT. Performed the experiments: SR TB. Analyzed the data: SR TB AT. Contributed reagents/materials/analysis tools: SR TB. Wrote the paper: SR AT.

References

1. Gerlach RG, Hensel M (2007) Protein secretion systems and adhesins: the molecular armory of Gram-negative pathogens. Int J Med Microbiol 297: 401–415.
2. Ma Q, Zhai Y, Schneider JC, Ramseier TM, Saier MH Jr (2003) Protein secretion systems of Pseudomonas aeruginosa and P fluorescens. Biochim Biophys Acta 1611: 223–233.
3. Jacquot J, Tabary O, Le Rouzic P, Clement A (2008) Airway epithelial cell inflammatory signalling in cystic fibrosis. Int J Biochem Cell Biol 40: 1703–1715.
4. Ahmad-Nejad P, Hacker H, Rutz M, Bauer S, Vabulas RM, et al. (2002) Bacterial CpG-DNA and lipopolysaccharides activate Toll-like receptors at distinct cellular compartments. Eur J Immunol 32: 1958–1968.
5. Tart AH, Wozniak DJ (2008) Shifting paradigms in Pseudomonas aeruginosa biofilm research. Curr Top Microbiol Immunol 322: 193–206.
6. Gomez MI, Prince A (2007) Opportunistic infections in lung disease: Pseudomonas infections in cystic fibrosis. Curr Opin Pharmacol 7: 244–251.

7. Smith EE, Buckley DG, Wu Z, Saenphimmachak C, Hoffman LR, et al. (2006) Genetic adaptation by Pseudomonas aeruginosa to the airways of cystic fibrosis patients. Proc Natl Acad Sci U S A 103: 8487–8492.
8. Baldwin MR, Barbieri JT (2005) The type III cytotoxins of Yersinia and Pseudomonas aeruginosa that modulate the actin cytoskeleton. Curr Top Microbiol Immunol 291: 147–166.
9. Cowell BA, Evans DJ, Fleiszig SM (2005) Actin cytoskeleton disruption by ExoY and its effects on Pseudomonas aeruginosa invasion. FEMS Microbiol Lett 250: 71–76.
10. Ball G, Durand E, Lazdunski A, Filloux A (2002) A novel type II secretion system in Pseudomonas aeruginosa. Mol Microbiol 43: 475–485.
11. Cianciotto NP (2005) Type II secretion: a protein secretion system for all seasons. Trends Microbiol 13: 581–588.
12. Pier GB (2007) Pseudomonas aeruginosa lipopolysaccharide: a major virulence factor, initiator of inflammation and target for effective immunity. Int J Med Microbiol 297: 277–295.
13. Beutler B, National Institutes of Health (2007) How we sense microbes. [Bethesda, Md.: National Institutes of Health.
14. Elson G, Dunn-Siegrist I, Daubeuf B, Pugin J (2007) Contribution of Toll-like receptors to the innate immune response to Gram-negative and Gram-positive bacteria. Blood 109: 1574–1583.
15. Schroder K, Irvine KM, Taylor MS, Bokil NJ, Le Cao KA, et al. (2012) Conservation and divergence in Toll-like receptor 4-regulated gene expression in primary human versus mouse macrophages. Proc Natl Acad Sci U S A.
16. Ramphal R, Balloy V, Huerre M, Si-Tahar M, Chignard M (2005) TLRs 2 and 4 are not involved in hypersusceptibility to acute Pseudomonas aeruginosa lung infections. J Immunol 175: 3927–3934.
17. Skerrett SJ, Wilson CB, Liggitt HD, Hajjar AM (2007) Redundant Toll-like receptor signaling in the pulmonary host response to Pseudomonas aeruginosa. Am J Physiol Lung Cell Mol Physiol 292: L312–322.
18. Apodaca G, Bomsel M, Lindstedt R, Engel J, Frank D, et al. (1995) Characterization of Pseudomonas aeruginosa-induced MDCK cell injury: glycosylation-defective host cells are resistant to bacterial killing. Infect Immun 63: 1541–1551.
19. Kierbel A, Gassama-Diagne A, Rocha C, Radoshevich L, Olson J, et al. (2007) Pseudomonas aeruginosa exploits a PIP3-dependent pathway to transform apical into basolateral membrane. J Cell Biol 177: 21–27.
20. Diggle SP, Stacey RE, Dodd C, Camara M, Williams P, et al. (2006) The galactophilic lectin, LecA, contributes to biofilm development in Pseudomonas aeruginosa. Environ Microbiol 8: 1095–1104.
21. Kostyk AG, Dahl KM, Wynes MW, Whittaker LA, Weiss DJ, et al. (2006) Regulation of chemokine expression by NaCl occurs independently of cystic fibrosis transmembrane conductance regulator in macrophages. Am J Pathol 169: 12–20.
22. Hasko G, Deitch EA, Nemeth ZH, Kuhel DG, Szabo C (2002) Inhibitors of ATP-binding cassette transporters suppress interleukin-12 p40 production and major histocompatibility complex II up-regulation in macrophages. J Pharmacol Exp Ther 301: 103–110.
23. Schroeder TH, Lee MM, Yacono PW, Cannon CL, Gerceker AA, et al. (2002) CFTR is a pattern recognition molecule that extracts Pseudomonas aeruginosa LPS from the outer membrane into epithelial cells and activates NF-kappa B translocation. Proc Natl Acad Sci U S A 99: 6907–6912.
24. Sun Y, Karmakar M, Taylor PR, Rietsch A, Pearlman E (2012) ExoS and ExoT ADP ribosyltransferase activities mediate Pseudomonas aeruginosa keratitis by promoting neutrophil apoptosis and bacterial survival. J Immunol 188: 1884–1895.
25. Shafikhani SH, Engel J (2006) Pseudomonas aeruginosa type III-secreted toxin ExoT inhibits host-cell division by targeting cytokinesis at multiple steps. Proc Natl Acad Sci U S A 103: 15605–15610.
26. Gruenheid S, Finlay BB (2003) Microbial pathogenesis and cytoskeletal function. Nature 422: 775–781.
27. Rottner K, Lommel S, Wehland J, Stradal TE (2004) Pathogen-induced actin filament rearrangement in infectious diseases. J Pathol 204: 396–406.
28. Aiello D, Williams JD, Majgier-Baranowska H, Patel I, Peet NP, et al. (2010) Discovery and characterization of inhibitors of Pseudomonas aeruginosa type III secretion. Antimicrob Agents Chemother 54: 1988–1999.
29. Rietsch A, Mekalanos JJ (2006) Metabolic regulation of type III secretion gene expression in Pseudomonas aeruginosa. Mol Microbiol 59: 807–820.
30. Goodman AL, Kulasekara B, Rietsch A, Boyd D, Smith RS, et al. (2004) A signaling network reciprocally regulates genes associated with acute infection and chronic persistence in Pseudomonas aeruginosa. Dev Cell 7: 745–754.
31. Feuillet V, Medjane S, Mondor I, Demaria O, Pagni PP, et al. (2006) Involvement of Toll-like receptor 5 in the recognition of flagellated bacteria. Proc Natl Acad Sci U S A 103: 12487–12492.
32. Mizel SB, Honko AN, Moors MA, Smith PS, West AP (2003) Induction of macrophage nitric oxide production by Gram-negative flagellin involves signaling via heteromeric Toll-like receptor 5/Toll-like receptor 4 complexes. J Immunol 170: 6217–6223.
33. Petrilli V, Dostert C, Muruve DA, Tschopp J (2007) The inflammasome: a danger sensing complex triggering innate immunity. Curr Opin Immunol 19: 615–622.
34. Kumagai Y, Takeuchi O, Akira S (2008) TLR9 as a key receptor for the recognition of DNA. Adv Drug Deliv Rev 60: 795–804.
35. Rocchetta HL, Burrows LL, Lam JS (1999) Genetics of O-antigen biosynthesis in Pseudomonas aeruginosa. Microbiol Mol Biol Rev 63: 523–553.
36. Jacobs DM, Morrison DC (1977) Inhibition of the mitogenic response to lipopolysaccharide (LPS) in mouse spleen cells by polymyxin B. J Immunol 118: 21–27.
37. Zhang G, Ghosh S (2001) Toll-like receptor-mediated NF-kappaB activation: a phylogenetically conserved paradigm in innate immunity. J Clin Invest 107: 13–19.
38. Koulenti D, Rello J (2006) Gram-negative bacterial pneumonia: aetiology and management. Curr Opin Pulm Med 12: 198–204.
39. Perez A, Davis PB (2004) Gene profile changes after Pseudomonas aeruginosa exposure in immortalized airway epithelial cells. J Struct Funct Genomics 5: 179–194.
40. Stotland PK, Radzioch D, Stevenson MM (2000) Mouse models of chronic lung infection with Pseudomonas aeruginosa: models for the study of cystic fibrosis. Pediatr Pulmonol 30: 413–424.
41. Ho PK, Hawkins CJ (2005) Mammalian initiator apoptotic caspases. FEBS J 272: 5436–5453.
42. Sakahira H, Enari M, Nagata S (1998) Cleavage of CAD inhibitor in CAD activation and DNA degradation during apoptosis. Nature 391: 96–99.
43. Ashida H, Mimuro H, Ogawa M, Kobayashi T, Sanada T, et al. (2011) Cell death and infection: a double-edged sword for host and pathogen survival. J Cell Biol 195: 931–942.
44. Fink SL, Cookson BT (2007) Pyroptosis and host cell death responses during Salmonella infection. Cell Microbiol 9: 2562–2570.
45. Miao EA, Rajan JV, Aderem A (2011) Caspase-1-induced pyroptotic cell death. Immunol Rev 243: 206–214.
46. Bortoluci KR, Medzhitov R (2010) Control of infection by pyroptosis and autophagy: role of TLR and NLR. Cell Mol Life Sci 67: 1643–1651.
47. Fleiszig SM, Evans DJ, Do N, Vallas V, Shin S, et al. (1997) Epithelial cell polarity affects susceptibility to Pseudomonas aeruginosa invasion and cytotoxicity. Infect Immun 65: 2861–2867.
48. Kang HR, Lee CG, Homer RJ, Elias JA (2007) Semaphorin 7A plays a critical role in TGF-beta1-induced pulmonary fibrosis. J Exp Med 204: 1083–1093.
49. Vestal DJ, Jeyaratnam JA (2011) The guanylate-binding proteins: emerging insights into the biochemical properties and functions of this family of large interferon-induced guanosine triphosphatase. J Interferon Cytokine Res 31: 89–97.
50. Nguyen TT, Hu Y, Widney DP, Mar RA, Smith JB (2002) Murine GBP-5, a new member of the murine guanylate-binding protein family, is coordinately regulated with other GBPs in vivo and in vitro. J Interferon Cytokine Res 22: 899–909.
51. Cannon CL, Kowalski MP, Stopak KS, Pier GB (2003) Pseudomonas aeruginosa-induced apoptosis is defective in respiratory epithelial cells expressing mutant cystic fibrosis transmembrane conductance regulator. Am J Respir Cell Mol Biol 29: 188–197.
52. Rajan S, Cacalano G, Bryan R, Ratner AJ, Sontich CU, et al. (2000) Pseudomonas aeruginosa induction of apoptosis in respiratory epithelial cells: analysis of the effects of cystic fibrosis transmembrane conductance regulator dysfunction and bacterial virulence factors. Am J Respir Cell Mol Biol 23: 304–312.
53. Blum ES, Abraham MC, Yoshimura S, Lu Y, Shaham S (2012) Control of nonapoptotic developmental cell death in Caenorhabditis elegans by a polyglutamine-repeat protein. Science 335: 970–973.
54. Long JS, Ryan KM (2012) New frontiers in promoting tumour cell death: targeting apoptosis, necroptosis and autophagy. Oncogene.
55. Wu W, Liu P, Li J (2011) Necroptosis: An emerging form of programmed cell death. Crit Rev Oncol Hematol.
56. Li Y, Arita Y, Koo HC, Davis JM, Kazzaz JA (2003) Inhibition of c-Jun N-terminal kinase pathway improves cell viability in response to oxidant injury. Am J Respir Cell Mol Biol 29: 779–783.
57. Bonny C, Oberson A, Negri S, Sauser C, Schorderet DF (2001) Cell-permeable peptide inhibitors of JNK: novel blockers of beta-cell death. Diabetes 50: 77–82.
58. Nishijima M, Hara-Kuge S, Takasuka N, Akagawa K, Setouchi M, et al. (1994) Identification of a biochemical lesion, and characteristic response to lipopolysaccharide (LPS) of a cultured macrophage-like cell mutant with defective LPS-binding. J Biochem 116: 1082–1087.
59. Schromm AB, Lien E, Henneke P, Chow JC, Yoshimura A, et al. (2001) Molecular genetic analysis of an endotoxin nonresponder mutant cell line: a point mutation in a conserved region of MD-2 abolishes endotoxin-induced signaling. J Exp Med 194: 79–88.
60. Ohki K, Amano F, Kohashi O (2001) Lipopolysaccharide (LPS) and zymosan-resistant mutant isolated from a macrophage-like cell line, WEHI-3, with a defective response to LPS under serum-free conditions. Immunol Cell Biol 79: 462–471.
61. Delude RL, Yoshimura A, Ingalls RR, Golenbock DT (1998) Construction of a lipopolysaccharide reporter cell line and its use in identifying mutants defective in endotoxin, but not TNF-alpha, signal transduction. J Immunol 161: 3001–3009.
62. Sen GC (2001) Viruses and interferons. Annu Rev Microbiol 55: 255–281.
63. Gough DJ, Levy DE, Johnstone RW, Clarke CJ (2008) IFNgamma signaling-does it mean JAK-STAT? Cytokine Growth Factor Rev 19: 383–394.

64. Hu X, Ivashkiv LB (2009) Cross-regulation of signaling pathways by interferon-gamma: implications for immune responses and autoimmune diseases. Immunity 31: 539–550.
65. Yamada K, Miyamoto K (2005) Basic helix-loop-helix transcription factors, BHLHB2 and BHLHB3; their gene expressions are regulated by multiple extracellular stimuli. Front Biosci 10: 3151–3171.
66. Johansen HK, Hougen HP, Rygaard J, Hoiby N (1996) Interferon-gamma (IFN-gamma) treatment decreases the inflammatory response in chronic Pseudomonas aeruginosa pneumonia in rats. Clin Exp Immunol 103: 212–218.
67. Murphey ED, Herndon DN, Sherwood ER (2004) Gamma interferon does not enhance clearance of Pseudomonas aeruginosa but does amplify a proinflammatory response in a murine model of postseptic immunosuppression. Infect Immun 72: 6892–6901.
68. Horvat RT, Parmely MJ (1988) Pseudomonas aeruginosa alkaline protease degrades human gamma interferon and inhibits its bioactivity. Infect Immun 56: 2925–2932.
69. Bach EA, Aguet M, Schreiber RD (1997) The IFN gamma receptor: a paradigm for cytokine receptor signaling. Annu Rev Immunol 15: 563–591.
70. Rupper AC, Cardelli JA (2008) Induction of guanylate binding protein 5 by gamma interferon increases susceptibility to Salmonella enterica serovar Typhimurium-induced pyroptosis in RAW 264.7 cells. Infect Immun 76: 2304–2315.
71. Gorbacheva VY, Lindner D, Sen GC, Vestal DJ (2002) The interferon (IFN)-induced GTPase, mGBP-2. Role in IFN-gamma-induced murine fibroblast proliferation. J Biol Chem 277: 6080–6087.
72. Guenzi E, Topolt K, Lubeseder-Martellato C, Jorg A, Naschberger E, et al. (2003) The guanylate binding protein-1 GTPase controls the invasive and angiogenic capability of endothelial cells through inhibition of MMP-1 expression. EMBO J 22: 3772–3782.
73. Messmer-Blust AF, Balasubramanian S, Gorbacheva VY, Jeyaratnam JA, Vestal DJ (2010) The interferon-gamma-induced murine guanylate-binding protein-2 inhibits rac activation during cell spreading on fibronectin and after platelet-derived growth factor treatment: role for phosphatidylinositol 3-kinase. Mol Biol Cell 21: 2514–2528.
74. Weinlander K, Naschberger E, Lehmann MH, Tripal P, Paster W, et al. (2008) Guanylate binding protein-1 inhibits spreading and migration of endothelial cells through induction of integrin alpha4 expression. FASEB J 22: 4168–4178.
75. Sellins KS, Cohen JJ (1987) Gene induction by gamma-irradiation leads to DNA fragmentation in lymphocytes. J Immunol 139: 3199–3206.
76. Karpinich NO, Tafani M, Rothman RJ, Russo MA, Farber JL (2002) The course of etoposide-induced apoptosis from damage to DNA and p53 activation to mitochondrial release of cytochrome c. J Biol Chem 277: 16547–16552.

15

Nitrous Oxide Production in Sputum from Cystic Fibrosis Patients with Chronic *Pseudomonas aeruginosa* Lung Infection

Mette Kolpen[1,2], Michael Kühl[3,4,5], Thomas Bjarnsholt[1,2], Claus Moser[1], Christine Rønne Hansen[6], Lars Liengaard[3], Arsalan Kharazmi[1], Tanja Pressler[6], Niels Høiby[1,2], Peter Østrup Jensen[1]*

1 Department of Clinical Microbiology, Rigshospitalet, Copenhagen, Denmark, **2** Department of International Health, Immunology and Microbiology, Faculty of Health Sciences University of Copenhagen, Copenhagen, Denmark, **3** Marine Biological Section, Department of Biology, University of Copenhagen, Helsingør, Denmark, **4** Plant Functional Biology and Climate Change Cluster, University of Technology Sydney, Sydney, Australia, **5** Singapore Centre on Environmental Life Sciences Engineering, Nanyang Technological University, Singapore, Singapore, **6** Copenhagen CF Centre, Rigshospitalet, Copenhagen, Denmark

Abstract

Chronic lung infection by *Pseudomonas aeruginosa* is the major severe complication in cystic fibrosis (CF) patients, where *P. aeruginosa* persists and grows in biofilms in the endobronchial mucus under hypoxic conditions. Numerous polymorphonuclear leukocytes (PMNs) surround the biofilms and create local anoxia by consuming the majority of O_2 for production of reactive oxygen species (ROS). We hypothesized that *P. aeruginosa* acquires energy for growth in anaerobic endobronchial mucus by denitrification, which can be demonstrated by production of nitrous oxide (N_2O), an intermediate in the denitrification pathway. We measured N_2O and O_2 with electrochemical microsensors in 8 freshly expectorated sputum samples from 7 CF patients with chronic *P. aeruginosa* infection. The concentrations of NO_3^- and NO_2^- in sputum were estimated by the Griess reagent. We found a maximum median concentration of 41.8 μM N_2O (range 1.4–157.9 μM N_2O). The concentration of N_2O in the sputum was higher below the oxygenated layers. In 4 samples the N_2O concentration increased during the initial 6 h of measurements before decreasing for approximately 6 h. Concomitantly, the concentration of NO_3^- decreased in sputum during 24 hours of incubation. We demonstrate for the first time production of N_2O in clinical material from infected human airways indicating pathogenic metabolism based on denitrification. Therefore, *P. aeruginosa* may acquire energy for growth by denitrification in anoxic endobronchial mucus in CF patients. Such ability for anaerobic growth may be a hitherto ignored key aspect of chronic *P. aeruginosa* infections that can inform new strategies for treatment and prevention.

Editor: Erich Gulbins, University of Duisburg-Essen, Germany

Funding: This work was funded by Faculty of Health and Medical Sciences, University of Copenhagen. The funders had no role in study design, data collection and analysis, decision to publish, or preparation of the manuscript.

Competing Interests: The authors have declared that no competing interests exist.

* E-mail: Peter.Oestrup.Jensen@regionh.dk

Introduction

Cystic fibrosis (CF) is an autosomal recessive disease. It is caused by mutations in the cystic fibrosis trans-membrane conductance regulator gene [1] affecting apical ion transport. In the lungs, the defective ion transport results in endobronchial accumulation of thick, viscous mucus that prevents mucociliar cleaning of the lungs, and increases susceptibility to chronic respiratory infections [2,3]. *Pseudomonas aeruginosa* is a Gram-negative, gamma proteobacterium, which dominates chronic lung infections in CF patients and is considered the most serious complication of CF [4,5]. The chronic *P. aeruginosa* lung infection in CF patients is characterized by presence of endobronchial biofilm aggregates surrounded by numerous polymorphonuçlear leukocytes (PMNs) [6,7]. Despite the bactericidal activity of the PMNs and intensive antibiotic therapy, these biofilms persist and grow in the endobronchial mucus of CF patients over many years [7,8]. *P. aeruginosa* can withstand the bactericidal activity of the PMNs by forming biofilms of the protective mucoid phenotype [9] and by quorum sensing (QS)-regulated production of leukolytic amounts of rhamnolipid [10–13]. The summoned PMNs produce reactive oxygen species (ROS) through a respiratory burst, which leads to intense depletion of molecular oxygen (O_2) [14], a common feature of infected endobronchial mucus in CF [6]. Biofilm formation may explain why *P. aeruginosa* survives the attacking PMNs, but it is not known how *P. aeruginosa* acquires the energy required for the observed growth in endobronchial secretions [8] when O_2 is absent. However, *P. aeruginosa* can grow anaerobically with alternative electron acceptors or by arginine fermentation [15], and it has been suggested that *P. aeruginosa* can respire by denitrification in anoxic CF mucus utilizing nitrate (NO_3^-) and nitrite (NO_2^-), which are both present in sufficient amounts [15,16]. Although the ability of *P. aeruginosa* to utilize reduction of NOx for anaerobic respiration is well known [17], denitrification in mucus and persistent biofilms present in the airways of CF patients remains to be demonstrated. Since N_2O is a natural intermediate belonging to the gases defining denitrification [17], we used electrochemical microsensors [18] to measure O_2 and

N_2O concentration gradients at high spatio-temporal resolution in freshly expectorated sputum from CF patients with chronic *P. aeruginosa* lung infection.

Further evidence for denitrification was obtained from nitrate (NO_3^-) and nitrite (NO_2^-) turnover measurements in the sputum samples. These measurements provided important new insights to the micro-environmental conditions and chemical dynamics associated with persistent *P. aeruginosa* lung infections in CF patients and indicate that nitrogen compounds can play an important role in the interaction between pathogenic bacteria and an active immune response.

Results

N_2O and O_2 in sputum from CF patients with chronic *P. aeruginosa* lung infection

Representative measurements of O_2 and N_2O in freshly expectorated sputum were acquired with O_2- and N_2O microsensors (Fig 1A). Measurements of O_2- and N_2O profiles in expectorated sputum from a CF patient with chronic *P. aeruginosa* lung infection showed the distribution of an upper oxygenated zone and a lower anoxic zone. The N_2O profile reached the maximal concentration of N_2O in the lower anoxic part of the sputum sample, suggesting that denitrification is mainly confined to the anoxic zone. A slow decline of O_2 was apparently detected above the sputum surface. This may be because the position of the sputum surface was estimated by visual inspection, which is associated with uncertainty due to small amounts of heterogeneous saliva (Fig 1B).

Sputum is composed of heterogeneously distributed bacterial aggregates surrounded by PMNs consuming O_2, and this respiratory burst creates local anoxic microenvironments in the sputum [14]. The metabolic mechanisms are thus compartmentalized according to the availability of O_2 with an oxygenated zone, wherein the majority of O_2 is reduced to superoxide by the summoned PMNs, and an anoxic zone, where *P. aeruginosa* can utilize nitrate as electron acceptor during oxidative phosphorylation (Fig. 1C).

NO_3^- and NO_2^- in sputum from CF patients with chronic *P. aeruginosa* lung infection

NO_3^- and NO_2^- concentrations in sputum samples were measured before N_2O profiling and 1 day later (Fig 2). The concentration of NO_3^- was significantly higher immediately before N_2O profiling as compared to 1 and 2 days after incubation indicating NO_3^- depletion due to ongoing denitrification (Fig 2A, B). The NO_2^- concentration was not changed significantly after one day (Fig 2C), but by including additional measurements of the NO_2^- concentration in 7 sputum samples a significantly decreased NO_2^- concentration was detected (Fig 2D).

Distribution of N_2O in sputum from CF patients with chronic *P. aeruginosa* lung infection

Vertical profiles of O_2 in sputum samples showed depletion of O_2, indicating the formation of anoxic zones below a mean depth of 3.1 mm (SD = 3.0 mm) from the sputum surface (Fig 3A) suggesting that the average depth of O_2 penetration of ~3 mm. A higher concentration of N_2O was observed in the anoxic zone as compared to the oxic zone ($p<0.026$, $n=8$) (Fig 3B). To verify that N_2O is related to *P. aeruginosa* we found significantly less N_2O in three control sputum samples from 1 CF patient and from 2

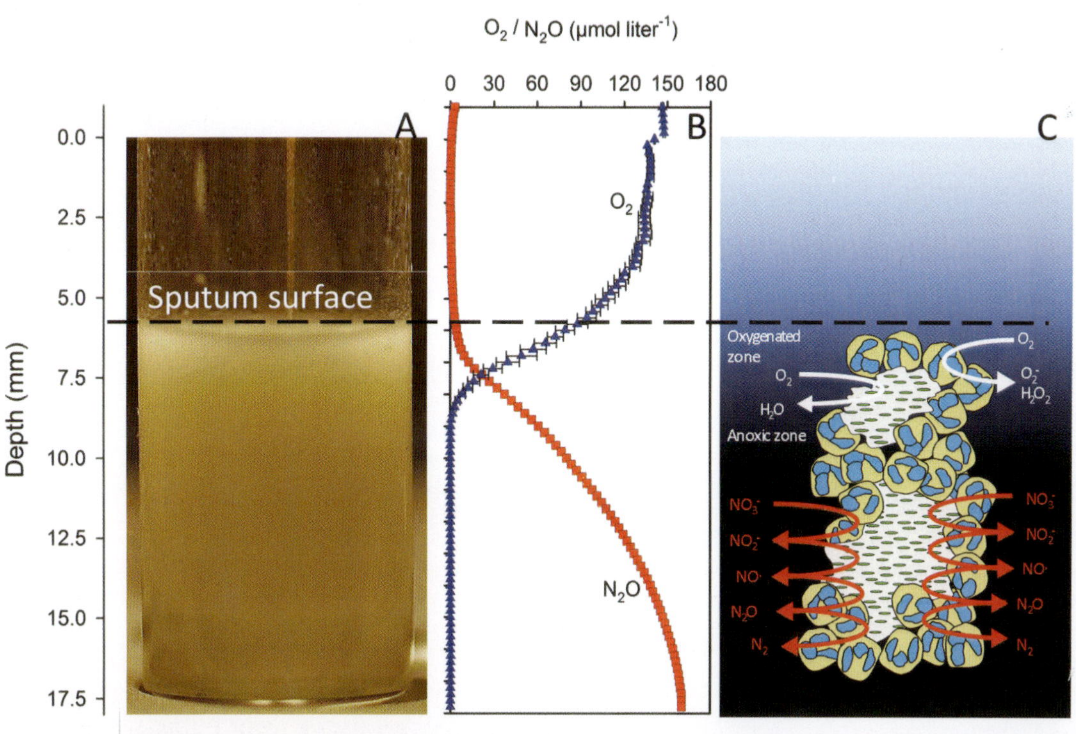

Figure 1. Microsensor measurements of chemical gradients in sputum. (A) Close up of a sputum sample from a cystic fibrosis patient with chronic *P. aeruginosa* lung infection with an inserted microsensor. (B) Representative microprofiles of N_2O and O_2 in a CF sputum sample. O_2 profiles are shown as the mean and SD of three microprofiles recorded in the beginning of the experiment and did not change significantly throughout the experimental period, while the N_2O profile represents the maximal N_2O levels measured about 6–7 h after beginning. (C) A schematic model of the involved PMN and biofilm processes in CF sputum explaining the microprofiles.

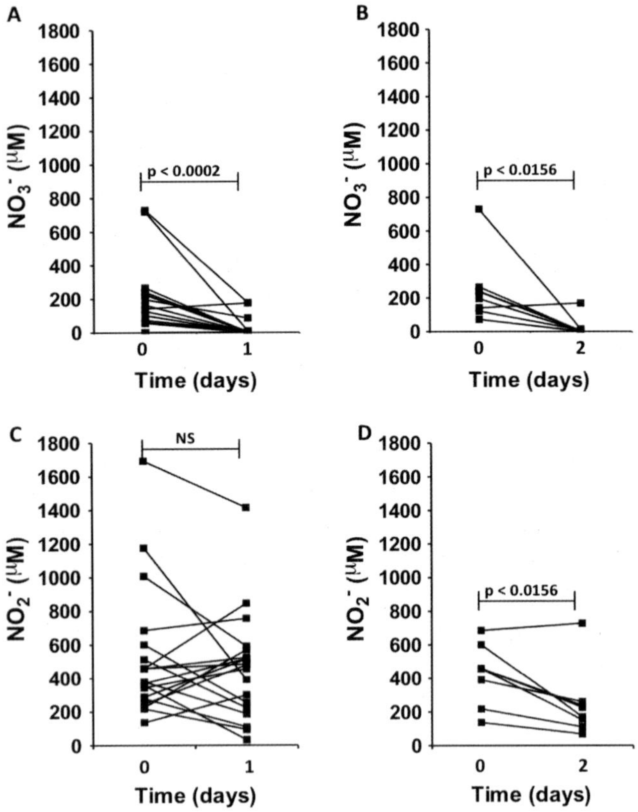

Figure 2. Consumption of NO3⁻ and NO2⁻ in sputum. (A, B) NO_3^- concentration in sputum samples from cystic fibrosis patients with chronic *P. aeruginosa* lung infection. (C, D) NO_2^- concentration in sputum samples from cystic fibrosis patients with chronic *P. aeruginosa* lung infection. Samples were collected immediately after expectoration and after 1 (n = 20) and 2 days (n = 7) of incubation. Data were analyzed by Wilcoxon signed rank test.

primary ciliary dyskinesia (PCD) patients without detectable *P. aeruginosa* ($p<0.030$).

Dynamics of N_2O in sputum from a CF patient with chronic *P. aeruginosa* lung infection

Figure 4 displays time series of representative N_2O profiles measured vertically through a sputum sample. The distribution of O_2 is displayed at 0 hr. During the initial measuring period, N_2O accumulated in the anoxic zone reaching a maximum concentration of 160 μM after 6.5 h incubation, which indicates ongoing production of N_2O. Within the subsequent 4 hours the accumulated N_2O decreased indicating consumption through reduction to N_2.

Rates of N_2O production and consumption in sputum samples

Measurements of the N_2O concentration dynamics over time in particular depths of a sputum sample showed an initial build-up of N_2O in layers below 7 mm (Fig. 5). In each layer, the slope of the net production curves was quasi-linear after ~180 min indicating a constant production of N_2O related to the particular layer and therefore that N_2O originates from immobile sources such as biofilm. The production ceased about 6–7 h after start of the sample incubation, and was then followed by a net consumption of N_2O over the following 4–5 h leading to N_2O depletion in the sputum sample after ~10–12 hours. In 4 sputum samples it was possible to estimate N_2O production and consumption rates (Table 1) and N_2O flux rates and cumulated emission (Figure 6) from measurements of such dynamic N_2O concentration microgradients. A substantial initial N_2O concentration was observed in the anaerobic zone of the remaining 4 assayed sputum samples. In these samples the N_2O concentration decreased steadily during incubation.

Discussion

The ability of microorganisms to exploit a wide range of electron acceptors for ATP generation by oxidative phosphorylation provides metabolic flexibility in transient environments as these organisms inhabit a variety of habitats ranging from soils, sediments to aquatic environments [19]. Even though several human pathogens, including *P. aeruginosa*, are equipped with the genetic setup for denitrification [20–22] including nitric oxide reductase (NOR) [22], we present the very first observations of N_2O production in clinical material from infected human airways demonstrating pathogenic metabolism based on denitrification. These data indicate that denitrification may serve as an alternative metabolic pathway allowing *P. aeruginosa* to thrive in O_2 depleted micro niches in the airways of CF patients. Besides our study, denitrification in humans has previously been demonstrated in human dental plaque [23] and has been related to infections of the gastrointestinal tract by the increased concentration of N_2O in exhaled breath from patients after oral intake of NO_3^- [24].

Seminal observations of O_2 depletion and the presence of OprF porin, which is involved in NO_3^- and NO_2^- diffusion, in habitats of *P. aeruginosa* during chronic lung infection of CF patients provided initial evidence for anaerobic respiration by denitrification [6,16]. To demonstrate denitrification we have included CF patients, who suffered from chronic *P. aeruginosa* infection in the endobronchial mucus as detected by routine culturing. We revealed a depletion of O_2 in CF sputum samples, which is in accordance with the steep O_2 gradients in endobronchial CF mucus [6] and due to O_2 consumption by activated PMNs for generation of ROS [14]. Our O_2 measurements in sputum confirmed the presence of O_2 concentration gradients reaching anoxia ~3 mm below the sputum surface.

The depletion of O_2 for microbial respiration in infected endobronchial CF mucus has motivated the present and several other studies of anaerobic metabolism by *P. aeruginosa* based on denitrification during chronic lung infection in CF. We demonstrated N_2O production and consumption in the sputum samples indicating the presence of active NOR and nitrous oxide reductase (N_2OR) for the reduction of nitric oxide (NO•) and N_2O [17]. Previously, NOR has been isolated from *P. aeruginosa* [25], the genes (*norCB*) have been sequenced [26] and functional NOR has been observed in clinical strains of *P. aeruginosa* by consumption of NO• [27].

In our study, the initial phase of N_2O production in the sputum samples was followed by a period of net N_2O consumption suggesting a depletion of NO• and a concomitant reduction of N_2O to N_2 by N_2OR. The N_2O consumption is in agreement with the demonstration of N_2OR activity and the identification of the *nos* genes in *P. aeruginosa* [28] as well as the induced genes for a N_2OR precursor in clinical isolates [29].

Our demonstration of significant N_2O production in sputum indicates ample presence of NO_3^- and NO_2^- that serve as electron acceptors for the denitrification pathway. We found high levels of NO_3^- and NO_2^- in the sputum, which are in agreement with previous findings [30–32]. It has been proposed that NO_3^-

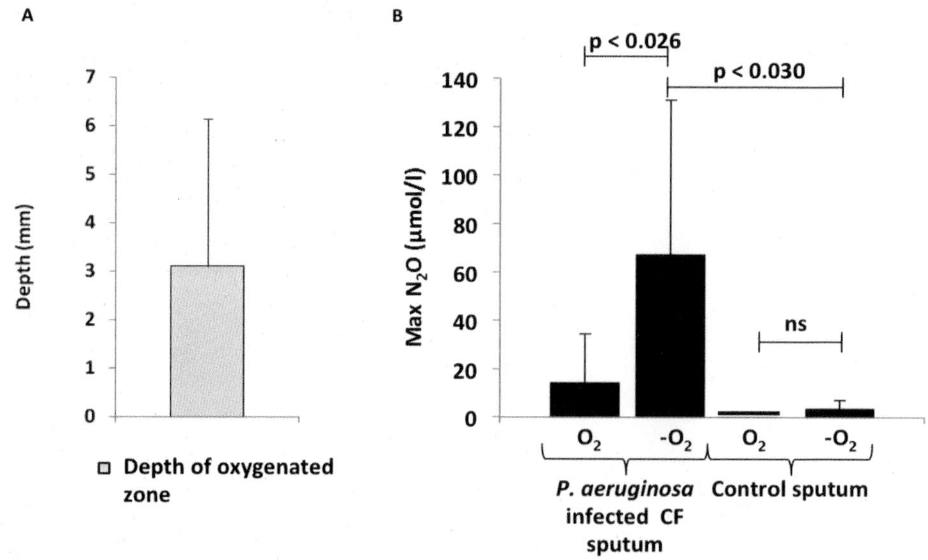

Figure 3. Distribution of O_2 and N_2O in sputum. (A) Depth of oxygenated zone in sputum samples from cystic fibrosis patients with chronic *P. eruginosa* lung infection (n = 8). (B) Maximal N_2O concentration in the oxic zone and anoxic zone in sputum samples from cystic fibrosis patients with chronic *P. aeruginosa* lung infection (n = 8). Control sputum without detectable *P. aeruginosa* was obtained from two PCD patients and one CF patient. Statistical analysis was performed by Student t-test.

and NO_2^- in CF sputum originates from the rapid reaction between superoxide (O_2^-) and NO• [15]. In this regard, we suggest the summoned activated PMNs [14] as a major source of O_2^-, while NO•, which is present in CF exhaled breath [33,34], may be produced by a variety of cells in the lungs. In fact, inhalation of NO• or incubation of sputum samples with NO• resulted in elevated levels of NO_3^- and NO_2^- in sputum from CF patients [35]. In addition, ongoing activity of the patients nitric oxide synthases was evidenced by the increased exhaled NO• from infected CF patients following supplementation with the substrate L-arginine [36,37].

As a consequence of our demonstration of N_2O production, we expected a consumption of the precursors NO_3^- and NO_2^-. Accordingly, NO_3^- was depleted in the sputum after incubation for 1 day, which likely is due to the membrane-bound nitrate reductase of *P. aeruginosa* [29]. NO_3^- consumption may also accompany assimilatory denitrification and ammonification resulting in the formation of ammonia (NH_4^+) [17], which has been detected in CF sputum [27]. However, assimilatory denitrification and ammonification does not involve production of N_2O [17,38,39] and NH_4^+ is also produced by several human cell types [40]. The concentration of NO_2^- was not changed during 1 day of incubation, but after 2 days of incubation the concentration of NO_2^- in the sputum was decreased significantly. This indicates that the production of NO• from NO_2^- is slower than the generation of NO_2^- resulting from reduction of NO_3^-. Indeed, during reduction of NO_3^- transient accumulation of NO_2^- is known from anaerobic cultures of *P. aeruginosa* growing by denitrification [16,41,42].

A further verification of ongoing dissimilatory denitrification in sputum is evident from the calculated rate of N_2O production (Fig. 6A), which easily can explain the depletion of NO_3^- during incubation (Fig. 2A). The depletion of NO_3^- in the sputum samples indicates that the NO_3^- in sputum samples is not replaced by the reaction between O_2^- and NO. This is possibly due to lack of contributions from immigrating PMNs and the epithelia as opposed to the conditions in the endobronchial mucus.

Since we calculated the rates of N_2O production by assuming linear changes between subsequent measurements in the beginning of incubation, the estimates are likely to reflect the situation in the endobronchial mucus, where reduced NO_3^- and NO_2^- is continuously being replaced as indicated by the high NO_3^- and NO_2^- content in fresh sputum. The estimated N_2O production, however, is calculated from the actual N_2O content and does not include the reduction of N_2O to N_2. Therefore, the actual rate of denitrification may be higher than our estimates.

We found the highest concentration of N_2O in the anoxic zone of the confined sputum samples indicating higher rate of denitrification without O_2 as previously demonstrated [43]. Accordingly, we suggest that the low concentration of N_2O found in the oxygenated zone is mainly due to diffusion from the active anoxic zone. Additionally, our estimate of the depth of the oxygenated zone implies that the bronchi, with diameters ranging from 0.8 to 13 mm [44,45], allow for numerous anoxic zones in the endobronchial mucus of the lungs and confirms the *in vivo* demonstration of O_2 depletion in the endobronchial mucus [6]. Consequently, our results propose the existence of several zones with N_2O production in the anoxic endobronchial mucus of the lungs of CF patients with chronic *P. aeruginosa* lung infection. However, such *in vivo* production of N_2O in CF patients still awaits direct experimental confirmation.

The involvement of denitrification enzymes as terminal oxidases that reduce nitrogen oxides in the highly branched respiratory chain of *P. aeruginosa* may enable anaerobic growth in the presence of nitrate or nitrite [19,46]. But the engagement of denitrification in *P. aeruginosa* may also contribute to virulence as evidenced by the finding of antibodies directed against components of denitrification in CF patients with *P. aeruginosa* lung infection [16,47] and the dependence on nitrite reductase for type III secretion [48]. In anaerobic cultures, denitrification promotes growth of *P. aeruginosa* [49], increases antibiotic tolerance of *P. aeruginosa* [50] and favors maintenance of the virulent mucoid phenotype [30].

A particular contribution to the pathogenesis of chronic lung infection in CF by NOR activity, is suggested by the induced *in vivo*

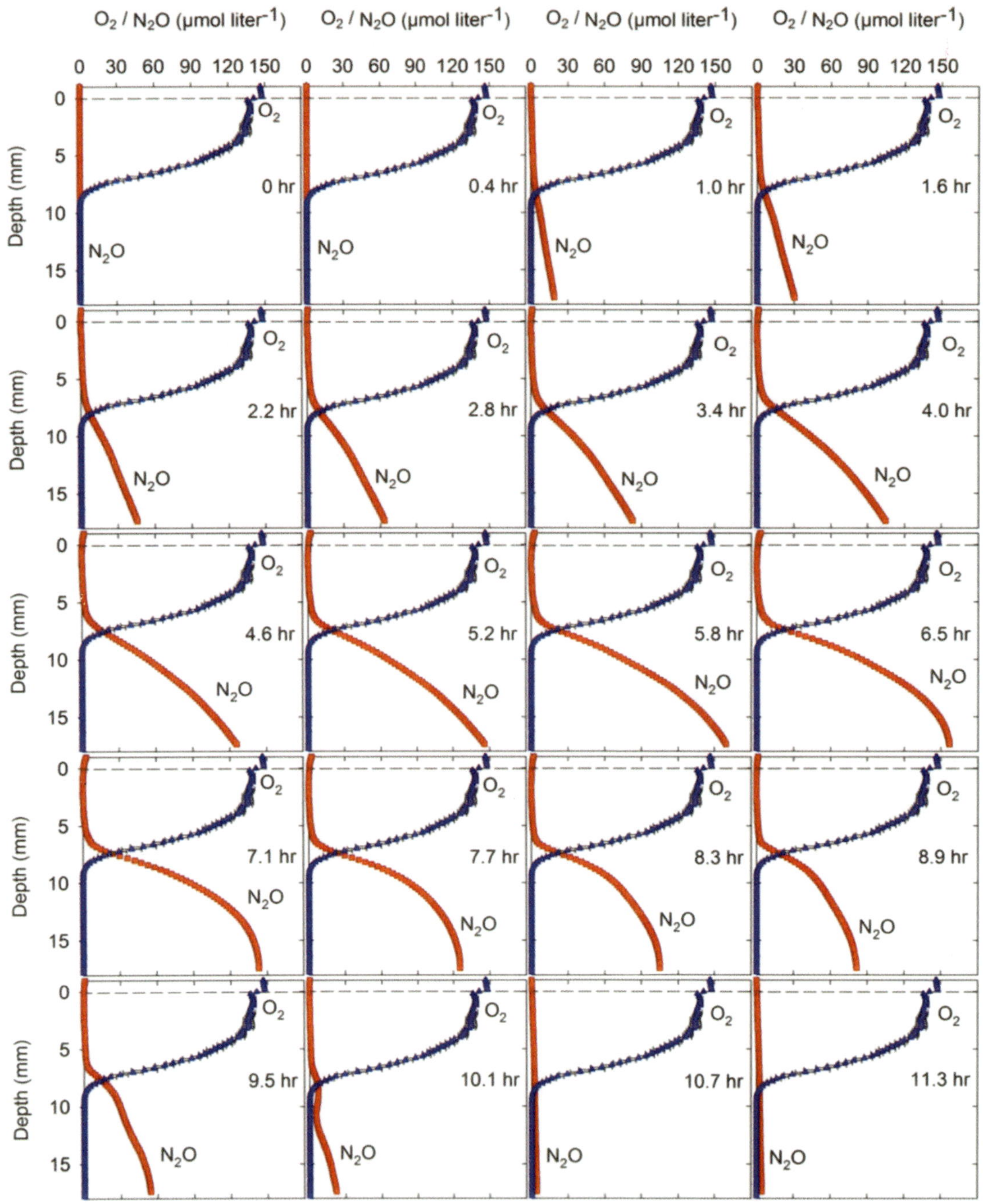

Figure 4. Generation and depletion of N_2O in sputum. Spatio-temporal dynamics of N_2O concentration profiles in a representative sputum sample from a cystic fibrosis patient with chronic *P. aeruginosa* lung infection showing initial accumulation of N_2O in the anoxic zone followed by total depletion. The O_2 concentration profile is shown as the mean and SD of three microprofiles recorded at the beginning of the experiment.

gene expression in clinical isolates [29] including the highly virulent mucoid isolates [51]. In this respect, the reduction of NO• to N_2O by active NOR may actually protect *P. aeruginosa* from the bactericidal action of NO• generated by the immune system. In fact, NOR-deficient *P. aeruginosa* is more susceptible to NO• generated by macrophages [52] and less virulent during infection of silkworm [53]. In addition, NOR activity increases the virulence of several pathogens [54–56].

In conclusion, this study points to the presence of anoxic microenvironments with strong spatio-temporal heterogeneity as well as a possible stratification of metabolic processes in the biofilm aggregates characteristic of chronic *P. aeruginosa* infections in the airways of CF patients. Such structural and metabolic heterogeneity may be a characteristic trait ensuring persistent infection. Indeed, spatio-temporal resolved measurements enabled the demonstrated of N_2O production in the anaerobic zones of freshly expectorated sputum samples from CF patients with chronic *P. aeruginosa* lung infection for the first time. Analysis of the N_2O production rates suggests ongoing generation of N_2O in the lungs of CF patients with chronic *P. aeruginosa* infection. N_2O production

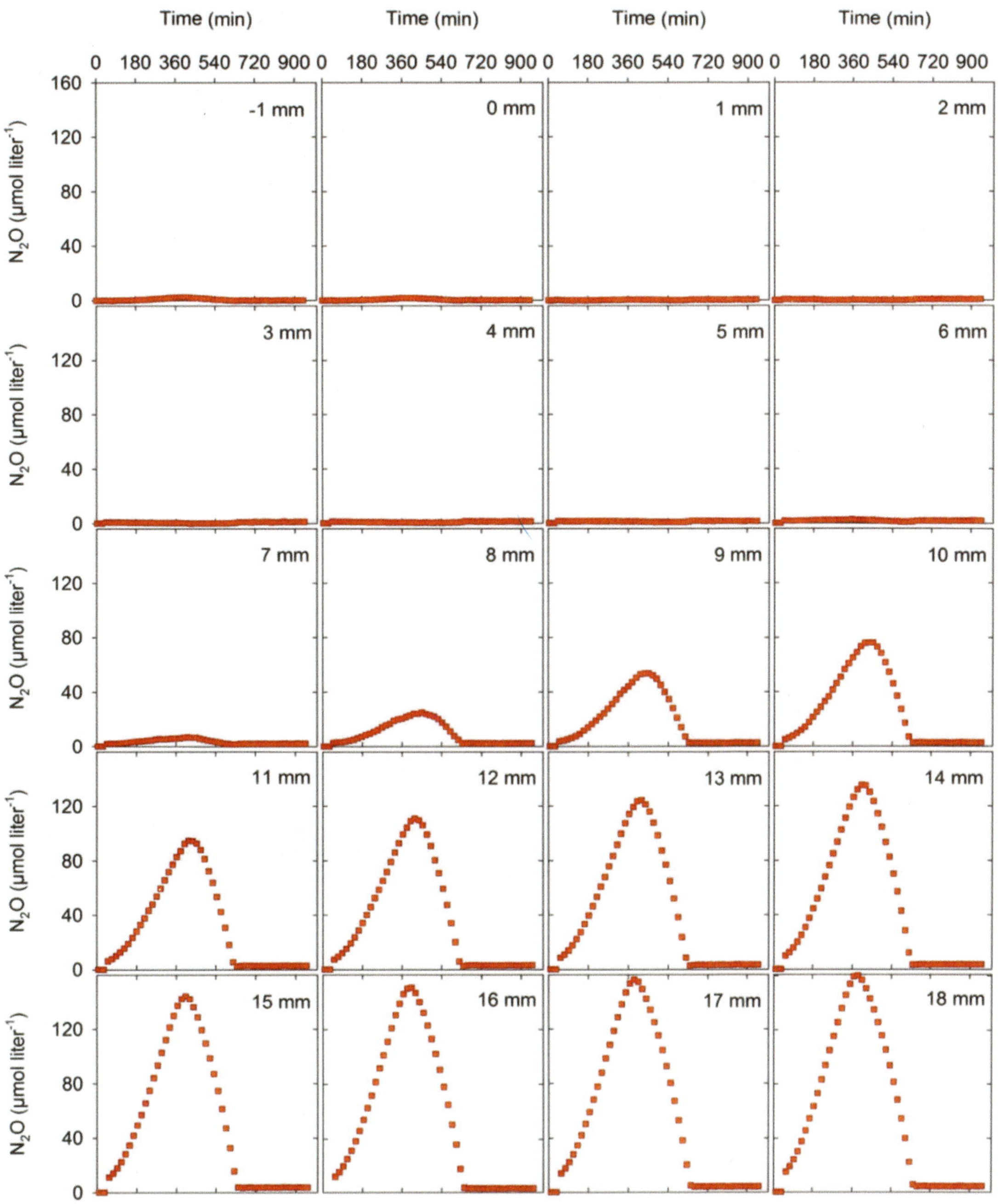

Figure 5. Rates of N2O production and consumption in sputum. Depth specific plots of N_2O concentration vs. time at particular measuring depths in the same sputum sample as displayed in Fig 4. Accumulation and thus net production of N_2O in all depths was observed until approximately 6 h, followed by net consumption of N_2O presumably due to depletion of nitrate around 6 h.

Table 1. N_2O production, consumption, max emission, and cumulated emission in 4 CF sputum samples.

	Net production rate (nmol $cm^{-3}min^{-1}$)	Net consumption rate (nmol $cm^{-3}min^{-1}$)	Max emission (nmol cm^{-2} min^{-1})	Cumulated emission (nmol cm^{-2})
Median	0.47	−0.39	5.06×10^{-5}	1.05×10^{-2}
Range	0.40–0.70	−0.77–−0.10	1.8×10^{-5}–6.78×10^{-5}	3.94×10^{-3}–1.46×10^{-2}

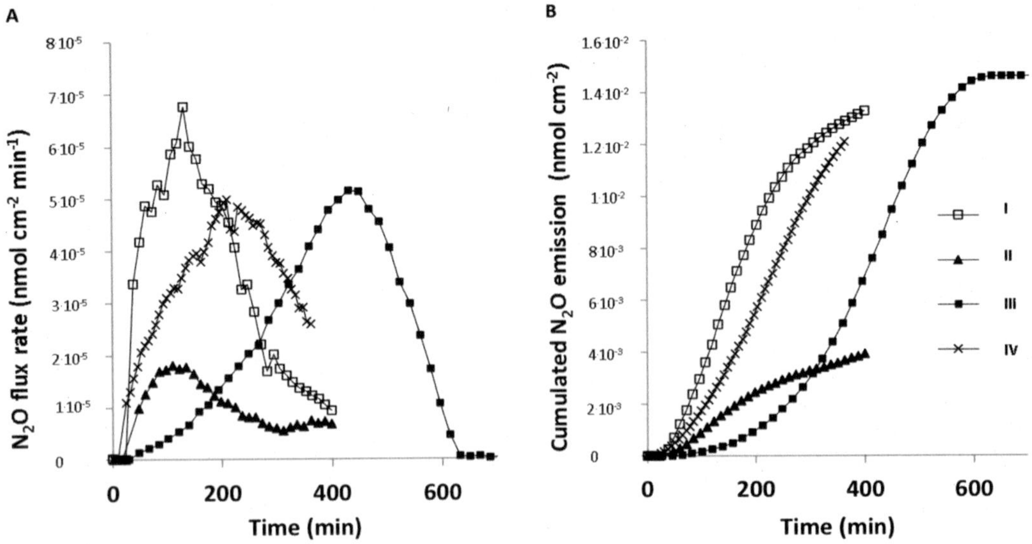

Figure 6. Efflux and cumulated emission of N_2O from sputum samples. (A) Estimated N_2O efflux rates in sputum samples from cystic fibrosis patients with chronic *P. aeruginosa* lung infection as calculated from N_2O microprofiles (n = 4). (B) Cumulated N_2O emission as calculated from N_2O microprofiles (n = 4). I, II, III and IV represents 4 different sputum samples.

by *P. aeruginosa* in this environment is associated with anaerobic growth, which can promote increased virulence and tolerance to antibiotic, as well as contribute to evasion of the host response. The chronic infected CF lung is in many ways a black box. By using the presented approach to elucidate the essential metabolites we may now open the black box and start mapping the micro-environment of infection which may inspire new strategies for prevention and treatment of chronic lung infections in CF.

Materials and Methods

Sputum Samples

As defined by the "Danish Act on Research Ethics Review of Health Research Projects" Section 2 the project does not constitute a health research project and was thus initiated without approval from The Committees on Health Research Ethics in the Capital Region of Denmark. Therefore, verbal informed consent was obtained using waiver of documentation of consent. The study was carried out on 21 anonymized samples of surplus expectorated sputum from 21 CF patients and 2 PCD patients (Table 2). Chronic *P. aeruginosa* infection was defined as the presence of *P. aeruginosa* in the lower respiratory tract at each monthly culture for >6 months, or for a shorter time in the presence of increased antibody response to *P. aeruginosa* (>2 precipitating antibodies, normal: 0–1) [57].

Microsensor Measurements of O_2 and N_2O. Each of 8 different sputum samples (1–2 ml) was added to a glass vial (35×12 mm) (Schuett Biotec, Germany) and allowed to settle for about 10 min. The glass vials were positioned in a heated metal rack, kept at 37°C. Vertical O_2-concentration profiles were recorded in the sputum with an amperometric O_2 microsensor (OX25, Unisense A/S, Århus, Denmark) mounted in a motorized PC-controlled profiling setup (MM33 and MC-232, Unisense A/S). Subsequently, vertical N_2O concentration profiles were recorded at defined time intervals for up to 12 hours with an amperometric N_2O microsensor [18] (N_2O-25, Unisense A/S) mounted in the micromanipulator.

The microsensors (tip diameter 25 µm) were connected to a picoammeter (PA2000, Unisense A/S) and positioned manually onto the upper surface of the sputum sample. Profile measurements were taken by movement of the sensor in vertical steps of 100 or 200 µm through the sputum sample. Positioning and data acquisition were controlled by dedicated software (Sensortrace Pro 2.0, Unisense A/S). The software was set to wait 3 seconds for the O_2-microprofile and 5 seconds for the N_2O-microprofile, before actual measurement and subsequent movement of the sensors to the next measuring depth. The interval between each cycle of profile measurements was 10 seconds.

The O_2-microsensor was linearly calibrated by measuring the sensor signal in an alkaline sodium ascorbate solution (zero O_2) and in air saturated free phosphate buffered saline (PBS) at experimental temperature and salinity. The O_2 concentration in air saturated water was determined from the known temperature and salinity according to [58]. The N_2O -microsensor was linearly calibrated according to [18] by measuring sensor signals in N_2O free PBS at experimental temperature and salinity and in PBS with sequential addition of a known volume of N_2O saturated PBS up

Table 2. Demographic data of the patients.

	CF patients		PCD patients
	Infectious status		
	P. aeruginosa	*S. aureus*	*H. influenzae*
Number (male)	20 (10)	1 (1)	2 (0)
Age (years)*	39 (24–50)	17	32 (27–36)
Duration of chronic infection (years)*, **	19 (4–38)		
FEV_1 (%)*	56 (23–96)	75	89 (70–109)
FVC (%)*	88 (46–139)	82	110 (95–125)

*Values are medians (range).
*Duration of chronic infection is only recorded for *P. aeruginosa* infections.
FEV_1, forced expiratory volume in 1 s.
FVC, forced vital capacity.

to a final concentration of 100 μM N_2O. The N_2O concentration in saturated PBS was determined according to [59].

NO_3^- and NO_2^- quantification. The concentration of NO_3^- and NO_2^- in sputum was measured in 20 samples. From each sputum sample, 0.1 ml was aspired with a syringe and was immediately diluted 10x in PBS and stored at -20°C for later analysis. The remaining sample was incubated in a glass vial at 37°C for 24 h before dilution 10x in PBS and storage at −20°C. The NO_3^- and NO_2^- levels in the sputum were measured using the Griess colorimetric reaction (no. 780001, Cayman Chemicals, USA) according to the manufacturer's recommendations. For this, sputum samples were transferred to a 96 well microtiter plate. NO_2^- concentration was estimated by addition of the Griess Reagent for 10 minutes, whereby NO_2^- was converted into a purple azo-compound, which was quantitated by the optical density at 540–550 nm measured with an ELISA plate reader (Thermo Scientific Multiskan EX, Thermo Fisher Scientific Inc, BioImage, Denmark). Total NO_3^- and NO_2^- levels were estimated by a two-step analysis process: The first step converted NO_3^- to NO_2^- utilizing NO_3^- reductase. After incubation for 2 hours, the next step involved the addition of the Griess Reagent, whereby NO_2^- was converted into a purple azo-compound. After incubation with Griess Reagent for 10 minutes, the optical density at 540–550 nm was measured with an ELISA plate reader (Thermo Scientific Multiskan EX, Thermo Fisher Scientific Inc, BioImage, Denmark). A NO_3^- standard curve was used for determination of total NO_3^- and NO_2^- concentration, while a NO_2^- standard curve was used for determination of NO_2^- alone. The concentration of NO_3^- was calculated as the difference between the NO_3^- concentration and the total NO_3^- and NO_2^- concentration.

Calculations of N_2O production rates. The local N_2O fluxes in sputum samples were calculated from the measured N_2O concentration gradient in the uppermost oxic sputum layer. It was assumed that no production or consumption of N_2O occurred in the presence of O_2. The flux was calculated using a modified version of Fick's 1st law of diffusion [60], where the slope of the profile in the sputum surface layer was calculated from the three uppermost measured concentrations (measurement a, b and c):

$$J=0.5\left[-D\frac{C_a-C_b}{x_a-x_b}\right]+0.5\left[-D\frac{C_b-C_c}{x_b-x_c}\right]$$

where J is the flux of N_2O (nmol N_2O cm^{-2} min^{-1}), D is the molecular diffusion coefficient of N_2O in water at 37°C (2.76×10^{-5} cm^2 s^{-1}) [61] and C is the concentration of N_2O (μmol $liter^{-1}$) at depth x_n, where n = a, b or c denote 3 subsequent depths of measurement. The cumulated N_2O emission was calculated by assuming linear changes between subsequent measurements. Net production and net consumption rates of N_2O in particular sputum layers were calculated from the slopes of linear increase and decrease of N_2O concentration at particular measuring depths in the sputum samples [62,63].

Statistical Analyses. Statistical significance was evaluated by Wilcoxon Signed Rank Test and by Students T-test. A p value <0.05 was considered statistically significant. The tests were performed with Prism 4.0c (GraphPad Software, La Jolla, California, USA).

Author Contributions

Conceived and designed the experiments: PØJ M. Kolpen M. Kühl. Performed the experiments: PØJ M. Kolpen M. Kühl CRH. Analyzed the data: PØJ M. Kolpen M. Kühl LL. Contributed reagents/materials/analysis tools: PØJ M. Kolpen M. Kühl CRH TP NH. Wrote the paper: PØJ M. Kolpen M. Kühl TB CM AK NH.

References

1. Riordan JR, Rommens JM, Kerem B, Alon N, Rozmahel R, et al. (1989) Identification of the cystic fibrosis gene: cloning and characterization of complementary DNA. Science 245: 1066–1073.
2. Knowles MR, Boucher RC (2002) Mucus clearance as a primary innate defense mechanism for mammalian airways. J Clin Invest 109: 571–577.
3. Boucher RC (2007) Evidence for airway surface dehydration as the initiating event in CF airway disease. J Intern Med 261: 5–16.
4. Koch C, Høiby N (1993) Pathogenesis of cystic fibrosis. Lancet 341: 1065–1069.
5. Koch C, Høiby N (2000) Diagnosis and treatment of cystic fibrosis. Respiration 67: 239–247.
6. Worlitzsch D, Tarran R, Ulrich M, Schwab U, Cekici A, et al. (2002) Effects of reduced mucus oxygen concentration in airway *Pseudomonas* infections of cystic fibrosis patients. J Clin Invest 109: 317–325.
7. Bjarnsholt T, Jensen PØ, Fiandaca MJ, Pedersen J, Hansen CR, et al. (2009) *Pseudomonas aeruginosa* biofilms in the respiratory tract of cystic fibrosis patients. Pediatr Pulmonol 44: 547–558.
8. Yang L, Haagensen JA, Jelsbak L, Johansen HK, Sternberg C, et al. (2008) In situ growth rates and biofilm development of *Pseudomonas aeruginosa* populations in chronic lung infections. J Bacteriol 190: 2767–2776.
9. Pedersen SS, Moller H, Espersen F, Sorensen CH, Jensen T, et al. (1992). Mucosal immunity to *Pseudomonas aeruginosa* alginate in cystic fibrosis. APMIS 100: 326–334.
10. Bjarnsholt T, Jensen PØ, Burmolle M, Hentzer M, Haagensen JA, et al. (2005) *Pseudomonas aeruginosa* tolerance to tobramycin, hydrogen peroxide and polymorphonuclear leukocytes is quorum-sensing dependent. Microbiology 151: 373–383.
11. Jensen PØ, Bjarnsholt T, Phipps R, Rasmussen TB, Calum H, et al. (2007) Rapid necrotic killing of polymorphonuclear leukocytes is caused by quorum-sensing-controlled production of rhamnolipid by *Pseudomonas aeruginosa*. Microbiology 153: 1329–1338.
12. van GM, Christensen LD, Alhede M, Phipps R, Jensen PØ, et al. (2009) Inactivation of the rhlA gene in *Pseudomonas aeruginosa* prevents rhamnolipid production, disabling the protection against polymorphonuclear leukocytes. APMIS 117: 537–546.
13. Alhede M, Bjarnsholt T, Jensen PØ, Phipps RK, Moser C, et al. (2009) *Pseudomonas aeruginosa* recognizes and responds aggressively to the presence of polymorphonuclear leukocytes. Microbiology 155: 3500–3508.
14. Kolpen M, Hansen CR, Bjarnsholt T, Moser C, Christensen LD, et al. (2010) Polymorphonuclear leucocytes consume oxygen in sputum from chronic *Pseudomonas aeruginosa* pneumonia in cystic fibrosis. Thorax 65: 57–62.
15. Hassett DJ, Cuppoletti J, Trapnell B, Lymar SV, Rowe JJ, et al. (2002) Anaerobic metabolism and quorum sensing by *Pseudomonas aeruginosa* biofilms in chronically infected cystic fibrosis airways: rethinking antibiotic treatment strategies and drug targets. Adv Drug Deliv Rev 54: 1425–1443.
16. Yoon SS, Hennigan RF, Hilliard GM, Ochsner UA, Parvatiyar K, et al. (2002) *Pseudomonas aeruginosa* anaerobic respiration in biofilms: relationships to cystic fibrosis pathogenesis. Dev Cell 3: 593–603. S1534580702002952 [pii].
17. Zumft WG (1997) Cell biology and molecular basis of denitrification. Microbiol Mol Biol Rev 61: 533–616.
18. Andersen K, Kjær T, Revsbech NP (2001) An oxygen insentitive microsensor for nitrous oxide. Sensors & Actuators B: Chemical 81: 42–48.
19. Richardson DJ (2000) Bacterial respiration: a flexible process for a changing environment. Microbiology 146 (Pt 3): 551–571.
20. Philippot L (2002) Denitrifying genes in bacterial and *Archaeal* genomes. Biochim Biophys Acta 1577: 355–376.
21. Philippot L (2005) Denitrification in pathogenic bacteria: for better or worst? Trends Microbiol 13: 191–192.
22. Zumft WG (2005) Nitric oxide reductases of prokaryotes with emphasis on the respiratory, heme-copper oxidase type. J Inorg Biochem 99: 194–215.
23. Schreiber F, Stief P, Gieseke A, Heisterkamp IM, Verstraete W, et al. (2010) Denitrification in human dental plaque. BMC Biol 8: 24.
24. Mitsui T, Kondo T (2004) Increased breath nitrous oxide after ingesting nitrate in patients with atrophic gastritis and partial gastrectomy. Clin Chim Acta 345: 129–133.
25. Hino T, Matsumoto Y, Nagano S, Sugimoto H, Fukumori Y, et al. (2010) Structural basis of biological N_2O generation by bacterial nitric oxide reductase. Science 330: 1666–1670.
26. Arai H, Igarashi Y, Kodama T (1995) The structural genes for nitric oxide reductase from *Pseudomonas aeruginosa*. Biochim Biophys Acta 1261: 279–284.
27. Gaston B, Ratjen F, Vaughan JW, Malhotra NR, Canady RG, et al. (2002) Nitrogen redox balance in the cystic fibrosis airway: effects of antipseudomonal therapy. Am J Respir Crit Care Med 165: 387–390.

28. SooHoo CK, Hollocher TC (1991) Purification and characterization of nitrous oxide reductase from *Pseudomonas aeruginosa* strain P2. J Biol Chem 266: 2203–2209.
29. Son MS, Matthews WJ Jr, Kang Y, Nguyen DT, Hoang TT (2007) In vivo evidence of *Pseudomonas aeruginosa* nutrient acquisition and pathogenesis in the lungs of cystic fibrosis patients. Infect Immun 75: 5313–5324.
30. Hassett DJ (1996) Anaerobic production of alginate by *Pseudomonas aeruginosa*: alginate restricts diffusion of oxygen. J Bacteriol 178: 7322–7325.
31. Jones KL, Hegab AH, Hillman BC, Simpson KL, Jinkins PA, et al. (2000) Elevation of nitrotyrosine and nitrate concentrations in cystic fibrosis sputum. Pediatr Pulmonol 30: 79–85.
32. Palmer KL, Brown SA, Whiteley M (2007) Membrane-bound nitrate reductase is required for anaerobic growth in cystic fibrosis sputum. J Bacteriol 189: 4449–4455.
33. Grasemann H, Michler E, Wallot M, Ratjen F (1997) Decreased concentration of exhaled nitric oxide (NO) in patients with cystic fibrosis. Pediatr Pulmonol 24: 173–177.
34. Linnane SJ, Keatings VM, Costello CM, Moynihan JB, O'Connor CM, et al. (1998) Total sputum nitrate plus nitrite is raised during acute pulmonary infection in cystic fibrosis. Am J Respir Crit Care Med 158: 207–212.
35. Ratjen F, Gartig S, Wiesemann HG, Grasemann H (1999) Effect of inhaled nitric oxide on pulmonary function in cystic fibrosis. Respir Med 93: 579–583.
36. Grasemann H, Grasemann C, Kurtz F, Tietze-Schillings G, Vester U, et al. (2005) Oral L-arginine supplementation in cystic fibrosis patients: a placebo-controlled study. Eur Respir J 25: 62–68.
37. Grasemann H, Tullis E, Ratjen F (2013) A randomized controlled trial of inhaled l-Arginine in patients with cystic fibrosis. J Cyst Fibros. Available: http://dx.doi.org/10.1016/j.jcf.2012.12.008.
38. Einsle O, Messerschmidt A, Stach P, Bourenkov GP, Bartunik HD, et al. (1999) Structure of cytochrome c nitrite reductase. Nature 400: 476–480.
39. Einsle O, Messerschmidt A, Huber R, Kroneck PMH, Neese F (2002) Mechanism of the six-electron reduction of nitrite to ammonia by cytochrome c nitrite reductase. J Am Chem Soc 124; 11737–11745.
40. Planelles G (2007) Ammonium homeostasis and human Rhesus glycoproteins. Nephron Physiol 105; 11–17.
41. Williams DR, Rowe JJ, Romero P, Eagon RG (1978) Denitrifying *Pseudomonas aeruginosa*: some parameters of growth and active transport. Appl Environ Microbiol 36: 257–263.
42. Hoffman LR, Richardson AR, Houston LS, Kulasekara HD, Martens-Habbena W, et al. (2010) Nutrient availability as a mechanism for selection of antibiotic tolerant *Pseudomonas aeruginosa* within the CF airway. PLoS Pathog 6: e1000712.
43. Thomas KL, Lloyd D, Boddy L (1994) Effects of oxygen, pH and nitrate concentration on denitrification by *Pseudomonas* species. FEMS Microbiol Lett 118: 181–186.
44. Seneterre E, Paganin F, Bruel JM, Michel FB, Bousquet J (1994) Measurement of the internal size of bronchi using high resolution computed tomography (HRCT). Eur Respir J 7: 596–600.
45. Hampton T, Armstrong S, Russell WJ (2000) Estimating the diameter of the left main bronchus. Anaesth Intensive Care 28: 540–542.
46. Arai H (2011) Regulation and Function of Versatile Aerobic and Anaerobic Respiratory Metabolism in *Pseudomonas aeruginosa*. Front Microbiol 2: 103.
47. Beckmann C, Brittnacher M, Ernst R, Mayer-Hamblett N, Miller SI, et al. (2005) Use of phage display to identify potential *Pseudomonas aeruginosa* gene products relevant to early cystic fibrosis airway infections. Infect Immun 73: 444–452.
48. Van Alst NE, Wellington M, Clark VL, Haidaris CG, Iglewski BH (2009) Nitrite reductase NirS is required for type III secretion system expression and virulence in the human monocyte cell line THP-1 by *Pseudomonas aeruginosa*. Infect Immun 77: 4446–4454.
49. Williams DR, Rowe JJ, Romero P, Eagon RG (1978) Denitrifying *Pseudomonas aeruginosa*: some parameters of growth and active transport. Appl Environ Microbiol 36: 257–263.
50. Borriello G, Werner E, Roe F, Kim AM, Ehrlich GD, et al (2004) Oxygen limitation contributes to antibiotic tolerance of *Pseudomonas aeruginosa* in biofilms. Antimicrob Agents Chemother 48: 2659–2664.
51. Lee B, Schjerling CK, Kirkby N, Hoffmann N, Borup R, et al (2011) Mucoid *Pseudomonas aeruginosa* isolates maintain the biofilm formation capacity and the gene expression profiles during the chronic lung infection of CF patients. APMIS 119: 263–274.
52. Kakishima K, Shiratsuchi A, Taoka A, Nakanishi Y, Fukumori Y (2007) Participation of nitric oxide reductase in survival of *Pseudomonas aeruginosa* in LPS-activated macrophages. Biochem Biophys Res Commun 355: 587–591.
53. Arai H, Iiyama K (2013) Role of nitric oxide-detoxifying enzymes in the virulence of *Pseudomonas aeruginosa* against the silkworm, *Bombyx mori*. Biosci Biotechnol Biochem 77: 198–200. DN/JST.JSTAGE/bbb/120656 [pii].
54. Shimizu T, Tsutsuki H, Matsumoto A, Nakaya H, Noda M (2012) The nitric oxide reductase of enterohaemorrhagic *Escherichia coli* plays an important role for the survival within macrophages. Mol Microbiol 85: 492–512.
55. Stevanin TM, Moir JW, Read RC (2005) Nitric oxide detoxification systems enhance survival of *Neisseria meningitidis* in human macrophages and in nasopharyngeal mucosa. Infect Immun 73: 3322–3329.
56. Loisel-Meyer S, Jimenez de Bagues MP, Basseres E, Dornand J, Kohler S, et al. (2006) Requirement of norD for *Brucella suis* virulence in a murine model of in vitro and in vivo infection. Infect Immun 74: 1973–1976.
57. Hoiby N (2000) Microbiology of cystic fibrosis. In: Hodson ME GD, editors. Cystic fibrosis. London, UK: Arnold. pp. 83–107.
58. Gundersen JK, Glud RN, Ramsing NB (1998) Predicting the signal of O_2 microsensors from physical dimensions, temperature, salinity, and O_2 concentration. Limnol Oceanogr 43: 1932–1937.
59. Weiss RF, Price BA (1980) Nitrous oxide solubility in water and seawater. Marine Chemistry 8: 347–359.
60. de Beer D, Stoodley P (2006) Microbial biofilms. In: Dworkin M, Falkow S, Rosenberg E, Schleifer KH, Stackebrandt E, editors. The Prokaryotes. New York: Springer Science. pp. 904–937.
61. Broecker WS, Peng TH (1974) Gas-exchange rates between air and sea. Tellus 26: 21–35.
62. Markfoged R, Nielsen LP, Nyord T, Ottosen LDM, Revsbech NP (2013) Transient N_2O accumulation and emission caused by O_2 depletion in soil after liquid manure injection. European journal of soil science 62: 541–550.
63. Liengaard L, Nielsen LP, Revsbech NP, Priemé A, Elberling B, et al. (2013) Extreme emission of N_2O from tropical wetland soil (Pantanal, South America). Frontiers in Microbiology 3: 433. doi: 10.3389/fmicb.2012.00433.

16

Hypoxia Modulates Infection of Epithelial Cells by *Pseudomonas aeruginosa*

Bettina Schaible[1,2], Siobhán McClean[3], Andrew Selfridge[1], Alexis Broquet[4], Karim Asehnoune[4,5], Cormac T. Taylor[1]✉, Kirsten Schaffer[6*]✉

1 UCD School of Medicine and Medical Science and The Conway Institute, University College Dublin, Dublin, Ireland, **2** School of Pharmacy, Queens's University, Belfast, United Kingdom, **3** Institute of Technology Tallaght, Dublin, Ireland, **4** Laboratoire UPRES EA 3826 «Thérapeutiques cliniques et expérimentales des infections», Faculté de médecine, Université de Nantes, Nantes, France, **5** Centre Hospitalier Universitaire de Nantes, Service anesthésie réanimation chirurgicale, Hôtel Dieu-HME, Nantes, France, **6** Department of Microbiology, St. Vincent's University Hospital, Dublin, Ireland

Abstract

Pseudomonas aeruginosa (P. aeruginosa) is an opportunistic pathogen commonly associated with lung and wound infections. Hypoxia is a frequent feature of the microenvironment of infected tissues which induces the expression of genes associated with innate immunity and inflammation in host cells primarily through the activation of the hypoxia-inducible factor (HIF) and Nuclear factor kappaB (NF-κB) pathways which are regulated by oxygen-dependent prolyl-hydroxylases. Hypoxia also affects virulence and antibiotic resistance in bacterial pathogens. However, less is known about the impact of hypoxia on host-pathogen interactions such as bacterial adhesion and infection. In the current study, we demonstrate that hypoxia decreases the internalization of *P. aeruginosa* into cultured epithelial cells resulting in decreased host cell death. This response can also be elicited by the hydroxylase inhibitor Dimethyloxallyl Glycine (DMOG). Reducing HIF-2α expression or Rho kinase activity diminished the effects of hypoxia on *P. aeruginosa* infection. Furthermore, in an in vivo pneumonia infection model, application of DMOG 48 h before infection with *P. aeruginosa* significantly reduced mortality. Thus, hypoxia reduces *P. aeruginosa* internalization into epithelial cells and pharmacologic manipulation of the host pathways involved may represent new therapeutic targets in the treatment of *P. aeruginosa* infection.

Editor: Jörn Karhausen, Duke University Medical Center, United States of America

Funding: This work was supported by grants from the Irish Research Council for Science, Engineering & Technology, and Science Foundation Ireland. The funders had no role in study design, data collection and analysis, decision to publish, or preparation of the manuscript.

Competing Interests: The authors have declared that no competing interests exist.

* E-mail: kirsten.e.schaffer@ucd.ie

✉ These authors contributed equally to this work.

Introduction

Lower respiratory tract infections are the leading cause of death among infectious diseases. Pulmonary infection with associated intra-alveolar exudates, edematous septal thickening and multiplying pathogens inhibit oxygen diffusion and result in decreased mucosal oxygenation leading to dysregulated gas exchange. *P. aeruginosa* is one of the major pathogens encountered in nosocomial infections causing severe lower respiratory tract infections, skin and soft tissue infections (especially in burn patients) and bacteremia in patients with leukemia, cancer or other immunosuppressive states. In addition *P. aeruginosa* is the main respiratory pathogen encountered in cystic fibrosis where it is associated with increased morbidity and mortality [1]. Hypoxia has been demonstrated in mucus filled airways of cystic fibrosis patients [2]. Treatment of *P. aeruginosa* infections is complicated by rising antimicrobial resistance, absence of an effective vaccine and by the lack of newer antimicrobial agents in development.

Prominent regions of hypoxia are common features of infected and inflamed tissues [3,4]. In infected tissues, oxygen consumption by bacterial pathogens and phagocytes exacerbates tissue hypoxia. Hypoxia is an important driver of innate immune and inflammatory gene expression in host cells through the activation of transcription factors including Nuclear Factor kappaB (NF-κB) and the Hypoxia inducible factor (HIF) [5,6,7]. Furthermore, it has recently become clear that hypoxia can also influence the expression of virulence and antibiotic resistance genes in invading pathogens such as *Shigella* and *Pseudomonas* species respectively [8,9]. However, despite the recognition that hypoxia independently affects both host and pathogen, less is known about how it impacts upon host-pathogen interactions such as adhesion and infection.

The Hypoxia inducible factor (HIF) is a master regulator of gene expression in metazoan cells exposed to hypoxia [10,11]. HIF consists of an oxygen-sensitive α-subunit and a constitutively expressed β-subunit. One of three isoforms of the HIF α-subunit bound to a single isoform of the HIF β-subunit constitutes dimeric HIF-1, HIF-2 or HIF-3 respectively [12]. HIF-1 and HIF-2 positively regulate the expression of discreet but overlapping cohorts of genes and demonstrate differential temporal dynamics [13]. HIF-3α is a negative regulator of HIF-1α and HIF-2α [14]. In the presence of sufficient oxygen (normoxia), HIF-α is degraded via hydroxylation by prolyl-hydroxylases (PHD) leading to ubiquitination by the von Hipple Lindau E3 ligase and degradation by the 26S proteasome [12]. The inhibition of the oxygen-dependent prolyl-hydroxylases in hypoxia leads to HIF stabilisation/transactivation with subsequent activation of HIF-dependent target genes. Three PHD isoforms have been identified to date. Among these, normoxic HIF-1α degradation is predominantly regulated by PHD 2. HIF plays a key role in immunity and inflammation by regulating events both in epithelial cells [15] and in immune cells including macrophages, neutrophils, T-cells and dendritic cells [16,17,18,19].

NF-κB consists of a family of transcription factors termed RelA (p65), RelB, c-Rel, p50 and p52 and is a master regulator of inflammation and innate immunity [20]. NF-κB is activated in response to hypoxia both in vitro and in vivo and contributes to the expression of inflammatory genes such as cyclooxygenase-2 (COX-2) [21,22]. It has recently become appreciated that the same oxygen-sensing hydroxylases that regulate HIF activity in hypoxia also control NF-κB activity during oxygen deprivation [23]. All three PHD isoforms have been implicated in the regulation of both HIF and NF-κB, however PHD2 is the primary isoform involved in the regulation of HIFα stability while PHD1 appears to be the main regulator of hypoxia-dependent NF-κB regulation [21]. Therefore, prolyl-hydroxylases play a central role in the regulation of immune gene expression in hypoxia.

Airway epithelial cells play an important role in host defence. Internalization of *P. aeruginosa* into airway epithelial cells has been demonstrated [24]. The role of bacterial internalization for progression of *P. aeruginosa* infection remains unclear. Here, we have investigated the effects of hypoxia on infection of epithelial cells with *P. aeruginosa* and discovered that activation of specific hypoxia sensitive pathways leads to decreased levels of bacterial internalization which promotes host cell survival. Indeed, it had been reported that activation of the HIF pathway increased epithelial cell barrier function in a *Clostridium difficile* toxin model [25]. A better understanding of the microenvironmental factors effecting host-bacterial interactions may reveal new therapeutic approaches to increasing host resistance against bacterial infection.

Materials and Methods

Ethics Statement

Mice used for in vivo experiments were treated in accordance with institutional policies and the guidelines stipulated by the animal welfare committee. The Committee of Animal Ethics of the University of Nantes approved all animal experimentation in this study.

Bacterial and cell culture

The *P. aeruginosa* strain ATCC 27853 and *E. coli* strain NCIB 9485 were purchased from ATCC (Manassus, VA). Clinical isolates used were derived from the sputa of cystic fibrosis patients chronically infected with *P. aeruginosa*. Bacteria were grown at 37°C on LB agar plates (Sigma-Aldrich, Dorset UK) or in liquid broths (Müller Hinton broth II, BD microbiology systems, Cockeysville MD) at 21% or 1% atmospheric oxygen. For heat-inactivation, bacteria in suspension were quantified and heat killed by exposure to 65°C for 2 h. To ensure that no living bacteria survived, 10 µl of the suspension was cultured on a LB agar plate and incubated overnight at 37°C.

A549 cells were grown in DMEM F12 Ham media (Sigma-Aldrich, Dorset UK) with 10% foetal calf serum (Gibco, Paisley, UK), 2 mM L-glutamine (Gibco, Paisley, UK), 100 U/ml penicillin and 100 µg/ml streptomycin (Gibco, Paisley, UK). Caco2 and MEF cells were cultured in DMEM media (Gibco, Paisley, UK) with 1% foetal calf serum, 100 U/ml penicillin and 100 µg/ml streptomycin. HepG2 wild type and cells stably transfected with shRNA sequences against HIF-1α and HIF-2α were a gift from Prof. B. Brüne (University of Frankfurt). Media for stably transfected HepG2 cells additionally contained 2 µg/ml puromycin dihydrochloride (Sigma-Aldrich, Dorset UK). 16HBE 14o- [26] and CFBE41o- cells (homozygous for ΔF508 mutation of the CFTR gene) were a gift of Prof. D. Gruenert (University of California, San Francisco) and were cultured in MEM with 10% FCS 2 mM L-glutamine and 100 U/ml penicillin/100 µg/ml streptomycin on a collagen/fibronectin/BSA coated surface.

Normoxic controls were cultured in 21% oxygen and 5% CO_2 in a humidified environment at 37°C. For culture in hypoxia, cells were transferred to a hypoxia chamber (Coy Laboratories, Grass Lake, MI; Ruskin Technologies, Leeds, U.K.) with a humidified atmosphere of 1% oxygen, 5% CO_2 and the balance N_2 at 37°C. At the onset of hypoxic exposure, the cell culture media was replaced with pre-equilibrated medium ensuring that the cells experienced an instantaneous drop in pO_2 levels.

Drugs and Reagents

To activate different TLR pathways, the following specific agonists were used; flagellin (from *S. thymimurium* 0.5 µg/ml, InvivoGen, San Diego, CA) for TLR5, Pam_3CysSK_4 (2 µg/ml, ECM microcollections, Tübingen, Germany) for TLR2 or LPS (*P. aeruginosa* derived, 0.5 µg/ml, Sigma-Aldrich, Dorset, UK) for TLR4. TNFα (10 ng/ml, Sigma-Aldrich, Dorset, UK) served as positive control. To mimic hypoxia, the pan-hydroxylase inhibitor Dimethyloxallyl Glycine (DMOG, Cayman Chemicals, Ann Arbor, MI) was used at 1 mM. Y27632 (Sigma-Aldrich, Dorset, UK) inhibited selective ROCK (Rho-associated coiled-coil forming protein serine/threonine kinase) at 10 µM. Inhibition of the NF-κB pathway was achieved by using Bay 11-7082 (Merck, Darmstadt Germany) at 10 µM, an inhibitor of IκBα phosphorylation. Controls were treated with the appropriate vehicle control.

Adhesion and Internalization Assays

A549 cells, MEF cells, 16HBE14o- and CFBE410- cells were seeded at 2×10^5 per well in 24 well plates (HepG2 cells at 6×10^5 per well). Before bacterial infection, cells were pre-incubated for 24 h in normoxia or hypoxia, in antibiotic free culture media pre-equilibrated to 1% or 21% oxygen respectively. Chemical inhibitors were added at the same time.

Bacteria were grown to mid log phase at an OD_{600} of 0.5–0.6. A549 cells and MEF cells were infected with bacteria at a MOI of 50:1 (or 16:1 for HepG2 cells). After incubation of infected cells for four hours (or indicated incubation time) under normoxic or hypoxic conditions, the medium was replaced with fresh medium containing 1 mg/ml amikacin (Sigma-Aldrich, Dorset UK) and 1 mg/ml ceftazidime (Sigma-Aldrich, Dorset UK) and cells were incubated for further 2 h in the presence of antibiotics to kill extracellular bacteria. Amikacin concentrations were increased to 4 mg/ml for experiments with clinical strains in hypoxia to reliably kill all extracellular bacteria. Inhibitors were added at every step during the experiment where media was replaced to maintain a constant concentration. After 2 h incubation in the presence of antibiotics, the media was removed and cells were washed three times with PBS. Fluid from the last washing step was plated on agar plates to document the absence of viable extracellular bacteria. After washing, 500 µl of cell-lysis buffer (PBS, 10 mM EDTA, 0.025%TritonX 100) was added for 20 min. The remainder of attached cells were scraped of the well and the lysate was plated on LB agar plates in duplicate. CFUs were counted after 24 h to 48 h incubation at 37°C.

To measure the number of adherent bacteria, cells were infected as for internalisation assays without the use of antibiotics to kill extracellular bacteria. After washing 3 times, cells were lysed as described above. The lysate, containing all cell associated bacteria (adherent and internalised), was plated on LB agar plates and quantified after 24 h incubation at 37°C. The number of adherent bacteria was calculated as the number of associated bacteria minus the number of internalized bacteria.

Lactate Dehydrogenase (LDH) assays

Cytotoxicity was determined by quantifying LDH released into cell culture media (Cytotoxicity Detection Kit, LDH, Roche, Dublin Ireland) via enzyme activity of LDH. After bacterial infection the complete cell culture media was removed for quantification of LDH released into the medium. To quantify total LDH, cells were lysed with Triton X (1% in serum free cell culture media) overnight at 4°C. 50 µl media or lysate were transferred with 50 µl of reaction mix in a 96 well plate and incubated at RT for 30 minutes in the dark. Absorbance was measured at 490 nm. Toxicity was calculated as LDH released into the medium as percentage of total LDH present in cells.

Western blotting and luciferase assay

Whole cell lysates were prepared as previously described [27,28]. The following antibodies were used for western blotting: p65, COX-2 (Santa Cruz Biotechnology. Santa Cruz, CA), HIF-1α (BD Transduction Laboratories, Oxford, UK), HIF-2α (Novus, St. Charles, MO) and β-actin (Sigma-Aldrich, Dorset, UK).

For luciferase reporter assays A549 cells were transfected with 125 ng pGL4.32[*luc2P*/NF-κB-RE/Hygro] luciferase reporter construct (Promega, Madison WI) and 25 ng pSV-β galactosidase vector (Promega, Madison WI). The following day the cells were pre-incubated for 24 h in either 21% oxygen or 1% oxygen and subsequently stimulated with specific ligands for TLR2, TLR4 and TLR5 for 6 h in the indicated oxygen concentration. Cells were washed with PBS and lysed with lysis buffer (Promega, Madison WI). Luciferase activity of the lysate was determined after adding luciferase substrate (Promega, Madison WI) by luminometry (Berthold Huntsville, AL).

Mouse pneumonia model

Six-week-old pathogen-free RjOrl:SWISS mice (CD-1 mice, weight 20–24 g) were purchased from Janvier Laboratories (Le Genest Saint Isle, France). Mice were maintained on a 12-hour light/dark cycle with access to food and water ad libitum. *P. aeruginosa* strain PAO1 was grown overnight in Brain Heart Infusion medium at 37°C under agitation. Immediately before use, the bacterial pellet (centrifuged at 1,000 g for 10 min) was washed twice using 0.9% NaCl. After the second wash, the pellet was resuspended in sterile saline buffer and the inoculum was calibrated by nephelometry (2×10^8 CFU/ml).

Mice were assigned to four groups (n = 10 per group): pneumonia alone (control group), DMOG treatment (8 mg/mouse, intraperitoneally) at the time of infection with *P. aeruginosa*, DMOG treatment 24 hours prior to infection and DMOG treatment 48 hours prior to infection. Pneumonia was induced as previously described [29]. Briefly, mice were anaesthetized with sevoflurane (Abbott, Chicago, IL, USA) and placed in dorsal recumbency. Transtracheal insertion of a 24-gauge feeding needle was used to inject 75 µl of a bacterial suspension adjusted to 2×10^8 CFU/ml (1.5×10^7 CFU/mouse). Survival was assessed twice per day up to 6 days following infection.

Statistical analysis

Data are presented as mean ± SEM for n independent experiments. Statistical analysis was carried out using unpaired student's t-test (Microsoft Excel 2010) or one-way analysis of variance ANOVA analysis with Tukey post test (Graph pad Prism 5 Software). Densitometry analysis was performed with Image J Software. Statistical significance was denoted as $p<0.05$. Hazard ratio for survival in the treated animal group versus the untreated group was calculated using GraphPad Prism software (San Diego, USA).

Results

Hypoxia decreases epithelial cell infection with *P. aeruginosa*

Adhesion and internalization are distinct events in the encounter between bacterial pathogens and host epithelial cells. Using antibiotic exclusion assay, we found that the internalization of *P. aeruginosa* greatly exceeds that of *Escherichia coli (E. coli)*, highlighting the invasive potential of *P. aeruginosa* for pulmonary epithelial cells (Figure S1). Furthermore, internalization of *P. aeruginosa* into A549 cells was decreased by 94.7±1.6% in hypoxia compared to normoxia (Figure 1A). Notably, a similar decrease in internalization was observed in epithelial cells which had been pre-incubated in hypoxia for 24 h (Figure 1A), indicating that the effects of hypoxia on infection are due for the most part to changes in host epithelial cells.

There was no difference in levels of adherence of *P. aeruginosa* to epithelial cells in hypoxia compared to normoxia (Figure 1B) demonstrating that decreased internalization is not a result of decreased bacterial adhesion.

The decreased numbers of internalized bacteria in hypoxia could be a result of decreased bacterial uptake into the host cell or increased intracellular killing. To determine which is the case, we performed a time course experiment assessing intracellular bacterial numbers at 30 minutes intervals following infection. In hypoxia, the number of internalized *P. aeruginosa* was decreased at all-time points from 1 to 4 hours post infection compared to normoxia (Figure 1C). We concluded that hypoxia decreased internalization rather than increased intracellular killing, as for increased intracellular killing we would have expected equal initial numbers of internalized bacteria in normoxia and hypoxia followed by a faster rate of decline in hypoxia. 24 h following infection the number of internalized bacteria had decreased from 100% to 9.6% in normoxia and from 13.8% to 1.5% in hypoxia (Figure 1D).

Next, we investigated the consequence of decreased bacterial uptake in hypoxia for host cell survival. *P. aeruginosa* is cytotoxic and capable of inducing death in epithelial cells [30]. To assess cytotoxicity in our model, we measured Lactate dehydrogenase (LDH) release following bacterial infection. 24 hours following infection, normoxic *P. aeruginosa* infected cells released significantly more LDH than hypoxic *P. aeruginosa* infected cells indicating decreased induction of cell death by *P. aeruginosa* infection under hypoxic conditions (Figure 1E). These data support a protective role for hypoxia in reducing epithelial cell infection by *P. aeruginosa*.

DMOG mimics the effects of hypoxia on *P. aeruginosa* infection of epithelial cells

To investigate the therapeutic potential of manipulating hypoxia sensitive pathways in *P. aeruginosa* infection, we tested the effect of the hydroxylase inhibitor DMOG on *P. aeruginosa* infection of epithelial cells. Because phenotypic differences in bacterial invasion and intracellular replication have been described for various *P. aeruginosa* strains, we investigated the impact of DMOG on the uptake of multiple strains. We used mucoid and non-mucoid *P. aeruginosa* isolates which we cultured from the sputa

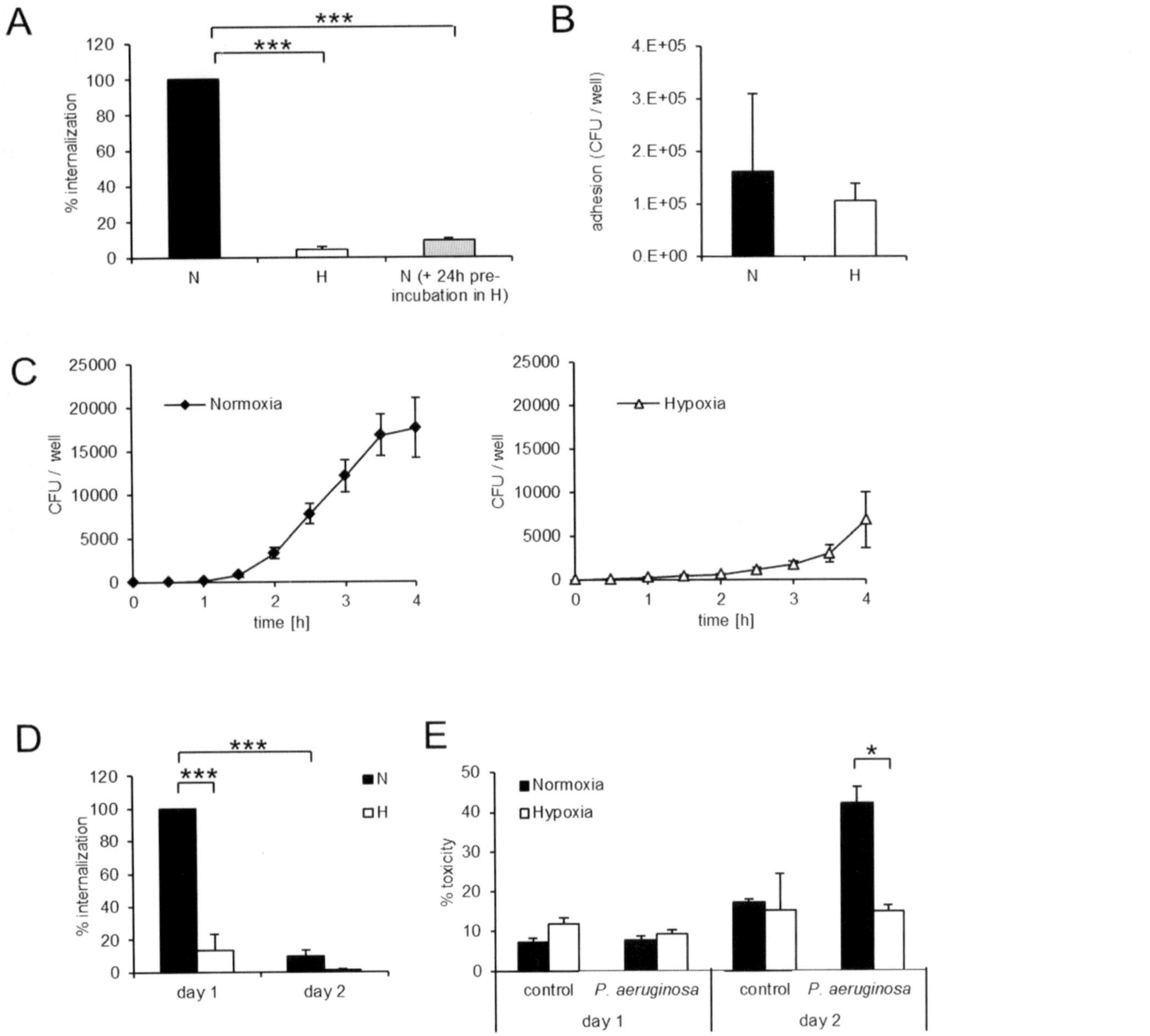

Figure 1. Hypoxia prevents internalization of *P. aeruginosa* into epithelial cells. A549 cells were infected with *P. aeruginosa* under normoxic (N) and hypoxic (H) conditions, after pre-incubation for 24 h in the respective environment for all experiments (A–E). A: Internalization of *P. aeruginosa* in normoxia, hypoxia and in normoxia after pre-incubation in hypoxia. B: Adhesion of *P. aeruginosa* in normoxia and hypoxia. C: Uptake of *P. aeruginosa* over time in normoxia and hypoxia. D: Internalization of *P. aeruginosa* directly after infection (day 1) or 24 h after infection (day 2). E: Cell toxicity of uninfected and *P. aeruginosa* infected cells was measured by LDH release directly after infection (day 1) or 24 h after infection (day 2). Data represent mean ± SEM of 3 independent experiments throughout (*$<$p 0.05; *** p$<$0.0001).

of cystic fibrosis patients. We also tested the effect of DMOG on uptake of *Burkholderia cenocepacia* (*B. cenocepacia*), an invasive pathogen also found in cystic fibrosis patients. We verified that bacterial multiplication took place in the presence of DMOG. Internalization of all *P. aeruginosa* strains and *B. cenocepacia* were significantly decreased in cells pre-treated with DMOG, indicating that mimicking hypoxia with pharmacologic hydroxylase inhibition may be a novel approach to preventing infection of pulmonary epithelial cells by *P. aeruginosa* and *B. cenocepacia* (Figure 2A–D).

Hypoxia amplifies *P. aeruginosa*-induced NF-κB activity but this does not account for decreased *P. aeruginosa* internalization

We next investigated potential mechanisms underpinning the effects of hypoxia on bacterial uptake into pulmonary epithelial cells. Because NF-κB is the master regulator of host innate immune responses to bacterial pathogens and up-regulation of NF-κB activity is associated with enhanced *P. aeruginosa* clearance from the lungs [31], we investigated whether hypoxia altered NF-κB activity in *P. aeruginosa* infected cells. Hypoxia amplified nuclear localization of NF-κB in *P. aeruginosa* infected pulmonary and colonic epithelial cells resulting in increased expression of the NF-κB target cyclooxygenase 2 (COX-2) (Figure 3A+S2).

To investigate whether hypoxia elicited increased NF-κB activity is equally mediated by all three major toll like receptors (TLRs), NF-κB-dependent luciferase reporter assays with selective TLR 2, 4 and 5 agonists were performed. In hypoxia, stimulation of TLR 5 by flagellin resulted in significantly higher NF-κB activity than stimulation of TLR 2 by Pam_3CysSK_4 or stimulation of TLR 4 by LPS (Figure 3B). We therefore concluded that TLR 5 mediated signalling is mainly responsible for increased nuclear translocation of p65.

We next investigated whether amplified NF-κB activity contributed to decreased bacterial internalization in hypoxia using two experimental approaches. First, bacterial internalization assays were performed in the presence of the NF-κB inhibitor BAY 11-7082. While BAY 11-7082 decreased *P. aeruginosa* internalization in normoxia, it did not impact upon hypoxia-induced decreases in internalization (Figure 3C). Second, to be able to investigate bacterial internalization in the presence of a complete knockdown of NF-κB, we performed internalization assays with IKK knockout mouse embryonic fibroblasts. *P. aeruginosa* internalization into mouse embryonic fibroblasts had been shown before [32]. Internalization of *P. aeruginosa* was diminished in IKK knockout cells and reversal of hypoxia-induced effects was not observed (Figure 3D). Thus, while hypoxia amplifies *P. aeruginosa* induced NF-κB activity, inhibiting NF-κB activity in hypoxia did not impact on decreased bacterial uptake indicating that the effects of hypoxia on *P. aeruginosa* uptake are independent of NF-κB.

HIF-2α partially mediates decreased bacterial internalization in hypoxia

We next investigated whether increased HIF activity may play a role in the decreased internalization of *P. aeruginosa* observed in hypoxia. Activation of HIF has been demonstrated for a variety of bacterial infections [33]. We tested the effects of depletion of HIF-1α or HIF-2α using HepG2 cells stably transfected with short hairpin plasmids. Analysis by densitometry revealed an 89% knockdown of HIF-1α expression and 79% knockdown of HIF-2α (Figure 4A). Bacterial internalization in normoxia was not affected by silencing HIF-1α or HIF-2α respectively (Figure 4B). Bacterial internalization into hypoxic control vector epithelial cells was reduced to 5.6%±0.8% of normoxic epithelial cells, whereas bacterial internalization into hypoxic HIF-2α knockdown cells was only reduced to 19.3%±0.7% of normoxic controls (Figure 4C) indicating that HIF-2α was participating in the hypoxia elicited effect.

Hypoxia enhances RhoA activity in *P. aeruginosa* infected cells and inhibition of this pathway partially normalizes decreased bacterial internalization

P. aeruginosa entry into cells is an actin-dependent process involving actin rearrangement regulated by Rho GTPases. Furthermore, *P. aeruginosa* exotoxins ExoS and ExoT have been demonstrated to affect Rho GTPase activity and inhibit bacterial internalization [34]. RhoA is a key regulator of the cytoskeleton of eukaryotic cells. RhoA activity increased in A549 cells in the presence of hypoxia upon infection with *P. aeruginosa* (Figure 5A).

Increased Rho activity leads to activation of downstream serine/threonine kinases (ROCK family). To determine the importance of Rho activity for decreased internalization in hypoxia, we performed internalization experiments in the presence of Y27632, a ROCK inhibitor [35]. Bacterial internalization in normoxia remained unchanged in the presence of Y27632, whereas Y27632 partially inhibited the reduced internalization observed in hypoxia (Figure 5B and 5C).

Stress fibre formation as a marker of cytoskeleton re-arrangement was increased in hypoxia and abolished by the ROCK

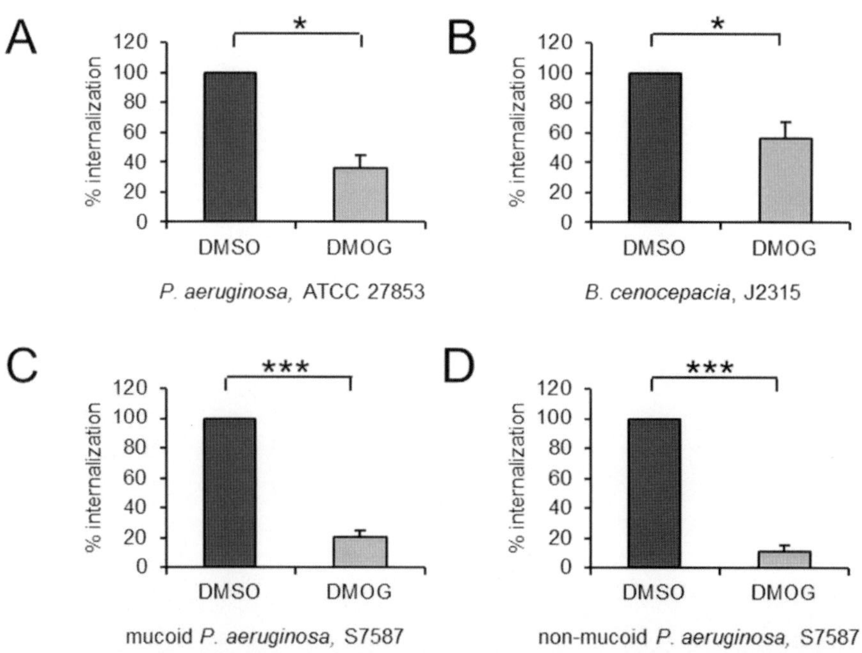

Figure 2. Bacterial internalization is decreased in DMOG treated cells. To mimic hypoxia, A549 cells were pre-treated with 1 mM of the pan-hydroxylase inhibitor DMOG or its' solvent DMSO for 24 h and throughout following infection with the *P. aeruginosa* reference strain ATCC 27853 (A), a CF pathogen *B. cenocepacia, J2315* (B) and two clinical *P. aeruginosa* isolates from CF patients, S7587, mucoid and non-mucoid *P. aeruginosa* (C and D). Data represent mean ± SEM of 3 independent experiments throughout (* $p<0.05$; *** $p<0.0001$).

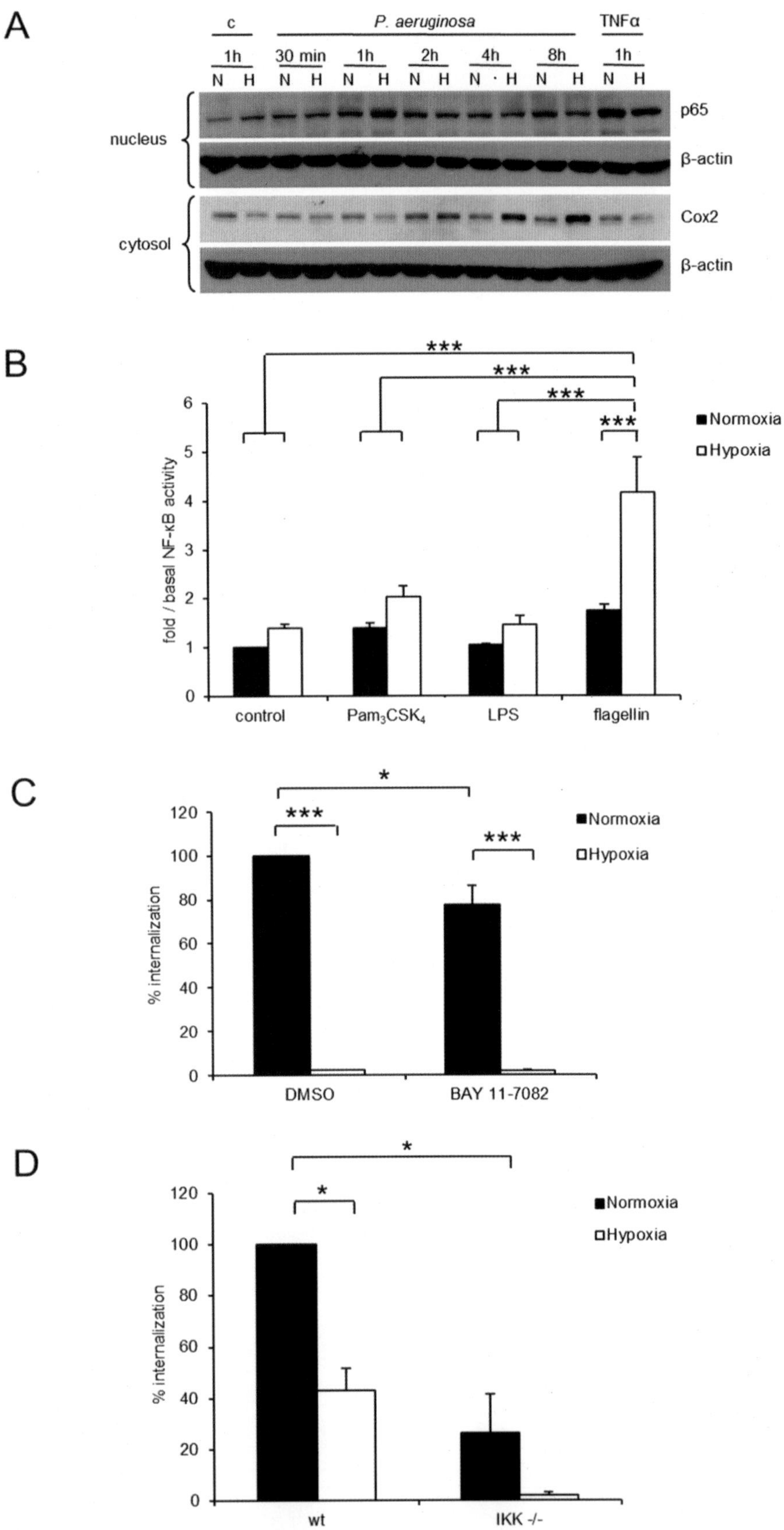

Figure 3. Hypoxia increases NF-κB activity in response to *P. aeruginosa* but silencing of NF-κB fails to normalize hypoxia induced decreased internalization. A: Protein levels of nuclear p65 and cytosolic Cox2 were investigated by immunoblot in A549 cells stimulated with heat inactivated *P. aeruginosa* in normoxia (N) and hypoxia (H) for the indicated times. B: NF-κB transcription factor activity was measured by a NF-κB

luciferase reporter assay in normoxic and hypoxic A549 cells stimulated with TLR ligands for TLR2 (Pam3CK4, 2 μg/ml), TLR4 (LPS, 0.5 μg/ml) and TLR5 (flagellin, 0.5 μg/ml). Data represent mean ± SEM of 6 independent experiments (*** $p<0.0001$). C: Intracellular *P. aeruginosa* in A549 cells in normoxia or hypoxia in the presence or absence of the NF-κB inhibitor BAY 11-7082 (10 μM) or its solvent DMSO were determined in an antibiotic protection assay. Data represent mean ± SEM of 4 independent experiments (* $p<0.05$, *** $p<0.0001$). D: Antibiotic protection assay with *P. aeruginosa* in MEF wt and IKK−/−cells under normoxic and hypoxic conditions. Data represent mean ± SEM of 2 independent experiments (* $p<0.05$).

inhibitor Y 27632 (Figure S3). Whereas hypoxia induced stress fibre formation was not attenuated in HIF-1α knockdown cells, stress fibre formation was decreased in hypoxia in HIF-2α knockdown cells suggesting different roles for the two HIF-α isoforms in cytoskeleton rearrangement (Figure S3).

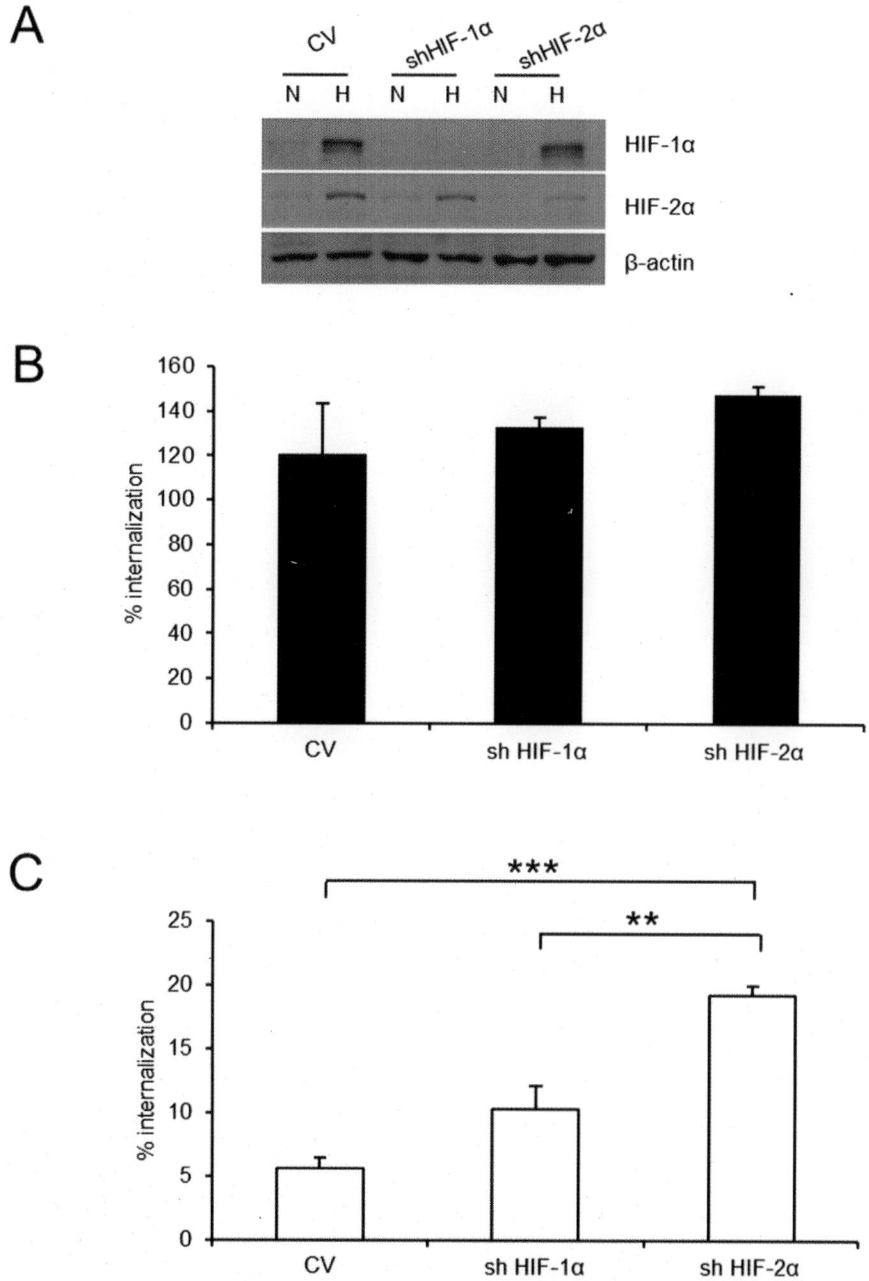

Figure 4. HIF-2α is partly responsible for decreased internalization of *P. aeruginosa* in hypoxia. A: Knock down of HIF-1α and HIF-2α protein in HepG2 cells stably expressing shRNA directed against HIF-1α and HIF-2α shown by immunoblot. B: Antibiotic protection assay in normoxia with *P. aeruginosa* in HepG2 cells (see A). Internalized *P. aeruginosa* are shown as % of normoxic control. Data represent mean ± SEM of 3 independent experiments. C: Antibiotic protection assay in hypoxia with *P. aeruginosa* in HepG2 cells (see A). Internalized *P. aeruginosa* are shown as % of normoxic control. Data represent mean ± SEM of 3 independent experiments (** $p<0.01$, *** $p<0.0001$).

Hypoxia decreases *P. aeruginosa* internalization independent of CFTR expression

The cystic fibrosis transmembrane conductance regulator protein (CFTR) has been postulated as an important regulator of pulmonary epithelial cell internalization of *P. aeruginosa* and the absence of a functional CFTR protein was associated with decreased *P. aeruginosa* internalization [36,37]. Decreased expression of CFTR in response to hypoxia has been observed in intestinal epithelial cells [38]. To investigate whether decreased *P. aeruginosa* internalization in hypoxia is dependent upon a functional CFTR, we investigated bacterial uptake in the bronchoepithelial cell line 16HBE 14o- and CFBE41o- cells (homozygous for ΔF508 mutation of the CFTR gene). Internalization of *P. aeruginosa* decreased to 29.7±9.6% of internalization into 16HBE 14o- cells in the absence of functional CFTR protein in CFBE41o-cells under normoxic conditions (Figure 6). Despite the overall decrease in internalized bacteria, the magnitude of the hypoxia elicited decreased internalization was comparable in the two cell lines: From 100% to 7.4±2.5% in 16HBE 14o- and from 100% to 1.3±0.6% in CFBE41o- cells, indicating that hypoxia decreases bacterial internalization independent of the presence of a functional CFTR (Figure 6).

DMOG decreases mortality in vivo in a pneumonia infection model

We next investigated whether the effects of prolyl-hydroxylase inhibition on bacterial internalization observed in vitro would impact on the course of infection in vivo. Mice were infected intratracheally with *P. aeruginosa*. DMOG was injected 48 h or 24 h before infection or simultaneous with *P. aeruginosa* infection. DMOG treatment on day 0 or 24 h before infection did not affect the survival rate of mice infected with *P. aeruginosa*. In contrast DMOG treatment 48 h before infection significantly increased survival of mice with a mortality of only 20% at 48 hpi and a final mortality rate of 30% compared to 80–100% in the other groups (hazard ratio for survival 3.533; 95% CI 1.185–16.81; p = 0.0270) (Figure 7).

Discussion

Epithelial cells are the first barrier encountered by bacterial pathogens and the interactions between bacteria and human epithelial cells are fundamental for the pathogenesis of bacterial infections. In bacterial infections, influx of inflammatory cells and multiplication of pathogens increases oxygen demands and hypoxia is subsequently a frequently encountered component of inflammatory environments in which infections take place. *P. aeruginosa* is the leading gram-negative pathogen in ventilator-associated pneumonia [39]. Intensive care mortality rates are significantly higher for bacteremic pneumonia compared to non-bacteremic pneumonia [40]. In the current study, we demonstrate that hypoxia strikingly attenuates internalisation of the human opportunistic pathogen *P. aeruginosa* into epithelial cells, potentially conferring increased resistance against bacterial invasion to epithelial cells. Hypoxia-induced decreases in internalization were not only observed in A549 pulmonary epithelial cells, but equally in 16 HBE 14o- human bronchoepithelial cells, an immortalized but non-transformed cell line retaining differentiated epithelial morphology and functions [26].

Despite phenotypic differences in invasion and intracellular replication among *P. aeruginosa* strains, all strains of *P. aeruginosa* were found to be capable of entering host cells in vitro [41,42]. Similarly in vivo, alveolar epithelial cells II were found to harbour intracellular *P. aeruginosa* in a murine infection model [43]. The

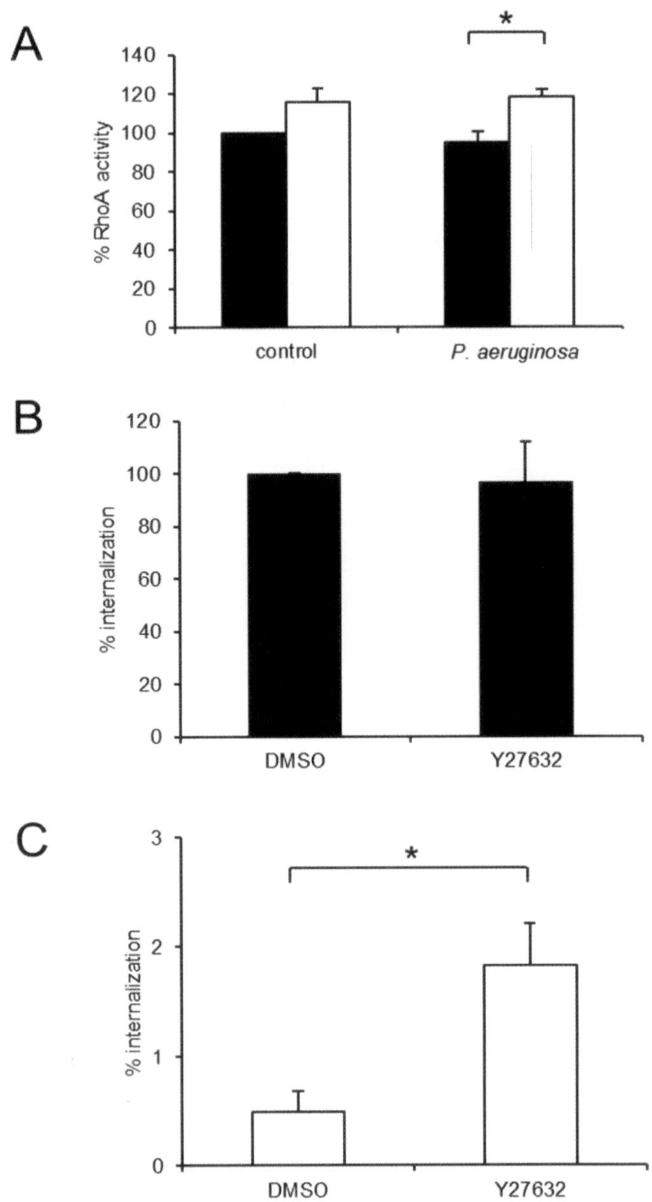

Figure 5. Increased RhoA activity in hypoxic, *P. aeruginosa* infected cells is partly responsible for decreased internalization of *P. aeruginosa* in hypoxia. A: Active RhoA (RhoA-GTP) was determined by ELISA in A549 cells pre-incubated in normoxia and hypoxia followed by infection with *P. aeruginosa*. Data represent mean ± SEM of 3 individual experiments (* $p<0.05$). B: Normoxic A549 cells were pre-treated with 10 μM Y27632 and throughout the following infection with *P. aeruginosa*. Internalized *P. aeruginosa* as % of normoxic control are shown. Data represent mean ± SEM of 5 individual experiments. C: Intracellular *P. aeruginosa* in A549 cells were determined in hypoxia with the same treatments as described in B. Internalized *P. aeruginosa* as % of normoxic control are shown. Data represent mean ± SEM of 5 individual experiments (* $p<0.05$).

pathophysiological consequences of *P. aeruginosa* internalisation into airway epithelial cells are unclear.

In this study LDH release was significantly increased in normoxic cells 24 h after infection compared to hypoxic cells. Invasive *P. aeruginosa* isolates were found to penetrate epithelial cell monolayers by either evoking epithelial cell death with subsequent disruption of monolayers or by transmigrating through epithelial

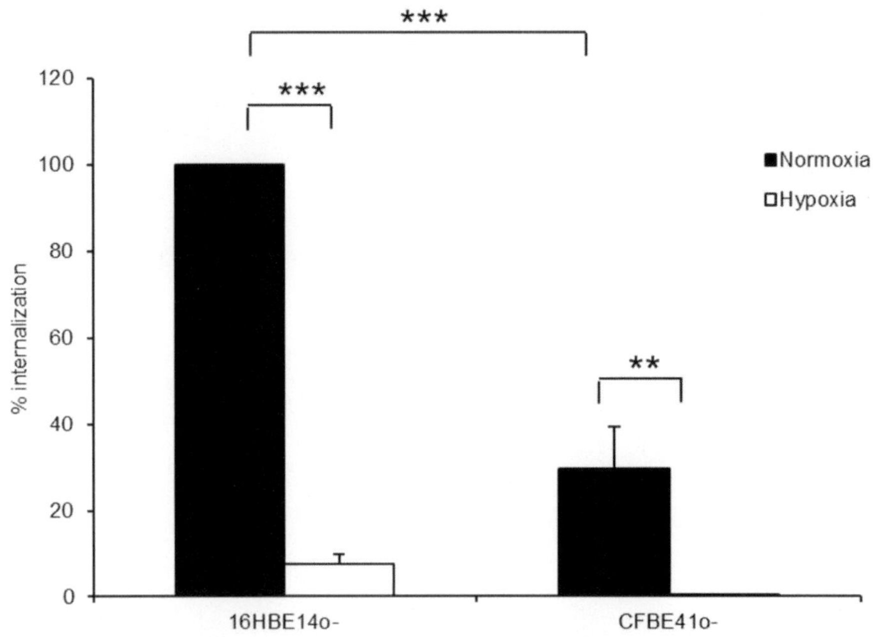

Figure 6. Decrease of intracellular *P. aeruginosa* in hypoxia is independent of CFTR. Intracellular *P. aeruginosa* were determined with an antibiotic exclusion assay in 16HBE14o- and CFBE41o- cells under normoxic and hypoxic conditions. Data represent mean ± SEM of 5 individual experiments (** $p<0.01$; *** $p<0.0001$).

cells [30]. Increased internalization resistance in response to hypoxia could therefore confer a cytoprotective effect upon epithelial cells and decrease transmigration of invasive bacteria. This is supported by our observation in vivo.

Hypoxia elicited decreased internalization was not restricted to the ATCC 27853 control strain, as two clinical *P. aeruginosa* isolates and a *B. cenocepacia* reference strain were equally impaired in their potential to internalize into pulmonary epithelial cells. Cystic fibrosis *P. aeruginosa* isolates have been found to attenuate virulence factor expression as part of immune evasion strategies in chronic infection [44]. Therefore it was not surprising that the absolute number of internalized bacteria was lower for the two CF isolates in comparison to the ATCC strain. Despite decreased numbers of internalized bacteria in normoxia, the relative decrease elicited by hypoxia was comparable for all clinical isolates, suggesting that rather than being a bacterial strain specific effect, decreased internalization was a host cell attributable phenomenon.

Two additional experimental observations suggested that hypoxia elicited epithelial cell responses are the major contributor to decreased bacterial internalization in hypoxia: 1. Pre-exposure of epithelial cells to hypoxia increased epithelial cell resistance to subsequent bacterial infection. 2. Applying Dimethyloxallyl Glycine (DMOG) decreased bacterial internalization. DMOG inhibits prolyl-hydroxylation of HIF-α subunits leading to increased HIF-α protein stability and increased transcriptional activity [45].

Epithelial cell signalling events elicited by bacterial internalization remain unclear. The two major transcription factors

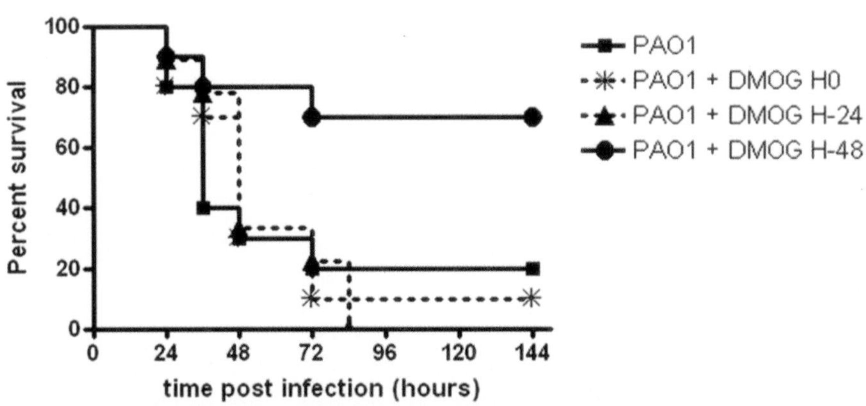

Figure 7. DMOG improves survival in a murine *P. aeruginosa* pneumonia model. Pneumonia was induced by instillation of 1.5×10^7 CFU/mouse of *P. aeruginosa*. Mice were assigned to four groups ($n=10$ per group): pneumonia alone (control group), DMOG treatment (8 mg/mouse, intraperitoneally) at the time of infection with *P. aeruginosa*, DMOG treatment 24 hours prior to infection and DMOG treatment 48 hours prior to infection. DMOG treatment 48 h before infection significantly increased survival of mice with a mortality of only 20% at 48 hpi and a final mortality rate of 30% compared to 80–100% in the other groups.

controlling hypoxia driven epithelial cell responses are NF-κB and HIF. Blocking NF-κB activity did not reverse decreased bacterial internalization in hypoxia. Increased HIF activity had been demonstrated for a variety of bacterial infections [33]. Although silencing of HIF-1α did not impact on bacterial internalization in hypoxia, silencing of HIF-2α partially restored bacterial internalization.

The inhibition of bacterial internalization by DMOG suggested that prolyl- hydroxylases would play an important part in the observed effect. Knockdown of prolyl-hydroxylases in HeLa cells resulted in activation of RhoA [46] and RhoA had been shown to be induced by hypoxia in mouse embryonic fibroblasts [47] and in renal cancer cells [48]. RhoA activity increased in pulmonary epithelial cells in the presence of hypoxia upon infection with *P. aeruginosa*. Inhibition of RhoA activity using an inhibitor partially restored *P. aeruginosa* internalization in hypoxia.

The cystic fibrosis transmembrane conductance regulator (CFTR) had been reported to function as an epithelial cell receptor facilitating internalization of *P. aeruginosa* into respiratory epithelial cells [37]. In pulmonary and intestinal epithelial cells, HIF has been reported to decrease CFTR expression [38,49], whereas hypoxia increased CFTR expression in corneal epithelial cells leading to increased *P. aeruginosa* binding and internalization [50]. Although bacterial internalization into bronchoepithelial cells was decreased, hypoxia still diminished bacterial internalization in the absence of functional CFTR suggesting that CFTR did not play a role in mediating decreased internalization in hypoxia. In the context of cystic fibrosis airway disease, absence of functional CFTR protein and presence of hypoxia in mucus filled airways could exert additive effects leading to complete inhibition of *P. aeruginosa* internalization.

In vivo HIF-1α deletion resulted in more severe *Clostridium difficile* toxin induced intestinal injury and inflammation [25]. In response to activation of the HIF pathway epithelial cells showed increased mucosal barrier function through activation of intestinal trefoil factor [51] and increased production of anti-inflammatory signalling molecules such as adenosine [52]. In the murine pneumonia model used in this study DMOG significantly decreased mortality in infected mice when given 48 h before *P. aeruginosa* infection. In contrast HIF increased translocation of Gram-positive bacteria through intestinal epithelial cells through upregulation of the platelet-activating factor receptor [53]. Differences in innate immunity responses against invading gram-negative and gram-positive pathogens were recently highlighted in a *C. elegans* model. Whether HIF upregulation in epithelial cells is protective or damaging for bacterial defence mechanisms, could depend on the type of bacterial pathogen (Gram-positive versus Gram-negative) and on the epithelial cell type involved. It is intriguing to speculate that stimulation of hypoxia dependent signalling pathways elicits protective mechanisms in pulmonary epithelial cells against invasion of pathogens. Empowering host defences could represent a novel strategy against bacterial pathogens which are challenging us with continuously increasing antimicrobial resistance.

In summary, we have shown that hypoxia or pharmacologic hydroxylase inhibition decreases internalization of *P. aeruginosa* into epithelial cells, attenuating cytotoxicity of *P. aeruginosa* infection. Decreased internalization was not *P. aeruginosa* strain specific and applied to the cystic fibrosis invasive pathogen *B. cenocepacia* as well. Decreased internalization in hypoxia was independent from NF-κB activity and CFTR expression. Both HIF2-α and RhoA are epithelial cell regulatory factors participating in this effect. In addition DMOG significantly improved survival in a murine *P. aeruginosa* pneumonia model.

Supporting Information

Figure S1 Internalization of *E. coli* in normoxia, hypoxia and in normoxia with cells pre-incubated in hypoxia. Antibiotic exclusion assays were performed with *E. coli* in A549 cells under normoxic and hypoxic conditions or in normoxia after hypoxic pre-incubation. Data are shown as % of intracellular normoxic *P. aeruginosa* and represent mean ± SEM of 3 individual experiments.

Figure S2 Enhanced NF-κB activity in intestinal epithelial cells in response to *P. aeruginosa* under hypoxic conditions. (A) Caco2 cells were incubated with heat inactivated *P. aeruginosa* in normoxia (N) and hypoxia (H). A representative immunoblot out of 3 independent experiments is shown.

Figure S3 Stress fibre formation is increased in hypoxia and attenuated by inhibiting RhoA or HIF-2α. HepG2 cells (wt, CV, shHIF1α, shHIF2α) were incubated in normoxia or hypoxia for 24 h, additionally wt cells were treated with 10 μM Y27632. The cells were stained for F-actin with Phalloidin. Green: Phalloidin, blue: Höchst, bar: 10 μm.

Acknowledgments

We gratefully thank Prof. B. Brüne for the stable transfected HepG2 cells.

Author Contributions

Conceived and designed the experiments: CTT KS. Performed the experiments: BS AS AB. Analyzed the data: BS AB CTT KS. Contributed reagents/materials/analysis tools: SM KA. Wrote the paper: BS CTT KS.

References

1. Spilker T, Coenye T, Vandamme P, LiPuma JJ (2004) PCR-based assay for differentiation of Pseudomonas aeruginosa from other Pseudomonas species recovered from cystic fibrosis patients. J Clin Microbiol 42: 2074–2079.
2. Worlitzsch D, Tarran R, Ulrich M, Schwab U, Cekici A, et al. (2002) Effects of reduced mucus oxygen concentration in airway Pseudomonas infections of cystic fibrosis patients. J Clin Invest 109: 317–325.
3. Colgan SP, Taylor CT (2010) Hypoxia: an alarm signal during intestinal inflammation. Nat Rev Gastroenterol Hepatol 7: 281–287.
4. Eltzschig HK, Carmeliet P (2011) Hypoxia and inflammation. N Engl J Med 364: 656–665.
5. Nizet V, Johnson RS (2009) Interdependence of hypoxic and innate immune responses. Nat Rev Immunol 9: 609–617.
6. Schaible B, Schaffer K, Taylor CT (2010) Hypoxia, innate immunity and infection in the lung. Respir Physiol Neurobiol 174: 235–243.
7. Taylor CT (2008) Interdependent roles for hypoxia inducible factor and nuclear factor-kappaB in hypoxic inflammation. J Physiol 586: 4055–4059.
8. Schaible B, Taylor CT, Schaffer K (2012) Hypoxia Increases Antibiotic Resistance in Pseudomonas aeruginosa through Altering the Composition of Multidrug Efflux Pumps. Antimicrob Agents Chemother 56: 2114–2118.
9. Marteyn B, West NP, Browning DF, Cole JA, Shaw JG, et al. (2010) Modulation of Shigella virulence in response to available oxygen in vivo. Nature 465: 355–358.
10. Semenza GL (2007) Hypoxia-inducible factor 1 (HIF-1) pathway. Sci STKE 2007: cm8.
11. Taylor CT (2008) Mitochondria and cellular oxygen sensing in the HIF pathway. Biochem J 409: 19–26.
12. Kaelin WG Jr, Ratcliffe PJ (2008) Oxygen sensing by metazoans: the central role of the HIF hydroxylase pathway. Mol Cell 30: 393–402.
13. Koh MY, Powis G (2012) Passing the baton: the HIF switch. Trends Biochem Sci 37: 364–372.

14. Maynard MA, Evans AJ, Shi W, Kim WY, Liu FF, et al. (2007) Dominant-negative HIF-3 alpha 4 suppresses VHL-null renal cell carcinoma progression. Cell Cycle 6: 2810–2816.
15. Karhausen J, Furuta GT, Tomaszewski JE, Johnson RS, Colgan SP, et al. (2004) Epithelial hypoxia-inducible factor-1 is protective in murine experimental colitis. J Clin Invest 114: 1098–1106.
16. Cramer T, Yamanishi Y, Clausen BE, Forster I, Pawlinski R, et al. (2003) HIF-1alpha is essential for myeloid cell-mediated inflammation. Cell 112: 645–657.
17. Naldini A, Morena E, Pucci A, Miglietta D, Riboldi E, et al. (2012) Hypoxia affects dendritic cell survival: role of the hypoxia-inducible factor-1alpha and lipopolysaccharide. J Cell Physiol 227: 587–595.
18. Walmsley SR, Print C, Farahi N, Peyssonnaux C, Johnson RS, et al. (2005) Hypoxia-induced neutrophil survival is mediated by HIF-1alpha-dependent NF-kappaB activity. J Exp Med 201: 105–115.
19. Jantsch J, Chakravortty D, Turza N, Prechtel AT, Buchholz B, et al. (2008) Hypoxia and hypoxia-inducible factor-1 alpha modulate lipopolysaccharide-induced dendritic cell activation and function. J Immunol 180: 4697–4705.
20. Hayden MS, Ghosh S (2012) NF-kappaB, the first quarter-century: remarkable progress and outstanding questions. Genes Dev 26: 203–234.
21. Taylor CT, Cummins EP (2009) The role of NF-kappaB in hypoxia-induced gene expression. Ann N Y Acad Sci 1177: 178–184.
22. Fitzpatrick SF, Tambuwala MM, Bruning U, Schaible B, Scholz CC, et al. (2011) An intact canonical NF-kappaB pathway is required for inflammatory gene expression in response to hypoxia. J Immunol 186: 1091–1096.
23. Cummins EP, Berra E, Comerford KM, Ginouves A, Fitzgerald KT, et al. (2006) Prolyl hydroxylase-1 negatively regulates IkappaB kinase-beta, giving insight into hypoxia-induced NFkappaB activity. Proc Natl Acad Sci U S A 103: 18154–18159.
24. Pielage JF, Powell KR, Kalman D, Engel JN (2008) RNAi screen reveals an Abl kinase-dependent host cell pathway involved in Pseudomonas aeruginosa internalization. PLoS Pathog 4: e1000031.
25. Hirota SA, Fines K, Ng J, Traboulsi D, Lee J, et al. (2010) Hypoxia-inducible factor signaling provides protection in Clostridium difficile-induced intestinal injury. Gastroenterology 139: 259–269 e253.
26. Cozens AL, Yezzi MJ, Kunzelmann K, Ohrui T, Chin L, et al. (1994) CFTR expression and chloride secretion in polarized immortal human bronchial epithelial cells. Am J Respir Cell Mol Biol 10: 38–47.
27. Taylor CT, Fueki N, Agah A, Hershberg RM, Colgan SP (1999) Critical role of cAMP response element binding protein expression in hypoxia-elicited induction of epithelial tumor necrosis factor-alpha. J Biol Chem 274: 19447–19454.
28. Bruning U, Cerone L, Neufeld Z, Fitzpatrick SF, Cheong A, et al. (2011) MicroRNA-155 promotes resolution of hypoxia-inducible factor 1alpha activity during prolonged hypoxia. Mol Cell Biol 31: 4087–4096.
29. Jacqueline C, Roquilly A, Desessard C, Boutoille D, Broquet A, et al. (2012) Efficacy of ceftolozane in a murine model of Pseudomonas aeruginosa acute pneumonia: in vivo antimicrobial activity and impact on host inflammatory response. J Antimicrob Chemother.
30. Hirakata Y, Finlay BB, Simpson DA, Kohno S, Kamihira S, et al. (2000) Penetration of clinical isolates of Pseudomonas aeruginosa through MDCK epithelial cell monolayers. J Infect Dis 181: 765–769.
31. Sadikot RT, Zeng H, Joo M, Everhart MB, Sherrill TP, et al. (2006) Targeted immunomodulation of the NF-kappaB pathway in airway epithelium impacts host defense against Pseudomonas aeruginosa. J Immunol 176: 4923–4930.
32. Evans DJ, Kuo TC, Kwong M, Van R, Fleiszig SM (2002) Mutation of csk, encoding the C-terminal Src kinase, reduces Pseudomonas aeruginosa internalization by mammalian cells and enhances bacterial cytotoxicity. Microb Pathog 33: 135–143.
33. Kempf VA, Lebiedziejewski M, Alitalo K, Walzlein JH, Ehehalt U, et al. (2005) Activation of hypoxia-inducible factor-1 in bacillary angiomatosis: evidence for a role of hypoxia-inducible factor-1 in bacterial infections. Circulation 111: 1054–1062.
34. Garrity-Ryan L, Kazmierczak B, Kowal R, Comolli J, Hauser A, et al. (2000) The arginine finger domain of ExoT contributes to actin cytoskeleton disruption and inhibition of internalization of Pseudomonas aeruginosa by epithelial cells and macrophages. Infect Immun 68: 7100–7113.
35. Uehata M, Ishizaki T, Satoh H, Ono T, Kawahara T, et al. (1997) Calcium sensitization of smooth muscle mediated by a Rho-associated protein kinase in hypertension. Nature 389: 990–994.
36. Bajmoczi M, Gadjeva M, Alper SL, Pier GB, Golan DE (2009) Cystic fibrosis transmembrane conductance regulator and caveolin-1 regulate epithelial cell internalization of Pseudomonas aeruginosa. Am J Physiol Cell Physiol 297: C263–277.
37. Pier GB, Grout M, Zaidi TS (1997) Cystic fibrosis transmembrane conductance regulator is an epithelial cell receptor for clearance of Pseudomonas aeruginosa from the lung. Proc Natl Acad Sci U S A 94: 12088–12093.
38. Zheng W, Kuhlicke J, Jackel K, Eltzschig HK, Singh A, et al. (2009) Hypoxia inducible factor-1 (HIF-1)-mediated repression of cystic fibrosis transmembrane conductance regulator (CFTR) in the intestinal epithelium. FASEB J 23: 204–213.
39. Hidron AI, Edwards JR, Patel J, Horan TC, Sievert DM, et al. (2008) NHSN annual update: antimicrobial-resistant pathogens associated with healthcare-associated infections: annual summary of data reported to the National Healthcare Safety Network at the Centers for Disease Control and Prevention, 2006–2007. Infect Control Hosp Epidemiol 29: 996–1011.
40. Magret M, Lisboa T, Martin-Loeches I, Manez R, Nauwynck M, et al. (2011) Bacteremia is an independent risk factor for mortality in nosocomial pneumonia: a prospective and observational multicenter study. Crit Care 15: R62.
41. Engel J, Balachandran P (2009) Role of Pseudomonas aeruginosa type III effectors in disease. Curr Opin Microbiol 12: 61–66.
42. Ha U, Jin S (2001) Growth phase-dependent invasion of Pseudomonas aeruginosa and its survival within HeLa cells. Infect Immun 69: 4398–4406.
43. Schmiedl A, Kerber-Momot T, Munder A, Pabst R, Tschernig T (2010) Bacterial distribution in lung parenchyma early after pulmonary infection with Pseudomonas aeruginosa. Cell Tissue Res 342: 67–73.
44. Mahenthiralingam E, Campbell ME, Speert DP (1994) Nonmotility and phagocytic resistance of Pseudomonas aeruginosa isolates from chronically colonized patients with cystic fibrosis. Infect Immun 62: 596–605.
45. Tian YM, Yeoh KK, Lee MK, Eriksson T, Kessler BM, et al. (2011) Differential sensitivity of hypoxia inducible factor hydroxylation sites to hypoxia and hydroxylase inhibitors. J Biol Chem 286: 13041–13051.
46. Vogel S, Wottawa M, Farhat K, Zieseniss A, Schnelle M, et al. (2010) Prolyl hydroxylase domain (PHD) 2 affects cell migration and F-actin formation via RhoA/rho-associated kinase-dependent cofilin phosphorylation. J Biol Chem 285: 33756–33763.
47. Greijer AE, van der Groep P, Kemming D, Shvarts A, Semenza GL, et al. (2005) Up-regulation of gene expression by hypoxia is mediated predominantly by hypoxia-inducible factor 1 (HIF-1). J Pathol 206: 291–304.
48. Turcotte S, Desrosiers RR, Beliveau R (2003) HIF-1alpha mRNA and protein upregulation involves Rho GTPase expression during hypoxia in renal cell carcinoma. J Cell Sci 116: 2247–2260.
49. Guimbellot JS, Fortenberry JA, Siegal GP, Moore B, Wen H, et al. (2008) Role of oxygen availability in CFTR expression and function. Am J Respir Cell Mol Biol 39: 514–521.
50. Zaidi T, Mowrey-McKee M, Pier GB (2004) Hypoxia increases corneal cell expression of CFTR leading to increased Pseudomonas aeruginosa binding, internalization, and initiation of inflammation. Invest Ophthalmol Vis Sci 45: 4066–4074.
51. Furuta GT, Turner JR, Taylor CT, Hershberg RM, Comerford K, et al. (2001) Hypoxia-inducible factor 1-dependent induction of intestinal trefoil factor protects barrier function during hypoxia. J Exp Med 193: 1027–1034.
52. Eltzschig HK (2009) Adenosine: an old drug newly discovered. Anesthesiology 111: 904–915.
53. Keely S, Glover LE, Weissmueller T, MacManus CF, Fillon S, et al. (2010) Hypoxia-inducible factor-dependent regulation of platelet-activating factor receptor as a route for gram-positive bacterial translocation across epithelia. Mol Biol Cell 21: 538–546.

Adaptation of *Pseudomonas aeruginosa* in Cystic Fibrosis Airways Influences Virulence of *Staphylococcus aureus In Vitro* and Murine Models of Co-Infection

Rossella Baldan[1], Cristina Cigana[2], Francesca Testa[1], Irene Bianconi[2], Maura De Simone[2], Danilo Pellin[3], Clelia Di Serio[3], Alessandra Bragonzi[2❡], Daniela M. Cirillo[1*❡]

1 Emerging Bacterial Pathogens Unit, San Raffaele Scientific Institute, Milan, Italy, **2** Infection and Cystic Fibrosis Unit, San Raffaele Scientific Institute, Milan, Italy, **3** University Centre for Statistics in the Biomedical Sciences, Università Vita-Salute San Raffaele, Milan, Italy

Abstract

Cystic fibrosis (CF) airways disease represents an example of polymicrobial infection whereby different bacterial species can interact and influence each other. In CF patients *Staphylococcus aureus* is often the initial pathogen colonizing the lungs during childhood, while *Pseudomonas aeruginosa* is the predominant pathogen isolated in adolescents and adults. During chronic infection, *P. aeruginosa* undergoes adaptation to cope with antimicrobial therapy, host response and co-infecting pathogens. However, *S. aureus* and *P. aeruginosa* often co-exist in the same niche influencing the CF pathogenesis. The goal of this study was to investigate the reciprocal interaction of *P. aeruginosa* and *S. aureus* and understand the influence of *P. aeruginosa* adaptation to the CF lung in order to gain important insight on the interplay occurring between the two main pathogens of CF airways, which is still largely unknown. *P. aeruginosa* reference strains and eight lineages of clinical strains, including early and late clonal isolates from different patients with CF, were tested for growth inhibition of *S. aureus*. Next, *P. aeruginosa/S. aureus* competition was investigated in planktonic co-culture, biofilm, and mouse pneumonia model. *P. aeruginosa* reference and early strains, isolated at the onset of chronic infection, outcompeted *S. aureus in vitro* and *in vivo* models of co-infection. On the contrary, our results indicated a reduced capacity to outcompete *S. aureus* of *P. aeruginosa* patho-adaptive strains, isolated after several years of chronic infection and carrying several phenotypic changes temporally associated with CF lung adaptation. Our findings provide relevant information with respect to interspecies interaction and disease progression in CF.

Editor: Nades Palaniyar, The Hospital for Sick Children and The University of Toronto, Canada

Funding: This study was supported to DMC and AB by Fondazione per la ricerca sulla Fibrosi Cistica (project FFC#9/2010). The funders had no role in study design, data collection and analysis, decision to publish, or preparation of the manuscript.

Competing Interests: The authors have declared that no competing interests exist.

* E-mail: cirillo.daniela@hsr.it

❡ These authors contributed equally to this work.

Introduction

Chronic airway infections and inflammation cause progressive lung disease and are the leading causes of mortality in patients with cystic fibrosis (CF) [1]. CF disease is characterized by the accumulation of secretion in the lungs and by a decreased mucociliary clearance that lead to an impaired ability to defeat bacterial infections. The viscous CF lung secretions provide an environment that protects bacteria from the assault of antibiotics and immune cells, thus favoring colonization and persistence. CF patients have a unique set of bacterial pathogens that are frequently acquired in an age dependent sequence [2]. The most frequently cultured organisms from the respiratory tract of young children are *Staphylococcus aureus* and non-typeable *Haemophilus influenzae*. Later, as the patient ages, infection progresses to involve opportunistic pathogens such as *Pseudomonas aeruginosa* and *Burkholderia cepacia*.

It is now becoming clear that the different bacteria coexisting in CF airways have a mutual interaction and contribute to the pathogenesis of the disease [3,4]. In a context that involves a complex polymicrobial community a single-species microbial analysis could be inadequate, as different microbes within the community can interact each other and the resulting infection pathogenesis differs from that in infections caused by the component species individually [3,5]. Chronic bacterial infections associated with CF lung disease have been studied by a range of culture-independent profiling methodologies [6–12], and each approach has revealed greater microbial diversity than was previously recognized. Overall, the results of these studies suggest that the polymicrobial nature of CF infections could play a key role in driving disease and response to therapy and, in turn, significantly impact upon clinical outcomes [1,7,13]. Nevertheless, very little is known about the role of interspecies interactions in the pathogenesis of the CF lung disease [14,15].

The Gram-positive bacterium *S. aureus* is the pathogen most commonly isolated in nasopharyngeal samples from young children with CF, and in the preantibiotic era, many CF patients succumbed to *S. aureus* infection [16]. Recent data demonstrate an increase in *S. aureus* infections in the CF population, not only in the US but also in Europe, with methicillin-resistant *S. aureus* (MRSA) strains being on the rise [17,18], reflecting the overall increase in prevalence and epidemiologic changes in the general population [19,20].

Of the multiple opportunistic bacteria that may infect CF patients, the Gram-negative bacterium *P. aeruginosa* is considered to be the most significant as it has clearly been linked to worsening of the pulmonary status [21]. Despite intensive antibiotic treatments, *P. aeruginosa* infections are difficult to eradicate [22]. The antibiotic treatment may favor the emergence of antimicrobial drug resistance. One of the most striking characteristics of *P. aeruginosa* chronic lung infection in CF patients is indeed the co-existence of multiple phenotypes that are highly resistant to any chemotherapy treatment [23].

Although *S. aureus* colonization/infection usually precedes chronic colonization of the respiratory tract by *P. aeruginosa*, it continues into adulthood, when 51% of patients become culture positive for *S. aureus* [24]. Both organisms are commonly co-isolated from CF respiratory cultures and it has been shown that risk factors for initial *P. aeruginosa* airway infection in patients with CF include *S. aureus* pre-colonization [25,26]. In addition, both species are able to shift between a planktonic (free-living) life style to surface-attached communities known as biofilms during chronic infections. In human diseases including CF, biofilm-related infections are directly correlated with dramatic increases in antibiotic resistance [27,28,29].

In this study, we aimed to explore the interactions between *S. aureus* and *P. aeruginosa* by using *in vitro* and murine models of pneumonia. During chronic infection, *P. aeruginosa* undergoes numerous selective pressures ranging from antibiotic treatments, host immune response and interactions with other microorganisms leading to the development of patho-adaptive lineages. The adaptation of *P. aeruginosa* to the CF niche selects for clones with reduced virulence in multi-hosts models [23,30]. We focused our attention on the reciprocal influence of *P. aeruginosa* and *S. aureus* and on understanding how *P. aeruginosa* adaptation to the CF lung may interfere with *S. aureus* interaction. Using a collection of longitudinal strains isolated from CF patients, we showed that *P. aeruginosa* strains out-competed *S. aureus*. This effect was associated with *P. aeruginosa* early strains, which in acute infection present higher virulence. On the contrary, *P. aeruginosa* late adapted strains showed reduced or abolished capacity to outcompete *S. aureus*. This work provides key results on lung pathogenicity caused by multi-bacterial infection.

Results

P. aeruginosa early and late clonal variants differently influence growth of *S. aureus*

Eight lineages of *P. aeruginosa* strains, including 12 early (early group) and 12 late (late group) clonal isolates from different patients with CF were tested for growth inhibition of *S. aureus* Newman and SH1000 strains on agar surfaces [25]. In particular, late *P. aeruginosa* strains selected for this study were collected over a period of 16.3 years and carried several patho-adaptive traits, including mucoid and hypermutable phenotypes (Table 1) as reported previously [23,31]. In addition, PAO1 and PA14 *P. aeruginosa* reference strains, which show phenotypic traits characteristic of early isolates [23], were also included.

As shown in Table 1, growth of *S. aureus* Newman and SH1000 strains was inhibited by PA14 and PAO1 *P. aeruginosa* reference strains and by 100% (12/12) and 91.6% (11/12) of *P. aeruginosa* early strains respectively in co-culture. The only exception was the strain KK1 which was previously described as different in terms of virulence potential from KK2, isolated at the same time point [23]. The strength of inhibition of *S. aureus* in some cases differed within clonal lineages (TR1 vs TR2; MF1 vs MF2; KK1 vs KK2).

Differently from *P. aeruginosa* early strains, 58.4% (7/12) of the late strains had no effect on growth of *S. aureus* Newman and SH1000 strains. These *P. aeruginosa* strains belonged to six different lineages (NN, BT, AA, TR, MF, KK) indicating presence of at least one *P. aeruginosa* strain unable to inhibit *S. aureus* growth in the majority of CF patients (75%: 6/8). The other two *P. aeruginosa* lineages (SG and BST) (25%: 2/8) inhibited *S. aureus* growth although to a lesser extent when compared to early strains. Late *P. aeruginosa* strains within the same lineage also differed with regard to the strength of *S. aureus* growth inhibition (SG57 vs SG58; BT72 vs BT73; TR66 vs TR67), indicating a diversification of the bacterial population during chronic infection as demonstrated for other virulence traits [23,32]. The average inhibition halo of late group was 11.6 mm versus Newman and 11.3 mm versus SH1000, while the average inhibition halo of early group was 18.3 mm versus Newman and 17.4 mm versus SH1000. Late group showed a statistically significant effect in reducing levels of inhibition (regression parameter = −6.76 versus Newman and regression parameter = −6.24 versus SH1000) with $p<0.01$ for both settings. This data indicated that, as a group, late *P. aeruginosa* strains differ significantly from early strains in their capacity to inhibit *S. aureus* growth, suggesting a trend of *P. aeruginosa* patho-adaptive variants to influence the growth of *S. aureus*.

On the contrary *S. aureus* did not exert any effect on the growth of *P. aeruginosa* (Table S1).

Competition between *S. aureus* and *P. aeruginosa* in planktonic co-cultures

Next, we investigated the interactions between *S. aureus* and *P. aeruginosa* in planktonic growth by comparing the growth kinetics of the two organisms in co-culture to those obtained in pure culture. One reference *P. aeruginosa* strain PA14 and a pair of sequential strains from patient AA were selected. Figure 1A shows the growth curves of the reference *S. aureus* Newman and *P. aeruginosa* PA14 strains in single and dual cultures. PA14 maintained the same growth rate in pure culture and in co-culture, and had a significant negative effect on the overall trend of the growth of Newman ($p<0.001$). In order to have a clear comprehension of the differences in growth between *S. aureus* and *P. aeruginosa*, we calculated the Competition Index (CI), that allows to compare the differences in growth curve of mixed cultures, and the CI-like index, the Relative Increase Ratio (RIR), that compares the growth curves of the two species in pure culture (see Materials and Methods). As shown in Figure 1B, the CI of PA14 versus Newman was significantly different from the RIR in late exponential phase (12 h, $p<0.001$) and stationary phase (24 h, $p<0.001$) of growth, suggesting an inhibitory effect of *P. aeruginosa* on *S. aureus*.

Next, we explored the effect of *P. aeruginosa* strains isolated at the onset of chronic colonization (early strains) or several years after acquisition (late strains) from CF patients on growth of *S. aureus*. A pair of well characterized *P. aeruginosa* clonal strains isolated from CF patient were selected: the AA2 early strain and AA43 late adapted strain carrying several phenotypic changes in virulence factor production, and patho-adaptive mutations within the genome temporally associated with CF lung infection [23,30,33]. The growth of Newman was significantly inhibited by the presence of the early AA2 strain ($p<0.001$), while AA2 strain was not affected from the presence of *S. aureus* (Figure 1C). The CI of AA2 versus Newman was significantly higher than the RIR in late exponential phase (8 h, $p<0.05$ and 12 h, $p<0.01$, Figure 1D) and in stationary phase (24 h, $p<0.01$). On the other hand, Newman and the late strain AA43 interfered each other in co-culture,

Table 1. *In vitro* growth inhibition of *S. aureus* and *P. aeruginosa*.

P. aeruginosa spot	*S. aureus* lawn (Newman) (inhibition halo)	*S. aureus* lawn (SH1000) (inhibition halo)
PAO1	strong (24.5 mm)	strong (20 mm)
PA14	strong (22 mm)	strong (19 mm)
SG1	strong (23.5 mm)	strong (22.5 mm)
SG57*	strong (23 mm)	strong (20.5 mm)
SG58*	weak (14.5 mm)	weak (15 mm)
NN2	weak (15 mm)	weak (14 mm)
NN83#*	no (9 mm)	no (9 mm)
BT1#	weak (15 mm)	weak (14.5 mm)
BT2	weak (15 mm)	weak (15 mm)
BT72*	no (9 mm)	no (9 mm)
BT73*	weak (13.5 mm)	weak (13 mm)
AA2	very strong (27 mm)	strong (20.5 mm)
AA43*	no (9 mm)	no (9 mm)
TR1	weak (13.5 mm)	weak (13.5 mm)
TR2	strong (20 mm)	strong (20 mm)
TR66*	weak (11.5 mm)	weak (11.5 mm)
TR67*	no (9 mm)	no (9 mm)
MF1	weak (15 mm)	strong (21 mm)
MF2#	strong (21 mm)	strong (18.5 mm)
MF51*	no (9 mm)	no (9 mm)
KK1	weak (12 mm)	no (9 mm)
KK2	very strong (27 mm)	very strong (26.5 mm)
KK71*	no (9 mm)	no (9 mm)
KK72*	no (9 mm)	no (9 mm)
BST2	weak (15 mm)	weak (14.5 mm)
BST44#*	weak (14.5 mm)	weak (12.5 mm)

Twenty-four *P. aeruginosa* isolates were collected from eight individuals with CF (SG, NN, BT, AA, TR, MF, KK, BST) at the onset of chronic colonization (numbered 1-2) or after 4.5–16.3 years of colonization (numbered 43-83). PAO1 and PA14 were included as reference strains. 5 µl spots of *P. aeruginosa* overnight cultures, normalized to 0.5 OD, were added to *S. aureus* lawn (normalized to 0.5 OD) on Mueller-Hinton agar and incubated overnight at 37°C. The table summarizes the results obtained: "weak inhibition" indicates an inhibition halo ≤15 mm; "strong inhibition" indicates an inhibition halo >15 mm and ≤25 mm; "very strong inhibition" indicates an inhibition halo >25 mm; "no inhibition" indicates absence of inhibition halo (9 mm is the diameter of the *P. aeruginosa* spot).
* Indicates mucoid phenotype.
\# Indicates hypermutable phenotype. For statistical analysis see "Results".

slightly but significantly reducing their growth rate compared to pure culture ($p<0.001$, Figure 1E). It is worth noting that AA43 inhibited the growth of Newman to a lower extent compared to AA2: while AA2 determined a reduction of 3, 5 and 6 log at 8, 12 and 24 h respectively, AA43 determined a reduction of less than 1 log at the same time points (Figure 1C and E). Being the competition reciprocal between the two species and considering their different growth rate in pure culture, the CI did not differ from the RIR (Figure 1F). Similar results were obtained using the same isolates of *P. aeruginosa*, AA2 and AA43, in co-culture with the reference *S. aureus* SH1000 (Figure S1) strengthening the results obtained with Newman. Taken together these data indicate that *P. aeruginosa* strains, including reference or those isolated at the early stage of chronic infection, can outcompete *S. aureus* in planktonic cultures. On the other hand, *P. aeruginosa* patho-adaptive strains lose this capacity over time.

S. aureus and *P. aeruginosa* interaction in biofilm

In order to understand if the reciprocal interaction among the two species could affect their capacity to produce biofilm, we quantified the biofilm biomass of individually cultured or co-cultured at a ratio 1:1 *S. aureus* and *P. aeruginosa* by staining with crystal violet. As shown in Figure 2, the results obtained from co-cultured pair of strains formed by Newman and PA14 revealed significantly lower level of biomass compared to Newman only (Newman vs Newman+PA14 $p<0.01$), but similar to that corresponding to PA14 alone. This data suggests an inhibitory effect exerted by *P. aeruginosa* on *S. aureus* biofilm formation. For clinical *P. aeruginosa* strains, while the OD value detected in the mixed biofilm formed by Newman and AA2 was not significantly different from both Newman and AA2 individually cultured, the OD value associated to the mixed biofilm formed by Newman and AA43 revealed significantly lower levels of biomass compared to both Newman (Newman vs Newman+AA43 $p<0.001$) and AA43 (AA43 vs Newman+AA43 $p<0.001$) individually cultured. This finding suggests a reciprocal interference of the two species, confirming the results of batch co-culture experiments.

We also determined the amount of viable bacteria of each species in both planktonic and sessile fractions in single and dual cultures. In co-culture, we noticed that all strains of *P. aeruginosa*

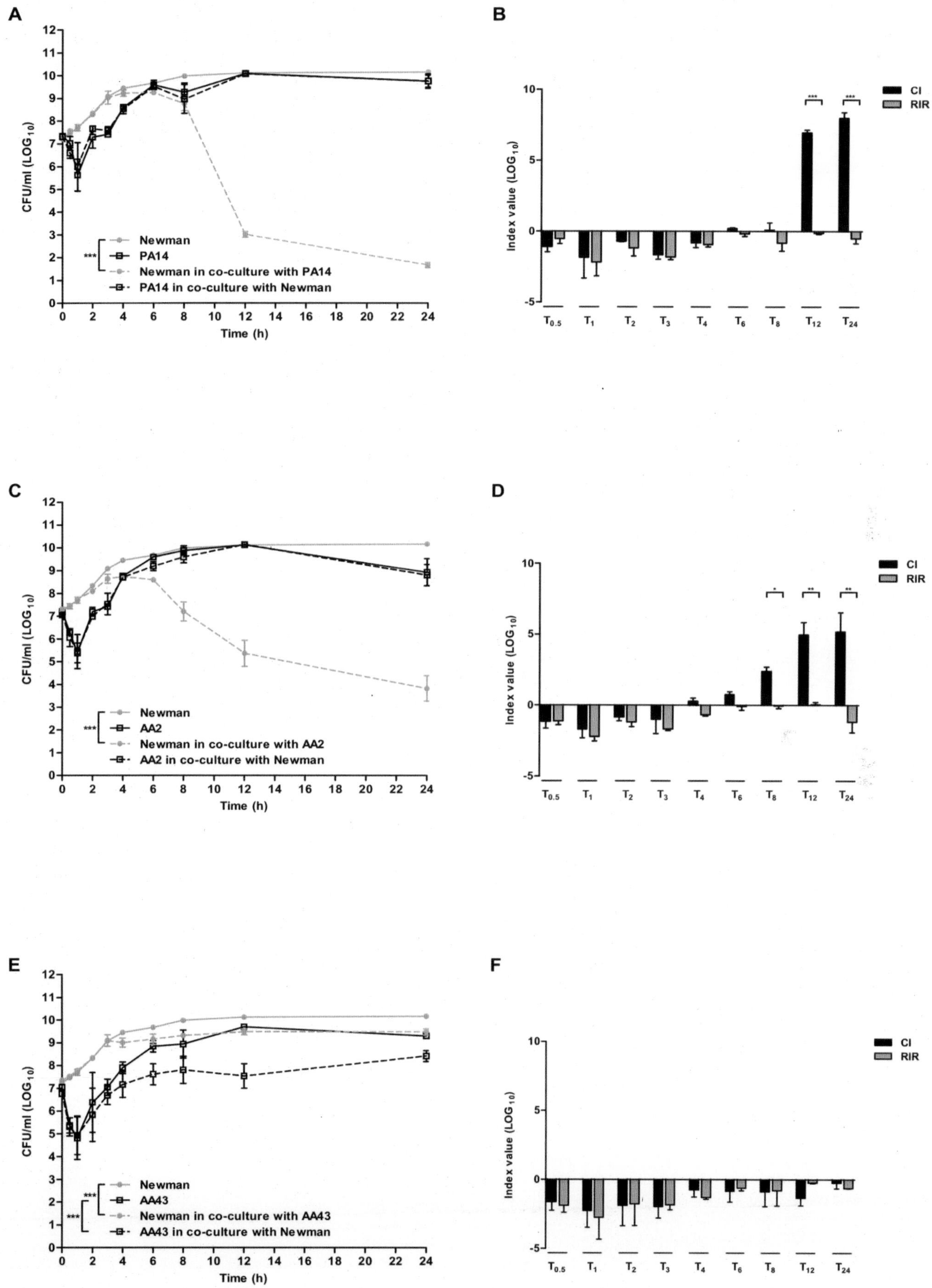
A
B
C
D
E
F
CFU/ml (LOG10)
Time (h)
Index value (LOG10)
Newman
PA14
Newman in co-culture with PA14
PA14 in co-culture with Newman
AA2
Newman in co-culture with AA2
AA2 in co-culture with Newman
AA43
Newman in co-culture with AA43
AA43 in co-culture with Newman
CI
RIR
***
T0.5
T1
T2
T3
T4
T6
T8
T12
T24

Figure 1. Single and dual species batch growth curves and competition index values. *S. aureus* strain (Newman) and *P. aeruginosa* strains (PA14 and two clinical early and late isolates from a CF patient AA2 and AA43) were grown for 24 hours in BHI in single culture and in co-culture after inoculation at equal ratio from mid-exponential phase pure cultures. Growth rate was monitored by colony count after plating on selective media for both species. Results are represented as the mean of values obtained from three independent experiments. The error bars indicate the standard deviations. A nonlinear mixed-effect model was fitted, using a four-parameters logistic regression function. Panel A: growth curves of Newman in pure culture and in co-culture with PA14; Panel B: Competition index (CI) and Relative Increase Ratio (RIR) calculated from single and dual cultures of Newman and PA14; Panel C: growth curves of Newman in pure culture and in co-culture with AA2; Panel D: CI and RIR calculated from single and dual cultures of Newman and AA2; Panel E: growth curves of Newman in pure culture and in co-culture with AA43; Panel F: CI and RIR calculated from single and dual cultures of Newman and AA43. Each value represents the mean of CI and RIR values from three independent experiments and the bars indicate standard deviation. Statistically significant differences in Student's t test and in nonlinear mixed-effect model are indicated by symbols when present: *: $p<0.05$; **: $p<0.01$; ***: $p<0.001$.

tested determined a reduction of the number of both sessile and planktonic Newman cells ($p<0.001$) (Figure 3A). In particular, the bacterial load of Newman in sessile fraction, when co-cultured with clinical early *P. aeruginosa* AA2, decreased of five log compared to pure culture, while the clonal late strain AA43 caused a lower (two log) reduction. A similar effect was observed also in planktonic fraction (Figure 3A) in agreement with batch co-culture data.

On the contrary, the presence of Newman had no effect on PA14 and AA2 growth in both planktonic and biofilm fractions, while it moderately inhibited the attachment to polystyrene and biofilm formation of the late *P. aeruginosa* strain AA43, confirming a reciprocal interaction between Newman and AA43 (Figure 3B, $p<0.001$).

Figure 4 shows the percentage of planktonic and sessile cells of the two species in single and dual cultures. While Newman in pure culture presented the highest percentage of sessile cells, in dual culture was negatively affected by the presence of PA14 and AA2, and the biofilm composition of the co-culture reflected that of *P. aeruginosa* in pure culture (Figure 4A and 4B). A reciprocal influence was evident only for the pair represented by Newman and the late strain AA43 (Figure 4C). It is worth noting that in single species biofilm, the mucoid AA43 strain, even if apparently displaying a lower biofilm biomass compared to AA2 after staining with crystal violet, presented a higher percentage of sessile cells compared to AA2 (5.7% vs 3.4% respectively).

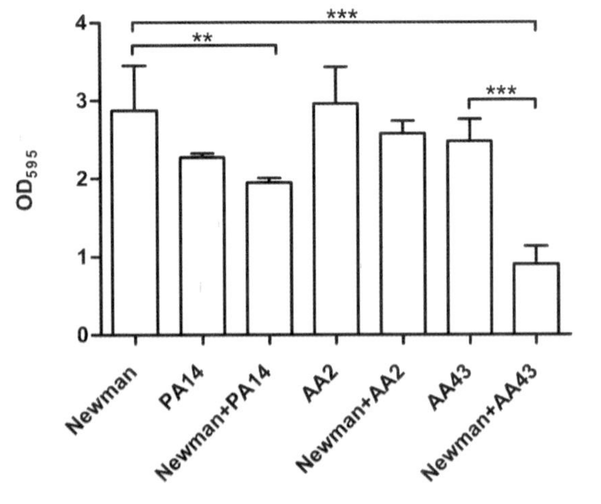

Figure 2. Biofilm formation by *S. aureus* and *P. aeruginosa* strains in single and dual cultures. Bacteria were grown overnight in 96-well flat-bottom microtiter plates in NB medium at 37°C either individually cultured or co-cultured at a 1:1 ratio. Biofilm biomass was quantified by staining with crystal violet and absorbance measurements at OD 595 nm. The values represent the means of three independent experiments, and the bars indicate standard deviation. Statistically significant differences in Student's t test are indicated by symbols when present: **: $p<0.01$; ***: $p<0.001$.

Competition between *P. aeruginosa* and *S. aureus* in a mouse model of acute lung infection

To test whether the observed differences in planktonic growth and biofilm formation *in vitro* would be relevant *in vivo*, a mouse model of acute pneumonia was used. Thus, we set up *in vivo* competition between *P. aeruginosa* and *S. aureus* in C57Bl/6NCrlBR mice challenged with 1×10^6 CFU of *S. aureus* and *P. aeruginosa* strains mixed together at a 1:1 ratio. Eighteen hours after infection, murine lungs were homogenized and plated. Differential CFU counting was performed to calculate the CI. Results show that *P. aeruginosa* reference strain PA14 and the early isolate AA2 outcompeted *S. aureus* strain Newman, as the CI, being significantly different from 1, indicated a competitive advantage of *P. aeruginosa* over *S. aureus* (PA14/Newman average CI = 5.0, $p<0.01$; AA2/Newman average CI = 3.3, $p<0.05$). Different results were obtained for the *P. aeruginosa* late isolate AA43 and Newman as the CI 18 hours after challenge was not significantly different from 1 (AA43/Newman CI = 0.9), indicating no competition in this case (Figure 5 and Table 2).

Discussion

The goal of this study was to investigate the influence of *P. aeruginosa* adaptation to the CF lung on interaction with *S. aureus* in co-culture, during biofilm formation and mouse lung infection, in order to gain important insight on the interplay occurring between the two main pathogens of CF airways, which is still largely unknown. For this purpose, we used a panel of deeply genetically and phenotypically characterized *P. aeruginosa* clonal strains isolated from CF patients at different time points during CF chronic lung infection [33,34].

We evaluated the inhibitory effect of eight *P. aeruginosa* lineages on *S. aureus*, including strains isolated both at early and late stage of chronic infection. A negative effect on *S. aureus* growth significantly associated with early-infecting *P. aeruginosa* strains was observed, while clonal late-infecting *P. aeruginosa* strains presented a significantly reduced or abolished virulence when co-cultivated with *S. aureus*. During chronic infection, *P. aeruginosa* undergoes adaptation to the CF lung, leading to patho-adaptive lineages that differ genotypically and phenotypically from the originally infecting strain. Such microevolution usually determines loss of motility, acquisition of mucoidy, antibiotic resistance and loss-of-function mutations in virulence genes, suggesting attenuation of virulence for CF adapted strains [30,35,36,37]. Here we demonstrated for the first time that *P. aeruginosa* virulence traits affect also the interaction with other CF-related pathogen as *S. aureus*. As described for other traits, intra-clonal variation was observed both in clonal *P. aeruginosa* early strains and late strains isolated at the same time from the CF patients. One of the most striking

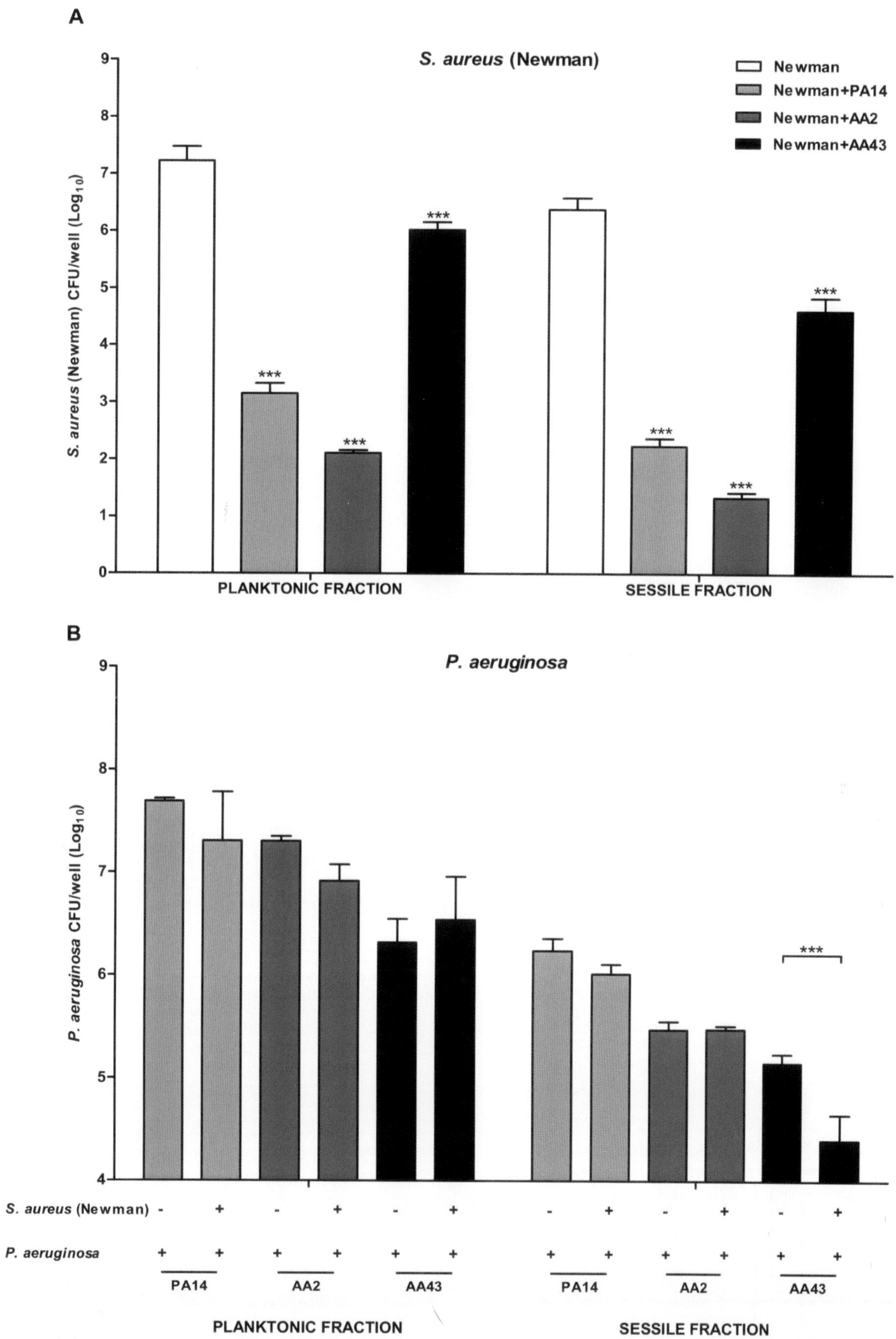
A
S. aureus (Newman)
Newman
Newman+PA14
Newman+AA2
Newman+AA43
S. aureus (Newman) CFU/well (Log10)
***
PLANKTONIC FRACTION
SESSILE FRACTION
B
P. aeruginosa
P. aeruginosa CFU/well (Log10)
S. aureus (Newman)
P. aeruginosa
PA14
AA2
AA43
PLANKTONIC FRACTION
SESSILE FRACTION

Figure 3. ***S. aureus*** **and** ***P. aeruginosa*** **planktonic and sessile cells in single and dual cultures.** Bacteria were grown overnight in 96-well flat-bottom microtiter plates in NB medium at 37°C either individually cultured or co-cultured at a 1:1 ratio. CFU counts were determined in both planktonic and sessile fractions. Panel A: planktonic (left) and sessile (right) cells of *S. aureus* strain Newman in pure culture and in co-culture with *P. aeruginosa* strains PA14, AA2 and AA43. Statistically significant differences are referred to Newman in pure culture. Panel B: planktonic (left) and sessile (right) cells of *P. aeruginosa* strains PA14, AA2 and AA43 in pure culture and in co-culture with *S. aureus* strain Newman. The values represent the means of three independent experiments, and the bars indicate standard deviation. Statistically significant differences in non-parametric Mann–Whitney test are indicated by symbols when present: **: $p<0.01$; ***: $p<0.001$.

characteristics of *P. aeruginosa* chronic lung infection in CF patients is the intense diversification of the bacterial population, leading to the co-existence of multiple phenotypes that may colonize different airways niches. Thus, the intra-clonal variation that we have observed is most likely the result of this process of genetic adaptation.

Under planktonic growth conditions, we have shown that both the reference *P. aeruginosa* strain PA14 and the clinical early strain AA2 strongly inhibited the growth of *S. aureus* during late logarithmic phase and stationary phase, without being influenced in their growth rate. Antagonism between microorganisms within a community could be attributed to simple competition for limited resources or to direct antagonistic effects [36]. There is evidence supporting antagonism between *P. aeruginosa* and *S. aureus*. Mashburn *et al.* demonstrated that *P. aeruginosa* can lyse *S. aureus* to use the iron released for its own growth [38]. Moreover, it has been reported that *S. aureus* is susceptible to an arsenal of respiratory inhibitors generated by *P. aeruginosa*, such as pyocyanin, hydrogen cyanide or alkyl-hydroxyquinoline N-oxides (HQNO), which are able to suppress the aerobic metabolism and growth of *S. aureus* [25,39]. Interestingly, the late *P. aeruginosa* strain AA43, clonal to AA2, inhibited the growth of *S. aureus* at a lower extent, compared to AA2 and was not able to outcompete it. Besides being less virulent, AA43 was also negatively affected by the presence of *S. aureus* as its growth rate was significantly slowed down by *S. aureus* cells.

Despite the increasing interest on the crucial role of biofilm in CF infections, interspecies interactions of different organisms in mixed species biofilms are still poorly understood [27]. Here we have shown that in co-culture biofilms all *P. aeruginosa* strains were able to outcompete *S. aureus* in both sessile and planktonic fractions and the composition of the population in mixed biofilms was determined by *P. aeruginosa*, albeit to different extent. Also under biofilm growth conditions, the clonal late *P. aeruginosa* strains AA43 presented a different behavior in the presence of *S. aureus* compared to the early AA2 strain. In single species biofilm, the mucoid AA43 strain, even if apparently displaying a lower biofilm biomass compared to AA2 after staining with crystal violet, presented a higher percentage of sessile cells compared to AA2. This difference in biofilm production reflects the well documented phenotypic changes occurring in *P. aeruginosa* during the establishment of chronic infection. Indeed, *P. aeruginosa* strains isolated from CF patients at early stage of chronic infection are generally non-encapsulated and express a variety of virulence factors, whereas *P. aeruginosa* isolates from late stage typically lack virulence factors and convert to a mucoid phenotype, associated with greater biofilm formation and resistance to phagocytosis [37]. In apparent contradiction, also the early strain AA2 was able to produce biofilm. This could be explained considering the complexity of the microbial interactions in the CF lung, the presence of a diverse community of *P. aeruginosa* strains, and the many factors contributing to the formation of the biofilm matrix of *P. aeruginosa*, besides alginate production. In addition not all adapted isolates are

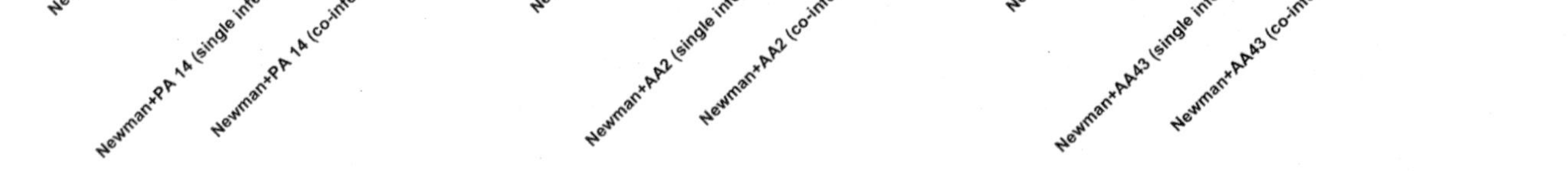

Figure 4. Percentage of planktonic and sessile cells in single and dual cultures. Bacteria were grown overnight in 96-well flat-bottom microtiter plates in NB medium at 37°C either individually cultured or co-cultured at a 1:1 ratio. CFU counts were determined in both planktonic and sessile fractions and the percentage of S. aureus and P. aeruginosa in the two fractions of single and dual cultures was calculated. Panel A: percentages of planktonic and sessile cells of Newman in single culture (first histogram), PA14 in single culture (second histogram), Newman and PA14 in ideal co-culture if the 2 species would not interfere each other (third histogram, percentages have been calculated considering the values of the first and second histograms), and Newman and PA14 in co-culture (fourth histogram). Panel B: percentages of planktonic and sessile cells of Newman in single culture (first histogram), AA2 in single culture (second histogram), Newman and AA2 in ideal co-culture if the 2 species would not interfere each other (third histogram, percentages have been calculated considering the values of the first and second histograms), and Newman and AA2 in co-culture (fourth histogram). Panel C: percentages of planktonic and sessile cells of Newman in single culture (first histogram), AA43 in single culture (second histogram), Newman and AA43 in ideal co-culture if the 2 species would not interfere each other (third histogram, percentages have been calculated considering the values of the first and second histograms), and Newman and AA43 in co-culture (fourth histogram). SA: S. aureus; PA: P. aeruginosa.

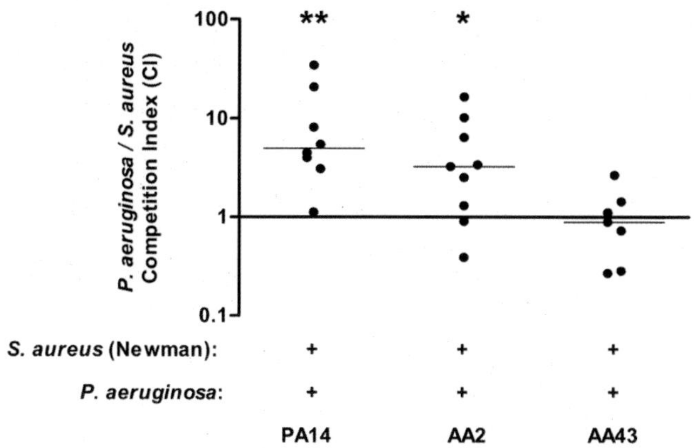

Figure 5. Competition between *P. aeruginosa* and *S. aureus* strains in a murine model of pneumoniae. Planktonic *S. aureus* strain Newman and *P. aeruginosa* clinical isolates AA2 and AA43 and reference strain PA14 were used to infect C57BL/6NCrlBR mice at a ratio of 1:1. After 18 hours of acute infection lungs homogenates were plated on selective plates to determine *S. aureus* and *P. aeruginosa* CFU. Each circle represents the CI for a single animal in each group. A CI value equal to 1 indicates equal competition of the two species; a CI value significantly <1 indicates a competitive advantage of *S. aureus* that outcompetes *P. aeruginosa*; a CI value significantly >1 indicates a competitive advantage of *P. aeruginosa* that outcompetes *S. aureus*. Wilcoxon signed rank test of the null hypothesis that the distribution of CI is symmetric about 1 was performed. Statistically significant differences are indicated by symbols when present: *: $p<0.05$; **: $p<0.01$. The data are pooled from two or three independent experiments.

mucoid and also early not adapted strains could produce biofilm exploiting other biofilm matrix molecules [40]. In agreement with data obtained in planktonic co-cultures, AA2 strongly inhibited the growth of *S. aureus* in mixed biofilm, without being affected. Qazi *et al.* demonstrated that factors related to biofilm formation are down-regulated in *S. aureus* in response to *P. aeruginosa* presence, consistently with our results [41]. Compared to AA2, *P. aeruginosa* AA43 inhibited *S. aureus* growth at lower extent, determining a reduction of *S. aureus* CFU count of about 1 and 2 log in planktonic and sessile fractions respectively, when measured against *S. aureus* individual biofilm. Moreover, the capacity to produce biofilm of AA43 was negatively affected by the presence of *S. aureus*, confirming its attenuated virulence and susceptibility to competitor organism.

Although several studies using *in vitro* models demonstrated an inhibitory effect of *P. aeruginosa* on the growth of also highly virulent *S. aureus* strains such as USA 300, in line with our results [27,42,43], *in vivo* models show contradictory results [42,44]. We further investigated *S. aureus*/*P. aeruginosa* reciprocal interaction setting up a murine model of acute lung co-infection. In agreement with *in vitro* data, the reference strain PA14 and the early CF clinical isolate AA2, after 18 hours of co-infection, inhibited *S. aureus*, while the late CF clinical isolate AA43 did not outcompete *S. aureus*.

It is known that environmental and early clinical isolates of *P. aeruginosa* are equipped with a repertoire of virulence factors and, among them, also substances with anti-bacterial activity, these factors are selected against during the adaptation process to the CF airways environment. The results obtained in the acute pneumonia model, in which an early isolate is able to inhibit the growth of another pathogen, while its clonal adapted strain is no longer able to do so, strengthen the loss of anti-bacterial factors during adaptation.

Our data underline the importance of bacterial interactions in lung infection and in particular of the complexity of the interactions of different pathogens that coexist in the CF airways. However, given the genetic adaptation process of *P. aeruginosa* that leads to the selection of different patho-adaptive variants, descending from the initial infecting clone, further combinations of clonal lineages of early and late isolates should be tested to strengthen our *in vivo* data. Moreover, considering that the adaptation process during chronic infection involves also *S. aureus*, other experiments using clinical early and late *S. aureus* strains as well as adapted phenotypes such as small colony variants should be performed. Our results showing the influence of adaptation on the reciprocal interactions between *S. aureus* and *P. aeruginosa* deserve further investigations including the host response and the effect of environmental conditions, such as microaerobic and anaerobic

Table 2. Colonization of murine lungs with S. aureus and P. aeruginosa reference and clinical strains in competition experiments.

	PA14/Newman (n = 9[a])	AA2/Newman (n = 9[a])	AA43/Newman (n = 9[a])
Mortality, % (no. of dead/total mice)	0 (0/9)	0 (0/9)	0 (0/9)
Co-infected[b], % (no. of co-infected/ surviving mice)	89 (8/9)	100 (9/9)	78 (7/9)
P. aeruginosa infected[c], % (no. of infected/ surviving mice)	100 (9/9)	100 (9/9)	78 (7/9)
S. aureus infected[d], % (no. of infected/ surviving mice)	89 (8/9)	100 (9/9)	78 (7/9)
Total cfu/lung[e]	3.3×10^4	6.7×10^3	5.8×10^3
P. aeruginosa cfu/lung[e]	2.9×10^4	4.5×10^3	2.7×10^3
S. aureus cfu/lung[e]	4.2×10^3	2.2×10^3	3.1×10^3
CI[f]	5.0	3.3	0.9

[a]Pooled mice, analyzed in two independent experiments.
[b]Co-infected mice, surviving after 18 hours from challenge.
[c]Number of pooled mice infected with *P. aeruginosa* after 18 hours.
[d]Number of pooled mice infected with *S. aureus* after 18 hours.
[e]Median values are reported.
[f]Competition Index.

conditions, on pathogens interactions, using both *in vitro* and *in vivo* models of chronic infection that better mirror the progression of CF lung disease.

Materials and Methods

Animals and ethics statement

Animal studies were conducted according to protocols approved by the San Raffaele Scientific Institute (Milan, Italy) Institutional Animal Care and Use Committee (IACUC, Number 444) and adhered strictly to the Italian Ministry of Health guidelines for the use and care of experimental animals. All efforts were made to minimize the number of animals used and their suffering.

Research on *P. aeruginosa* bacterial isolates from the individuals with CF has been approved by the responsible physician at the CF center at Hannover Medical School, Germany. All patients gave informed consent before the sample collection. Approval for storing of biological materials was obtained by the Hannover Medical School, Germany.

Bacterial strains

For *S. aureus*, Newman and SH1000 reference strains, were used in the study [45,46]. Two *P. aeruginosa* reference strains, PA14 [47] and PAO1 [48], and 8 clonal lineages of *P. aeruginosa* clinical strains from CF patients (AA, SG, NN, BT, TR, MF, KK, BST), including strains isolated at the onset of chronic colonization (early: AA2, SG1, NN2, BT1, BT2, TR1, TR2, MF1, MF2, KK1, KK2, BST2) or several years after acquisition and before patient's death (late: AA43, SG57, SG58, NN83, BT72, BT73, TR66, TR67, MF51, KK71, KK72, BST44) were used in this study [23]. Clonality of strains, assessed by Pulsed Field Gel Electrophoresis and multiple phenotypic traits, including motility, mucoid phenotype, *LasR* phenotype, and pyocyanin secretion, have been determined and previously reported [23,32].

S. aureus growth inhibition on agar surface

S. aureus cultures (Newman and SH1000) grown overnight in Luria-Bertani broth (LB, Difco^{TM}) were normalized to 0.5 OD_{600} and uniformly spread on Mueller-Hinton agar plate (MH, Difco^{TM}) by using a cotton swab. Then 5 µl of *P. aeruginosa* culture, grown overnight in LB broth and normalized to 0.5 OD_{600}, were added to the *S. aureus* lawn followed by incubation overnight at 37°C [25]. The same procedure was performed spotting *S. aureus* culture on *P. aeruginosa* lawn. The following *P. aeruginosa* clonal lineages, including early and late clinical strains, were tested: AA, SG, NN, BT, TR, MF, KK and BST (for details see paragraph "Bacterial strains"). As *P. aeruginosa* reference strains we used PA14 and PAO1. The inhibition score was defined as follows: "no inhibition" when no halo was observed around the spot of *P. aeruginosa* that measures 9 mm; "weak inhibition" indicated an inhibition halo $\leq$15 mm; "strong inhibition" indicated an inhibition halo >15 mm and $\leq$25 mm; "very strong inhibition" indicated an inhibition halo >25 mm. The choice for inhibition strength ranges was based on preliminary assays performed using the lawn of about 30 *S. aureus* strains (including both reference and clinical strains of different origin) and spotting about 60 *P. aeruginosa* strains (both reference and clinical strains) on the different lawns.

Planktonic mono-culture and co-culture growth curves

All growth curves were performed in 30 ml of nutrient-rich not selective medium, Brain-Heart Infusion broth (BHI, Difco^{TM}), at 37°C with shaking (180 rpm). The following strains were tested: *S. aureus* (Newman, SH1000), *P. aeruginosa* (PA14, AA2 and AA43). Strains were grown overnight in BHI and subcultured in fresh medium for 2.5 hours to reach the mid-exponential phase of growth. Bacteria were centrifuged, pellet was resuspended in fresh medium and the OD_{600} was measured to adjust the concentration of bacteria. For co-cultures each pair of *S. aureus* and *P. aeruginosa* strains were inoculated at equal ratio (1 OD_{600}, optical density) from mid-exponential phase pure cultures and incubated at 37°C for 24 hours. Pure cultures of each organism were used for comparative purposes. At different time points (0, 0.5, 1, 2, 3, 4, 6, 8, 12 and 24 hours), samples were taken, serially diluted in sterile phosphate-buffered saline (PBS) and plated onto Mannitol Salt agar (MSA, Difco^{TM}) and Pseudomonas Isolation agar (PIA, Difco^{TM}) to discriminate the two bacterial species. The agar plates were incubated for 24 hours at 37°C and colony forming units (CFU) were enumerated. Each experiment was repeated three times independently. The competition index (CI) for mixed culture was calculated as *P. aeruginosa*-to-*S. aureus* ratio within the output sample, divided by the corresponding ratio for the input (inoculum at time t = 0), as described by Macho and colleagues [49]. To allow an easier comparison between the variations observed in single versus mixed cultures a CI-like index, the Relative Increase Ratio (RIR) was calculated as *P. aeruginosa*-to-*S. aureus* ratio within the output sample, divided by the corresponding ratio in the inoculum, using growth results from pure cultures [49]. As the RIR is calculated on the results obtained from single growth curves, only a CI that differs statistically from the RIR of the same time-point can be considered a result of a significant competition between the species [49].

Biofilm production

Biofilm production in static conditions was visualized by crystal violet (CV) staining as previously described [34]. The following *S. aureus* and *P. aeruginosa* strains were tested: Newman, PA14, AA2 and AA43. Strains were grown overnight in Nutrient Broth (NB, Difco^{TM}) and subcultured in fresh medium for 2.5 hours to reach the mid-exponential phase of growth. Bacteria were centrifuged, pellet was washed with PBS, resuspended in fresh medium and the OD_{600} was measured to adjust the concentration of bacteria [34]. Experiments were performed in triplicate and repeated three times independently. The data were then averaged and the standard deviation was calculated.

To correlate the growth in the planktonic fraction with biofilm formation, the planktonic cell fractions, which were transferred to new microtiter plates, were quantified by plating serial dilutions on MSA and PIA agar plates. To enumerate the sessile cells of *S. aureus* and *P. aeruginosa*, the wells were rinsed three times with 200 µl of PBS to remove non-adherent and weakly adherent bacteria. Then, the biofilm was removed by scraping the surface of each well with 1 ml PBS and the recovered cells were suspended by vortexing for 30 sec. The number of sessile cells was determined by plating serial dilutions on MSA and PIA agar plates. To ensure the complete detachment of the bacteria, CV (1%) assay was performed on each of the wells scraped, and absorbance determined at 595 nm.

Mouse model of acute lung single and co-infection

Experiment of acute infection with *S. aureus* and *P. aeruginosa* strains were performed using C57Bl/6NCrlBR male mice (20–22 gr), purchased by Charles River, with minor modification to previous published protocols [20,30]. For the co-infections, *P. aeruginosa* referent strain PA14 and clinical isolates AA2 and AA43, and *S. aureus* referent strain Newman, grown at middle exponential phase, were recovered by centrifugation and resuspended in PBS to the desired sub-lethal dose for infection of 1×10^6 CFU both for *P. aeruginosa* and *S. aureus* and mixed together at a ratio of 1:1.

C57Bl/6NCrlBR mice were anesthetized by an intraperitoneal injection of a solution of 2.5% Avertin (2,2,2-tribromethanol, 97%; Sigma Aldrich) in 0.9% NaCl and administered in a volume of 0.015 mlg^{-1} body weight. Trachea was directly visualized by a ventral midline incision, exposed and intubated with a sterile, flexible 22-g cannula (Becton, Dickinson, Italy) attached to a 1 ml syringe. Co-infection was established with a 60 µl inoculum implanted via the cannula into the lung, with both lobes inoculated. Mice were also infected with 1×10^6 CFU of planktonic *P. aeruginosa* or *S. aureus* for comparative purposes.

After 18 hours from infection, mice were euthanized and murine lungs were aseptically excised, homogenized and plated onto MSA and PIA plates for differential CFU counting. The competition index (CI) was calculated as the ratio of *P. aeruginosa* to *S. aureus* bacteria recovered from the murine lungs after 18 hours from infection adjusted by the input ratio that was inoculated in each animal (*in vivo* CI). A CI value equal to 1 indicates equal competition of the two species; a CI value significantly <1 indicates a competitive advantage of *S. aureus* that outcompetes *P. aeruginosa*; a CI value significantly >1 indicates a competitive advantage of *P. aeruginosa* that outcompetes *S. aureus*.

Statistical analysis

In vitro agar growth inhibition data were analyzed by means of a LME (Linear Mixed effect model) separated for Newman and SH1000. Response variable was inhibition and covariates were groups (early versus late) and a random effect on patient to account for lineages heterogeneity. To analyze batch co-culture data reported in Figure 1A, 1C, 1E the CFU/ml values were transformed using a log10 function. Data retrieved from single and co-culture experiments showed a similar starting point (estimated by intercept parameter A) and different behavior in some settings over time , leading to different plateau values (estimated by parameter B) at the end of the follow-up period. This suggested to use a nonlinear mixed-effect model (ref), (with the non-linearity described by a four-parameters logistic regression function) to estimate the log10(CFU/ml) trend, modelled as it follows: $A+B/\{1+\exp[(C-x)/\exp(D)]\}$.

This kind of model is widely used for growth curve modeling. Since the parameter A represents horizontal asymptote relative to the starting point, we assign a random effect (representing the heterogeneity among experiments) on this parameter to include heterogeneity among experiments. Parameter B represents the horizontal asymptote relative to the final plateau; we studied the possible influence of single/co-culture (described by its indicator variable), in order to test the hypothesis of different plateau at the end of the follow up. This represents the main effect of interest and its significance was tested comparing likelihood with and without it. Parameter C is the inflection point and has been estimated using a maximum likelihood principle. Parameter D is strictly connected to the so called scale parameter and represents the growth rate of the logistic function. A fixed effect common for single single and co-culture was estimated. RIR and CI indexes were analyzed using Student's t-test and the null hypothesis: mean CI was not significantly different from mean RIR [49]. *In vitro* biofilm data (OD values) were analyzed using Two-tailed Student's t-test [34]. CFU biofilm data were analyzed by means of Mann–Whitney test, a non-parametric procedure to evaluate a null hypothesis that two populations are the same against an alternative that one population tends to have larger values than the other. Competition index (CI) of *in vivo* experiments was calculated adapting the methods previously published [20]. To assess bacterial competition Wilcoxon signed rank test of the null hypothesis that the distribution of CI is symmetric about 1 was used. Significance was set at the usual level 0.05. All statistical analyses were performed using R 2.15.2 (http://www.R-project.org/).

Supporting Information

Table S1 ***In vitro*** **growth inhibition of** ***P. aeruginosa*****.**

Figure S1 Single and dual species batch growth curves and competition index values. S. aureus strain (SH1000) and P. aeruginosa strains (PA14 and two clinical early and late isolates from a CF patient AA2 and AA43) were grown for 24 hours in BHI in single culture and in co-culture after inoculation at equal ratio from mid-exponential phase pure cultures. Growth rate was monitored by colony count after plating on selective media for both species. Results are represented as the mean of values obtained from three independent experiments. The error bars indicate the standard deviations. A nonlinear mixed-effect model was fitted, using a four-parameters logistic regression function. Panel A: growth curves of SH1000 in pure culture and in co-culture with PA14; Panel B: Competition index (CI) and Relative Increase Ratio (RIR) calculated from single and dual cultures of SH1000 and PA14; Panel C: growth curves of SH1000 in pure culture and in co-culture with AA2; Panel D: CI and RIR calculated from single and dual cultures of SH1000 and AA2; Panel E: growth curves of SH1000 in pure culture and in co-culture with AA43; Panel F: CI and RIR calculated from single and dual cultures of SH1000 and AA43. Each value represents the mean of CI and RIR values from three independent experiments and the bars indicate standard deviation. Statistically significant differences in Student's t test and in nonlinear mixed-effect model are indicated by symbols when present: *: $p<0.05$; ***: $p<0.001$.

Acknowledgments

The authors thank Barbara Sipione for her technical support. The authors thank B. Tummler, Klinische Forschergruppe, OE 6710, Medizinische Hochschule Hannover, Hannover, Germany, for supplying the *P. aeruginosa* strains from CF patients and Prof. BC. Kahl, Institut für Medizinische Mikrobiologie Universitätskliniken Muenster, Germany for supplying *S. aureus* strains.

Author Contributions

Conceived and designed the experiments: RB IB CC AB DMC. Performed the experiments: RB FT MDS IB CC. Analyzed the data: RB FT IB CC DP CDS. Contributed reagents/materials/analysis tools: CDS DMC AB. Wrote the paper: RB CC IB DP CDS AB DMC.

References

1. Sibley CD, Rabin H, Surette MG (2006) Cystic fibrosis: a polymicrobial infectious disease. Future Microbiol 1: 53–61.
2. Cystic Fibrosis Foundation Patient Registry: Annual Data Report 2008. Available: http://www.cff.org. Accessed 2014 Feb 12.
3. Rogers GB, Hoffman LR, Whiteley M, Daniels TW, Carroll MP, et al. (2010) Revealing the dynamics of polymicrobial infections: implications for antibiotic therapy. Trends Microbiol 18(8):357–64.
4. Hibbing ME, Fuqua C, Parsek MR, Peterson SB (2010) Bacterial competition: surviving and thriving in the microbial jungle. Nat Rev Microbiol 8(1):15–25.

5. Ryan RP, Fouhy Y, Garcia BF, Watt SA, Niehaus K, et al. (2008) Interspecies signalling via the *Stenotrophomonas maltophilia* diffusible signal factor influences biofilm formation and polymyxin tolerance in *Pseudomonas aeruginosa*. Mol Microbiol 68:75–86.
6. Nocker A, Burr M, Camper AK (2007) Genotypic microbial community profiling: a critical technical review. Microb Ecol 54:276–289.
7. Rogers GB, Carroll MP, Bruce KD (2009) Studying bacterial infections through culture-independent approaches. J Med Microbiol 58:1401–1418.
8. Sibley CD, Parkins MD, Rabin HR, Duan K, Norgaard JC, et al. (2008) A polymicrobial perspective of pulmonary infections exposes an enigmatic pathogen in cystic fibrosis patients. Proc Natl Acad Sci U S A 105:15070–15075.
9. Bittar F, Richet H, Dubus JC, Reynaud-Gaubert M, Stremler N, et al. (2008) Molecular detection of multiple emerging pathogens in sputa from cystic fibrosis patients. PLoS One 3:e2908.
10. Bouchara JP, Hsieh HY, Croquefer S, Barton R, Marchais V, et al. (2009) Development of an oligonucleotide array for direct detection of fungi in sputum samples from patients with cystic fibrosis. J Clin Microbiol 47:142–152.
11. Armougom F, Bittar F, Stremler N, Rolain JM, Robert C, et al. (2009) Microbial diversity in the sputum of a cystic fibrosis patient studied with 16S rDNA pyrosequencing. Eur J Clin Microbiol Infect Dis 28:1151–1154.
12. Ecker DJ, Sampath R, Massire C, Blyn LB, Hall TA, et al. (2008) Ibis T5000: a universal biosensor approach for microbiology. Nat Rev Microbiol 6:553–558.
13. Rogers GB, Stressmann FA, Walker AW, Carroll MP, Bruce KD (2010) Lung infections in cystic fibrosis; deriving clinical insight from microbial complexity. Exp Rev Mol Diag 10:187–196.
14. Brogden KA, Guthmiller JM, Taylor CE (2005) Human polymicrobial infections. Lancet 365(9455):253–255. 6.
15. Peters BM, Jabra-Rizk MA, O'May GA, Costerton JW, Shirtliff ME (2012) Polymicrobial interactions: impact on pathogenesis and human disease. Clin Microbiol Rev 25(1):193–213.
16. Döring G (1997) *Staphylococcus aureus* in cystic fibrosis: implications for prognosis and treatment. Pediatr Pulmonol Suppl 16:235–6.
17. Razvi S, Quittell L, Sewall A, Quinton H, Marshall B, et al. (2009) Respiratory microbiology of patients with cystic fibrosis in the United States, 1995 to 2005. Chest 136(6):1554–60.
18. Goss CH, Muhlebach MS (2011) Review: *Staphylococcus aureus* and MRSA in cystic fibrosis. J Cyst Fibros 10(5):298–306.
19. Johnson AP (2011) Methicillin-resistant *Staphylococcus aureus*: the European landscape. J Antimicrob Chemother 66 Suppl 4:iv43–iv48.
20. Baldan R, Testa F, Lorè NI, Bragonzi A, Cichero P, et al. (2012) Factors contributing to epidemic MRSA clones replacement in a hospital setting. PLoS One 7(8):e43153.
21. Ratjen F, McColley SA (2012) Update in cystic fibrosis 2011. Am J Respir Crit Care Med 1;185(9):933–6.
22. Döring G, Hoiby N, Consensus Study Group (2004) Early intervention and prevention of lung disease in cystic fibrosis: a European consensus. J Cyst Fibros 3(2):67–91.
23. Bragonzi A, Paroni M, Nonis A, Cramer N, Montanari S, et al. (2009) *Pseudomonas aeruginosa* microevolution during cystic fibrosis lung infection establishes clones with adapted virulence. Am J Respir Crit Care Med 15;180(2):138–45.
24. Jarry TM, Cheung AL (2006) *Staphylococcus aureus* escapes more efficiently from the phagosome of a cystic fibrosis bronchial epithelial cell line than from its normal counterpart. Infect Immun 74(5):2568–77.
25. Hoffman LR, Deziel E, D'Argenio DA, Lepine F, Emerson J, et al. (2006) Selection for *Staphylococcus aureus* small-colony variants due to growth in the presence of *Pseudomonas aeruginosa*. Proc Natl Acad Sci USA 103(52):19890–19895.
26. Maselli J, Sontag MK, Norris JM, MacKenzie T, Wagener JS, et al. (2003) Risk factors for initial acquisition of *Pseudomonas aeruginosa* in children with cystic fibrosis identified by newborn screening. Pediatr Pulmonol 35(4):257–262.
27. Yang L, Liu Y, Markussen T, Høiby N, Tolker-Nielsen T, et al. (2011) Pattern differentiation in co-culture biofilms formed by *Staphylococcus aureus* and *Pseudomonas aeruginosa*. FEMS Immunol Med Microbiol 62(3):339–47.
28. Høiby N, Bjarnsholt T, Givskov M, Molin S, Ciofu O (2010) Antibiotic resistance of bacterial biofilms. Int J Antimicrob Agents 35(4):322–32.
29. Lipuma JJ (2010) The changing microbial epidemiology in cystic fibrosis. Clin Microbiol Rev 23:299–323.
30. Lorè NI, Cigana C, De Fino I, Riva C, Juhas M, et al. (2012) Cystic fibrosis-niche adaptation of *Pseudomonas aeruginosa* reduces virulence in multiple infection hosts. PLoS One 7(4):e35648.
31. Montanari S, Oliver A, Salerno P, Mena A, Bertoni G, et al. (2007) Biological cost of hypermutation in *Pseudomonas aeruginosa* strains from patients with cystic fibrosis. Microbiology 153(Pt 5):1445–54.
32. Bragonzi A, Wiehlmann L, Klockgether J, Cramer N, Worlitzsch D, et al. (2006) Sequence diversity of the mucABD locus in *Pseudomonas aeruginosa* isolates from patients with cystic fibrosis. Microbiology 152(Pt 11):3261–9.
33. Cigana C, Curcurù L, Leone MR, Ieranò T, Lorè NI, et al. (2009) *Pseudomonas aeruginosa* exploits lipid A and muropeptides modification as a strategy to lower innate immunity during cystic fibrosis lung infection. PLoS One 23;4(12):e8439.
34. Bragonzi A, Farulla I, Paroni M, Twomey KB, Pirone L, et al. (2012) Modelling co-infection of the cystic fibrosis lung by Pseudomonas aeruginosa and Burkholderia cenocepacia reveals influences on biofilm formation and host response. PLoS One 7(12):e52330.
35. Bianconi I, Milani A, Cigana C, Paroni M, Levesque RC, et al. (2011) Positive signature-tagged mutagenesis in *Pseudomonas aeruginosa*: tracking patho-adaptive mutations promoting airways chronic infection. PLoS Pathog 3;7(2):e1001270.
36. Harrison F (2007) Microbial ecology of the cystic fibrosis lung. Microbiology 153(Pt 4):917–23.
37. Folkesson A, Jelsbak L, Yang L, Johansen HK, Ciofu O, et al. (2012) Adaptation of *Pseudomonas aeruginosa* to the cystic fibrosis airway: an evolutionary perspective. Nat Rev Microbiol 10(12):841–51.
38. Mashburn LM, Jett AM, Akins DR, Whiteley M (2005) *Staphylococcus aureus* serves as an iron source for *Pseudomonas aeruginosa* during in vivo coculture. J Bacteriol 187(2):554–66.
39. Biswas L, Biswas R, Schlag M, Bertram R, Götz F (2009) Small-colony variant selection as a survival strategy for *Staphylococcus aureus* in the presence of *Pseudomonas aeruginosa*. Appl Environ Microbiol 75(21):6910–2.
40. Mann EE, Wozniak DJ (2012) *Pseudomonas* biofilm matrix composition and niche biology. FEMS Microbiol Rev 36(4):893–916.
41. Qazi S, Middleton B, Muharram SH, Cockayne A, Hill P, et al. (2006) N-acylhomoserine lactones antagonize virulence gene expression and quorum sensing in *Staphylococcus aureus*. Infect Immun 74(2):910–9.
42. Pastar I, Nusbaum AG, Gil J, Patel SB, Chen J, et al. (2013) Interactions of methicillin resistant *Staphylococcus aureus* USA300 and *Pseudomonas aeruginosa* in polymicrobial wound infection. PLoS One 8(2):e56846.
43. Qin Z, Yang L, Qu D, Molin S, Tolker-Nielsen T (2009) *Pseudomonas aeruginosa* extracellular products inhibit staphylococcal growth, and disrupt established biofilms produced by *Staphylococcus epidermidis*. Microbiology 155(Pt 7):2148–56.
44. Dalton T, Dowd SE, Wolcott RD, Sun Y, Watters C, et al. (2011) An *in vivo* polymicrobial biofilm wound infection model to study interspecies interactions. PLoS One 6(11):e27317.
45. Baba T, Bae T, Schneewind O, Takeuchi F, Hiramatsu K (2008) Genome sequence of *Staphylococcus aureus* strain Newman and comparative analysis of staphylococcal genomes: polymorphism and evolution of two major pathogenicity islands. J Bacteriol 190(1):300–10.
46. Horsburgh MJ, Aish JL, White IJ, Shaw L, Lithgow JK, et al. (2002) SigmaB modulates virulence determinant expression and stress resistance: characterization of a functional rsbU strain derived from *Staphylococcus aureus* 8325-4. J Bacteriol 184(19):5457–67.
47. Liberati NT, Urbach JM, Miyata S, Lee DG, Drenkard E, et al. (2006) An ordered, nonredundant library of *Pseudomonas aeruginosa* strain PA14 transposon insertion mutants. Proc Natl Acad Sci U S A 21;103(8):2833–8.
48. Stover CK, Pham XQ, Erwin AL, Mizoguchi SD, Warrener P, et al. (2000) Complete genome sequence of *Pseudomonas aeruginosa* PAO1, an opportunistic pathogen. Nature 406(6799):959–64.
49. Macho AP, Zumaquero A, Ortiz-Martín I, Beuzón CR (2007) Competitive index in mixed infections: a sensitive and accurate assay for the genetic analysis of *Pseudomonas syringae*-plant interactions. Mol Plant Pathol 8(4):437–50.pone.0089614.

18

Biophysical Characterisation of Calumenin as a Charged F508del-CFTR Folding Modulator

Rashmi Tripathi[1,2]*, Nathalie Benz[1,3], Bridget Culleton[5¤], Pascal Trouvé[1], Claude Férec[1,2,5,6]

1 INSERM UMR1078, Brest, France, **2** Université de Bretagne Occidentale, Faculté de Medecine et des sciences de la santé, Brest, France, **3** Association Gaétan Saleün, Brest, France, **4** Department of Biology, National University of Ireland, Maynooth, Maynooth, Co Kildare, Ireland, **5** Hôpital Morvan, Laboratoire de Génétique Moléculaire et d'Histocompatibilité, Brest, France, **6** Etablissement Français du Sang-Bretagne, Brest, France

Abstract

The cystic fibrosis transmembrane regulator (CFTR) is a cyclic-AMP dependent chloride channel expressed at the apical surface of epithelial cells lining various organs such as the respiratory tract. Defective processing and functioning of this protein caused by mutations in the CFTR gene results in loss of ionic balance, defective mucus clearance, increased proliferation of biofilms and inflammation of human airways observed in cystic fibrosis (CF) patients. The process by which CFTR folds and matures under the influence of various chaperones in the secretory pathway remains incompletely understood. Recently, calumenin, a secretory protein, belonging to the CREC family of low affinity calcium binding proteins has been identified as a putative CFTR chaperone whose biophysical properties and functions remain uncharacterized. We compared hydropathy, instability, charge, unfoldability, disorder and aggregation propensity of calumenin and other CREC family members with CFTR associated chaperones and calcium binding proteins, wild-type and mutant CFTR proteins and intrinsically disordered proteins (IDPs). We observed that calumenin, along with other CREC proteins, was significantly more charged and less folded compared to CFTR associated chaperones. Moreover like IDPs, calumenin and other CREC proteins were found to be less hydrophobic and aggregation prone. Phylogenetic analysis revealed a close link between calumenin and other CREC proteins indicating how evolution might have shaped their similar biophysical properties. Experimentally, calumenin was observed to significantly reduce F508del-CFTR aggregation in a manner similar to AavLEA1, a well-characterized IDP. Fluorescence microscopy based imaging analysis also revealed altered trafficking of calumenin in bronchial cells expressing F508del-CFTR, indicating its direct role in the pathophysiology of CF. In conclusion, calumenin is characterized as a charged protein exhibiting close similarity with IDPs and is hypothesized to regulate F508del-CFTR folding by electrostatic effects. This work provides useful insights for designing optimized synthetic structural correctors of CFTR mutant proteins in the future.

Editor: Vladimir N. Uversky, University of South Florida College of Medicine, United States of America

Funding: The authors thank the Association Gaétan Saleün, the French foundation Vaincre la Mucoviscidose, Conseil Général de Bretagne (http://www.conseil-general.com/conseil-regional/conseil-regional-bretagne.htm) and Inserm (http://www.inserm.fr) for their financial support. BC was funded by an Irish Research Council EMBARK post-graduate fellowship. The funders had no role in study design, data collection and analysis, decision to publish, or preparation of the manuscript.

Competing Interests: The authors have declared that no competing interests exist.

* Email: rashmi_tripathi81@hotmail.com

¤ Current address: Megazyme International Ireland, Bray Business Park, Bray, Co. Wicklow, Ireland

Introduction

Cystic fibrosis (CF) is the most common autosomal recessive genetic disorder affecting one in every 2000–3000 neonates in the Caucasian population, caused by loss of function mutations in the cystic fibrosis transmembrane regulator gene [1]. This gene encodes a chloride channel with two nucleotide binding domains (NBDs) 1 and 2, a regulatory domain (R) and the membrane spanning domains (MSDs) 1 and 2. The interfaces between NBDs and MSDs are formed by the cytoplasmic loops (CLs) 1–4. Individual domains form loosely folded conformations co-translationally, while post-translational processing results in the formation of higher ordered tertiary structures (for review see [2]). Its function as an ATP-gated ion channel following R-domain phosphorylation by cAMP-dependent protein kinase (PKA) is dependent on ATP binding at two composite sites (site 1 consisting of NBD1 Walker motifs and signature motif of NBD2 and site 2 comprising the NBD2 Walker motifs and the NBD1 signature motif [3]).

Nearly 2000 sequence variants of this gene have been identified so far in CF patients (Cystic Fibrosis Mutation Database:). These mutations have been grouped into six different classes and affect protein synthesis, trafficking, regulation, conductance, splicing or transcription and protein stability of the CFTR chloride channel respectively [4]. In the most commonly occurring F508del mutation, which accounts for nearly two thirds of mutated alleles in CF patients, native NBD-CL4 and CL1 interaction is disrupted, compromising CFTR domain assembly and maturation [2,5,6]. As a result, ATP-dependent relay of conformational changes of NBDs and MSDs involved in chloride channel gating are affected along with CFTR biogenesis [7]. Besides regulating chloride transport, CFTR loss of function also hampers other physiological processes regulated by this channel, such as sodium transport, ATP transport, vesicular transport, acidification of intracellular organelles and bicarbonate-chloride exchange [8–10]. The most common clinical symptoms of CF include chronic lung infection, pancreatic insufficiency, male infertility and reduced life expectancy (39 years at an average), with lung disease being the most common cause of morbidity in CF patients [11].

Recently, calumenin, belonging to the CREC (abbreviation for Cab45, reticulocalbin, ERC-45 and calumenin) family of low affinity calcium binding proteins containing multiple EF-hands, has been identified as a putative G551D-CFTR (Gly to Asp mutation at position 551) chaperone [12]. This CFTR mutation, located in the NBD, is known to cause gating defects [13] and is observed in approximately 5% of CF cases, with a severe clinical phenotype [11,12]. Besides associating specifically with G551D-CFTR, calumenin is also predicted to interact with wild-type CFTR [12]. Evidence for this interaction has been provided using co-immunoprecipitation and surface plasmon resonance, which we believe is insufficient to conclude that the interaction between calumenin and CFTR is 'direct' in the cellular environment. Nevertheless, we assume that calumenin lies in close proximity to CFTR, or at least exists in the same protein complex and hypothesize that it might have an effect on CFTR folding. Besides calumenin, RCN1 and RCN2 are the other two CREC proteins that have been identified as interacting partners of wild-type and F508del-CFTR, with RCN1 being enriched in the wild-type CFTR associated proteome and RCN2 being enriched in both the wild-type and F508del-CFTR associated proteomes [14].

Currently, the biophysical properties and functions of calumenin as a chaperone remain unknown. The aim of our study was to investigate the biophysical features of the calumenin amino acid sequence, test its effects on the folding dynamics of F508del-CFTR protein in the presence of calcium, MgATP and ethylenediaminetetraacetic acid (EDTA) and analyze its intra-cellular distribution in human CFBE41o- bronchial cells expressing wild-type or F508del-CFTR. We analyzed various parameters (such as hydropathy, instability, charge, unfoldability, state of disorder and aggregation propensity) of calumenin, along with other CREC family members, CFTR associated chaperones (such as HSC70, HSP40, AHA1 etc.), calcium binding proteins (such as calgranulin, PSOR1, PDCD6), wild-type and mutant CFTR sequences (F508del-CFTR, G551D-CFTR) and five previously described intrinsically disordered proteins (IDPs) [15–17]. IDPs were included as a control group in our analysis, since they are characterized by a high state of disorder in their polypeptide sequences [15,18]. This property, along with protein flexibility, has also been observed in some chaperones such as HSP70 and is believed to aid in their molecular recognition properties [19,20].

We report that calumenin and other CREC family members are significantly more charged and less folded compared to conventional CFTR associated chaperones. In contrast to wild-type and mutant CFTR proteins, calumenin along with other CREC proteins, showed significantly less hydropathy and aggregation propensity. Phylogenetic analysis revealed common ancestry of CREC proteins and similarity with both chaperones and calcium binding proteins. In order to investigate the underlying molecular mechanism of calumenin action, *in vitro* protein-folding experiments were performed which demonstrated a reduction in F508del-CFTR aggregation by calumenin in the presence of calcium, MgATP and EDTA. Similar anti-aggregation properties were observed for AavLEA1, a well-characterized IDP described previously in literature [17,21]. Imaging analysis revealed that in CFBE41o- cells expressing wild-type CFTR, calumenin demonstrated extensive localization in the endoplasmic reticulum (ER) and Golgi compartments. These results are consistent with its role as a secretory protein [22]. Unlike the CFTR [23], it was largely excluded from EEA1 containing endocytic vesicles suggesting that its association with CFTR might be restricted to specific intracellular compartments and that the two proteins might undergo dissociation during its secretion. Moreover, in a large proportion of cells expressing F508del-CFTR, it was translocated to the cytoplasm and the nucleus and exhibited increased retention in the endocytic pathway, indicating altered physiology of mutant cells. Overall, our results draw a correlation between the computationally predicted physicochemical similarity of calumenin with disordered proteins and their experimentally determined *in vitro* anti-aggregation activity. We also discuss the implications of these findings in designing optimized synthetic correctors of mutant CFTR proteins in the future.

Materials and Methods

Bioinformatics

Calumenin, along with other CFTR interacting proteins with chaperone functions, calcium binding properties or those belonging to the CREC family were selected from the dataset published by Wang et al. in 2006 [14]. We decided to incorporate two other CREC proteins RCN3 and SDF4 in the dataset for comparison as well. Five proteins previously described as being intrinsically disordered [15–17] along with wild-type CFTR and its mutant variants F508del-CFTR, G551DCFTR were also included. Measurements for various biophysical parameters such as hydropathy, given by GRAVY scores (Grand average of hydropathy), instability, unfoldability, charge, disorder (IUPRED scores) and aggregation propensity were performed for all the proteins using the ProtParam tool (http://web.expasy.org/protparam/) [24], FoldIndex (http://bip.weizmann.ac.uk.il/fldbin/findex) [25], IUPRED server (http://iupred.enzim.hu) [26,27] and Aggrescan server (http://bioinf.uab.es/aggrescan/) [28]. IUPRED and aggregation scores were normalized for protein length. Table S1 shows the raw scores. Phylogenetic tree construction was performed after multiple sequence alignment using CLUSTAL omega [29], version 1.2.0, with five iterations (for guide tree construction and HMM profiling). Aligned sequences were used for tree construction in the PHYLIP format using CLUSTALW2 program with UPGMA clustering method, distance correction and percent identity matrix parameter being true [30].

Statistical analysis

All statistical analysis was performed using R 3.0.1 statistical package. Data normality was assessed using the Shapiro-Wilk test and depending upon whether data was observed to be normal or not, ANOVA or Kruskal-Wallis test was performed to estimate whether the mean difference observed between different protein classes was significant enough. Post-hoc analysis was carried out using either the Tukey's test or Mann-Whitney test with Bonferroni correction. Principal component analysis and hierarchial clustering were performed to observe the correlations between different biophysical parameters and the distribution of proteins across the first two components that describe the maximum variation in the data. Principal component analysis (PCA) applies orthogonal transformation to convert a set of observations of possibly correlated variables into a set of values of uncorrelated variables called principal components. The number of principal components is less than or equal to the number of original variables. This transformation is defined in such a way that the first principal component has the largest possible variance and each succeeding component in turn has the highest variance possible under the constraint that it is orthogonal to (i.e., uncorrelated with) the preceding components. Hierarchial clustering further highlights the variation observed between various proteins on the PCA map, where the sum of the within-cluster inertia are calculated for each partition. The suggested partition is the one with the higher relative loss of inertia (i(clustersn+1)/ i(cluster n)). The absolute loss of inertia (defined as the squared distance between clusters) (i(cluster n)-i(cluster n+1)) is plotted with the tree.

Cloning of AavLEA1

The *AavLEA1* gene was cloned as described in Goyal *et al.* [31] with minor modifications at the NUI Maynooth, Ireland. Briefly, the gene was amplified from cDNA (prepared using SuperScript III RT (Invitrogen)) according to Goyal *et al.* and cloned into the pET15b vector (Novagen) on the *NdeI/BamHI* sites coding for AavLEA1 protein and a N-terminal His6 tag. The vector was then transformed into BL21 (DE3) cells. The plasmid has been deposited in Addgene plasmid reference database (reference number: 53093).

F508del-CFTR anti-aggregation assay

Pure recombinant human calumenin was obtained from Prospec (Israel) and purified full length F508del-CFTR [32] was a generous gift from Prof. Robert Ford (University of Manchester, UK). AavLEA1 was purified using Ni-NTA Fast Start kit (Qiagen) from BL21 (DE3) *E.coli* cells containing pET15b-AavLEA1 according to the manufacturer's instructions and dialyzed extensively into water. Proteins were concentrated using Vivaspin6 protein concentrators, 3 kDa (Sartorius Stedim Biotech). Protein concentrations were determined by plotting a standard curve using different concentrations of bovine serum albumin and Folin's reagent, by measuring absorbance at 660 nm of reaction mixtures after incubation at 37°C for 20 minutes in the dark. F508del-CFTR protein aggregation assay to monitor formation of off-pathway species were initiated by rapid dilution of F508del-CFTR in 6 M GuHCl to a final concentration of 1 μM into pre-warmed (37°C) folding mix (Buffer R: 100 mM Tris-HCl, pH 7.4, 0.385 M L-arginine-HCl, 2 mM EDTA, 10 mM dithiothreitol and 25 mM GuHCl). In experiments containing Calumenin or AavLEA1, a final concentration of 0.5 μM of protein in Buffer C (20 mM imidazole, pH 7.0, 2 mM magnesium acetate, 10 mM $(NH_4)_2SO_4$, 25 mM KCl, 1 mM dithiothreitol) was added. BSA was used as a negative control at 0.5 μM concentration. MgATP was used at a final concentration of 50 μM. $CaCl_2$ was used at 0.75 mM and 2 mM final concentration. EDTA was used at a final concentration of 5 mM. Total reaction volume used was 100 μl. Aggregation was followed over time at 37°C by turbidity measured at 405 nm in a Biophotometer (eppendorf). Multiple measurements were made to ensure consistency in readings (three consecutive identical readings were considered reliable).

Immunofluorescence

CFBE41o- wild-type or F508del airway epithelial lines [33,34] were maintained in Eagle's minimum essential medium (Lonza) with 10% FBS (PAA), 1X L-glutamine and 0.3 mg/ml hygromycin (Invitrogen) at 37°C and 5% CO_2. Before imaging, cells were seeded on 20 mm diameter cover slips and incubated at 37°C until a confluence of 50-60% was obtained. Fixation was carried out in 4% paraformaldehyde for 10 minutes. After fixation and three 5 minutes washes with PBS-T (1X Phosphate buffered saline with 0.1% Tween), cells were permeabilised with 0.5% Triton X-100 in PBS for 4 minutes. After 5-minutes washes with PBS-T, non-specific binding was prevented by blocking with 2% BSA in 1X PBS, for 30 minutes at room temperature. Primary antibody against calumenin (H40, Santa Cruz) was applied for 2 hours at room temperature. After three 5 minutes washes with PBS-T, cells were incubated with Alexa fluor 488 goat anti-rabbit IgG (Molecular probes) secondary antibody diluted 1:1000 in 2% BSA for 1 hour 30 minutes. After three 5-minute washes with PBS-T, second labeling against PDI (Protein Disulphide Isomerase, Invitrogen), Golgi marker (abcam ab27043) or EEA1 (BD Biosciences, 610457) was performed using antibody at 1:1000 concentration in 2% BSA in 1X PBS for 12 hours at 4°C. After three 5-minute washes with PBS-T, cells were incubated with anti-mouse Texas Red (Molecular probes) secondary antibody (1:1000 dilution in 2% BSA). For CFTR staining, cells were grown on 18 mm coverslips, fixed with 3% paraformaldehyde in TBS for 20 min at room temperature, then rinsed in TBS, permeabilized with 0.10% Triton X-100 in TBS for 10 min, and rinsed again with TBS. The samples were then stained as follows: after fixation, nonspecific sites were blocked with TBS containing 1% goat serum for 60 min at room temperature, then the cells were stained with primary antibody [anti-CFTR antibody H-182 (Santa-Cruz Biotechnology), 1:100] for 90 min at room temperature and rinsed four times in TBS containing 1% goat serum. Next, samples were incubated with the goat anti-rabbit secondary antibody conjugated to Alexa Fluor 488 (1:800) for 60 min at room temperature. After five washes with 1% goat serum, second labelling against EEA1 was performed using antibody at 1:1000 concentration in 1% goat serum for 90 min at room temperature. The cells were then rinsed four times with 1% goat serum and incubated with the goat anti-mouse secondary antibody conjugated to Cy3 (1:800) for 60 min at room temperature. After five final washes, samples were mounted in VectaShield + DAPI (VECTOR Laboratories Inc., Burlingame, CA), dried, and viewed with AxioStar plus microscope (100X oil, Carl Zeiss GmbH, Jena, Germany). Negative controls were also performed by omitting the primary antibodies. Visualization of all images was performed using Axio Vision Rel. 4.8 software. Pearson's correlation coefficient for colocalisation was estimated using JACoP package on ImageJ [35].

Results

Calumenin and other CREC family proteins are significantly more charged and less folded compared to other CFTR associated chaperones

In order to investigate the specific biophysical properties of calumenin as a putative CFTR chaperone, we decided to compare various biophysical parameters such as protein hydropathy (GRAVY), unfoldability, aggregation propensity, charge, instability and disorder of calumenin and other CREC family members with previously described CFTR associated chaperones and calcium binding proteins (See Methods and Table S1). CFTR variants (wild type, F508del, G551D) and intrinsically disordered proteins (IDPs) were also used in this analysis due to their extremely high and low hydropathy values respectively. The high hydrophobicity of CFTR and its mutant sequences is due to the presence of transmembrane segments in their amino acid sequences [36]. IDPs have also been previously characterized by high charge and unfoldedness in their polypeptide sequences [18,37].

As can be observed, a majority of proteins in our dataset demonstrate a GRAVY (grand average hydropathy) score below zero. This score is a useful predictor of protein hydropathy or hydrophobicity, where positive scores indicate that proteins are highly hydrophobic and negative scores reflect protein hydrophilicity. CFTR proteins, being bona fide membrane proteins, demonstrate the highest mean GRAVY scores, while IDPs demonstrate the lowest mean GRAVY scores. An overall significant difference was detected between all the protein classes (ANOVA, $F(4,24) = 8.82$,p-value<0.001). However, Tukey's post-hoc analysis revealed that CREC proteins, including calumenin, showed significantly lower GRAVY scores compared to CFTR proteins (p-value<0.01), while no significant difference was observed between CREC proteins and other protein classes. Similar analysis was performed for other parameters including unfoldability, aggregation, instability, charge and disorder (IUPRED). Figure 1 depicts the box-plots showing the overall distribution of data belonging to different protein classes for all the biophysical parameters analysed. Significant differences in mean scores were detected for unfoldability (ANOVA, $F(4,24) = 9.47$, p-value<0.001), aggregation propensity (ANOVA, $F(4,24) = 16.31$,$p<0.001$), charge (KW test, Chi-squared value $= 13.63$, $d.f = 4.0$, p-value<0.01) and disorder (IUPRED) (KW test, Chi-squared value $= 17.32$, $d.f = 4.0$, p-value<0.01). As can be observed, CREC proteins, including calumenin, were less folded compared to CFTR proteins and chaperones (Tukey's post-hoc test, p-values<0.001 and <0.01 respectively). They were also less aggregation prone compared to CFTR proteins (Tukey's post-hoc test, p-value<0.001). In this respect, they were found to be similar to IDPs, which also showed significantly less aggregation propensity compared to CFTR proteins (Tukey's post-hoc test, p-value <0.001). IDPs were also observed to be significantly more disordered compared to chaperones (Mann-Whitney test with Bonferonni correction, p-value<0.05). Interestingly, we observed that calumenin, along with other CREC proteins possessed a significantly greater amount of charge compared to the chaperone group (Mann-Whitney test with Bonferonni correction, p-value$<$ 0.05). No significant difference was observed between different protein groups with respect to their instability values.

All the pair-wise correlation plots are shown in Figure 2. Table 1 (shown in Figure 2) depicts significant pair-wise correlation values observed in our dataset between different biophysical parameters. As can be observed GRAVY scores show a high degree of correlation with protein unfoldability (Adjusted R-squared value: 0.95, p-value<0.001) and aggregation propensity (Adjusted R-squared value:0.93, p-value<0.001). Unfoldability and disorder (IUPRED) were found to be moderately correlated with aggregation propensity (Adjusted R-squared values: 0.85,0.74 respectively, p-values<0.001 and <0.001 respectively). The only variable observed to be weakly correlated with charge was protein unfoldability (Adjusted R-squared value: 0.48, p-value<0.001).

In order to discern the biophysical landscape of different classes of proteins analysed, multivariate principal component analysis and hierarchial clustering were carried out. As observed in Figure 3A, the first two principal components are represented on the x and y axes respectively and cover 67.98% and 17.15% of the total variance observed in our dataset. The variables factor map (Figure 3B) gives directionality to different biophysical parameters as observed on the PCA plot. As can be observed calumenin lies in the region corresponding to high charge, along with other CREC family members RCN1, RCN2, RCN3 and SDF4. Interestingly, other calcium associated proteins such as calnexin and CALGRANB also cluster in this region. CFTR variants are observed in the region corresponding to high GRAVY, unfoldability and aggregation propensity. Strikingly, we observe a large variation in the physicochemical characteristics of CFTR associated chaperones. Most of the disordered proteins in our dataset lie in the region corresponding to high disorder, except for ArLEA1A, which was observed to cluster with other CFTR associated chaperones on the PCA plot.

Hierarchial clustering (Figure 4) further revealed the presence of four related clusters obtained from the factor map, with all the CREC proteins partitioned in a single cluster with calnexin. Calumenin is observed to be most similar to RCN1 protein. Disordered proteins and CFTR variants also cluster separately. Interestingly, we observed considerable similarity between chaperones HSP90A and HSP40 and calcium binding proteins CALGRANB and PSOR1 respectively. Overall, our combined PCA and hierarchial clustering results demonstrate similarity in the biophysical properties of calumenin and other CREC proteins which distinguishes them from other CFTR associated chaperones, disordered proteins and CFTR variants.

Phylogenetic analysis of CREC proteins reveals common ancestry and similarity with chaperones and calcium binding proteins

In order to establish a relationship between the biophysical properties of CREC proteins, chaperones, calcium binding proteins, IDPs and CFTR variants and their evolutionary relatedness, we aligned their sequences using Clustal omega [29] and constructed a phylogenetic tree using UPGMA clustering method [30,38]. Figure 5 shows that the CREC proteins share common ancestry and show close relatedness with other chaperones and calcium binding proteins such as HSP90A, Calpastatin and CALGRANB. Calumenin protein is observed to lie closest to RCN1 and RCN3. These results demonstrate correlation between the biophysical properties of calumenin and its phylogeny. Common evolutionary origins are also observed for heat shock family of chaperones (HSPA5, HSPA1L, HSC70 and HSP70), CFTR variants, CCT3/CCT4 and late embryogenesis abundant proteins ArLEA1A/AavLEA1. Interestingly, we observed a close relationship between IDPs (LEA proteins AavLEA1 and ArLEA1A, RYBP, Calpastatin, 4EBP1) and chaperone proteins. These results demonstrate similarity between chaperones and IDP sequences and corroborate previous findings that have shown that chaperones are also characterised by a state of disorder in their protein sequences, which helps in the molecular recognition of their targets [39].

Calumenin and AavLEA1 reduce F508del-CFTR aggregation

In order to elucidate the specific molecular function of calumenin, an *in vitro* F508del-CFTR folding assay was devised. A similar CFTR-NBD domain folding assay based on the defective folding kinetics of NBD domain has previously shown the anti-aggregation properties of HSC70 as a CFTR chaperone [40]. The principle on which this assay is based is the following. Proteins are initially denatured and refolded in a test tube at 37°C by consecutive addition of GuHCl, a denaturing agent, and a renaturation buffer. In the absence of chaperones, regions of a particular polypeptide sequence containing hydrophobic amino acids like tryptophan undergo 'hydrophobic collapse' resulting in the formation of large sized aggregates, which in turn can be monitored by an increase in turbidity at ~400 nm. Addition of folding factors like chaperones to the reaction mix, can redirect the folding route of a protein by preventing "hydrophobic collapse" and formation of large aggregates.

We initially performed a test experiment to monitor the kinetics of aggregate formation of purified F508del-CFTR and observed

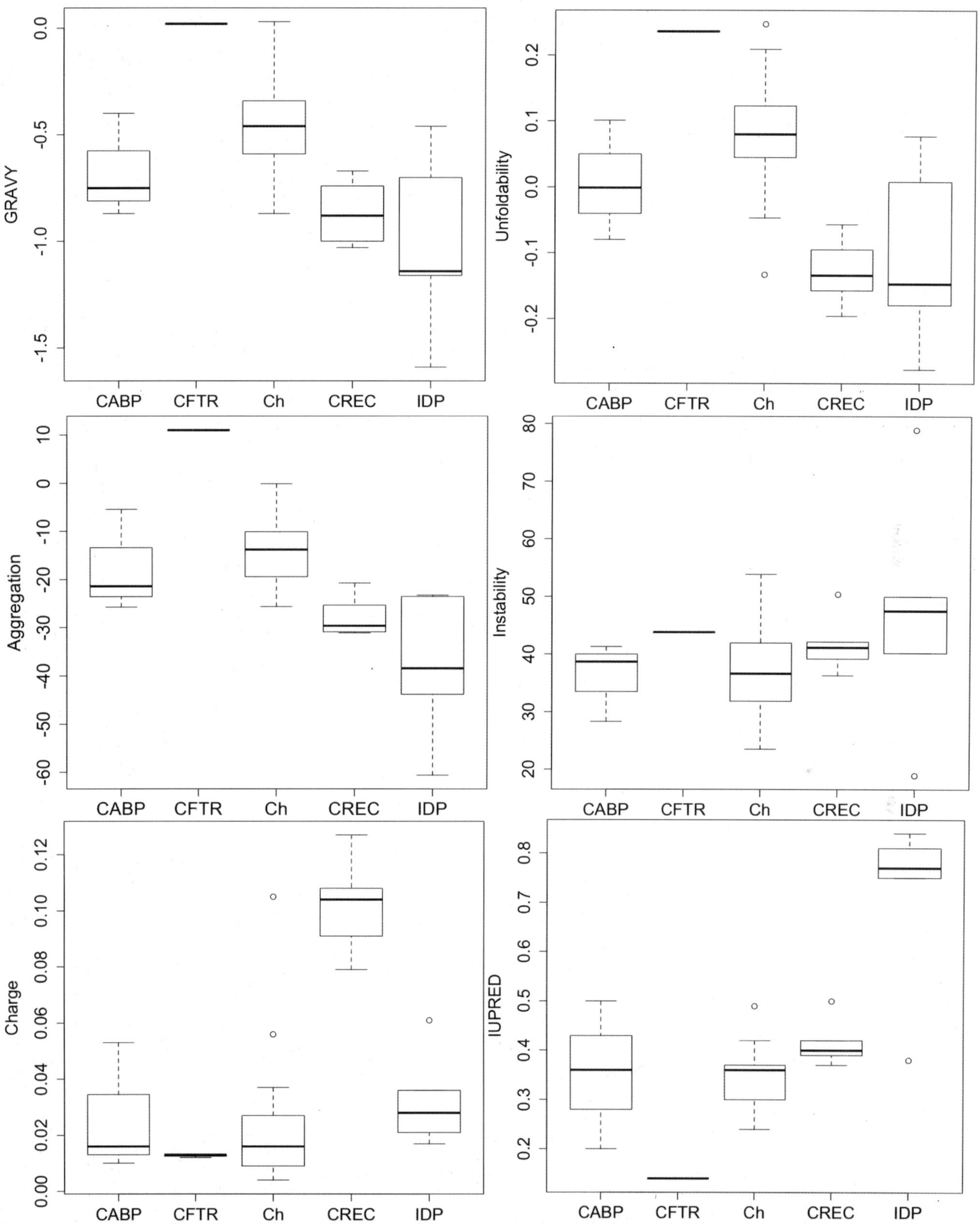

Figure 1. Box-plots showing GRAVY, Unfoldability, Aggregation, Instability, Charge and IUPRED (disorder) measurements. Protein groups used in this analysis are the following: Calcium binding proteins (CABP), CFTR wild-type and mutant (F508del and G551DCFTR) proteins (CFTR), chaperones (Ch), CREC proteins (CREC) and intrinsically disordered proteins (IDP). CREC proteins demonstrated significantly lower hydropathy (GRAVY) scores compared to CFTR proteins (p-value<0.01). These proteins also showed lesser unfoldability compared to CFTR proteins (p-value<0.001) and chaperones (p-value<0.01). In terms of aggregation, CREC proteins posses significantly less proportion of aggregation prone residues in their sequences compared to calcium binding proteins and CFTR proteins (p-values<0.01 and <0.001 respectively). No significant difference

between groups was observed for Instability scores. CREC proteins showed a significantly greater amount of charge compared to chaperones (p-value<0.05). IDPs were also significantly more disordered compared to chaperones (p-value<0.05).

slower aggregation kinetics during the first ten minutes of addition of GuHCl and renaturation buffer at 37°C, followed by an exponential increase in aggregation between 15–20 minutes and saturation between 20–30 minutes. In a control sample without any protein, no exponential increase in aggregation was noted. Following, the initial establishment of this assay, the effect of

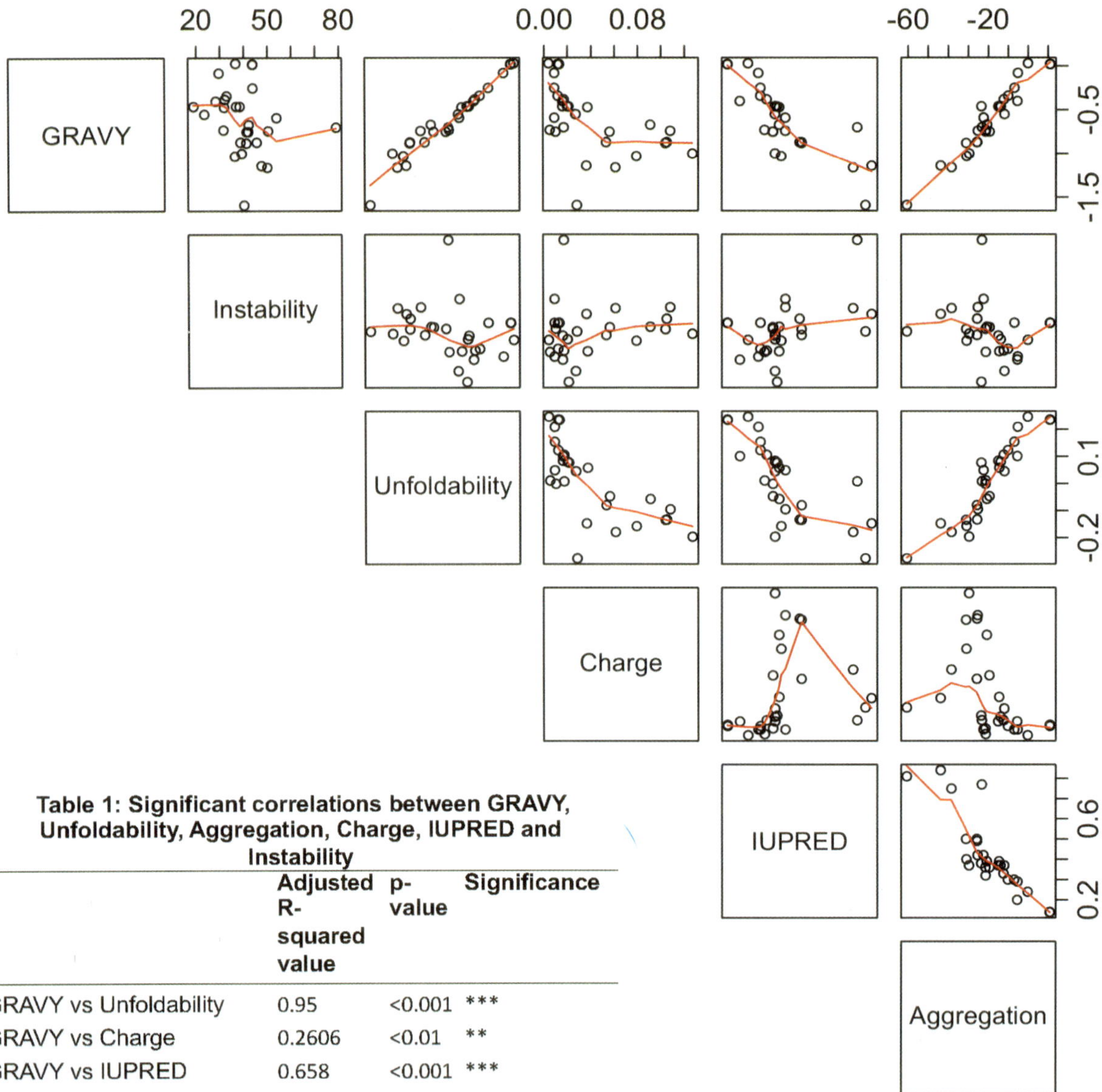

Table 1: Significant correlations between GRAVY, Unfoldability, Aggregation, Charge, IUPRED and Instability

	Adjusted R-squared value	p-value	Significance
GRAVY vs Unfoldability	0.95	<0.001	***
GRAVY vs Charge	0.2606	<0.01	**
GRAVY vs IUPRED	0.658	<0.001	***
GRAVY vs Aggregation	0.926	<0.001	***
Instability vs Unfoldability	0.29	<0.01	**
Instability vs IUPRED	0.1788	<0.05	*
Unfoldability vs Charge	0.4766	<0.001	***
Unfoldability vs IUPRED	0.5563	<0.001	***
Unfoldability vs Aggregation	0.8528	<0.001	***
Charge vs Aggregation	0.1788	<0.05	*
IUPRED vs Aggregation	0.7451	<0.001	***

Figure 2. Correlation plots for GRAVY, Unfoldability, Aggregation, Instability, Charge and IUPRED (disorder). In each plot, the y-axis is represented by the score highlighted in each row of the matrix, while it's corresponding x-axis is depicted by parameters described in the rows above or below it. Table 1 shows the pair-wise correlation values for all the parameters analyzed.

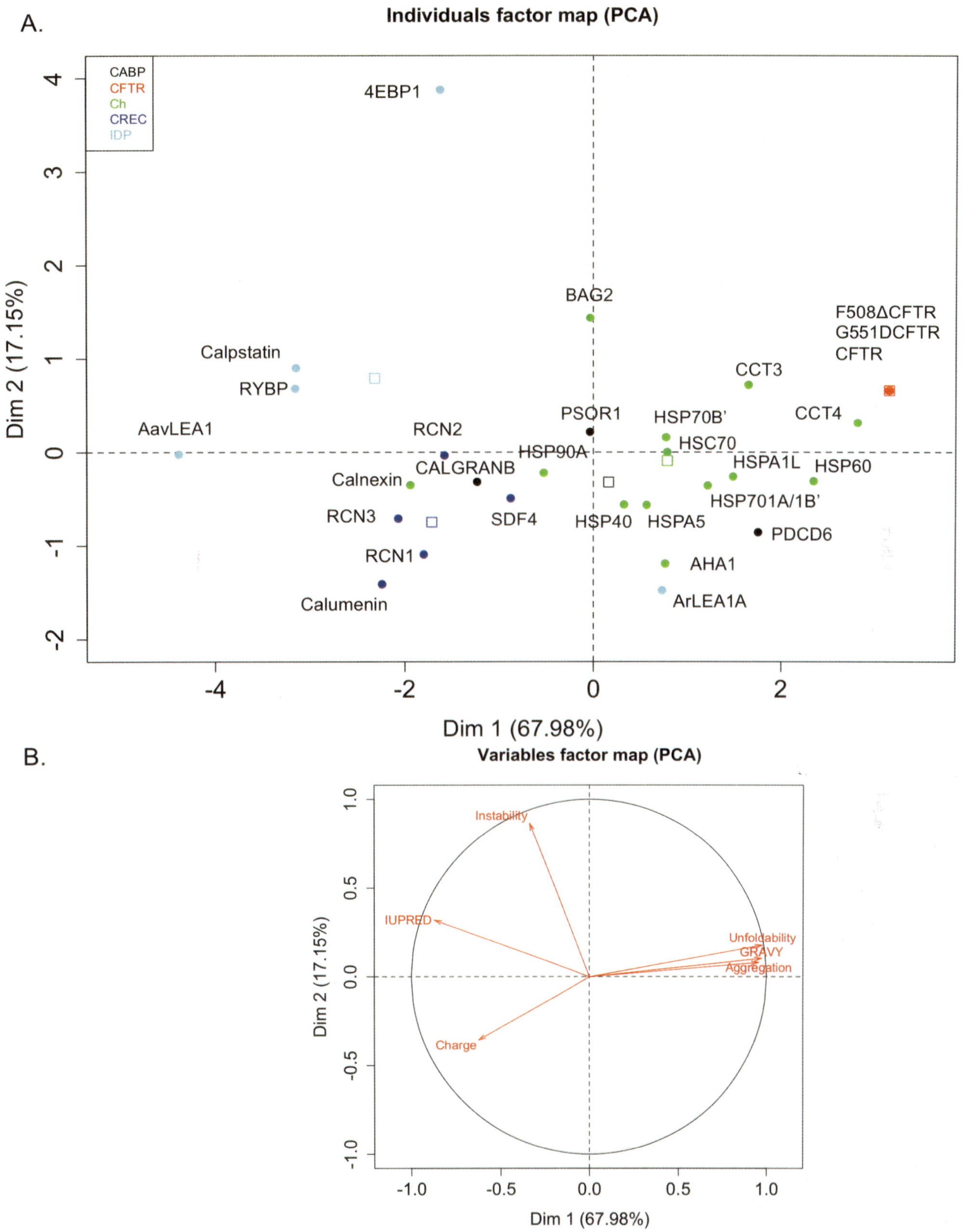

Figure 3. Principal component analysis draws correlations between different biophysical parameters for different protein categories. Multivariate data (Table S1) was scaled and transformed into different components in such a way that the first principal component has the largest possible variance and each succeeding component in turn has the highest variance possible under the constraint that is orthogonal to it (i.e., uncorrelated with) the preceding components. **A.** The first two principal components are represented on the x and y axes respectively and cover 67.98% and 17.15% of the total variance observed in our dataset. **B.** The variables factor map gives directionality to different biophysical parameters

as observed on the PCA plot. Each filled circle represents a unique protein. The color legend is described on the top left corner (CABP (black): Calcium binding proteins, CFTR (red): CFTR variants, Ch (green): Chaperones, CREC (blue): CREC proteins, IDP (cyan): intrinsically disordered proteins). As can be observed calumenin lies in the region corresponding to high charge, along with other CREC family members RCN1, RCN2, RCN3 and SDF4. Unfilled open boxes in various colours depict positions of different protein classes on the PCA map.

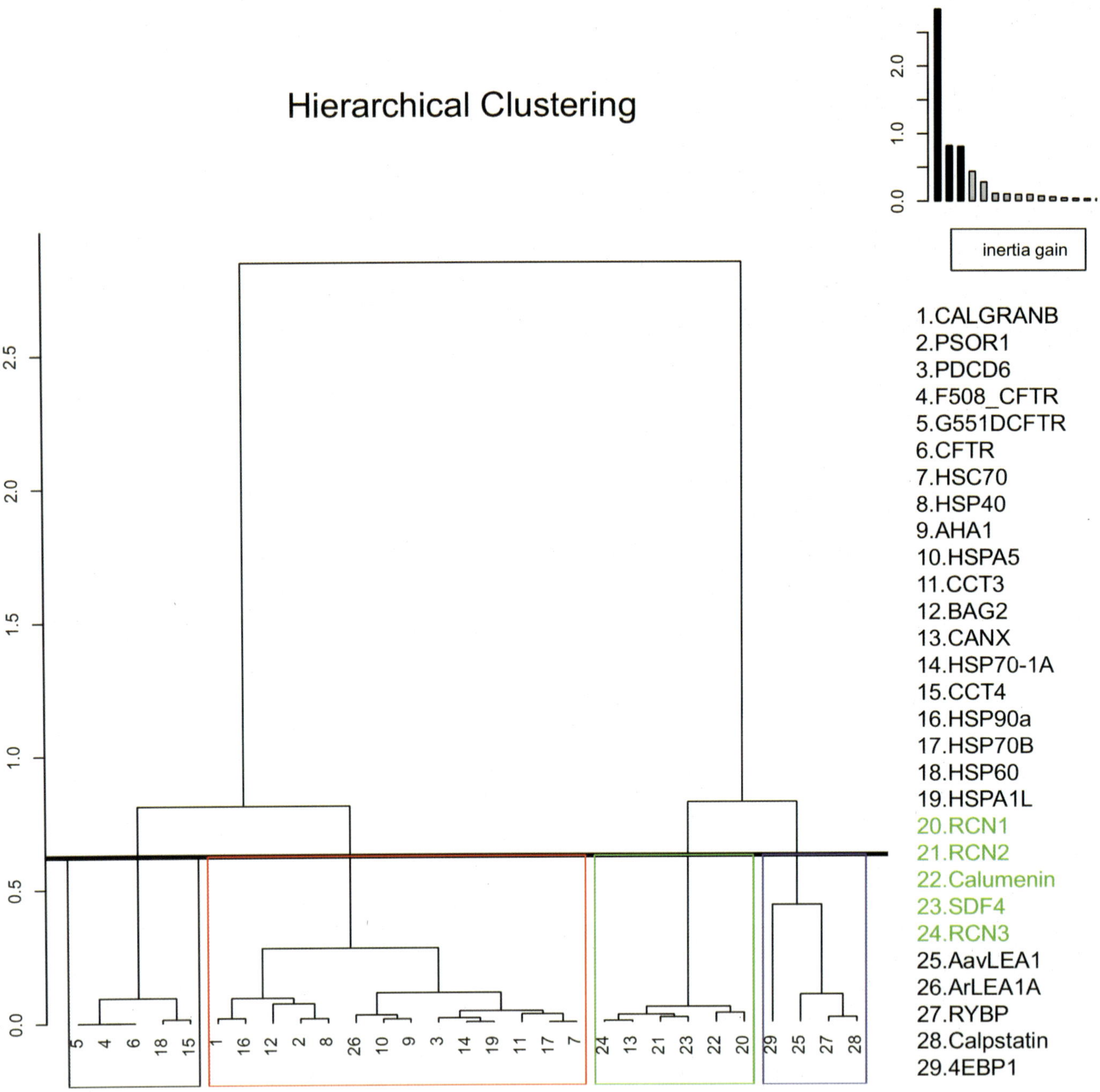

Figure 4. Hierarchial clustering of proteins based on their biophysical features. Sequential clustering was performed by computing the Euclidean distance matrix and by following the Ward's criterion after data transformation during PCA. A dendrogram was drawn, where each vertical line represents a cluster and a horizontal line connecting between any two vertical lines represents the merger of clusters, where its height is related to the dissimilarity measure between the merged clusters. Inertia is defined as multidimensional variance and can be decomposed as variance observed "between" and "within" different clusters, where Ward criterion aims to minimize the increase or "gain" of "within inertia". As can be observed on the plot on the top right hand corner, a step-wise decrease in inertia was performed until no further decrease was observed for different clusters. CREC proteins are observed in a single cluster (green) along with calnexin, chaperones and calcium binding proteins are observed to be inter-related in a separate cluster (red), while CFTR proteins (black) and disordered proteins cluster separately (blue). CREC proteins are shown in green text.

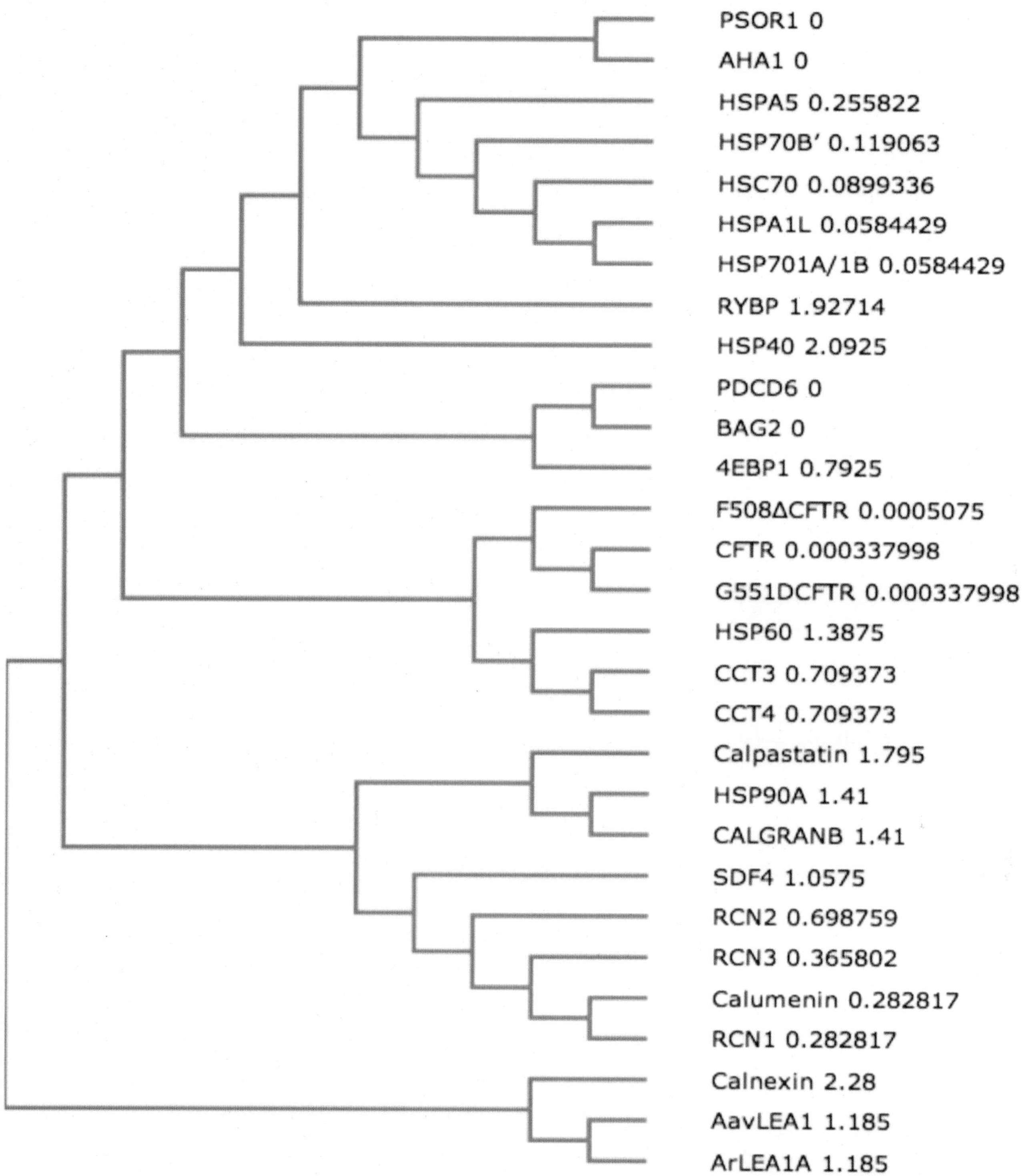

Figure 5. Phylogenetic tree. A cladogram was constructed after multiple sequence alignment of all the protein sequences using Clustal omega. Common evolutionary ancestry is observed for CREC proteins. The evolutionary distance is depicted next to each branch, where 0 indicates collapsing of the two branches into a single node.

adding calumenin in a 2:1 stochiometric ratio (F508del-CFTR: Calumenin) was investigated. As can be observed (Figure 6), calumenin alone was able to reduce F508del aggregation by ~33%.

Since calumenin is a known calcium binding protein, addition of 2 mM calcium to the reaction mixture was observed to reduce aggregation by ~83%. In contrast, low calcium (0.75 mM), was observed to promote aggregation by ~44%. Further addition of MgATP, reduced F508del-CFTR aggregation by ~75% (for 0.75 mM calcium) and ~86% (for 2 mM calcium). The most dramatic anti-aggregation effect (~92% reduction) was observed upon addition of EDTA to the F508del-CFTR and calumenin reaction mixture.

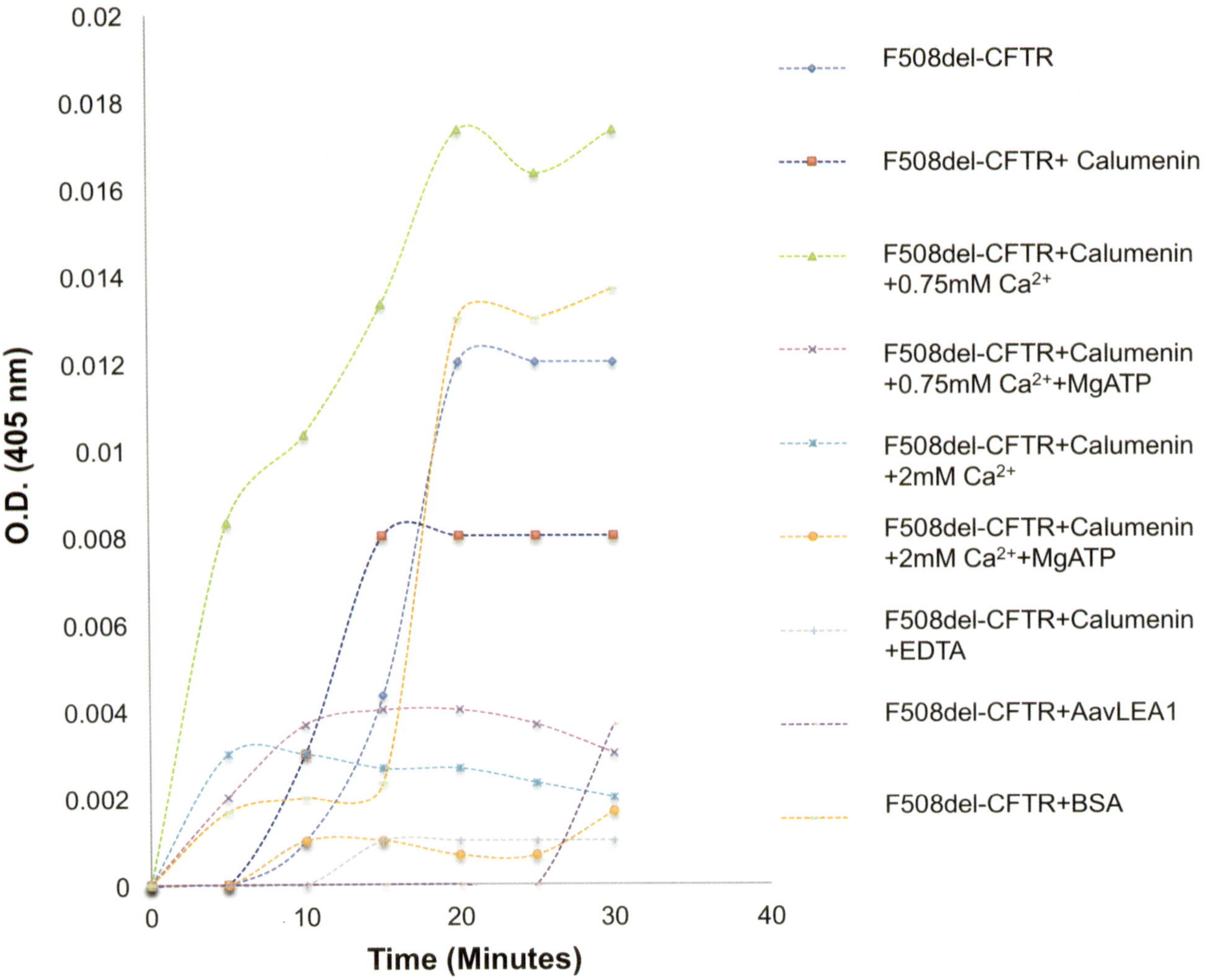

Figure 6. F508del-CFTR folding assay. Proteins were denatured and renatured in a test tube at 37°C resulting in the formation of large sized aggregates whose formation was monitored by an increase in turbidity at 405 nm. F508del-CFTR aggregation was observed to follow a typical 'S-curve'. Addition of calumenin to the reaction mixture was observed to reduce F508del aggregation by ~33%. 2 mM calcium further reduced aggregation substantially by ~83%. In contrast, 0.75 mM calcium was observed to promote aggregation (by ~44%). Further addition of MgATP, reduced F508del-CFTR aggregation by ~75% (for 0.75 mM calcium) and ~86% (for 2 mM calcium). Calumenin with EDTA had the maximum effect (~92% reduction) in reducing aggregation. AavLEA1, and IDP, prevented F508del-CFTR aggregation at early time points. Bovine serum albumin (BSA) was used as a negative control in our reactions.

Recently, a family of intrinsically disordered proteins called late embryogenesis abundant (LEA) proteins have been shown to broadly reduce the aggregation of proteins found in anhydrobiotic organisms and of proteins containing polyglutamine repeats [21]. We questioned whether addition of AavLEA1, an LEA protein found in the anhydrobiotic nematode *Aphenlenchus avenae* [41] could also inhibit formation of F508del-CFTR aggregates. As can be observed in Figure 6, addition of AavLEA1 to the folding mix also reduced F508del-CFTR aggregation by ~69%. These results support previous observations which have described the importance of disorder in chaperone sequences that might play a role in their protein-folding functions.

Calumenin trafficking is altered in bronchial cells expressing F508del-CFTR

In order to understand the physiological significance of the CFTR-calumenin interaction, we performed intra-cellular localization analysis of calumenin in immortalized human bronchial CFBE41o- epithelial cell line homozygous for F508del mutation or expressing wild-type CFTR. Wild-type CFTR is known to traffic through the ER and the Golgi, to reach the plasma membrane, where its concentration is maintained at a steady state by endocytic recycling through EEA1 containing vesicles, while the F508del mutation is known to increase CFTR retention in the ER and decrease its stability at the membrane by increasing its turnover through EEA1 vesicles [23,42,43].

On the other hand, calumenin and its fifteen protein isoforms of varying lengths, demonstrate complex intra-cellular localization patterns in the secretory pathway, cytoplasm and the nucleus [22,44]. It is currently not known, whether calumenin, like CFTR, might recycle through EEA1 containing endocytic vesicles as well. Previous research has shown calumenin to localize in the ER in both wild-type and G551DCFTR expressing cells using an antibody towards a single epitope [12], which we now know is present in four out of the fifteen calumenin isoforms- b,3,5 and 13 (See multiple sequence alignment of isoforms in the File S1).

Subtle sequence variations of this epitope sequence are also detected in isoforms such as a/c,4,6,7,8,9,10,11,14 and 15 hinting towards significant cross reactivity of this antibody for fourteen out of the fifteen isoforms. However, given the limited availability of antibodies for detection of different isoforms and the technical difficulty involved in raising isoform specific antibodies, we decided to investigate the localization pattern of calumenin and its isoforms in both CFBE41o- wild-type and F508del cells using the antibody currently available to us.

Figure 7 shows calumenin and PDI (ER marker)/Golgi/EEA1(endocytic vesicle marker) staining in CFBE41o- wild type or F508del cells. Individual nuclei were stained using DAPI. CFBE41o- cells were also analyzed for CFTR accumulation in EEA1 vesicles. Table S2 depicts the Pearson's correlation coefficient values between the green and red channels for different intra-cellular markers. In CFBE41o- cells expressing wild-type CFTR, a majority of cells showed vesicular distribution of calumenin (~75%) indicating its presence in the ER and Golgi compartments, although a few cells also demonstrated its presence in the cytoplasm and nucleus. The Pearson's correlation values observed for calumenin and ER/Golgi markers (Figured 7A and B) were high (0.857 and 0.581 respectively). In contrast, the presence of calumenin in EEA1 vesicles was low (Figure 7C) (Pearson's correlation coefficient: 0.083). CFTR protein showed greater accumulation in EEA1 containing vesicles, compared to calumenin (Figure 7D) (Pearson's correlation coefficient: 0.287). These results are consistent with previous findings, which have also shown the localization of CFTR in EEA1 vesicles [24].

In CFBE cells homozygous for the F508del-CFTR mutation, a majority of cells (~90%) exhibited displacement of calumenin from the secretory pathway to the cytoplasm and the nucleus (Figures 8A–D). This correlated with a marked reduction in the Pearson's correlation coefficient value for calumenin in the Golgi vesicles (0.328), while there was little change observed for its localization in the ER (0.805) (Figures 8A and B), indicating defective trafficking of calumenin through the secretory pathway. Additionally, we also observed enhanced accumulation of both calumenin and CFTR in EEA1 containing endocytic vesicles (Pearson's correlation coefficients: 0.195 and 0.503 respectively) (Figures 8C and D). Overall, our imaging data suggests abnormal trafficking of calumenin isoforms in bronchial cells expressing F508del-CFTR, compared to cells expressing wild-type CFTR. The implications of these findings are further discussed below.

Discussion

Calumenin is a calcium binding CREC protein with multiple EF-hands that undergoes secretion [22] and has recently been found to be associated with G551DCFTR protein [12]. It has been hypothesized to function as a putative CFTR chaperone, however so far its biophysical properties have remained uncharacterized. In this study we have drawn comparisons between calumenin, including other CREC proteins, and proteins previously known to act as CFTR associated chaperones and calcium binding proteins. The composition of different protein sequences in our dataset has been deduced using various parameters such as hydropathy (GRAVY), unfoldability, aggregation propensity, instability, charge and disorder by applying bioinformatics based prediction tools such as ProtParam [24], FoldIndex [25], IUPRED [26,27] and Aggrescan [28]. These tools have proved valuable in characterizing the functions of numerous novel proteins in the past [45–48].

In our data, we observed high correlation between GRAVY, unfoldability and aggregation scores, however only a moderate correlation was noticed between unfoldability and disorder. Similar correlations between these parameters have been observed in previous studies [45,46,49]. Intrinsically disordered proteins (IDPs) [15] were used as a control group in our analysis, since it has been previously proposed that some chaperones are also characterized by a state of disorder [19] and unfoldedness [50], which might help in their molecular recognition properties. For example, Reichmann *et al.* have recently described the unfolded nature of Hsp33 chaperone, an oxidative stress sensor whose unfoldability allows it to stabilize other partially folded client proteins during stressed conditions [50]. It was hypothesized that this comparison might help elucidate whether calumenin and CREC proteins are similar to disordered proteins with respect to their sequence composition.

Our results reveal that calumenin (along with other CREC proteins) is significantly more charged, less folded, hydrophobic and aggregation prone compared to other CFTR associated chaperones. In this respect, its biophysical profile tends to be more closely aligned with IDPs. Our experimental results demonstrating anti-aggregation effects of calumenin and AavLEA1, an IDP belonging to the family of LEA proteins, on F508del-CFTR folding kinetics tend to support this hypothesis. Based on these results, we propose that calumenin might act as a charged, relatively unfolded chaperone of F508del-CFTR. It is possible that it might have an effect on the folding of wild-type CFTR protein as well.

Since calumenin is a known calcium binding protein, similar to other CREC family members, we decided to investigate whether addition of low (0.75 mM) or high amounts of (2 mM) Ca^{2+} ions to the folding mix had any effects on it chaperone activity. Our data showed that a low concentration of Ca^{2+} ions promoted F508del-CFTR aggregation while a higher concentration (2 mM), inhibited aggregation. These results suggest that calumenin could function both as a positive or negative regulator of F508del-CFTR folding and aggregation in the presence of low or high concentrations of Ca^{2+} ions respectively. We can extrapolate our *in vitro* results for calcium dependent F508del-CFTR folding modulation by calumenin, with known *in vivo* changes in ER calcium stores observed in nasal epithelial cells of CF patients. An expansion of the ER and an increased mobility of Ca^{2+} ions in short term (6–11 days) cultures of nasal epithelial cells has been previously reported and is hypothesized to be an adaptive response to chronic infection and inflammation observed in CF patients [51]. In long term cultures (30–40 days), a reversal of this phenotype is observed. One can therefore propose a model whereby calumenin might exert its anti-aggregation effects in the presence of high amounts of Ca^{2+} ions to minimize F508del-CFTR misfolding and aggregation in CF cells during inflammation. However, prolonged inflammation and ER stress are expected to decrease ER calcium levels [52], thereby promoting F508del-CFTR aggregation in the presence of calumenin in the longer term.

The anti-aggregation activity of calumenin was also found to be dependent on the presence of MgATP, where it was observed to synergistically reduce F508del-CFTR aggregation with both low and high amounts of calcium. It is possible that binding of calcium and MgATP to the calumenin-CFTR complex might induce changes in protein conformation that could prevent the 'hydrophobic collapse' of F508del-CFTR protein. Indeed, calcium has been shown to induce the α-helical folding and compaction of another CREC protein, RCN1 [53], while.binding of MgATP to the CFTR NBD domain has been known to influence its dimerization and gating function [54].

Lastly, addition of EDTA, a chelating agent, to the folding mix with calumenin, resulted in the most dramatic reduction in

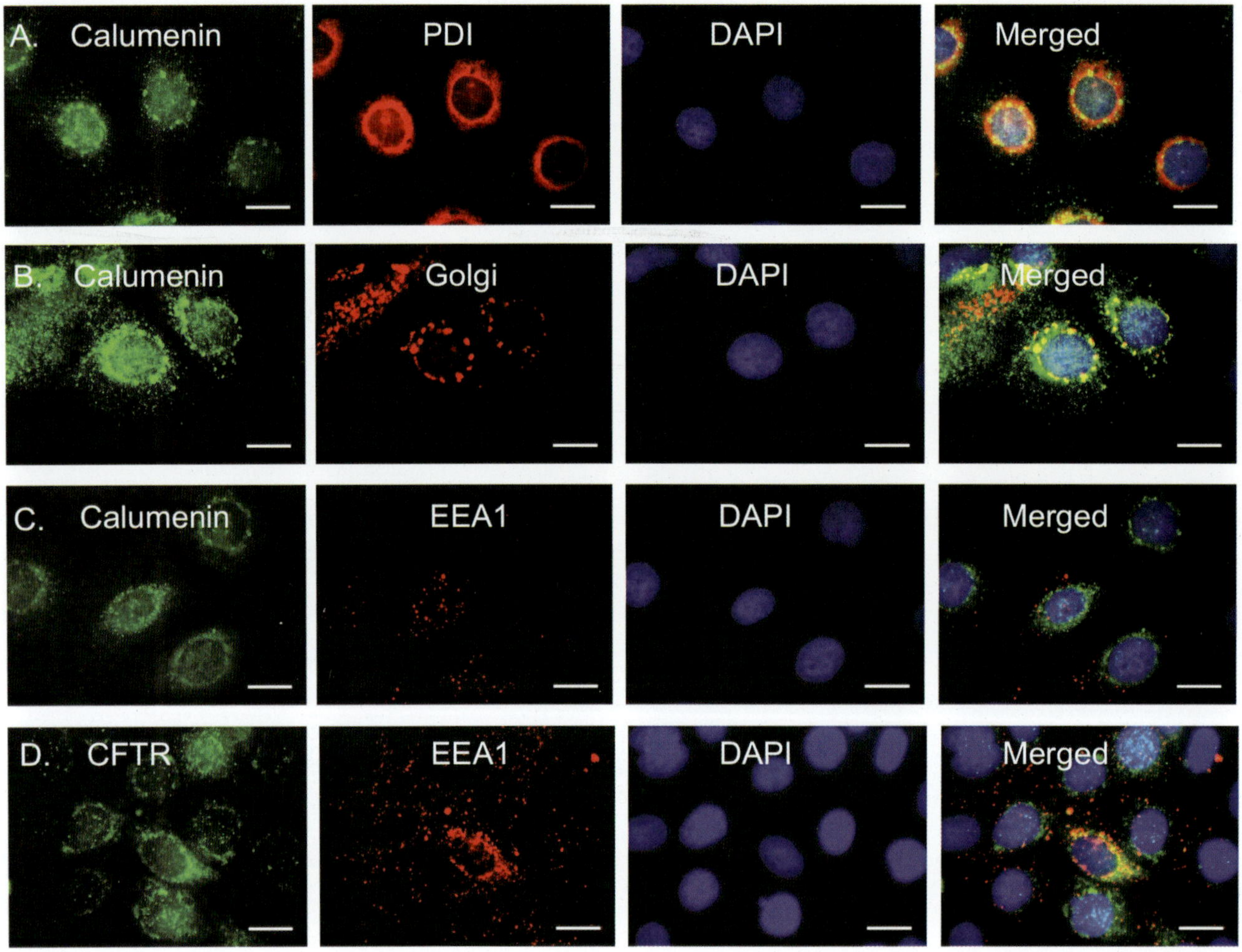

Figure 7. Calumenin trafficking in CFBE41o- cells expressing wild-type CFTR. Calumenin or CFTR (green) in CFBE41o- wild-type or F508del cells were visualized using fluorescence microscopy. Second labeling was performed for either PDI (an ER marker). Golgi marker or EEA1 (marker for endosomal vesicles) (red). The nuclei were stained blue with DAPI. Colocalisation of green and red pixels was detected in merged images (yellow). **A.** Calumenin and PDI (for ER staining) **B.** Calumenin and Golgi and **C.** Calumenin and EEA1 in CFBE41o- wild-type cells. **D.** CFTR and EEA1 in CFBE41o- wild-type cells. Scale bar: 20 μm.

F508del-CFTR aggregation kinetics. EDTA is expected to sequester all the positively charged ions such as Mg^{2+} and Ca^{2+} from the reaction mix, thereby allowing calumenin to acquire its native state. Buffer C used in our F508del-CFTR folding assay, indeed contained 2 mM Mg^{2+} ions, which could have inhibited the intrinsic anti-aggregation properties of calumenin, dependent on the high amount of charge in its sequence.

Our *in vitro* aggregation results could be further confirmed by *in vivo* analytical techniques such as fluorescence recovery after photobleaching (FRAP) [55] and Förster resonance energy transfer (FRET) [56] to monitor F508del-CFTR aggregation and interaction with calumenin respectively.

Immunofluorescence imaging of CFBE41o- cells expressing wild-type CFTR revealed that calumenin accumulated in the ER and Golgi compartments as previously reported [22]. This was evident by the high Pearson's correlation coefficient values observed for calumenin and ER/Golgi markers. Interestingly, calumenin was observed to be retro-translocated to the cytoplasm and the nucleus in the majority of CFBE cells expressing F508del-CFTR. We propose there could be three possible explanations for this observed phenomenon. (1) This might be a consequence of the unfolded protein response [57] triggered in cells expressing misfolded proteins that allows them to be cleared by the ER associated degradation machinery [58]. (2) Calumenin might be mobilized from the ER in response to intra-cellular Ca^{2+} signaling, that has been found to be increased in cells expressing F508del-CFTR [59]. (3) Calumenin might undergo alternative splicing into various isoforms that might in turn translocate to the cytoplasm and nucleus [22,44]. Alternative splicing of XBP1 transcript mediated by inositol receptor endonuclease 1 (IRE1) has been shown to be triggered during the unfolded protein response triggered in response to misfolded proteins in the endoplasmic reticulum [60]. Calumenin isoforms could also be potentially phosphorylated and translocated into the nucleus [44] where they might elicit changes in gene expression. Previously it has been shown that calreticulin, another calcium sensitive chaperone in the ER, can affect the protein levels of myocyte enhancer factor (MEF) 2C, a cardiac specific transcription factor involved in cardiac development [61]. We can also expect significant heterogeneity in distribution of various calumenin isoforms in human bronchial cells as has been demonstrated for a number of calcium regulated proteins in the endoplasmic reticulum [62].

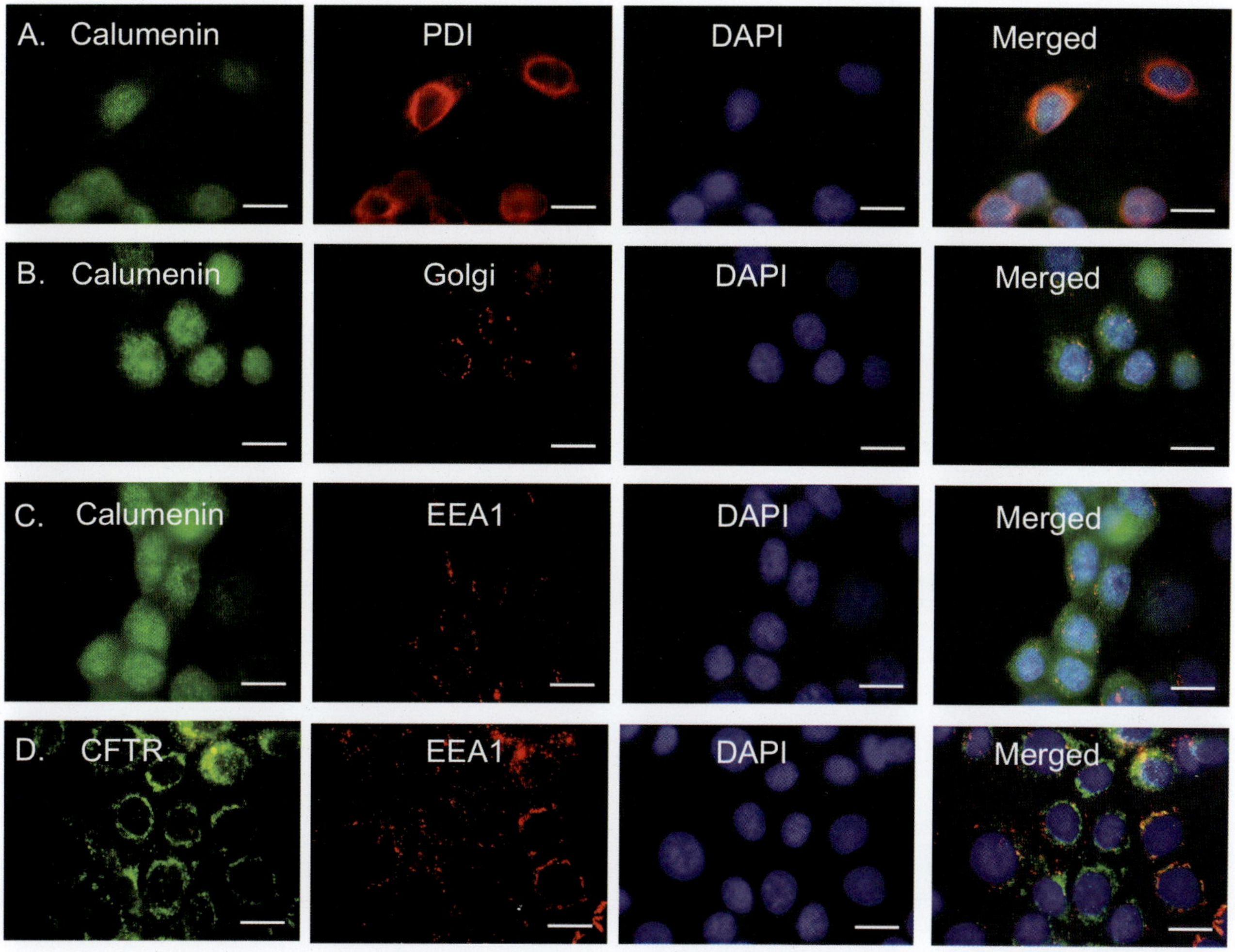

Figure 8. Calumenin trafficking is altered in CFBE41o- cells expressing F508del-CFTR. Calumenin or CFTR (green) in CFBE41o- wild-type or F508del cells were visualized using fluorescence microscopy. Second labeling was performed for either PDI (an ER marker). Golgi marker or EEA1 (marker for endosomal vesicles) (red). The nuclei were stained blue with DAPI. Colocalisation of green and red pixels was detected in merged images (yellow). **A.** Calumenin and PDI (for ER staining) **B.** Calumenin and Golgi and **C.** Calumenin and EEA1 in CFBE41o- cells expressing F508del-CFTR. **D.** CFTR and EEA1 in CFBE41o- cells expressing F508del-CFTR. Scale bar: 20 μm.

Since CFTR is maintained at a steady state in the plasma membrane by endocytic recycling through EEA1 containing vesicles and the F508del mutation is known to decrease its stability at the membrane by increasing its turn-over through these vesicles [23,42,43], it was decided to compare endocytic trafficking of calumenin in both the wild-type CFTR and F508del-CFTR expressing CFBE41o- cells. It was hypothesized that if the calumenin-CFTR interaction was strong, we would expect equal localization of calumenin and CFTR in EEA1 vesicles.

Our data revealed that calumenin localization in EEA1 containing vesicles was substantially reduced compared to CFTR in both wild-type and F508del cells. These results suggest that calumenin, might not be as efficiently recycled in the endocytic pathway, as compared to CFTR. We speculate that the low pH of the secretory vesicles (~5.5) compared to the ER (~7) might result in conformational changes of calumenin, which has an isoelectric point (pI) of ~4.4, allowing it to detach from the CFTR complex and undergo further processing required for its function as a secretory protein. The low pH of the secretory vesicles is known to induce conformational changes in protein structures resulting in the formation of aggregates [63] or novel protein-protein interactions required for vesicular sorting [64]. However, in cells expressing F508del-CFTR, calumenin showed increased accumulation in EEA1 vesicles, suggesting its increased endocytic uptake in CF cells.

Currently, it is not clear how calumenin-CFTR interaction might contribute towards the observed pathophysiology of cystic fibrosis. On one hand, we can speculate that calumenin might prevent deleterious misfolding and aggregation of F508del-CFTR, and possibly G551DCFTR, to a certain extent, as part of the cell's innate defense mechanism in the short term. However, given that we observe a translocation of calumenin in the cytoplasm and the nucleus in a majority of F508del-CFTR expressing cells, indicates that its potentially beneficial effect in regulating F508del-CFTR folding might be compromised due to its displacement from the ER in the longer term. Previously, it has been suggested that depletion of ER calcium by inhibitors of calcium pumps such as thapsigargin, allows misfolded F508del-CFTR to proceed to the membrane more efficiently by releasing it from its associated calcium dependent chaperones [65]. We speculate that calumenin might also inhibit F508del-CFTR trafficking in a manner similar to other calcium dependent chaperones and therefore its association with CFTR might be deleterious to the cell.

Given the paucity of cellular chaperones (including calumenin) in countering the negative effects of F508 deletion in CF patients, one can envisage designing superior synthetic peptides with optimized biophysical parameters that might be able to structurally correct the F508del folding defect. Since calumenin has been characterized as a charged, F508del-CFTR folding modulator in this paper, optimising the quantity of charge in peptide sequences, could be one strategy to induce correct folding of protein sequences. Further insights into the design parameters for such peptides are gained by the observation that certain suppressor mutations such as G550E and I539T can partially rescue the F508del-CFTR to the cell surface [6]. Both these mutations involve a substitution of a polar amino acid with a hydrophobic amino acid. One can imagine that it might be possible to design peptides with optimal hydrophobic content in their sequence composition and specificity towards the NBD1 domain to correct the F508del-CFTR folding defect during the early stages protein translation in the ER in a similar manner [66].

An alternative strategy could involve designing peptides that might prevent the association of chaperones with mutant CFTR, thereby enabling it to traffic more efficiently through the secretory pathway. A similar chaperone displacement strategy has been previously applied by expressing the NBD1 plus the regulatory domain fragment in human airway cells [67] which partially restored F508del-CFTR trafficking and functions. Increasing the amount of disorder in peptide sequences could also prevent deleterious chaperone associations with F508del-CFTR. Additionally, such peptides could potentially also serve as synthetic "molecular shields" [16] by preventing the aggregation of misfolded mutant CFTR molecules. Our results regarding the anti-aggregation activity of AavLEA1, an IDP, lend further support to this hypothesis. Bioinformatics based selection and screening of combinatorial peptide libraries [68,69] could be potentially applied to synthesize peptides with maximum structural correction efficiencies of mutant CFTR proteins. It would be exciting to test this approach in the future as a potential therapeutic strategy in CF.

Supporting Information

Table S1 GRAVY, Instability, Unfoldability, Charge, IUPRED and Aggregation scores of proteins used in our analysis.

Table S2 Pearson's correlation coefficient values between red and green channels.

File S1 Multiple sequence alignment of calumenin isoforms.

Acknowledgments

We would like to thank members of INSERM UMR1078 for their help during various stages of this study especially Dr. Chandran Ka. We would also like to thank Phillippe Elies and Gérard Sinquin from the Plateforme d'Imagerie et de Mesures en Microscopie, UBO. Drs. Stijn van Dongen and Anton Enright from the European Bioinformatics Institute and Prof. Mark Blondel have provided useful advice and suggestions.

Author Contributions

Conceived and designed the experiments: RT PT. Performed the experiments: RT NB. Analyzed the data: RT. Contributed reagents/materials/analysis tools: PT BC CF. Wrote the paper: RT.

References

1. Lao O, Andrés AM, Mateu E, Bertranpetit J, Calafell F (2003) Spatial patterns of cystic fibrosis mutation spectra in European populations. Eur J Hum Genet 11: 385–394.
2. Lukacs GL, Verkman AS (2012) CFTR: folding, misfolding and correcting the ΔF508 conformational defect. Trends Mol Med 18: 81–91.
3. Vergani P, Lockless SW, Nairn AC, Gadsby DC (2005) CFTR channel opening by ATP-driven tight dimerization of its nucleotide-binding domains. Nature 433: 876–880.
4. Zielenski J (2000) Genotype and phenotype in cystic fibrosis. Respiration 67: 117–133.
5. Du K, Lukacs GL (2009) Cooperative Assembly and Misfolding of CFTR Domains In Vivo. Mol Biol Cell 20: 1903–1915.
6. Hoelen H, Kleizen B, Schmidt A, Richardson J, Charitou P, et al. (2010) The primary folding defect and rescue of ΔF508 CFTR emerge during translation of the mutant domain. PLoS One 5: e15458.
7. Serohijos AWR, Aleksandrov AA, He L, Cui L, Dokholyan N V, et al. (2008) Phenylalanine-508 mediates a cytoplasmic – membrane domain contact in the CFTR 3D structure crucial to assembly and channel function. Proc Natl Acad Sci 105: 3256–3261.
8. Reisin IL, Prat AG, Abraham E, Amaran JF, Gregoryn RJ, et al. (1994) The cystic fibrosis transmembrane conductance regulator is a dual ATP and chloride channel. J Biol Chem 269: 20584–20591.
9. Stutts MJ, Canessa CM, Olsen JC, Hamrick M, Cohn JA, et al. (1995) CFTR as a cAMP-dependent regulator of sodium channels. Science (80) 269: 847–850.
10. Mehta A (2005) CFTR: more than just a chloride channel. Pediatr Pulmonol 39: 292–298.
11. O'Sullivan BP, Freedman SD (2009) Cystic fibrosis. Lancet 373: 1891–1904.
12. Teng L, Kerbiriou M, Taiya M, Le Hir S, Mignen O, et al. (2012) Proteomic identification of calumenin as a G551D-CFTR associated protein. PLoS One 7: e40173.
13. Bompadre SG, Sohma Y, Li M, Hwang T-C (2007) G551D and G1349D, two CF-associated mutations in the signature sequences of CFTR, exhibit distinct gating defects. J Gen Physiol 129: 285–298.
14. Wang X, Venable J, LaPointe P, Hutt DM, Koulov A V, et al. (2006) Hsp90 cochaperone Aha1 downregulation rescues misfolding of CFTR in cystic fibrosis. Cell 127: 803–815.
15. Tompa P (2002) Intrinsically unstructured proteins. Trends Biochem Sci 27: 527–533.
16. Chakrabortee S, Tripathi R, Watson M, Schierle GS, Kurniawan DP, et al. (2012) Intrinsically disordered proteins as molecular shields. Mol Biosyst 8: 210–219.
17. Pouchkina-Stantcheva NN, McGee BM, Boschetti C, Tolleter D, Chakrabortee S, et al. (2007) Functional divergence of former alleles in an ancient asexual invertebrate. Science 318: 268–271.
18. He B, Wang K, Liu Y, Xue B, Uversky VN, et al. (2009) Predicting intrinsic disorder in proteins: an overview. Cell Res 19: 929–949.
19. Kovacs D, Tompa P (2012) Diverse functional manifestations of intrinsic structural disorder in molecular chaperones. Biochem Soc Trans 40: 963–968.
20. Bardwell JCA, Jakob U (2013) Conditional disorder in chaperone action. Trends Biochem Sci 37: 517–525.
21. Chakrabortee S, Meersman F, Kaminski Schierle GS, Bertoncini CW, McGee B, et al. (2010) Catalytic and chaperone-like functions in an intrinsically disordered protein associated with desiccation tolerance. Proc Natl Acad Sci U S A 107: 16084–16089.
22. Wang Q, Feng H, Zheng P, Shen B, Chen L, et al. (2012) The intracellular transport and secretion of calumenin-1/2 in living cells. PLoS One 7: e35344.
23. Gentzsch M, Chang X, Cui L, Wu Y, Ozols V V, et al. (2004) Endocytic trafficking routes of wild type and ΔF508 cystic fibrosis transmembrane conductance regulator. Mol Biol Cell 15: 2684–2696.
24. Gasteiger E, Hoogland C, Gattiker A, Duvaud S, Wilkins MR, et al. (2005) Protein identification and analysis tools on the ExPASy server. John M Walk Proteomics Protoc Handbook, Humana Press (2005): 571–607.
25. Prilusky J, Felder CE, Zeev-Ben-Mordehai T, Rydberg EH, Man O, et al. (2005) FoldIndex: a simple tool to predict whether a given protein sequence is intrinsically unfolded. Bioinformatics 21: 3435–3438.
26. Dosztányi Z, Csizmók V, Tompa P, Simon I (2005) The pairwise energy content estimated from amino acid composition discriminates between folded and intrinsically unstructured proteins. J Mol Biol 347: 827–839.
27. Dosztányi Z, Csizmok V, Tompa P, Simon I (2005) IUPred: web server for the prediction of intrinsically unstructured regions of proteins based on estimated energy content. Bioinformatics 21: 3433–3434.
28. Conchillo-Solé O, de Groot NS, Avilés FX, Vendrell J, Daura X, et al. (2007) AGGRESCAN: a server for the prediction and evaluation of "hot spots" of aggregation in polypeptides. BMC Bioinformatics 8: 65.
29. Sievers F, Wilm A, Dineen D, Gibson TJ, Karplus K, et al. (2011) Fast, scalable generation of high-quality protein multiple sequence alignments using Clustal Omega. Mol Syst Biol 7: 539.

30. McWilliam H, Li W, Uludag M, Squizzato S, Park YM, et al. (2013) Analysis Tool Web Services from the EMBL-EBI. Nucleic Acids Res 41: W597–600.
31. Goyal K, Tisi L, Basran A, Browne J, Burnell A, et al. (2003) Transition from natively unfolded to folded state induced by desiccation in an anhydrobiotic nematode protein. J Biol Chem 278: 12977–12984.
32. O'Ryan L, Rimington T, Cant N, Ford RC (2012) Expression and purification of the cystic fibrosis transmembrane conductance regulator protein in Saccharomyces cerevisiae. J Vis Exp: 1–7.
33. Cozens AL, Yezzi MJ, Kunzelmann K, Ohrui T, Chin L, et al. (1994) CFTR expression and chloride secretion in polarized immortal human bronchial epithelial cells. Am J Respir Cell Mol Biol 10: 38–47.
34. Bruscia E, Sangiuolo F, Sinibaldi P, Novelli G (2002) Isolation of CF cell lines corrected at ΔF508-CFTR locus by SFHR-mediated targeting. Gene Ther: 683–685.
35. Bolte S, Cordelières FP (2006) A guided tour into subcellular colocalization analysis in light microscopy. J Microsc 224: 213–232.
36. Choi MY, Partridge AW, Daniels C, Du K, Lukacs GL, et al. (2005) Destabilization of the transmembrane domain induces misfolding in a phenotypic mutant of cystic fibrosis transmembrane conductance regulator. J Biol Chem 280: 4968–4974.
37. Uversky VN, Gillespie JR, Fink AL (2000) Why are "natively unfolded" proteins unstructured under physiologic conditions? Proteins 41: 415–427.
38. Larkin MA, Blackshields G, Brown NP, Chenna R, McGettigan PA, et al. (2007) Clustal W and Clustal X version 2.0. Bioinformatics 23: 2947–2948.
39. Bardwell JCA, Jakob U (2012) Conditional disorder in chaperone action. Trends Biochem Sci 37: 517–525.
40. Strickland E (1997) The molecular chaperone Hsc70 assists the in vitro folding of the N-terminal nucleotide-binding domain of the cystic fibrosis transmembrane conductance regulator. J Biol Chem 272: 25421–25424.
41. Browne J, Tunnacliffe A, Burnell A (2002) Plant desiccation gene found in a nematode. Nature 416: 2002.
42. Prince LS, Workman RB, Marchase RB (1994) Rapid endocytosis of the cystic fibrosis transmembrane conductance regulator chloride channel. Proc Natl Acad Sci 91: 5192–5196.
43. Lukacs GL, Chang X, Bear C, Kartner N, Mohamed A, et al. (1993) The ΔF508 mutation decreases the stability of cystic fibrosis transmembrane conductance regulator in the plasma membrane. J Biochem 268: 21592–21598.
44. Feng H, Chen L, Wang Q, Shen B, Liu L, et al. (2013) Calumenin-15 facilitates filopodia formation by promoting TGF-β superfamily cytokine GDF-15 transcription. Cell Death Dis 4: e870.
45. Boschetti C, Pouchkina-Stantcheva N, Hoffmann P, Tunnacliffe A (2011) Foreign genes and novel hydrophilic protein genes participate in the desiccation response of the bdelloid rotifer Adineta ricciae. J Exp Biol 214: 59–68.
46. Neira JL, Contreras LM, de los Paños OR, Sánchez-Hidalgo M, Martínez-Bueno M, et al. (2010) Structural characterisation of the natively unfolded enterocin EJ97. Protein Eng Des Sel 23: 507–518.
47. Graña-Montes R, Sant'anna de Oliveira R, Ventura S (2012) Protein aggregation profile of the human kinome. Front Physiol 3: 438.
48. Graña-Montes R, Sant'Anna de Oliveira R, Ventura S (2012) Protein aggregation profile of the human kinome. Front Physiol 3: 438.
49. Kumar V, Punetha A, Sundar D, Chaudhuri TK (2012) In silico engineering of aggregation-prone recombinant proteins for substrate recognition by the chaperonin GroEL. BMC Genomics 13 Suppl 7: S22.
50. Reichmann D, Xu Y, Cremers CM, Ilbert M, Mittelman R, et al. (2013) Order out of disorder: working cycle of an intrinsically unfolded chaperone. Cell 148: 947–957.
51. Ribeiro CMP, Paradiso AM, Carew MA, Shears SB, Boucher RC (2005) Cystic fibrosis airway epithelial Ca^{2+} signaling: the mechanism for the larger agonist-mediated Ca^{2+} signals in human cystic fibrosis airway epithelia. J Biol Chem 280: 10202–10209.
52. Mekahli D, Bultynck G, Parys JB, De Smedt H, Missiaen L (2011) Endoplasmic-reticulum calcium depletion and disease. Cold Spring Harb Perspect Biol 3.
53. Suzuki N, Ban S, Itoh E, Chen S, Imai F, et al. (2014) Calcium-dependent structural changes in human reticulocalbin-1. J Biochem 155: 281–293.
54. Hwang TC, Sheppard DN (2009) Gating of the CFTR Cl- channel by ATP-driven nucleotide-binding domain dimerisation. J Physiol 587: 2151–2161.
55. Fua L, Sztula E (2009) ER-associated complexes (ERACs) containing aggregated cystic fibrosis transmembrane conductance regulator (CFTR) are degraded by autophagy. Eur J Cell Biol 88: 215–226.
56. Qadri YJ, Cormet-Boyaka E, Rooj AK, Lee W, Parpura V, et al. (2012) Low temperature and chemical rescue affect molecular proximity of DeltaF508-cystic fibrosis transmembrane conductance regulator (CFTR) and epithelial sodium channel (ENaC). J Biol Chem 287: 16781–16790.
57. Ellgaard L, Helenius A (2003) Quality control in the endoplasmic reticulum. Nat Rev Mol Cell Biol 4: 181–191.
58. Farinha CM, Amaral MD (2005) Most F508del-CFTR is targeted to degradation at an early folding checkpoint and independently of calnexin. Mol Cell Biol 25: 5242–5252.
59. Martins JR, Kongsuphol P, Sammels E, Dahimène S, Aldehni F, et al. (2011) F508del-CFTR increases intracellular Ca^{2+} signaling that causes enhanced calcium-dependent Cl^{-} conductance in cystic fibrosis. Biochim Biophys Acta 1812: 1385–1392.
60. Calfon M, Zeng H, Urano F, Till JH, Hubbard SR, et al. (2002) IRE1 couples endoplasmic reticulum load to secretory capacity by processing the XBP-1 mRNA. Nature 415: 92–96.
61. Hattori K, Nakamura K, Hisatomi Y, Matsumoto S, Suzuki M, et al. (2007) Arrhythmia induced by spatiotemporal overexpression of calreticulin in the heart. Mol Genet Metab 91: 285–293.
62. Papp S (2003) Is all of the endoplasmic reticulum created equal? The effects of the heterogeneous distribution of endoplasmic reticulum Ca^{2+}-handling proteins. J Cell Biol 160: 475–479.
63. Hyun Yoo S (1996) Protein Chemistry and Structure: pH and and Ca^{2+}-dependent aggregation property of secretory vesicle matrix proteins and the potential role of Chromogranins A and B in secretory vesicle biogenesis. J Biol Chem 271: 1558–1565.
64. Hyun Yoo S (1994) pH-dependent interaction of chromogranin A with integral membrane proteins of secretory vesicle including 260-kDa protein reactive to inositol 1,4,5-trisphosphate receptor antibody. J Biol Chem 269: 12001–12006.
65. Egan ME, Glöckner-Pagel J, Ambrose C, Cahill PA, Pappoe L, et al. (2002) Calcium-pump inhibitors induce functional surface expression of Delta F508-CFTR protein in cystic fibrosis epithelial cells. Nat Med 8: 485–492.
66. Johnson AE, Waes MA Van (1999) A Dynamic Gateway at the ER Membrane. Annu Rev Cell Dev Biol: 799–842.
67. Sun F, Mi Z, Condliffe SB, Bertrand CA, Gong X, et al. (2008) Chaperone displacement from mutant cystic fibrosis transmembrane conductance regulator restores its function in human airway epithelia. FASEB J 22: 3255–3263.
68. Maillard N, Clouet A, Darbre T, Reymond J-L (2009) Combinatorial libraries of peptide dendrimers: design, synthesis, on-bead high-throughput screening, bead decoding and characterization. Nat Protoc 4: 132–142.
69. Rathinakumar R, Wimley WC (2008) Biomolecular engineering by combinatorial design and high-throughput screening: small, soluble peptides that permeabilize membranes. J Am Chem Soc 130: 9849–9858.

Emergence of Carbapenem Resistance Due to the Novel Insertion Sequence IS*Pa*8 in *Pseudomonas aeruginosa*

Randal C. Fowler, Nancy D. Hanson*

Creighton University School of Medicine, Department of Medical Microbiology and Immunology, Center for Research in Anti-Infectives and Biotechnology, Omaha, Nebraska, United States of America

Abstract

Chronic lung infections due to the persistence of *Pseudomonas aeruginosa* in cystic fibrosis patients are typically associated with the emergence of antibiotic resistance. The purpose of this study was to investigate the mechanisms responsible for the emergence of carbapenem resistance when a clinical isolate of *P. aeruginosa* collected from a patient with cystic fibrosis was challenged with meropenem. Nine carbapenem-resistant mutants were selected with subinhibitory concentrations of meropenem from a clinical isolate of *P. aeruginosa* and characterized for carbapenem resistance. Increased carbapenem MICs were associated with the identification of the novel insertion sequence IS*Pa*8 within *oprD* or its promoter region in all the mutants. The position of IS*Pa*8 was different for each of the mutants evaluated. In addition, Southern blot analyses identified multiple copies of IS*Pa*8 within the genomes of the mutants and their parent isolate. These data demonstrate that transposition of IS elements within the *Pseudomonas* genome can influence antibiotic susceptibility. Understanding the selective pressures associated with the emergence of antibiotic resistance is critical for the judicious use of antimicrobial chemotherapy and the successful treatment of bacterial infections.

Editor: Ruth Hall, The University of Sydney, Australia

Funding: This work was supported in part by a research grant from Johnson and Johnson Pharmaceutical Research and Development and by Creighton University. The funders had no role in study design, data collection and analysis, decision to publish, or preparation of the manuscript.

Competing Interests: This work was supported in part by a research grant from Johnson and Johnson Pharmaceutical Research. There are no patents, products in development, or marketed products to declare. This does not alter the authors' adherence to all the PLOS ONE policies on sharing data and materials, as detailed online in the guide for authors.

* E-mail: ndhanson@creighton.edu

Introduction

Carbapenems such as imipenem, meropenem, and doripenem are frequently used as last resort drugs for the treatment of multidrug-resistant *P. aeruginosa* infections. *P. aeruginosa* is the predominate pathogen in chronic respiratory infections in patients with cystic fibrosis. The most formidable characteristic of *P. aeruginosa* is the rapid development of resistance during therapy to multiple antibiotics including the carbapenems, making eradication of this microorganism from the airways of cystic fibrosis patients difficult if not impossible [1,2]. Although the carbapenems remain a viable therapeutic option, their usage carries an increased risk for developing carbapenem resistance thereby reducing their efficacy [3–9].

P. aeruginosa can employ a combination of plasmid-encoded and/or chromosomally-encoded mechanisms to evade carbapenem therapy. However, in non-carbapenemase-producing *P. aeruginosa*, meropenem and doripenem resistance is associated with the overexpression of the *mexAB-oprM* efflux pump with concomitant loss of the carbapenem-specific porin OprD [10,11], while imipenem resistance has only been associated with the down-regulation of OprD [10,12]. Mutations such as nucleotide substitutions, deletions, and insertion sequence (IS) elements within the *oprD* gene or its promoter region can decrease or cause a loss of OprD production, resulting in significant reductions in susceptibility of *P. aeruginosa* to carbapenem antibiotics [13–17]. Furthermore, IS21 disruption of the efflux regulator *mexR* has been associated with decreased β-lactam susceptibility due to increased expression of the efflux pump *mexAB-oprM* [18]. These data in addition to other studies highlight the various roles IS elements play in promoting the emergence of antibiotic resistance [19].

In this study, we challenged a carbapenem susceptible *P. aeruginosa* isolate collected from a cystic fibrosis patient with subinhibitory concentrations of meropenem and investigated the molecular mechanisms associated with the emergence of carbapenem resistance.

Methods

Strains and Culture Conditions

P. aeruginosa isolate PA42 was isolated from a sputum culture of a 20 year-old patient with cystic fibrosis from the Pediatrics Pulmonology Cystic Fibrosis Clinic at the University of Nebraska Medical Center. Gram staining revealed that PA42 had a rounded cell morphology compared to the laboratory isolate PAO1 (Figure S1). PA42 was identified as *P. aeruginosa* using the Vitek 2 System. In addition, the sequence data for *oprF* and *oprD* showed 100% and 92% identities to the sequenced strain *P. aeruginosa* PAO1 (GenBank Accession No. AE004091.2).

Bacterial Susceptibility

PAO1 and PA443, an isolate collected from a cystic fibrosis patient, were susceptible to all anti-pseudomonal agents tested and were used as comparator isolates. Susceptibility of the *P. aeruginosa* isolates to imipenem, meropenem, and doripenem was determined using agar dilution methodology according to the Clinical Laboratory Standards Institute (CLSI) [20]. Quality control strains *E. coli* ATCC 25922, *E. coli* ATCC 35218, and *P. aeruginosa* ATCC 27853 were included in susceptibility testing experiments.

Generation of Isogenic Mutants

Parent isolate PA42 was challenged with subinhibitory concentrations of meropenem during log-phase growth to generate an isogenic panel of carbapenem-resistant mutants. *P. aeruginosa* cells were harvested by centrifugation, resuspended in sterile saline, and diluted to achieve populations of 10^7, 10^8, and 10^9 cfu/mL. Diluted cultures were inoculated into sets of Mueller-Hinton agar plates containing 0.25 μg/mL or 0.5 μg/mL of meropenem. After 24 h of incubation at 37°C, individual colonies were selected at random from each meropenem plate and putative mutants were evaluated for a ≥4-fold increase in meropenem MIC by agar dilution in accordance with CLSI guidelines [20].

PCR and Sequencing

Genomic DNA was prepared from all bacterial isolates as previously described [21]. PCR was conducted in a final volume of 50 μL with 2 units of High-Fidelity Platinum® Taq Polymerase (Invitrogen, Carlsbad, CA), 3% DMSO, and primers that flanked either *oprD* or *oprF* (Table S1). The amplification conditions were 95°C for 5 min followed by 25 cycles at 95°C for 30 s, 56°C for 30 s, and 72°C for 3 min. A combination of primers specific for *oprD* and IS*Pa8* were used in a PCR using a 52°C annealing temperature to determine the location of IS*Pa8* with respect to the *oprD* gene in the isogenic mutants (Table S1). PCR products were column purified using a Millipore Amicon® Ultra Ultracel® 50 K filter (Millipore, Billerica, MA, USA) and sequenced by ACGT, Inc. (Wheeling, IL).

Real Time RT-PCR

RNA was isolated from cultures grown to mid-log phase and gene expression was evaluated by real time RT-PCR as previously described [22]. The expression of *mexA* for PA42 and its isogenic mutants was compared to PAO1 and represented as a ratio (fold-change). Expression studies were performed in triplicate with independent bacterial cultures and the relative expression of *mexA* was determined by averaging the results from three independent RNA extractions.

Outer Membrane Protein Analysis

Outer membrane proteins were isolated and resolved in an 11% SDS–PAGE with a constant current of 25 mA [23]. Proteins were stained with coomassie blue R-250 and photographed using the Molecular Imager® Gel Doc XR+ System with Image Lab Software.

Pulsed Field Gel Electrophoresis and Southern Hybridization

Pulsed field gel electrophoresis (PFGE) analysis was performed on *P. aeruginosa* genomic DNA digested with *Spe*I as previously described [24]. Southern hybridizations were performed on restricted genomic DNA using methods described by Sambrook and Russell [25]. A 182 bp DIG-labeled probe specific for IS*Pa8* was synthesized with primers ISPa8F2 and ISPa8R2 (Table S1) using a Roche PCR DIG Probe Synthesis Kit (Roche, Penzberg, Germany) and column purified. The restricted genomic DNA was vacuum blotted to a positively charged nylon membrane and hybridization was carried out with a Roche DIG Nucleic Acid Detection Kit (Roche, Penzberg, Germany) as instructed by the manufacturer.

Results

In vitro Meropenem Mutant Selection and Susceptibilities

Clinical isolate PA42 was challenged with subinhibitory levels of meropenem. Mutants were isolated from meropenem agar plates and evaluated for carbapenem susceptibilities and mechanisms of carbapenem resistance. The mutational frequency of PA42 challenged with 0.25 μg/mL (⅛ the MIC) of meropenem ranged from 1×10^{-7} to 9×10^{-7}, while the mutational frequency was 8×10^{-9} with 0.5 μg/mL (¼ the MIC) of meropenem. In comparison to PA42, the MICs of imipenem and doripenem were 32-fold and 16-fold higher for the selected mutants 711M, 714M, 811M, 812M, 925M, and 927M, while a 4- to 8-fold increase in doripenem MICs and an 8- to 16-fold increase in imipenem MICs were observed for mutants 922M and 924M, respectively. In addition, all the isogenic mutants had a meropenem MIC of 16 μg/mL (Table 1).

Mechanisms Associated with Carbapenem Resistance

Previous studies have shown that a loss of the OprD porin is the most common mechanism associated with reduced susceptibility to the carbapenems in *P. aeruginosa* [2,13,14]. It is possible that the elevated carbapenem MICs for the isogenic mutants was associated with mutations within *oprD* that were selected during meropenem exposure (Table 1). To determine whether nucleotide changes within *oprD* had occurred, the *oprD* gene and its flanking regions were amplified by PCR and sequenced. Parent isolate PA42 generated a PCR product of the predicted size (1586 bp) (Figure 1) and sequence analysis of the *oprD* gene from PA42 showed 99% similarity to *oprD* from *P. aeruginosa* LESB58 (GenBank Accession No. FM209186.1) and 92% similarity to *oprD* from *P. aeruginosa* PAO1 (GenBank Accession No. AE004091.2). Surprisingly, the PA42 mutants amplified a much larger PCR product (~3000 bp) than the PCR product for PA42, which suggested the presence of a large insertion within the *oprD* gene (Figure 1). Sequence analysis of mutant 712M revealed the presence of a 1324 bp IS element located within the *oprD* gene (Accession No. KC710194). The IS element was identified as having 96% similarity to IS*Pa8* (http://www-IS.biotoul.fr) and was flanked by 19 bp imperfect terminal inverted repeats. An open reading frame within IS*Pa8* was found to encode a 364 amino acid protein having 84% identity to a putative transposase in *Pseudoxanthomonas suwonensis* (GenBank Accession No. CP002446.1). PCR analysis using a combination of IS*Pa8* and *oprD*-specific primer sets listed in Table S1 revealed that IS*Pa8* had also inserted within *oprD* or its promoter region in the other isogenic mutants (Figure 1). To identify the insertion site and confirm the IS element was IS*Pa8*, a single sequence reaction was performed using primers listed in Table S1. PCR and sequence analysis determined that the disruption of *oprD* in eight mutants was due to IS*Pa8* insertion, while the insertion of IS*Pa8* was found 57 bp upstream of the translational start codon of *oprD* in mutant 922M. Although inactivation of the *oprD* gene in the isogenic mutants was due to IS*Pa8*, the position and orientation of this IS element was different with respect to *oprD* (Figure 2).

Meropenem and doripenem resistance can emerge through a combination of down-regulation or loss of OprD in the outer membrane and an up-regulation of MexAB-OprM in non-metallo-β-lactamase producing *P. aeruginosa* isolates [2,11]. To account for the higher MICs of meropenem and doripenem in the isogenic mutants, we compared the relative transcript levels of

Table 1. Carbapenem susceptibility and gene expression data for *P. aeruginosa* isolates.

Isolate	Phenotype[a]	Selective Agent[b]	Mutant Frequency	MIC (μg/mL)[c]			Relative *mexA* expression ± SD
				IPM	MEM	DOR	
PAO1	WT	–	–	2	0.5	0.5	1.00
PA443	CF	–	–	2	0.25	0.25	0.85±0.20
PA42	P	–	–	0.5	2	0.25	3.99±1.23
711M	M	0.25	9×10^{-7}	16	16	4	3.57±1.10
712M	M	0.25	9×10^{-7}	8	16	8	3.62±0.74
714M	M	0.25	9×10^{-7}	16	16	4	5.46±1.35
811M	M	0.25	1×10^{-7}	16	16	4	4.95±0.85
812M	M	0.25	1×10^{-7}	16	16	4	4.14±1.99
922M	M	0.5	8×10^{-9}	4	16	1	3.12±0.38
924M	M	0.5	8×10^{-9}	8	16	2	4.89±1.48
925M	M	0.5	8×10^{-9}	16	16	4	4.02±1.73
927M	M	0.5	8×10^{-9}	16	16	4	4.57±1.32

[a]WT, wild-type isolate; CF, clinical isolate from cystic fibrosis patient; P, parent isolate; M, mutant of PA42.
[b]Subinhibitory concentration (μg/mL) of meropenem used for mutant selection.
[c]IPM, imipenem; MEM, meropenem; DOR, doripenem.

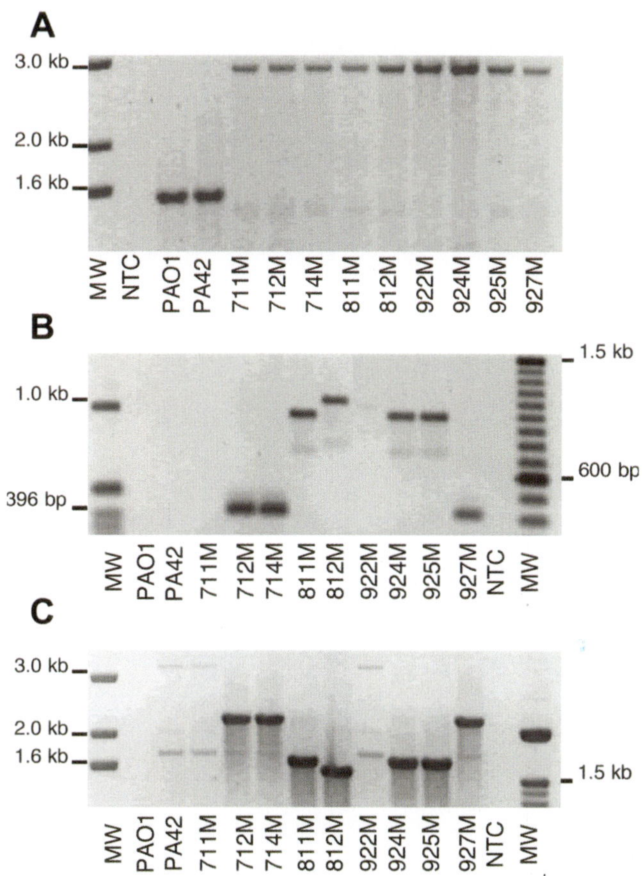

Figure 1. PCR amplification of *oprD* and IS*Pa8* from carbapenem-resistant mutants of *P. aeruginosa*. (A) Primers that flanked the *oprD* gene were used to PCR-amplify the *oprD* gene giving an expected PCR product size is 1586 bp. Each lane is labeled with its respective DNA ladder (1 kb DNA ladder, Invitrogen), no template control (NTC), or *P. aeruginosa* isolate. (B) PCR amplification of IS*Pa8* within the *oprD* gene in the nine carbapenem-resistant mutants. Primers ISPa8F1 and OprDRTR3 were used to map the approximate location of the IS*Pa8* within the *oprD* gene. The smaller PCR products indicate IS*Pa8* has inserted near the 3′ end of *oprD*, while larger PCR products indicate IS*Pa8* is inserted near the 5′ end. No PCR product was observed for mutant 711M. (C) Primers OprDRTF2 and ISPa8R2 were used to confirm the location of IS*Pa8* within the *oprD* gene in the nine isogenic mutants. Non-specific bands were amplified in PA42, mutant 711M, and mutant 922M suggesting that multiple IS*Pa8* elements may be present within the genome. To confirm that IS*Pa8* had inserted within the *oprD* gene or its flanking regions in mutants 711M and 922M, PCR products for these mutants shown in (A) were sequenced using primers OprDRTF2 or ISPa8F1.

mexA in the isogenic mutants, their parent PA42, and a fully susceptible cystic fibrosis isolate PA443 to *mexA* transcript levels in PAO1. *mexA* expression was 4-fold higher in PA42 than PAO1 and PA443, indicating that *mexA* expression was already elevated above "wild-type" levels observed for PAO1 and PA443. However, *mexA* transcript levels were similar among the isogenic mutants and their parent, PA42 suggesting that *mexA* expression did not change upon meropenem selection (Table 1).

Outer Membrane Profiles of PA42 and Isogenic Mutants

The inactivation of *oprD* by IS*Pa8* suggested that the OprD protein was no longer produced. Therefore, the presence of OprD in the outer membrane was analyzed in the isogenic mutants. The outer membrane profiles for PA42 and its mutants showed that OprD was produced in PA42 but not in the isogenic mutants (Figure 3). The loss of OprD correlated with the insertional inactivation of the *oprD* gene by IS*Pa8* and the reduced carbapenem susceptibility in the isogenic mutants. In addition to the loss of OprD in the mutants, parent isolate PA42 and the isogenic mutants did not produce the major outer membrane protein OprF (Figure 3). To investigate the potential source of IS*Pa8* on the chromosome of PA42, we sought to identify whether the loss of OprF was also the result of IS*Pa8* insertion within the *oprF* gene. To test this hypothesis, the *oprF* gene and its flanking regions were PCR amplified and sequenced. PCR amplification of *oprF* from PA42 generated a much larger product (~3000 bp) than the predicted 1672 bp product from PAO1 (Figure 4). Sequence analysis of *oprF* for PA42 identified the insertion of IS*Pa8* 31 nucleotides upstream of the translational start codon of *oprF* (Accession No. KC710195). The disruption of the *oprF* promoter region by IS*Pa8* in parent isolate PA42 correlated with a 50-fold decrease in *oprF* expression compared to *oprF* expression in PAO1 (data not shown). Additionally, the rounded cell shape observed for PA42 could be linked to the loss of OprF as previously reported [26–28]. Subsequently, amplification of the *oprF* gene in the isogenic mutants resulted in PCR products that were ~1,400 bp larger than expected (Figure 4). OprF was absent or produced at low levels in the outer membranes of PA42 and its mutants (Figure 3). Taken together, these data indicated that IS*Pa8* remained upstream of *oprF* during meropenem exposure and was responsible for the lack of OprF production in PA42 and the isogenic mutants.

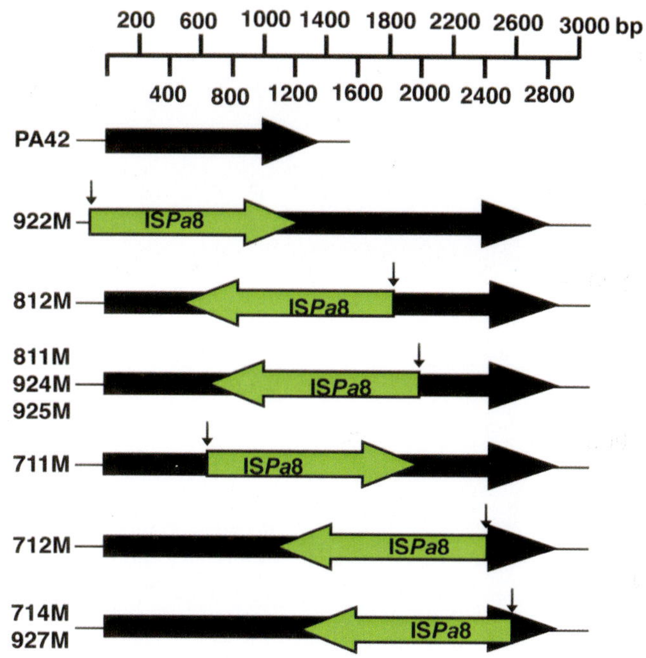

Figure 2. Insertion sites of IS*Pa8* with respect to the *oprD* gene in PA42 and nine isogenic mutants. The solid black arrows represent the *oprD* gene while the green arrows represent the location and orientation of IS*Pa8* within *oprD*. The downward arrow indicates the predicted insertion site of IS*Pa8* within *oprD* as determined by sequence analysis.

PFGE Patterns and IS*Pa8* Copy Number

To determine the copy number of IS*Pa8* in PA42 and its mutants, PFGE and Southern blot experiments were performed.

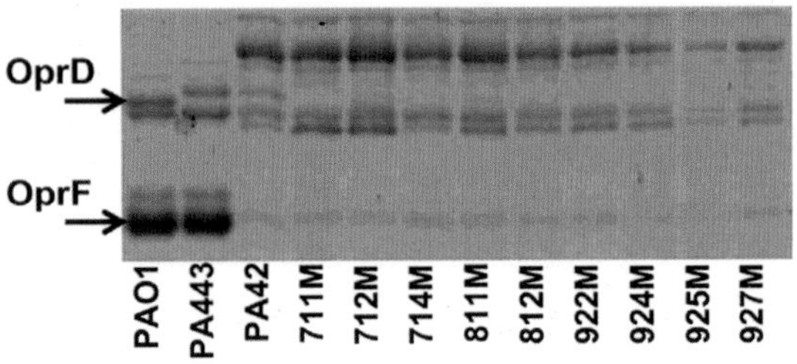

Figure 3. Outer membrane analysis of *P. aeruginosa* PA42 and nine isogenic mutants. Outer membrane profiles were analyzed for the presence of the porin, OprD. PAO1 and a fully susceptible cystic fibrosis isolate, PA443, were included as positive controls. The locations of OprD and OprF proteins are indicated.

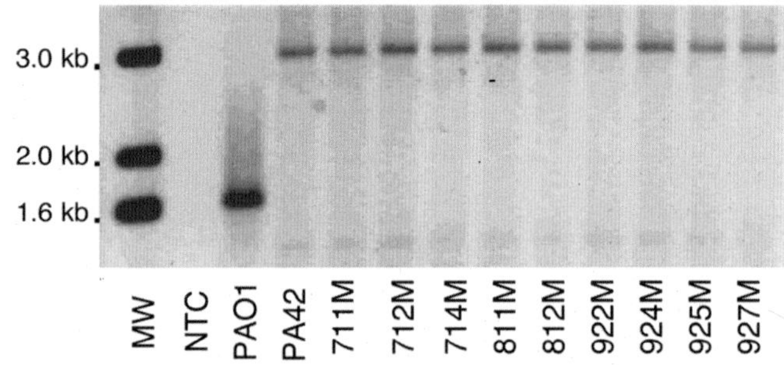

Figure 4. PCR amplification of the *oprF* gene in PAO1, PA42, and nine isogenic mutants. The expected PCR product size is 1,672 bp. Each lane is labeled with its respective DNA ladder (1 kb DNA ladder, Invitrogen), no template control (NTC), or *P. aeruginosa* isolates.

As anticipated, PA42 and its mutants were highly related by PFGE as indicated by their indistinguishable PFGE patterns (Figure 5, Figure S2). Surprisingly, Southern blot analysis revealed multiple hybridization signals for IS*Pa8* in PA42 and mutant 812M demonstrating that multiple copies of IS*Pa8* exist in their genomes (Figure 5). Note that in Figure 5 the DIG-probe was highly specific for IS*Pa8* as no hybridization signal was observed in the IS*Pa8*-negative control PAO1. Multiple copies of IS*Pa8* were also observed in the genomes of the other mutants (Figure S2). However, we could not differentiate the number of hybridization signals between PA42 and each mutant due to the high copy number (>20 copies) of the IS*Pa8* within their genomes as illustrated in the analysis of PA42 and mutant 812M (Figure 5).

Discussion

Carbapenem resistance poses a major therapeutic challenge for the treatment of *P. aeruginosa* infections, particularly in patients with cystic fibrosis. Our current understanding of the mechanisms responsible for carbapenem resistance consists of an interplay between the over-expression of *mexAB-oprM* and the down-regulation of the porin, OprD [2,10,11]. The most common mechanism of imipenem resistance is the absence of OprD production which can result from mutations, insertions, and/or deletions in the *oprD* gene as well as the down-regulation of *oprD* transcription [13–17]. In this study, the insertion of a novel IS element, identified as IS*Pa8*, within the *oprD* gene was associated with the emergence of carbapenem resistance in *P. aeruginosa* mutants selected with subinhibitory levels of meropenem. These findings are in agreement with other investigations where IS element insertion has been linked to a decrease in carbapenem susceptibility and loss of OprD production. These observations indicate that the *oprD* gene and/or its promoter region may serve as a hot spot in the genome for IS element insertion [15–17,29].

The loss of OprD in the outer membrane has been shown to decrease the susceptibility of *P. aeruginosa* by 4- to 16-fold for imipenem, compared to 4- to 32-fold for meropenem and 8- to 32-fold for doripenem [11,30], while up-regulation of *mexAB-oprM* expression increased the MICs of meropenem and doripenem from 0.12–0.5 μg/mL to 4 μg/mL [11]. However, a concomitant loss of OprD and up-regulation of this efflux pump can increase the MIC of meropenem above "wild-type" levels (~16 μg/mL) [10]. In this study, meropenem resistance (16 μg/mL) among the isogenic mutants resulted from increased *mexA* transcript levels that preceded meropenem exposure in addition to a loss of OprD through insertional disruption by IS*Pa8* allowing for the selection of the meropenem mutants. Interestingly, the parent isolate from which carbapenem-resistant mutants were selected showed a 4-fold increase in *mexA* expression compared *mexA* expression in PAO1 which correlated with the MIC of meropenem (2 μg/mL). However, meropenem selection did not modify the expression of *mexA* in the isogenic mutants compared to the parent isolate PA42, suggesting that *mexA* expression may have reached an expression threshold sufficient to achieve high meropenem MICs (Table 1). However, as previous described [10], it is the combination of increased *mexA* expression and loss of OprD as displayed in these isogenic mutants that resulted in the MICs of doripenem and meropenem to increase above the resistance breakpoint, while the loss of OprD alone was responsible for the reduction in susceptibility to imipenem in these mutants. These data demonstrate that OprD-mediated resistance is not always the first step

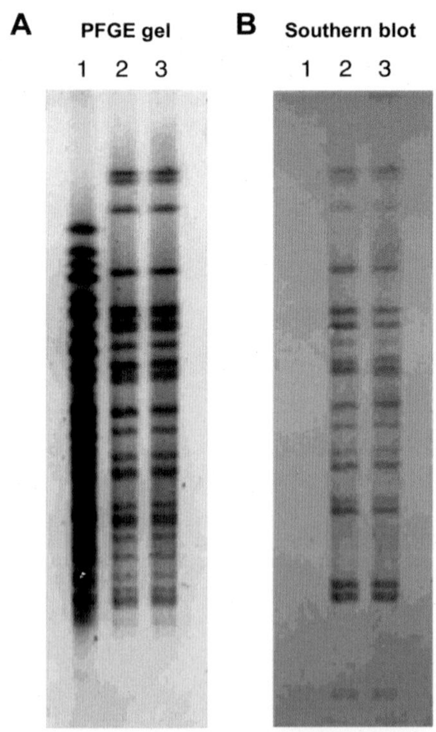

Figure 5. Pulsed Field Gel Electrophoresis and Southern blot analyses using IS*Pa8*-specific probe. (A) PFGE gel of *Spe*I chromosomal digests of wild-type strain PAO1, parent isolate PA42, and mutant 812M visualized using SYBR gold. (B) Southern blot of the gel depicted in Figure 5(A) using an IS*Pa8*-specific probe. Lane 1, PAO1 (negative control); lane 2, parent isolate PA42; lane 3, mutant 812M.

toward carbapenem resistance as has been previously suggested [10,11]. Taken together, these data further support that a combination of chromosomally-encoded resistance mechanisms are necessary to achieve meropenem and/or doripenem MICs above the resistance breakpoint.

Transposable elements such as IS elements can promote the adaptation and survival of Gram-negative bacteria under different environmental niches through the disruption of genes and genomic rearrangements. This form of adaptation has been well documented in clinical isolates of *P. aeruginosa* that have developed resistance to β-lactam antibiotics [15–19]. Moreover, IS elements modulate genomic plasticity and participate in the evolution of *P. aeruginosa* isolates within the lung environment of patients with cystic fibrosis through genetic rearrangements [31]. The presence of multiple copies of IS*Pa*8 in the host chromosome of PA42 suggests that it may have played an important role in the evolution of this clinical isolate. Recently, Doumith *et al* suggested that bacterial chromosomes may contain multiple copies of IS elements and their insertion into porin genes may be selected under antibiotic pressure [32]. To our knowledge, our study is the first to provide support that when a selective pressure is applied to a bacteria with multiple copies of an IS element, antibiotic-resistant mutants with insertional disruptions in porin genes will be selected for within the bacterial population. Interestingly, multiple insertion events of IS*Pa*8 occurred within the *oprD* gene or promoter region among the meropenem selected mutants, which may be a reflection of the host genome containing several copies of the IS*Pa*8 element (Figure 2). These data suggest that *P. aeruginosa* isolates with a high copy number of IS elements within its genome could lead to the emergence of antibiotic resistance. This observation could have serious implications in clinical practice where carbapenem monotherapy is used as the primary treatment of *P. aeruginosa* infections. Ruiz-Martinez *et al* reported a similar finding where imipenem monotherapy was used to treat a fully susceptible *P. aeruginosa* infection in a patient, which resulted in the selection of an imipenem-resistant variant due to the inactivation of the *oprD* gene by IS*Pa*133 [29]. Taken together, these data indicate that the selective pressure exerted by a carbapenem can select mutants from *P. aeruginosa* isolates that contain multiple copies of IS element in the genome thereby allowing for the rapid development carbapenem resistance.

This study serves as an important reminder that monotherapy, particularly with a carbapenem, may not always be appropriate for treating *P. aeruginosa* infections as it can readily develop resistance to antibiotics. Although IS elements have been shown to influence the genetic and phenotypic characteristics of bacteria as described in this study, little is known about what stimulates their transposition. Therefore, future studies looking to identify factors that influence the mobilization and insertion of IS elements could contribute significantly to our current knowledge of mechanisms involved in the emergence of antibiotic resistance and the evolution of *P. aeruginosa*.

Supporting Information

Figure S1 Macroscopic and microscopic analysis of *P. aeruginosa* isolates PAO1 and PA42. Macroscopic analysis of PAO1 grown on blood agar shows a non-mucoid phenotype while PA42 was mucoid when grown on blood agar. Gram-staining revealed characteristic Gram-negative rods for PAO1 and unique Gram-negative cocci for PA42 at 40X and 100X objectives.

Figure S2 Pulsed Field Gel Electrophoresis and Southern blot analyses using IS*Pa*8-specific probe. (A) PFGE gel of *Spe*I chromosomal digests of wild-type strain PAO1, parent isolate PA42, and eight carbapenem-selected mutants visualized using SYBR gold. Lane 1, size standard *Staphylococcus aureus* NCTC 8325; lane 2, negative control PAO1; lane 3, parent isolate PA42; lane 4, mutant 711M; lane 5, mutant 712M; lane 6, mutant 714M; lane 7, mutant 811M; lane 8, mutant 922M; lane 9, mutant 924M; lane 10, mutant 925M; lane 11, mutant 927M. (B) Southern blot of the gel depicted in Figure S2(A) using an IS*Pa*8-specific probe. Lane 1, size standard *Staphylococcus aureus* NCTC 8325; lane 2, negative control PAO1; lane 3, parent isolate PA42; lane 4, mutant 711M; lane 5, mutant 712M; lane 6, mutant 714M; lane 7, mutant 811M; lane 8, mutant 922M; lane 9, mutant 924M; lane 10, mutant 925M; lane 11, mutant 927M.

Table S1 Primers used in this study.

Acknowledgments

We thank Richard Goering for his contribution to the collection and interpretation of data.

Author Contributions

Conceived and designed the experiments: RCF NDH. Performed the experiments: RCF. Analyzed the data: RCF NDH. Contributed reagents/materials/analysis tools: NDH. Wrote the paper: RCF NDH.

References

1. George AM, Jones PM, Middleton PG (2009) Cystic fibrosis infections: Treatment strategies and prospects. FEMS Microbiol Lett. 300: 153–164. doi: 10.1111/j.1574-6968.2009.01704.x.
2. Lister PD, Wolter DJ, Hanson ND (2009) Antibacterial-resistant *Pseudomonas aeruginosa*: Clinical impact and complex regulation of chromosomally encoded resistance mechanisms. Clin Microbiol Rev. 22: 582–610. doi:10.1128/CMR.00040-09.
3. Carmeli Y, Troillet N, Eliopoulos GM, Samore MH (1999) Emergence of antibiotic-resistant *Pseudomonas aeruginosa*: Comparison of risks associated with different antipseudomonal agents. Antimicrob Agents Chemother 43: 1379–1382.
4. Lepper PM, Grusa E, Reichl H, Hoqel J, Trautmann M (2002) Consumption of imipenem correlates with beta-lactam resistance in *Pseudomonas aeruginosa*. Antimicrob Agents Chemother 46: 2920–2925. doi: 10.1128/AAC.46.9.2920-2925.2002.
5. Andrade SS, Jones RN, Gales AC, Sader HS (2003) Increasing prevalence of antimicrobial resistance among *Pseudomonas aeruginosa* isolates in latin american medical centres: 5 year report of the SENTRY antimicrobial surveillance program (1997–2001). J Antimicrob Chemother 52: 140–141. doi: 10.1093/jac/dkg270.
6. Cao B, Wang H, Sun H, Zhu Y, Chen M (2004) Risk factors and clinical outcomes of nosocomial multi-drug resistant *Pseudomonas aeruginosa* infections. J Hosp Infect 57: 112–118. doi:10.1016/j.jhin.2004.03.021.
7. Hsueh PR, Chen WH, Luh KT (2005) Relationships between antimicrobial use and antimicrobial resistance in Gram-negative bacteria causing nosocomial infections from 1991–2003 at a university hospital in Taiwan. Int J Antimicrob Agents 26: 463–472. doi:10.1016/j.ijantimicag.2005.08.016.
8. Fujimura S, Nakano Y, Sato T, Shirahata K, Watanabe A (2007) Relationship between the usage of carbapenem antibiotics and the incidence of imipenem-resistant *Pseudomonas aeruginosa*. J Infect Chemother 13: 147–150. doi: 10.1007/s10156-007-0507-x.
9. Pluss-Suard C, Pannatier A, Kronenberg A, Muhlemann K, Zanetti G (2013) Impact of antibiotic use on carbapenem resistance in *Pseudomonas aeruginosa*: Is there a role for antibiotic diversity? Antimicrob Agents Chemother doi:10.1128/AAC.01348-12.
10. Kohler T, Michea-Hamzehpour M, Epp SF, Pechere JC (1999) Carbapenem activities against *Pseudomonas aeruginosa*: Respective contributions of OprD and efflux systems. Antimicrob Agents Chemother 43: 424–427.
11. Livermore DM (2002) Of *Pseudomonas*, porins, pumps and carbapenems. J Antimicrob Chemother. 47: 247–250.

12. Ochs MM, McCusker MP, Bains M, Hancock REW (1999) Negative regulation of the *Pseudomonas aeruginosa* outer membrane porin OprD selective for imipenem and basic amino acids. Antimicrob Agents Chemother 43: 1085–1090.
13. Pai H, Kim J-W, Kim J, Lee JH, Choe KW, et al. (2001) Carbapenem resistance mechanisms in *Pseudomonas aeruginosa* clinical isolates. Antimicrob Agents Chemother 45: 480–484.
14. Pirnay JP, De Vos D, Mossialos D, Vanderkelen A, Cornelis P, et al. (2002) Analysis of the *Pseudomonas aeruginosa oprD* gene from clinical and environmental isolates. Environ Microbiol 4: 872–882.
15. Wolter DJ, Hanson ND, Lister PD (2004) Insertional inactivation of *oprD* in clinical isolates of *Pseudomonas aeruginosa* leading to carbapenem resistance. FEMS Microbiol Lett 236: 137–143.
16. Evans JC, Segal H (2007) A novel insertion sequence, ISPA26, in *oprD* of *Pseudomonas aeruginosa* is associated with carbapenem resistance. Antimicrob Agents Chemother 51: 3776–3777.
17. Diene SM, L'homme T, Bellulo S, Stremler N, Dubus J, et al. (2013) IS*Pa*46, a novel insertion sequence in the *oprD* porin gene of an imipenem-resistant *Pseudomonas aeruginosa* isolate from a cystic fibrosis patient in marseille, France. Int J Antimicrob Agents 42: 268–271.
18. Boutoille D, Corvec S, Caroff N, Giraudea C, Espaze E, et al. (2004) Detection of an IS21 insertion sequence in the *mexR* gene of *Pseudomonas aeruginosa* increasing beta-lactam resistance. FEMS Microbiol Lett. 230: 143–146.
19. Depardieu F, Podglajen I, Leclercq R, Collatz E, Courvalin P (2007) Modes and modulations of antibiotic resistance gene expression. Clin Microbiol Rev 20: 79–114. doi: 10.1128/CMR.00015-06.
20. Clinical and Laboratory Standards Institute (2012) Performance Standards for Antimicrobial Susceptibility Testing: Twenty-Second Informational Supplement. CLSI document M100-S22. CLSI, Wayne, PA, USA.
21. Schmidtke AJ, Hanson ND (2006) Model system to evaluate the effect of *ampD* mutations on AmpC-mediated beta-lactam resistance. Antimicrob Agents Chemother 50: 2030–2037. doi:10.1128/AAC.01458-05.
22. Wolter DJ, Black JA, Lister PD, Hanson ND (2009) Multiple genotypic changes in hypersusceptible strains of *Pseudomonas aeruginosa* isolated from cystic fibrosis patients do not always correlate with the phenotype. J Antimicrob Chemother 64: 294–300. doi: 10.1093/jac/dkp185. Epub 2009 May 25.
23. Wolter DJ, Smith-Moland E, Goering RV, Hanson ND, Lister PD (2004) Multidrug resistance associated with *mexXY* expression in clinical isolates of *Pseudomonas aeruginosa* from a Texas hospital. Diagn Microbiol Infect Dis 50: 43–50.
24. Goering R, Ribot E, Gerner-Smidt P (2011) Pulsed-field gel electrophoresis: Laboratory and epidemiologic considerations for interpretation of data. In: Persing D, Tenover F, Tang Y, et al, editors. Molecular Microbiology. Washington, DC: ASM. p. 167–177.
25. Sambrook J, Russell D (2001) Molecular Cloning – A Laboratory Manual. Cold Spring Harbor, NY: Cold Spring Harbor Laboratory Press.
26. Woodruff WA, Hancock RE (1989) *Pseudomonas aeruginosa* outer membrane protein F: Structural role and relationship to the *Escherichia coli* OmpA protein. J Bacteriol 171: 3304–3309.
27. Rawling EG, Brinkman FS, Hancock RE (1998) Roles of the carboxy-terminal half of *Pseudomonas aeruginosa* major outer membrane protein OprF in cell shape, growth in low-osmolarity medium, and peptidoglycan association. J Bacteriol 180: 3556–3562.
28. Freulet-Marriere MA, El Hamel C, Chevalier S, Dé E, Molle G, et al. (2000) Evidence for association of lipopolysaccharide with *Pseudomonas fluorescens* strain MF0 porin OprF. Res Microbiol 151: 873–876. doi.org/10.1016/S0923-2508(00)01154-2.
29. Ruiz-Martinez L, Lopez-Jimenez L, d'Ostuni V, Fuste E, Vinuesa T, et al. (2011) A mechanism of carbapenem resistance due to a new insertion element (ISPa133) in *Pseudomonas aeruginosa*. Int Microbiol 14: 51–58.
30. Sakyo S, Tomita H, Tanimoto K, Fujimoto S, Ike Y (2006) Potency of carbapenems for the prevention of carbapenem-resistant mutants of *Pseudomonas aeruginosa*: The high potency of a new carbapenem doripenem. J Antibiot (Tokyo) 59: 220–228. doi:10.1038/ja.2006.31.
31. Kresse AU, Blocker H, Romling U (2006) ISPa20 advances the individual evolution of *Pseudomonas aeruginosa* clone C subclone C13 strains isolated from cystic fibrosis patients by insertional mutagenesis and genomic rearrangements. Arch Microbiol 185: 245–254. doi: 10.1007/s00203-006-0089-5.
32. Doumith M, Ellington MJ, Livermore DM, Woodford N (2009) Molecular mechanisms disrupting porin expression in ertapenem-resistant *Klebsiella* and *Enterobacter spp.* clinical isolates from the UK. J Antimicrob Chemother 63: 659–667. doi: 10.1093/jac/dkp029.

A novel *Pseudomonas aeruginosa* Bacteriophage, Ab31, a Chimera Formed from Temperate Phage PAJU2 and *P. putida* Lytic Phage AF: Characteristics and Mechanism of Bacterial Resistance

Libera Latino[1,2], Christiane Essoh[1,2], Yann Blouin[1,2], Hoang Vu Thien[3], Christine Pourcel[1,2]*

1 Univ Paris-Sud, Institut de Génétique et Microbiologie, UMR 8621, Orsay, France, **2** CNRS, Orsay, France, **3** Hôpital Armand Trousseau, Assistance Publique-Hôpitaux de Paris (APHP), Bactériologie, Paris, France

Abstract

A novel temperate bacteriophage of *Pseudomonas aeruginosa,* phage vB_PaeP_Tr60_Ab31 (alias Ab31) is described. Its genome is composed of structural genes related to those of lytic *P. putida* phage AF, and regulatory genes similar to those of temperate phage PAJU2. The virion structure resembles that of phage AF and other lytic *Podoviridae* (*S. enterica* Epsilon 15 and *E. coli* phiv10) with similar tail spikes. Ab31 was able to infect *P. aeruginosa* strain PA14 and two genetically related strains called Tr60 and Tr162, out of 35 diverse strains from cystic fibrosis patients. Analysis of resistant host variants revealed different phenotypes, including induction of pigment and alginate overproduction. Whole genome sequencing of resistant variants highlighted the existence of a large deletion of 234 kbp in two strains, encompassing a cluster of genes required for the production of CupA fimbriae. Stable lysogens formed by Ab31 in strain Tr60, permitted the identification of the insertion site. During colonization of the lung in cystic fibrosis patients, *P. aeruginosa* adapts by modifying its genome. We suggest that bacteriophages such as Ab31 may play an important role in this adaptation by selecting for bacterial characteristics that favor persistence of bacteria in the lung.

Editor: Mark J. van Raaij, Centro Nacional de Biotecnologia - CSIC, Spain

Funding: LL holds a PhD fellowship co-financed by the Direction Générale de l'Armement (DGA) and by the Paris Saclay "Initiative d'excellence" (IDEX). The funders had no role in study design, data collection and analysis, decision to publish, or preparation of the manuscript.

Competing Interests: The authors have declared that no competing interests exist.

* E-mail: christine.pourcel@u-psud.fr

Introduction

Cystic fibrosis (CF) is one of the most common life-threatening, autosomal recessive genetic diseases in Caucasian children. This is due to mutations that occur in a single gene encoding the CF transmembrane regulator. The life expectancy of CF patients is above all related to the development of lung disease: the persistence of abundant mucous secretion in the lungs leads to chronic coughing at a young age, followed by frequent lung infections [1]. The microorganisms that colonize the CF patients' lungs belong to various bacterial genera. For 30% of CF patients, the predominant bacterial species during early life is *Staphylococcus aureus*, whereas in early adolescence, chronical infection with *Pseudomonas aeruginosa* is common: up to 80% of adult CF patients are colonized by this pathogen [2]. Later during colonization of the lungs, non-motile, anaerobic, mucoid variants of *P. aeruginosa* form a biofilm, a structure that confers resistance to several antimicrobial agents [3]. Usually, the microorganisms account for less than 10% of the dry weight of the biofilm, while 90% is composed of bacterially-produced extracellular polymeric substances (EPS) that form a matrix in which the bacterial cells are embedded [4].

The most abundant component of the EPS produced by *P. aeruginosa* is a polyanionic alginate, a copolymer of mannuronic and glucuronic acids [5]. Typically, *P. aeruginosa* mucoid strains arise in the lungs of CF patients due to mutations in the *mucA* gene or when MucA is degraded by regulated intramembrane proteolysis [6]. Conversion of non-mucoid *P. aeruginosa* strains to mucoid variants can also be the consequence of selective pressure operated by bacteriophages [7,8]. Recent studies have shown that bacteriophages can drive the emergence of numerous variants with enhanced virulence potential [9,10].

The majority of *Pseudomonas* tailed phages belong to the order Caudovirales with three main families. Strictly lytic phages are found among the *Myoviridae* with a long contractile tail, and the *Podoviridae* with a short tail, whereas members of the *Siphoviridae* are temperate phages, implying the possibility to undergo lytic or lysogenic interactions with their host [11]. The most striking feature emerging from phage genome comparative analyses is that they are extensively mosaic, with different segments having distinct evolutionary histories. A simple general explanation is that horizontal genetic exchanges play a dominant role in shaping these genome architectures [12,13]. Gene modules are exchanged using host- or phage-encoded recombination machinery. Although some phages can switch host using different mechanisms, the host preferences represent a significant barrier to genetic exchange. Moreover, phages infecting a common host can also exhibit substantial diversity, creating additional barriers to genetic exchange [12,13]. Horizontal gene transfer and the pattern of vertical, divergent evolution of phage genomes has led to the definition of different phage genera, and consequently, to a classification based on criteria related to phage genome organization and replication strategy [11]. Despite rapid phage evolution and the short generation time, viral genomes can be stably maintained over ecologically significant time and distance, and this allows their classification. Viral species can be identified and they appear to be globally widespread. Indeed, related members of specific genera with sequence identity up to 99%, can be isolated from different habitats across the globe [14,15]. The part of the phage genome that varies greatly within each genus is confined to genes encoding the metabolic conversion proteins (early region) and the tail spikes, indicating a local adaptation necessary to infect specific hosts in specific environmental conditions.

In the present study we describe a new phage, vB_PaeP_-Tr60_Ab31, whose genome is the result of recombination between two phages belonging to two different families. This phage exerts a selective pressure on *P. aeruginosa*, which could be deleterious to chronically infected patients.

Materials and Methods

Ethics Statement

The present project is in compliance with the Helsinki Declaration (Ethical Principles for Medical Research Involving Human Subjects). Strains were collected from sputum as part of the patients' usual care, without any additional sampling. The ethic committee "Comité Consultatif pour la Protection des Personnes dans la Recherche Biomédicale (CCPPRB) Ile-De-France", who was consulted, specifically approved this study, and declared that patient informed consent was not needed.

Bacterial Strains

The two reference *P. aeruginosa* strains UCBPP-PA14 [16] and PAO1 [17] were purchased from the "Collection de l'Institut Pasteur" (CIP, Paris, France), and C50 was a gift of U. Römling (Karolinska Institute, Sweden) [18]. The other strains were isolated from sputum of French CF patients, and were previously genotyped using Variable number of tandem repeats (VNTR) analysis (MLVA) [19,20]. Strains were considered to belong to the same clonal complex when they shared at least 10 VNTR size alleles out of 15. Serological typing was performed using 4 polyvalent and 16 monovalent antisera (Bio-Rad), as described [21]. Briefly, the slide agglutination procedure was performed on 24 h cultures of *P. aeruginosa*: one loop (0.01 ml) of bacterial culture (approximately 3×10^6 CFU) was mixed with one drop (0.01 ml) of each antiserum (firstly the four polyvalent sera, then the four monovalent sera, corresponding to the positive polyvalent serum). The slide was gently shaken with a rotary movement, and the mixture was examined with the naked eye over a dark surface. A positive reaction was defined as the appearance of agglutination in a maximum of 2 min.

Phage Amplification and Purification

Phages were amplified on fresh LB agar plates at a ratio of 1 phage for 1000 bacteria. An overnight culture of bacteria grown in LB medium was concentrated 10 times in saline magnesium (SM) phage buffer (50 mM Tris-HCl pH 7.5, 100 mM NaCl, 8.1 mM $MgSO_4$, 0.01% gelatin). Phages were added and, after 15 min of incubation at room temperature, the mixture was poured onto a round plate together with 4 ml of soft agar. After complete bacterial lysis ($\approx$ 8 h), 5 ml of SM phage buffer supplemented with a drop of chloroform were added to the recovered soft agar, containing phage particles. After centrifugation, the supernatant was filtered through a 0.22-µm pore size membrane, and kept at 4°C.

Small Drop and Double Agar Plate Assay

For the small drop assay, 50 µl of 10X concentrated *P. aeruginosa* overnight culture were added to 4 ml molten soft agar (0.7%), and poured over an LB agar plate. Then, 10 µl of serially diluted test lysate were spotted onto the bacterial lawn. For the double agar plaque assay, a mixture of 50 µl of bacterial suspension and 10 µl of phages at ten-fold serial dilutions was kept for 15 min at room temperature, and then poured onto a solid agar plate with 4 ml of soft agar. Plates were inverted and incubated overnight at 37°C.

Liquid Infection

LB medium (10 ml), supplemented with 10 mM $CaCl_2$, was inoculated at 2.5% with an overnight culture of the indicator strain, and incubated at 37°C. When an OD_{600} of 0.6 was reached, phage suspensions at different multiplicities of infection (M.O.I.) were added. The OD_{600} was periodically measured, and when a significant reduction of the culture density was recorded, 50 µl of chloroform were added in order to facilitate bacterial lysis and release of phages. The suspension was centrifuged at 2,500×*g* for 10 min at 4°C to eliminate bacterial debris, and the supernatant was filtered through a 0.22 µm filter.

Electron Microscopy Examination

Phage preparations were stained with 2% potassium phosphotungstate (pH 7.0), and then visualized using an EM208S transmission electron microscope (FEI, Eindhoven, The Netherlands) operating at 80 kV.

Isolation of Resistant Bacteria

Putative resistant bacteria were isolated by simply picking bacterial colonies growing inside the lysis zone of a small drop assay, and streaking them onto new plates. Putative resistant bacteria were also recovered at the end of the liquid infections, by directly streaking 1 µl of the phage-bacterial mixture on a solid agar plate. Up to twenty colonies were picked and challenged with phages through the small drop assay. Some of them were susceptible to phage Ab31, and were thereafter called "non-resistant". Thermolysates of both resistant and non-resistant strains were prepared by resuspending a colony in 100 µl of water, heating at 95°C for 10 min, followed by cooling on ice for 5 min. Centrifugation was performed at 2,500×*g* for 10 min at 4°C to pellet cell debris, and 2 µl of the supernatant were used for PCR amplification.

Phage DNA Purification

Phage DNA was purified using a rapid method adapted from [22], as described in [14]. Briefly, phages were amplified on fresh LB agar plates for 8 h at 37°C, then 5 ml of SM buffer were added to the plate, followed by overnight incubation at 4°C. The buffer was transferred to a tube, and bacterial debris were pelleted by centrifugation at 2,500×*g* for 10 min at 4°C. A mixture of 0.2 ml 2 M Tris-HCl pH 7.5, 0.4 ml 0.5 M EDTA, 0.2 ml 10% SDS and 10 µl diethylpyrocarbonate was added to 4 ml of supernatant. Following incubation at 65°C for 30 min, the tube was cooled on ice, and 1 ml of 5 M KOH was added. After 1 h incubation on ice, centrifugation was performed at 25,000×*g* for 20 min at 4°C. DNA contained in the supernatant was precipitated with 2 vol of absolute ethanol, pelleted by centrifugation, washed twice with 70% ethanol, dried and dissolved in 0.4 ml of TE buffer (10 mM

Tris-HCl pH 7.5, 1 mM EDTA). Bacterial DNA was purified using the classical CTAB (cetyl-trimethylammonium bromide)-phenol extraction method as described [19]. Purified DNA was resuspended in TE buffer. The quality and concentration of DNA was measured using a ND-1000 Spectrophotometer (NanoDrop®, Labtech, Palaiseau, France).

Sequencing

Whole genome sequencing was performed by the CNRS sequencing facility in Gif sur Yvette (IMAGIF) using the Illumina platform (Illumina Genome Analyzer IIx). Assembly of short sequence reads was performed using BioNumerics tools (Applied Maths, Sint-Martens-Latem, Belgium) as described [14]. The phage genome was annotated automatically using the BaSyS annotation tools [23]. Bacterial genome contigs were annotated using BioNumerics annotation tools. Detailed methods are available on the website http://bacteriophages.igmors.u-psud.fr.

The annotated Ab31 phage sequence has been deposited at EMBL-EBI under accession number HG798806. Total reads of bacterial genome sequences have been deposited at EMBL-EBI under accession number PRJEB5001.

PCR Detection of Phage DNA

Oligonucleotides selected to test for the presence of phage DNA in resistant bacteria and to analyze the deletions in bacterial genomes, are listed in Table 1. PCR was performed using purified DNA and Taq polymerase as recommended by the supplier (VWR, Strasbourg France). PCR products were analyzed on 2% agarose gels in 0.5X TBE buffer.

Results

Ab31 Virulence Spectrum

P. aeruginosa phage vB_PaeP_Tr60_Ab31, subsequently called Ab31, was isolated in Abidjan (Ivory Coast) as part of a study to determine the phage diversity in waste water of this city [Essoh *et al.* submitted]. Ab31 was originally enriched on *P. aeruginosa* strain PA14, and subsequently amplified in this strain or in Tr60 (both of serotype O10). A total of 36 *P. aeruginosa* strains were tested for their susceptibility to the phage, including strains from the most frequently encountered clonal complexes in CF patients, PA14 and C50 [24], and reference strain PAO1 (Table 2). Six strains were shown to belong to the PA14 clonal complex (Tr60, Tr162, C7-11, C5-17, C9-12 and C8-12), and seven strains (Tr60, Tr162, C1-3, C3-1, C3-11, C4-14 and C9-5) were of serotype O10. The latter strains were selected in case the host O antigen would serve as a receptor for the phage, as described for *Vibrio cholera* phage VP4 [25]. Ab31 was responsible for complete lysis of Tr60 and Tr162, two non-mucoid strains with the same genotype, isolated from two CF patients at a one year interval, in the same hospital [19]. With the other strains no significant signs of lysis were detected.

Table 1. List of primers used for PCR amplification.

Phage Ab31	
Ab31-Reg1-F	GACTCAGACCACTGAGATGA
Ab31-Reg1-R	ACGTGTTGGCAGTTGTAGAA
Ab31-Term-F	TACAACGCGGATATCCGTGT
Ab31-Term-R	TGCTCCCTCTGATGGACAAA
P. aeruginosa	
PaTr60_Del22kb_F	TCATCCACTGTACGCCGCCG
PaTr60_Del22kb_R	CCGTTCCTGATGCTCGACCAGT
PaTr60_Del11kb_F	GACCATGACCTTGTCGCCAT
PaTr60_Del11kb_R	AGGAGGAAATGGGTGCGGAA
Porin1_PaerDel234_F	GAAATAGAGATTGCGCAGGC
Porin1_PaerDel234_R	CACCTTCGACGAGAGACACA
CupA_Paer_F	AGGATCGTCGGCGAGTAGTA
CupA_Paer_R	CTCTATAGCGGCTACTACAC
Porin2_PaerDel234_F	CTCAAGGACATCTACCGACA
Porin2_PaerDel234_R	AAGTCGCCGATCTGGATGAA
PaerDel234_Flank_F	TCCATCGCCTGCATGGCTTC
PaerDel234_Flank_R	CGGCATAACTTCAATCAGGC

Phage Characteristics

The morphology of phage Ab31 was determined by transmission electron microscopy (Fig. 1). The phage possesses an icosahedral head with a diameter of approximately 60 nm, and a short non-contractile tail. Moreover, the subterminal tail spikes were similar to those of phage AF of *P. putida* [26].

Infections in solid agar plates and in liquid medium were performed to analyse the Ab31 multiplication characteristics. When a phage suspension was analyzed on indicator strains using the double agar plaque assays, small clear plaques without a halo were observed. Dot assay revealed a clear zone with only a few small resistant colonies. Since it was known that many phages require $CaCl_2$ to adsorb on the bacterial surface, the infection in liquid medium was performed using LB supplemented or not with 10 mM of $CaCl_2$. Upon infection at an M.O.I. of 0.01, in the presence of 10 mM $CaCl_2$, production of PFUs was stimulated 100-fold. In these conditions, the adsorption time was 4 min and the burst size was 30–50 phages per cell.

Infection in liquid LB medium at an M.O.I. of 0.1 never led to a complete clearing of the bacterial culture (Fig. 2), but we observed that not all the bacteria that survived after infection were resistant, when later challenged with Ab31. This resembles the phenomenon of persistence, in which a subset of an isogenic bacterial population occurring within a susceptible population, tolerates antibiotics [27].

Interestingly, we observed that phage infection led to a change in color of the bacterial culture from yellowish-green to green. It is likely that the presence of the phage affects the production of the pyoverdine, a virulence factor of *P. aeruginosa* [28].

Genome Characteristics

The Ab31 genome encompasses 45,550 bp, and the overall GC-content is ≈ 57%, which is lower than that of the *P. aeruginosa* PA14 genome (66.3% G+C), a characteristic shared by other *P. aeruginosa* phages [29]. Comparing the virtual gel obtained by *in silico* restriction endonuclease analysis with the experimental restriction enzyme banding pattern (Fig. 3), it was possible to establish that Ab31 DNA is apparently circular. Indeed, the number of fragments expected from *in silico* digestion of the circular Ab31 DNA with *Eco*RI, *Hind*III, *Sma*I, *Ssp*I, *Cla*I, *Sal*I and *Sph*I was 17, 12, 12, 6, 18, 23 and 19 respectively, perfectly matched, in number and in size, with the bands obtained by experimental agarose electrophoresis. Ab31 DNA digestion using *Not*I and *Pvu*II, from which 3 and 2 fragments, respectively, were expected using *in silico* digestion analysis, produced many faint bands in addition to the expected ones. This phenomenon, which

Table 2. List of the strains used and susceptibility to Ab31.

Strain	Description	Serotype[a]	Source or reference	Ab31 growth[b]
PA14	Sequenced	10	[16]	C+++
PAO1	Sequenced	5	[17]	0
C50	Clone C	UN	[18]	0
Tr60	PA14-clone	10	[19]	C+++
Tr162	PA14-clone	10	[19]	C+++
C7-11	PA14-clone	15	[14,20]	trace
C5-17	PA14-clone	17	[14,20]	0
C9-12	PA14-clone	17	[14,20]	0
C8-12	PA14-clone	6	[14,20]	trace
C1-1		5	[14,20]	0
C1-2		3	[14,20]	0
C1-3		10	[14,20]	0
C1-11	Mucoid	15	[14,20]	trace
C1-14		1	[14,20]	0
C2-10		4	[14,20]	0
C2-18		12	[14,20]	0
C3-1		10	[14,20]	0
C3-2		13	[14,20]	trace
C3-11		10	[14,20]	0
C3-15		17	[14,20]	0
C3-16		1	[14,20]	0
C3-18		16	[14,20]	0
C3-19		6	[14,20]	0
C4-14		10	[14,20]	0
C5-2		17	[14,20]	0
C5-13		17	[14,20]	0
C7-6		3	[14,20]	0
C8-5		5	[14,20]	0
C8-7		12	[14,20]	0
C8-14		1	[14,20]	0
C8-15	Mucoid	1	[14,20]	0
C8-20		2	[14,20]	0
C9-5		10	[14,20]	0
C9-11		17	[14,20]	0
C9-17		17	[14,20]	0
C10-5		UN	[14,20]	0

[a]UN, unknown.
[b]5 μL of Ab31 stock suspension (≈ 10^8 PFU/ml) were spotted on *P. aeruginosa* lawns. C+++, complete clearing; trace, a few individual plaques; 0, a turbid spot where the pipette tip touched the agar.

was observed repeatedly, indicates the existence of a non-specific digestion also called relaxed sequence recognition or star activity [30].

Overall the Ab31 genome did not align with any known phage sequence. However, at the nucleotide level it showed some rare regions of homology with structural genes of phage AF [26] and of a prophage of *P. putida* GB-1 strain [CP000926-1] (up to 70% DNA-DNA similarity), and with genes involved in replication in phage PAJU2 [31] (from 85 to 97%). At the protein level it was possible to observe additional similarities with AF (shown in red on Fig. 4) and PAJU2 (shown in blue in Fig. 4). AF and PAJU2 are two lambdoid phages whose genomes are respectively 42,689 bp and 46,872 bp long. Attempts to localize the genome ends by PCR analysis were not successful, as expected if the genome adopts a circular configuration. Therefore we were not able to determine the position of the first nucleotide, and we decided to assign it by comparison with the related phage AF.

In the Ab31 genome, 69 putative "open reading frames" (ORFs) were identified. Thirty five ORFs were transcribed on the positive strand (Fig. 4). On the basis of sequence similarity comparisons in the GenBank database, 25 ORFs could be assigned to putative functions. The majority of the other ORFs

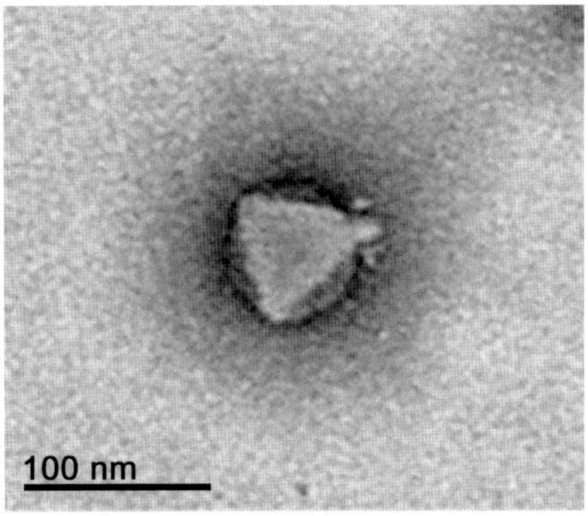

Figure 1. Electron microscopy analysis of phage Ab31. Scale bar represents 100 nm.

exhibited similarity to uncharacterized bacterial or phage proteins. No tRNA genes were predicted.

Nucleotide position 1 was 60 bp upstream of the ATG codon of a putative protein containing a Helix Turn Helix domain, and sharing similarities with the small terminase subunit encoded by *Escherichia coli* phage phiv10 [32] and *Salmonella enterica* phage epsilon 15 [33]. A putative phage large terminase subunit, encoded immediately downstream of the predicted first coding sequence, shared similarities (maximal identity of 77%, E-value lower than e-200) with a prophage-encoded sequence located within the *S. enterica* serovar Wandsworth str. A4-580 genome. The terminase genes constitute the packaging module typically located at the beginning of the so-called late region of the phage genome. A large part of the late region usually encodes the morphogenesis proteins, whereas genes located in the early region are necessary to initiate the phage multiplication cycle. Following phage adsorption to the bacterial surface, early genes are injected first and, in some phages, they allow complete injection of the phage genome [34]. Phage Ab31 showed high similarity in the late region with the podovirus AF of *P. putida* and the prophage of *P. putida* strain GB-1: indeed, eight coding sequences reported in Fig. 4 resembled those of phage AF. These included the putative major capsid protein (maximal identity of 75%, E-value of 8e-180), internal virion protein B (maximal identity of 35%, E-value of 4e-6), the structural lysozyme (maximal identity of 33%, E-value of 8e-32) and the tail spike protein (maximal identity of 40%, E-value of 4e-37). Moreover, three hypothetical proteins located in the same region showed similarities with hypothetical proteins gp4, gp9 and gp12 of phage AF.

The second major block of genes of the Ab31 genome, downstream of the putative tail spike coding region, constitutes the so-called early/middle region. Twenty-three putative and hypothetical proteins encoded by genes located in this region shared similarities with the *P. aeruginosa* siphovirus PAJU2, showing maximal identity percentages that vary from 39% to 100%. This region starts with a putative acetyl-transferase sharing 46% identity with the PAJU2 acetyl-transferase (E-value lower than e-200), and a putative PAJU2-like integrase (identity 99% with PAJU2; E-value lower than e-200). Other related proteins included putative replication proteins O and P, NinB protein, phage antitermination protein Q and endolysin (Fig. 4).

Bacterial Resistance

Different conditions were used for infecting bacteria, in order to favor different resistance mechanisms. Most of the resistant and/or lysogenic bacteria were obtained from typical infection at 37°C in liquid medium of *P. aeruginosa* strains PA14, Tr60 and Tr162, at an M.O.I. of 1, 0.1 or 0.01. Some resistant Tr60 bacteria were also recovered from an infection in liquid medium performed at 42°C at an M.O.I. of 1. In this experiment the incubation was prolonged for 72 h, and the phage suspension was added each 24 h at the same M.O.I., for a total of three infections. Ab31-resistant variants of PA14 and Tr162 were also recovered from infections performed on solid agar plates at 37°C or 30°C, using a small drop plaque assay, and extending the incubation for 72 h in order to allow the growth of resistant bacteria inside the lysis zone. With the different approaches, about 80% (91 out of 114) of recovered bacteria were confirmed to be resistant to the phage. A majority of the resistant bacteria obtained from plates formed mucoid colonies, with entire margins and smooth surfaces, a particular characteristic often

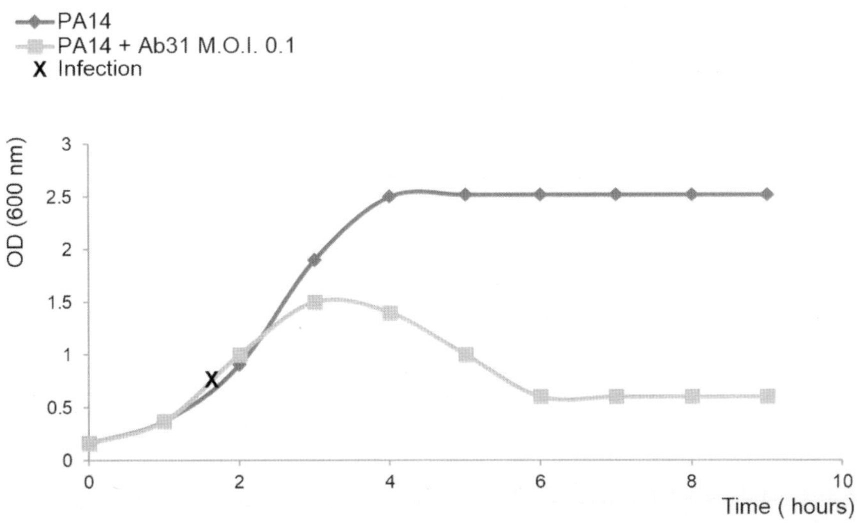

Figure 2. Growth curve of uninfected PA14 (dark grey curve) and of PA14 infected by Ab31 at an M.O.I. of 0.1 (light grey curve).

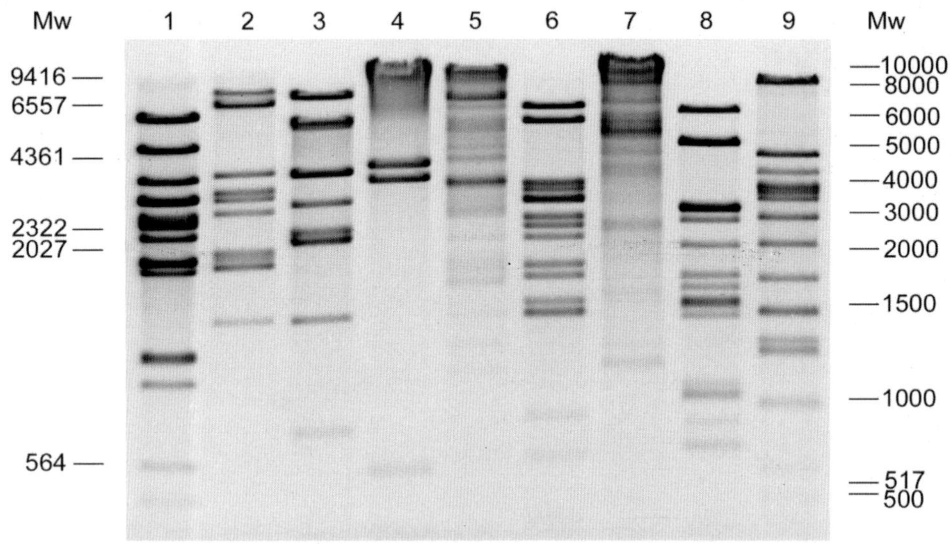

Figure 3. Restriction enzyme analysis of the Ab31 genome. Ab31 phage DNA (2 µg) digested with *EcoRI* (1), *HindIII* (2), *SmaI* (3), *SspI* (4), *NotI* (5), *ClaI* (6), *PvuII* (7), *SalI* (8) and *SphI* (9) were analyzed by electrophoresis on a 0.8% agarose gel. On the left the λDNA/*HindIII* and on the right 1 kbp ladder are reported and they were used as molecular weight markers (Mw).

observed with *P. aeruginosa* strains isolated from sputa of CF patients [Sousa, 2013 #1739]. In contrast, non-resistant bacterial strains derived from the same experiment showed a non-mucoid phenotype and shared the same morphological characteristics with the wild type uninfected bacterial strain. From infected bacteria incubated on plates at 30°C, some mucoid resistant variants showing a brown pigmentation were also isolated. Ten resistant isolates were serotyped to check whether a switch had occurred, but they were all serotype O10 like the parental strains.

In order to test for the existence of lysogens, the presence of the phage DNA was searched in the Ab31-resistant bacteria after two passages on solid agar medium. Two regions of the phage genome were amplified, designated as RegI and Term, and predicted to produce 550 bp and 600 bp long amplicons respectively. The results for some of the resistant isolates and for Ab31 phage DNA used as a control, are shown in Fig. 5. When the DNA of the resistant bacteria was amplified using the RegI (Fig. 5A) or Term primers (Fig. 5B), a band of the expected size was detected with every tested isolate except for Tr60-100A. This Ab31-resistant variant was derived from infection in liquid medium at 37°C at an M.O.I. of 0.1. All the resistant variants from solid infection were positive for phage DNA, whereas only 40% of resistant from liquid infection contained phage DNA. The isolates showing a brown pigmentation were not lysogenized.

Bacterial Genome Sequence Analysis

In order to study the basis of the resistance and to identify the possible integration site of the phage genome in the bacterial chromosome, the original Tr60 strain and four Ab31 resistant variants were chosen for whole genome sequencing. Tr60-10A and Tr60-100B were two putative lysogenic bacteria derived from infection in liquid medium at an M.O.I. of 1 and 0.1, respectively. Tr60-100A was a non-lysogenic isolate derived from infection in liquid medium performed at an M.O.I. of 0.1. PA14-P1 was a putative lysogenic bacteria. Tr60-10A and Tr60-100A showed a mucoid phenotype. The bacterial draft genomes were assembled and partially annotated using *P. aeruginosa* PA14 as a reference [16,35].

Upon alignment of the sequenced genomes, two deletions were found in the *P. aeruginosa* Tr60 genome as compared to that of PA14. The first deletion encompassed approximately 22 kbp (coordinates 1919495 to 1941370). It started with 2.5 kbp of DNA of unknown function and ended inside a gene encoding a pirin-like protein (ORF PA14_22080 to ORF PA14_22280), and also contained genes for a resolvase and a recombinase. The second deletion encompassed approximately 11 kbp, and covered exactly the sequence of the Pf1 prophage of *P. aeruginosa* PA14 (Genbank: AY324828). Both deletions were identified in Tr60, in all Tr60 variants that were sequenced and in the genome of reference strain PAO1. The existence of the two deletions was confirmed by PCR in Tr60 and its Ab31-resistant variants using primers localised in the flanking regions (Table 1; Fig. 6). The deletions were also observed in Tr162 and in PAO1, as expected. In addition to the two deleted regions, approximately 215 "single nucleotide polymorphisms" (SNPs) were found when the genome sequences of Tr60 and PA14 were compared.

We then looked at the differences between Tr60 and its Ab31-resistant variants. A deletion of about 234 kbp was found in Tr60-10A and Tr60-100A, two mucoid variants obtained from different infections performed with the same Tr60 bacterial culture. Using *P. aeruginosa* PA14 as a reference genome, 175 coding sequences were found to lie within this region (Table 3, genome coordinates approximately 3190870 and 3424480 in PA14). Some of these coded for enzymes involved in amino acid uptake or biosynthesis, for glucose metabolism and for transmembrane proteins. No homologous genes were found in the other regions of the bacterial genome except for the porins. A cluster of five genes involved in the CupA fimbrial organelle assembly was possibly relevant to phage resistance: the chaperone CupA1, the fimbrial subunit CupA2, the usher CupA3, CupA4, an atypical adhesin, and the chaperone CupA5 [36]. Primer pairs were selected within this region (in two porin-encoding genes and in the *cupA4* gene), and in the flanking sequences, in order to confirm the existence of the deletion by PCR amplification. When amplification was performed with primers localised inside the region of deletion, an amplicon was observed for all the samples tested except for Tr60-10A and Tr60-100A (the result for *cupA* is shown on Fig. 7A). In

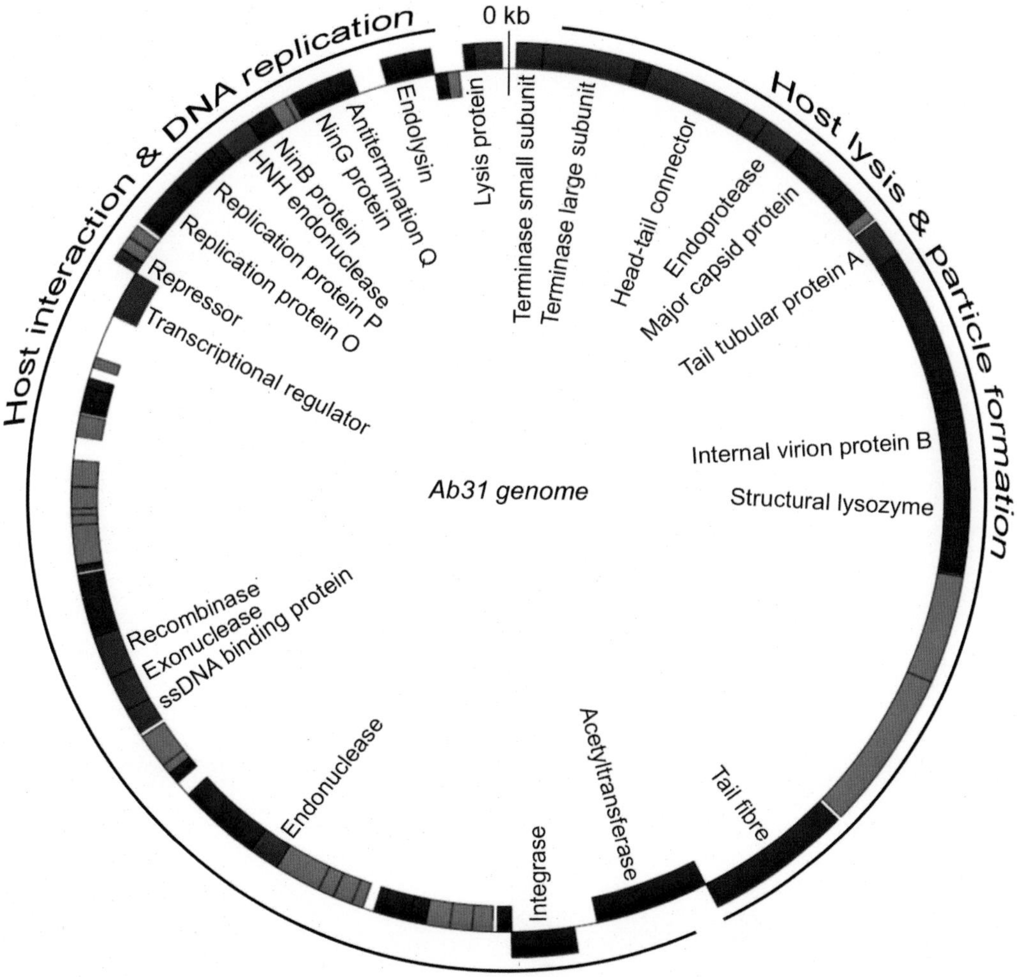

Figure 4. Annotation of the Ab31 genome. The Ab31 hypothetical terminal ends are at the 1 position. The morphogenesis module includes proteins similar to those encoded by phage AF (red), whereas the replication, recombination and lysis modules consist of genes similar to those of phage PAJU2 (blue). Genes encoding hypothetical proteins which have homologies with other phages are shown in purple color. Genes encoding hypothetical proteins of unknown function are shown in green color.

contrast, amplification with the Flank234 primers, localised on both sides of the deleted region, produced a 600 bp amplicon only for Tr60-10A and Tr60-100A (Fig. 7B). In order to check whether the deletion was pre-existing in a subpopulation of the Tr60 culture before phage infection, 94 bacterial colonies were picked and PCR was performed on thermolysates with the Flank 234 and porin primers. The results showed that none of the isolates were deleted for the 234 kbp region (data not shown).

Compared to Tr60, Tr60-10A and Tr60-100A showed approximately the same amount of SNPs (respectively 29 and 26). The mutations occurred in the same coding sequences for both resistant bacteria. In particular, mutations were found in a

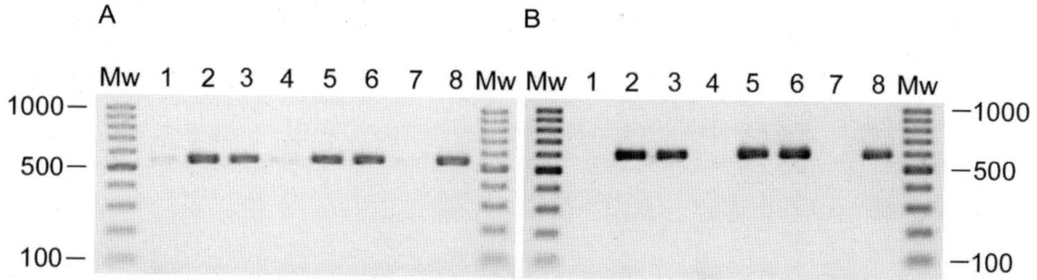

Figure 5. PCR detection of the Ab31 genome in resistant bacteria using Reg1 (A) and Term primers (B). Tr60-E (5) and PA14-P1 (6) are derived from infection on solid agar plates at 37°C and 30°C, respectively. Tr60-10A (2), Tr60-100B (3) and Tr60-100A (4) are derived from an infection assay performed at 37°C in liquid medium at an M.O.I. of 0.1. PA14 (7), Tr60 (1) and Ab31 (8) are used as negative and positive controls, respectively. Samples were run on a 2% agarose gel for 45 min at 135 V. Mw, 100 bp ladder molecular weight markers.

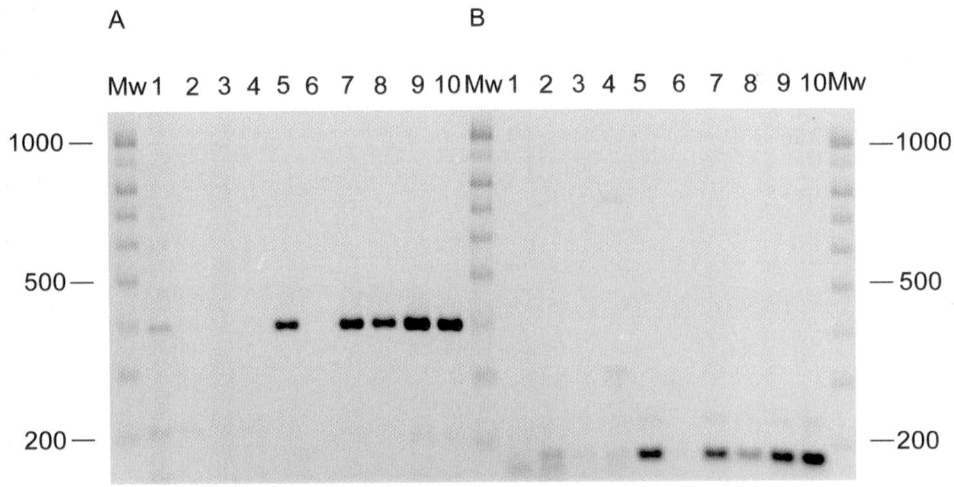

Figure 6. PCR investigation of the 11 kbp (A) and 22 kbp (B) deletions observed in Tr60. C9-12 (1), C5-17 (2), C7-11 (3), C8-12 (4), PAO1 (5), PA14 (6), Tr162 (7), Tr60 (8), Tr60-10A (9), Tr60-100A (10). Samples were run in a 2% agarose gel for 45 min at 135 V. Mw, 100 bp ladder molecular weight markers.

transcriptional regulator, in the NADH dehydrogenase I subunit F, the pyoverdine biosynthesis protein PvcA, phenazine biosynthesis protein PhzD, C32 tRNA thiolase and in an MFS transporter. Specific mutations in a gene for an Usher protein and in a gene for a lipase chaperone, were detected in Tr60-10A and Tr60-100A, respectively. The sequence of the Tr60-100B isolate was compared with that of Tr60, and no SNPs were found.

The PA14-P1 genome showed 129 SNPs as compared to PA14. They affected genes encoding the hemolysin activator, the pyochelin synthase, an RNA methyltransferase, an acetyltransferase, the pyoverdin synthase, and several membrane proteins, including multidrug efflux pumps, type III secretion system proteins and an ABC transporter.

Search for the Phage Integration Site

To identify integrated Ab31 genomes, we first searched for phage reads among the three isolates found to possess phage DNA by PCR, but they were detected only in Tr60-100B. We then looked for phage-bacteria hybrid sequences among the total reads obtained for this isolate. The hybrid reads centered on a 64 bp region found at position 4552973–4553038 in the *P. aeruginosa* PA14 genome (and also in the Tr60 genome), and at position 21471–21534 on the Ab31 genome. These regions correspond in PA14 to the serine tRNA gene (PA14_51230) localized downstream of a glycosyltransferase gene, and, in the Ab31 genome, to a region that covers part of the phage integrase and part of a non-coding sequence upstream of this gene (Fig. 8).

Discussion

Phage Ab31 is a temperate phage genomically related to both the virulent podovirus AF phage of *P. putida* and the temperate siphovirus phage PAJU2 of *P. aeruginosa*. The Ab31 virion structure resembles that of phage AF, *S. enterica* phage Epsilon 15 and *E. coli* phage phiv10, with similar spikes, previously shown to bind and cleave the O-antigen component of the host's cell surface lipopolysaccharide [37]. Some *Pseudomonas* phages can diffuse through alginate present in *Pseudomonas* biofilms [38] owing to a depolymerizing enzyme that is part of the phage particles. One of the most significant examples of such an activity has been reported for phage AF. A halo surrounds the AF plaques at 30°C, due to an EPS-degrading activity within the tail spikes [26]. We did not see such a halo around Ab31 plaques, whatever the strain used or the temperature. Alignment of the tail spike protein sequences of phage Ab31 and phage AF showed limited homology only at the N-terminus (Fig. 9). Conservation of the N-terminal part is necessary for association of the spikes with the tail structure, whereas the C-terminal part of the spike protein, involved in recognition of and binding to the cell receptor, shows the highest level of variation [39,40,41]. This finding provides evidence that bacteria and bacteriophages have co-evolved in order to overcome the barriers that are imposed by one on the other. Recent observations suggest that bacterial resistance to phages in cystic fibrosis patients evolves with the duration of colonization [42]. The infection by Ab31 causes a slight change in the colour of the bacterial culture from yellowish-green to green, as also observed with phage PAJU2 [43]. Mutation in genes for pyoverdine biosynthesis were identified in some resistant isolates, but further analyses are necessary to determine their significance.

Among the diverse strains tested, Ab31 is specific for PA14 and for Tr60 and Tr162, two strains genetically close to PA14, and isolated from French CF patients in the same hospital. Other strains belonging to the same clonal complex but isolated at other locations were found to be resistant to Ab31, as were strains with the same O serotype. Sequencing of Tr60 revealed the presence of two regions of deletion, one of which corresponds to prophage Pf1, also designated Pf5 in the PA14 genome [44]. It was previously shown that Pf4, a Pf1-like prophage in PAO1, mediated the formation of small-colony variants, and was also a factor contributing to the bacterial virulence, but this was not confirmed for Pf5 in PA14 [45,46]. The 22 kbp region corresponding to the second deletion encodes a resolvase and a recombinase, proteins that usually participate in DNA transfer.

Differences in the bacterial response to phage infection were observed in this study depending on the infection method used. From the infection on solid agar plate, clear lysis zones were observed, an indication that most cells were killed, whereas in liquid culture complete lysis was never obtained. This observation may be related to the formation of pseudolysogens after bacterial infection. The genomes of two sequenced Ab31-resistant variants (Tr60-10A and PA14-P1), shown to contain phage DNA when analysed by PCR, surprisingly did not contain phage reads. A

Table 3. List of coding sequences (CDS) and their position in the 234 kbp deleted region.

CDS	Position	Product
1	87..1418	amino acid permease
2	1482..2921	gamma-aminobutyraldehyde dehydrogenase
3	2967..4220	diaminobutyrate–2-oxoglutarate aminotransferase
4	4267.5229	dehydrogenase
5	- strand (5522..7501)	acetate permease
6	- strand (7558..9828)	acyl-CoA synthetase
7	- strand (9291..10061)	dehydrogenase
8	- strand (10058..11284)	acyl-CoA dehydrogenase
9	- strand (11634..12851)	FadE36, aminoglycoside phosphotransferase
10	12886..14838	propionate catabolism operon regulator
11	- strand (14904..15443)	hypothetical protein
12	- strand (15466..17769)	paraquat-inducible protein B
13	- strand (17762..18619)	paraquat-inducible protein A
14	- strand (19040..20638)	aldehyde dehydrogenase
15	- strand (20752..21747)	hypothetical protein
16	- strand (21775..22950)	hypothetical protein
17	- strand (22981..24408)	MFS transporter
18	- strand (24489..25907)	porin
19	- strand (25912..26925)	4-hydroxythreonine-4-phosphate dehydrogenase
20	- strand (26922..27881)	hypothetical protein
21	- strand (27874..29298)	MFS transporter
22	29301..30479	hypothetical protein
23	30464.32554	hypothetical protein
24	32544..33569	LysR family transcriptional regulator
25	33651..34127	hypothetical protein
26	34342..35232	ABC transporter substrate-binding protein
27	35313..36029	amino acid permease
28	36031..36708	amino acid ABC transporter permease
29	- strand (36724..37608)	hypothetical protein
30	- strand (37734..39329)	signal transduction protein
31	- strand (39418..40800)	dehydrogenase
32	- strand (40640..41758)	hypothetical protein
33	- strand (41808..43745)	TetR family transcriptional regulator
34	- strand (42545..44821)	hydrogen cyanide synthase HcnC
35	- strand (43801..45267)	hydrogen cyanide synthase HcnB
36	- strand (45192..45626)	hydrogen cyanide synthase HcnA
37	45789..47114	adenylate cyclase
38	- strand (47111..47767)	hypothetical protein
39	- strand (48272..49708)	carboxylate-amine ligase
40	48802..51048	hypothetical protein
41	50993..51982	hypothetical protein
42	- strand (51966..52247)	hypothetical protein
43	52256..52957	hypothetical protein
44	- strand (52961..55336)	sensor/response regulator hybrid
45	56396..56686	hypothetical protein
46	- strand (56717..57031)	hypothetical protein
47	- strand (56994..57581)	hypothetical protein
48	- strand (57371..58447)	hypothetical protein
49	- strand (59123..60370)	hypothetical protein
50	- strand (59701..60759)	hypothetical protein

Table 3. Cont.

CDS	Position	Product
51	- strand (60474..61766)	hypothetical protein
52	- strand (61900..62265)	hypothetical protein
53	62570..64174	glycogen synthase
54	64033..65925	glycosyl hydrolase
55	65918..67972	4-alpha-glucanotransferase
56	67752..70745	maltooligosyl trehalose synthase
57	71060..73210	glycosyl hydrolase
58	76155..77918	cardiolipin synthase 2
59	76625..78910	hypothetical protein
60	- strand (78912..81272)	glycogen branching protein
61	- strand (81107..84409)	trehalose synthase
62	- strand (84420..86534)	hypothetical protein
63	- strand (86558..87439)	KU domain-containing protein
64	- strand (87462..87704)	hypothetical protein
65	- strand (87718..88263)	hypothetical protein
66	- strand (88437..90566)	hydroperoxidase II
67	- strand (90647..90814)	hypothetical protein
68	91301..91711	hypothetical protein
69	- strand (91718..94156)	glycogen phosphorylase
70	- strand (94209..94496)	hypothetical protein
71	94740..94928	hypothetical protein
72	- strand (94948..95991)	short-chain dehydrogenase
73	- strand (95834..96352)	ompetence-damaged protein
74	- strand (96363..96608)	metallothionein
75	- strand (96913..99468)	ATP-dependent DNA ligase
76	- strand (99453..100118)	hypothetical protein
77	99851..100615	hypothetical protein
78	- strand (101068..102432)	transporter
79	- strand (102461..103387)	hypothetical protein
80	- strand (103126..104031)	EAL domain-containing protein
81	- strand (103980..104669)	chaperone CupA5
82	- strand (104683..108297)	fimbrial subunit CupA4
83	- strand (106041..108659)	usher
84	- strand (108643..109476)	chaperone CupA2
85	110882..112108	fimbrial subunit CupA1
86	112535..113170	hypothetical protein
87	- strand (113206..114660)	aldehyde dehydrogenase
88	- strand (114676..116313)	dehydrogenase
89	- strand (116418..117350)	LysR family transcriptional regulator
90	- strand (117387..118523)	hypothetical protein
91	118649.119554	LysR family transcriptional regulator
92	119600..120130	hypothetical protein
93	120147..121259	hypothetical protein
94	- strand (121794..122870)	O6-methylguanine-DNA methyltransferase
95	123062..124045	hypothetical protein
96	- strand (124030..124896)	hypothetical protein
97	- strand (124934..125998)	LysR family transcriptional regulator
98	126034..127413	major facilitator transporter
99	127438..128667	porin

Table 3. Cont.

CDS	Position	Product
100	128700..129443	LamB/YcsF family protein
101	129529..131091	hypothetical protein
102	131159.131635	hypothetical protein
103	- strand (131654..133426)	thiamine pyrophosphate protein
104	133525..133995	hypothetical protein
105	- strand (134394..136025)	short chain dehydrogenase
106	- strand (135137..136177)	esterase
107	- strand (136077..137552)	flavin-binding monooxygenase
108	137699..138733	AraC family transcriptional regulator
109	138861..139727	hypothetical protein
110	- strand (139729..141048)	transmembrane sensor protein
111	- strand (141294..142682)	MFS transporter
112	- strand (142477..144135)	permease
113	- strand (144849..147995)	TonB-dependent receptor
114	- strand (147592..148680)	hypothetical protein
115	- strand (148424..149845)	hypothetical protein
116	- strand (149077..150093)	hydrolase
117	- strand (150527..152425)	asparagine synthetase, glutamine-hydrolysing
118	- strand (152447..153649)	ring-hydroxylating dioxygenase, large terminal
119	- strand (153923..154405)	leucine-responsive regulatory protein
120	154451..155173	kynurenine formamidase, KynB
121	155177..156427	kynureninase
122	155773..157989	amino acid permease
123	158230..160149	hypothetical protein
124	160165..162093	hypothetical protein
125	- strand (162130..163506)	transcriptional regulator
126	163546..163755	hypothetical protein
127	163932..165599	hypothetical protein
128	- strand (165992..168586)	sensory box protein
129	- strand (168758..171127)	elongation factor G
130	171142..173784	TonB dependent receptor
131	173892..175688	carbamoyl transferase
132	175732..176895	MFS transporter
133	176840..177565	hydrolase
134	176941..178200	hypothetical protein
135	178277..180169	copper resistance protein A
136	179851..181221	copper resistance protein B
137	- strand (181241..182575)	hypothetical protein
138	- strand (182667..183848)	pyridoxal-phosphate dependent protein
139	- strand (183994..185604)	ABC transporter ATP-binding protein
140	- strand (185606..186622)	ABC transporter permease
141	- strand (186624..187697)	peptide ABC transporter permease
142	- strand (187699..189507)	ABC transporter substrate-binding protein
143	- strand (189511..192537)	TonB-dependent receptor
144	- strand (192730..193722)	LysR family transcriptional regulator
145	193773..195158	major facilitator transporter
146	- strand (195165..196064)	DNA-binding transcriptional regulator CynR
147	- strand (197377..198330)	Fe2+-dicitrate sensor, membrane protein
148	- strand (198327..199004)	RNA polymerase sigma factor

Table 3. Cont.

CDS	Position	Product
149	199037..201157	hypothetical protein
150	203113..204468	hypothetical protein
151	204410..204787	hypothetical protein
152	204854..206836	hypothetical protein
153	- strand (208017..209408)	serine/threonine transporter SstT
154	- strand (209734..211104)	amino acid permease
155	- strand (211261..212637)	glutamine synthetase
156	213047..213901	hypothetical protein
157	213157..214200	hypothetical protein
158	- strand (214325..215800)	hypothetical protein
159	- strand (215925..216731)	hypothetical protein
160	217181..218839	thiamine pyrophosphate protein
161	- strand (218847..220016)	hypothetical protein
162	- strand (219521..220477)	hypothetical protein
163	- strand (220564..222048)	transcriptional regulator
164	222029..222676	hypothetical protein
165	- strand (222751..223581)	hypothetical protein
166	- strand (223074..223547)	transcriptional regulator
167	223638..224072	hypothetical protein
168	223754..225226	bile acid/Na+ symporter family transporter
169	225251..227203	ring-cleaving dioxygenase
170	- strand (225281..226636)	glutathione reductase
171	- strand (227385..228275)	UTP-glucose-1-phosphate uridylyltransferase
172	- strand (228272..229873)	nucleotide sugar dehydrogenase
173	- strand (230015..230575)	transcriptional regulator
174	230812..232002	periplasmic multidrug efflux lipoprotein
175	232018..233901	multidrug efflux protein

possible explanation could be that the phage genome did not integrate in the bacterial chromosome but was retained in a small proportion of cells after infection. Indeed, there is evidence that some of the putative lysogenic bacteria lose the phage genome after several replatings. In contrast, Tr60-100B is a true lysogenic variant. The phage integrated within the bacterial genome through a site-specific recombination process using the shared 64 bp sequence, as shown for PAJU2 [43].

In this study, mucoid variants of *P. aeruginosa* Tr60 and PA14 were obtained after infection of the host in liquid medium. These variants were stably resistant to the phage, although they were not lysogenic. Miller *et al.* showed that temperate phages with elongated heads and flexible tails (similar to PAJU2 virions), induced from CF-associated *P. aeruginosa* strains, were capable of converting non-mucoid strains to the mucoid phenotype [8]. We may hypothesize that the presence of the phage induced a stress that caused mutations in genes involved in alginate production. An alternative explanation could be that the phage selected a subpopulation of mucoid bacteria, with the mucoid layer inhibiting early stages of infection. MucA is a negative regulator of alginate production through sequestration of AlgU, the primary sigma factor responsible for the expression of the alginate biosynthetic operon from the algD promoter [47]. Alternatively, conversion to mucoidy can occur when MucA is degraded by regulated intramembrane proteolysis operated by AlgW [6]. The activation of AlgW, and the consecutive proteolysis of MucA, is thought to be in response to extracellular stress, as well as the accumulation of misfolded envelope proteins. Interestingly, genome sequencing of two non-pigmented mucoid Ab31-resistant variants (Tr60-10A and Tr60-100A) revealed that no modifications of proteins involved in the alginate biosynthesis occurred. Among the Ab31 resistant variants we also obtained brown-colored, mucoid variants of PA14. The pigment which likely corresponds to pyomelanin, accumulated when the plates were kept at room temperature. It was shown that pyomelanin production is due to loss of the homogentisate gene, *HmgA* and this favors persistence in the lung of CF patients [48].

Notably, two mucoid variants of Tr60 carry a large deletion of 234 kbp corresponding to, among others, genes coding for proteins necessary to assemble a fimbrial organelle. This gene cluster which encodes components of the chaperone-usher pathway and a fimbrial unit, participates in biofilm formation [36,49]. Conceivably fimbriae could be involved in phage adsorption but further investigation is required to confirm or refute this hypothesis. Other deleted genes that might act as phage receptors, are those for two porins, and one being a member of the LamB/YcsF family protein. Previous studies have shown that an outer membrane porin encoded by the *ompLC* gene in *Edwardsiella*

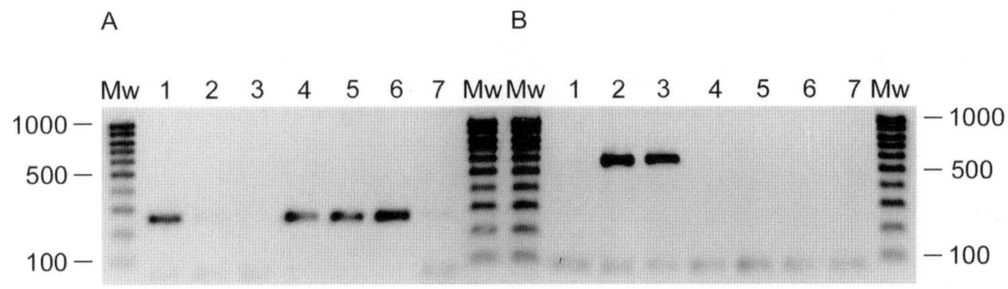

Figure 7. PCR investigation of the 234 kb deletion on Ab31 resistant bacteria using CupA (A) and Flank234 primers (B). Tr60 (1), Tr60-10A (2), Tr60-100A (3), Tr60-100B (4), PA14-P1 (5), PA14 (6), Negative control (7). The experimental conditions are those of Fig.5.

ictaluri is required for phage sensitivity [50], while LamB is the receptor for *Escherichia coli* bacteriophage λ. LamB was shown to be sufficient to confer λ phage sensitivity upon transformation of the *lamB* gene into bacteria of different species [51,52].

Since the two resistant isolates, in addition to the 234 kbp deletion, show a few nucleotide differences (≈ 40 SNPs) with Tr60, two hypotheses could be formulated to explain the origin of the deletion. It is possible that a variant subpopulation with the 234 kbp deletion preexisted in the Tr60 stock suspension, and that the phage infection led to its selection. We could not detect such variants by PCR analysis on 94 isolated colonies or on total DNA extracted from a Tr60 culture. Another possible explanation is that phage infection promoted rearrangement of the host genome. This hypothesis is supported by the finding that at both ends of the 234 kbp region present in the original Tr60 strain, there are sequences of 10 bp in length (ctcggcatga and ctcggcgatga) that differ by a single nucleotide insertion. Notably a similar sequence (c-cggcatga) was detected in the phage Ab31 genome at the end of the gene encoding an acetyl-transferase, upstream of the phage integrase. The 10 bp sequence "ctcggcgatga" constitutes the junction of the deleted region on the resistant bacterial genome. Moreover, the sequence upstream the 234 kbp region encodes several proteins involved in transposition, including a bacterial transposase. This suggests that the origin of the deletion in Tr60 was most probably a recombination and/or transposition event in which the phage was also involved. Large genomic deletions have been observed during early stage adaptation of *P. aeruginosa* in CF patients, but none were as large as 234 kbp, which represents about 3.6% of the genome [24,53]. Rau and colleagues described a deletion of 148 kbp, encompassing the *cupA* cluster [53]. It is not known whether the presence of phages could play a role in the induction of such deletions. Ab31-resistant strain PA14-P1 showed no deletion corresponding to those which characterize Tr60-10A and Tr60-100A. A number of mutations in different genes were observed, but at this time it is impossible to know which one is responsible for phage resistance.

Looking at the Ab31 genome sequence it is possible to distinguish two main modules. The first, showing homologies with the AF phage genome, covers the so-called late region and contains sequences encoding the structural proteins of the phage, such as those for capsid, tail-to-head connector, tail and tail spikes. The second Ab31 genomic region encodes proteins involved in recombination and replication of the phage genome, and constitutes the so-called early/middle region. This contains several genes that show similarities with those of PAJU2 explaining why, although phage Ab31 shows a morphology typical of the virulent AF podovirus, it behaves as a temperate phage capable of lysogenizing *P. aeruginosa* strains. Indeed, the Ab31 insertion site in

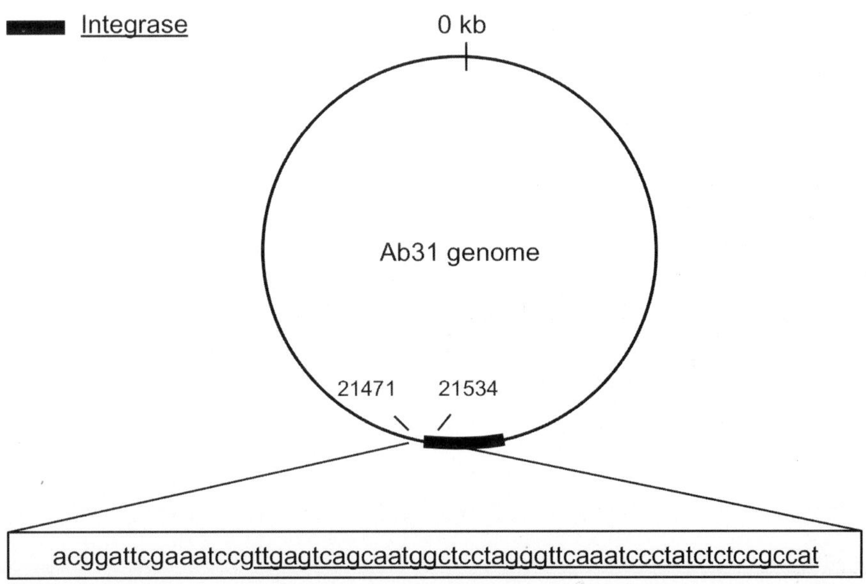

Figure 8. Schematic representation of the Ab31 insertion region. A 64 bp sequence is shared by the phage and the *P. aeruginosa* Tr60 genome. The portion of the shared region that overlaps with the phage integrase encoding gene is underlined.

```
Ab31_Spike      LTVSTTDSVIEYEGNGVTTAFPVPFKFPANG--DLVVTQVYNDVSTTLSLGANYSVVGAG
AF_Spike        MTVSSSASTASFPGNGVTTVFPLPFRFFSNSDVEVSLLNVASGVVTPQSIGTNYTLSGAG
                :***:: *. .: ******.**:**:* :*.  :: : :* ..* *. *:*:**:: ***

Ab31_Spike      -----AQAGGAVIVNIPTPAGATLSISRSLAAVQETDLRNQGRYFAETHESVFDYLTMLI
AF_Spike        DPEVDGNANSTLTMLVAPPPGVTLIVERVMDAVQQTDIINQARFFPEIHENVFDRLVMLI
                     .:*..:: : :..*.*.** :.* : ***:**: **.*:*.* **.*** *.***

Ab31_Spike      QQGFSGLSRALRRPIGKDYFDAENRRISNVSDPVLSQDAVTRKWSEEYFSDLISDIQGPV
AF_Spike        QQNASVIGRALLRPIGKDYFDALGYRIANLHDPIGSQDAATMAYVQQAIAALLEIGSGSA
                **. * :.*** ********** . **:*: **: ****.* : :: :: *:. .*..

Ab31_Spike      NNAQNVLYVD-GDGISTTVQKGIIKQFTSVSDVRGKAGDKDGDQAVLLGYYQDSPGVGGG
AF_Spike        NNAANVLYVPNGPNPTPLTVQNRLRQAIFLDDYKTTVVDGVTSNQVDLENALLACTTKGA
                *** ***** * . :. . :. ::* :.* : .. * .: * * : . *.

Ab31_Spike      NLYWDSLSVEPDNGGSVFAVTGVPNGRWKRDITHGVWAEWFGARNDGTDAAGTTAAVWAA
AF_Spike        DLFWP---------------------------------------DPVPRVSTSPLPT
                :*:*                                        .. .::: .:

Ab31_Spike      IIALRHDPETIVQYIGGPTVTAYASGRLNFGNGVFALQPDSFDITQDLGLTIVGQGFRGK
AF_Spike        LHTVRHVGPGAIKADG---LTFYVDPKYAQQNVIYMAPGGTGDGLSPSRPLNGFNGTLAA
                : ::**      ::   *   :* *.. :     * ::    .: *  .        :*  .

Ab31_Spike      NQAMKAATTLLCKGVSSGFFFRHYGNGARNLTFKDMDVVYENSDFTGDIVESLTSPGLTL
AF_Spike        LKNYAPLKSRWTVEGSAGTYFEDVQFPNYLASSHDNYLAWNFPAPAGLRAEPGTYPAILS
                 :   . .:          *:* :*..       : :*  :.:: .  :*  .*. * *.:

Ab31_Spike      ER--TRLGCYGGLLGTRVQTARSCIRPTFDEFLRCEDVVFDGAQNGFWSDGARTVPGLSF
AF_Spike        GIGNTALTGFHTGIGNRMTVNNLCVANFYDNSLTNVRQVRRGIAVGAYST-LFLVNCASQ
                     * *  :   :*.*: . . *:   :*: *       *   *   * :*     *   *

Ab31_Spike      GGWGTTLMNCTFYDIANVMIHHAANRGRSIVNVIGCAFNPINISPARCFDITNIEGINVT
AF_Spike        GNGLSNLAALPSGTLIITGGRHKGSRYGIDNTAGRCSMTATTTTYAVVEDALEYG-----
                *.  :.*   .   :  .  :* ..*      ..  *::.. . : *   *  :

Ab31_Spike      GNQFTPGTGSQPTQEWIRLLGSTGAMDGNTFSGPSSKLGTIGGVDPSSIRFSNNRVSCQG
AF_Spike        ---LYEKHDASTVSDYTEWRNNGKHPAAVLYGAAIFAYKSNASVDTRGNKFYANNICWN-
                   :    .:....:: .  ..     .  :...        : ..**. . :*  *.:. :

Ab31_Spike      GLVVSGGIFTGSGNEYSIADHGVDVSPVAITTLDIGPDIFKSGVSGNSYRISADSSLLGG
AF_Spike        ---ARGGFVADNPDIPDVYGTGVDANTRRFLCRGGGGDDLQTYRAN--RPAEISTRYTGG
                   . **:.:.. :  .: . ***... :   . * * :::  :.       . .:   **

Ab31_Spike      RINYIFEQDNSNSKFSNVSSRVSIDNVDRRISTIG---SLPSTASPYFSGRTYNVTVAGT
AF_Spike        STTSTTDVVLLNQIAEIREGYLANNDQSLRIRLIGRAQVADALITPQLRVNGSGVITLGT
                 .  :    *.  .  .. :: :: . **  **        :  :* :  .  .* . **

Ab31_Spike      FTLPT----PIPGIRLRVMKSTATALTVSTTSGSNILVGASSARTSAVATAAEIGPAIEF
AF_Spike        YRITAGKYGEIRLVVRPNIARTAFSVEFSCTDAVQNLGAAVGQIITTTTDLTVATLQVEV
                : :.:    *  :   : ** :: .* *.. : * .* .   ::.:  :    :*.

Ab31_Spike      VAFSSTSWMAQVLSGSWSFS-
AF_Spike        AGRADAGGTASFLTCMVDLLG
                .. :.:.  *..*:   .:
```

Figure 9. Alignment of the spike protein sequence of phages Ab31 and AF.

P. aeruginosa is the same as in PAJU2. Phages AF and PAJU2 infect *P. putida* and *P. aeruginosa*, respectively. These bacterial species are closely related, and phage genome exchanges probably occurred during infection of a lysogenic host by the virulent phage. As a result of their mosaic structure, some temperate phage genomes can migrate between unrelated bacteria [54]. Although genetically distant, phages AF and PAJU2 share a lambdoid genome organization which could favor genetic replacement (modular exchanges of gene blocks) [55,56]. Similar events seem to occur between D3112-like phages morphologically identical to phage lambda, and the transposable coliphage Mu belonging to the *Myoviridae* family [57]. Several types of recombination events are thought to build phage genomes. There are examples of conserved sequences at gene boundaries that could serve to target homologous recombination at these positions, via transposition or site-specific recombination [13]. However a major contributor to phage genome building is illegitimate recombination, or recombination between short conserved sequences (a few bases), coupled with functional selection of genes [13,58].

Conclusion

Our observations show that phage Ab31 is the result of a rare recombination event between genomes of two unrelated bacteriophages, normally infecting different bacterial species. It is capable of forming lysogens but its genome can also apparently persists unintegrated for a long time in the bacterial cells, with accompanying repression of virulence functions thus allowing the bacteria to escape lysis. In addition, we show that the phage exerts strong pressure on the bacteria by selecting for variants with new phenotypes, possibly improving their adaptation to chronic lung infection.

Acknowledgments

We are grateful to Barry Holland and Gilles Vergnaud for their comments on and corrections of the manuscript. This work has benefited from the facilities and expertise of the high throughput electron microscopy and sequencing platform of IMAGIF (Centre de Recherche de Gif - www.imagif.cnrs.fr).

Author Contributions

Conceived and designed the experiments: CE HVT CP. Performed the experiments: LL CE YB. Analyzed the data: LL CE YB CP. Contributed reagents/materials/analysis tools: CE HVT. Wrote the paper: LL YB CP.

References

1. Penketh AR, Wise A, Mearns MB, Hodson ME, Batten JC (1987) Cystic fibrosis in adolescents and adults. Thorax 42: 526–532.
2. Brussow H (2012) *Pseudomonas* biofilms, cystic fibrosis, and phage: a silver lining? MBio 3.
3. Hogardt M, Heesemann J (2010) Adaptation of *Pseudomonas aeruginosa* during persistence in the cystic fibrosis lung. Int J Med Microbiol 300: 557–562.
4. Flemming HC, Wingender J (2010) The biofilm matrix. Nat Rev Microbiol 8: 623–633.
5. Schurks N, Wingender J, Flemming HC, Mayer C (2002) Monomer composition and sequence of alginates from *Pseudomonas aeruginosa*. Int J Biol Macromol 30: 105–111.
6. Qiu D, Eisinger VM, Rowen DW, Yu HD (2007) Regulated proteolysis controls mucoid conversion in *Pseudomonas aeruginosa*. Proc Natl Acad Sci U S A 104: 8107–8112.
7. Al-Dujaili AH, Harris DM (1975) *Pseudomonas aeruginosa* infection in hospital: a comparison between 'infective' and 'environmental' strains. J Hyg (Lond) 75: 195–201.
8. Miller RV, Rubero VJ (1984) Mucoid conversion by phages of *Pseudomonas aeruginosa* strains from patients with cystic fibrosis. J Clin Microbiol 19: 717–719.
9. Hosseinidoust Z, Tufenkji N, van de Ven TG (2013) Predation in homogeneous and heterogeneous phage environments affects virulence determinants of *Pseudomonas aeruginosa*. Appl Environ Microbiol 79: 2862–2871.
10. Hosseinidoust Z, van de Ven TG, Tufenkji N (2013) Evolution of *Pseudomonas aeruginosa* virulence as a result of phage predation. Appl Environ Microbiol 79: 6110–6116.
11. Ceyssens PJ, Lavigne R (2010) Bacteriophages of *Pseudomonas*. Future Microbiol 5: 1041–1055.
12. Hatfull GF (2008) Bacteriophage genomics. Curr Opin Microbiol 11: 447–453.
13. Hatfull GF, Hendrix RW (2011) Bacteriophages and their genomes. Curr Opin Virol 1: 298–303.
14. Essoh C, Blouin Y, Loukou G, Cablanmian A, Lathro S, et al. (2013) The Susceptibility of *Pseudomonas aeruginosa* Strains from Cystic Fibrosis Patients to Bacteriophages. PLoS One 8: e60575.
15. Lu S, Le S, Tan Y, Zhu J, Li M, et al. (2013) Genomic and proteomic analyses of the terminally redundant genome of the *Pseudomonas aeruginosa* phage PaP1: establishment of genus PaP1-like phages. PLoS One 8: e62933.
16. Rahme LG, Stevens EJ, Wolfort SF, Shao J, Tompkins RG, et al. (1995) Common virulence factors for bacterial pathogenicity in plants and animals. Science 268: 1899–1902.
17. Holloway BW (1955) Genetic recombination in *Pseudomonas aeruginosa*. J Gen Microbiol 13: 572–581.
18. Romling U, Wingender J, Muller H, Tummler B (1994) A major *Pseudomonas aeruginosa* clone common to patients and aquatic habitats. Appl Environ Microbiol 60: 1734–1738.
19. Vu-Thien H, Corbineau G, Hormigos K, Fauroux B, Corvol H, et al. (2007) Multiple-locus variable-number tandem-repeat analysis for longitudinal survey of sources of *Pseudomonas aeruginosa* infection in cystic fibrosis patients. J Clin Microbiol 45: 3175–3183.
20. Llanes C, Pourcel C, Richardot C, Plesiat P, Fichant G, et al. (2013) Diversity of beta-lactam resistance mechanisms in cystic fibrosis isolates of *Pseudomonas aeruginosa*: a French multicentre study. J Antimicrob Chemother 68: 1763–1771.
21. Brokopp CD, Gomez-Lus R, Farmer JJ, 3rd (1977) Serological typing of *Pseudomonas aeruginosa*: use of commercial antisera and live antigens. J Clin Microbiol 5: 640–649.
22. Cameron JR, Philippsen P, Davis RW (1977) Analysis of chromosomal integration and deletions of yeast plasmids. Nucleic Acids Res 4: 1429–1448.
23. Van Domselaar GH, Stothard P, Shrivastava S, Cruz JA, Guo A, et al. (2005) BASys: a web server for automated bacterial genome annotation. Nucleic Acids Res 33: W455–459.
24. Cramer N, Klockgether J, Wrasman K, Schmidt M, Davenport CF, et al. (2011) Microevolution of the major common *Pseudomonas aeruginosa* clones C and PA14 in cystic fibrosis lungs. Environ Microbiol 13: 1690–1704.
25. Xu J, Zhang J, Lu X, Liang W, Zhang L, et al. (2013) O antigen is the receptor of *Vibrio cholerae* serogroup O1 El Tor typing phage VP4. J Bacteriol 195: 798–806.
26. Cornelissen A, Ceyssens PJ, Krylov VN, Noben JP, Volckaert G, et al. (2012) Identification of EPS-degrading activity within the tail spikes of the novel *Pseudomonas putida* phage AF. Virology.
27. Balaban NQ, Merrin J, Chait R, Kowalik L, Leibler S (2004) Bacterial persistence as a phenotypic switch. Science 305: 1622–1625.
28. Crosa JH (1989) Genetics and molecular biology of siderophore-mediated iron transport in bacteria. Microbiol Rev 53: 517–530.
29. Kwan T, Liu J, Dubow M, Gros P, Pelletier J (2006) Comparative genomic analysis of 18 *Pseudomonas aeruginosa* bacteriophages. J Bacteriol 188: 1184–1187.
30. Wei H, Therrien C, Blanchard A, Guan S, Zhu Z (2008) The Fidelity Index provides a systematic quantitation of star activity of DNA restriction endonucleases. Nucleic Acids Res 36: e50.
31. Uchiyama J, Rashel M, Takemura I, Kato S, Ujihara T, et al. (2012) Genetic characterization of *Pseudomonas aeruginosa* bacteriophage KPP10. Arch Virol 157: 733–738.
32. Perry LL, SanMiguel P, Minocha U, Terekhov AI, Shroyer ML, et al. (2009) Sequence analysis of *Escherichia coli* O157:H7 bacteriophage PhiV10 and identification of a phage-encoded immunity protein that modifies the O157 antigen. FEMS Microbiol Lett 292: 182–186.
33. Kropinski AM, Kovalyova IV, Billington SJ, Patrick AN, Butts BD, et al. (2007) The genome of epsilon15, a serotype-converting, Group E1 *Salmonella enterica*-specific bacteriophage. Virology 369: 234–244.
34. Roos WH, Ivanovska IL, Evilevitch A, Wuite GJ (2007) Viral capsids: mechanical characteristics, genome packaging and delivery mechanisms. Cell Mol Life Sci 64: 1484–1497.
35. Lee DG, Urbach JM, Wu G, Liberati NT, Feinbaum RL, et al. (2006) Genomic analysis reveals that *Pseudomonas aeruginosa* virulence is combinatorial. Genome Biol 7: R90.
36. Ruer S, Stender S, Filloux A, de Bentzmann S (2007) Assembly of fimbrial structures in *Pseudomonas aeruginosa*: functionality and specificity of chaperone-usher machineries. J Bacteriol 189: 3547–3555.

37. Jiang X, Jiang H, Li C, Wang S, Mi Z, et al. (2011) Sequence characteristics of T4-like bacteriophage IME08 benome termini revealed by high throughput sequencing. Virol J 8: 194.
38. Hanlon GW, Denyer SP, Olliff CJ, Ibrahim LJ (2001) Reduction in exopolysaccharide viscosity as an aid to bacteriophage penetration through *Pseudomonas aeruginosa* biofilms. Appl Environ Microbiol 67: 2746–2753.
39. Steven AC, Trus BL, Maizel JV, Unser M, Parry DA, et al. (1988) Molecular substructure of a viral receptor-recognition protein. The gp17 tail-fiber of bacteriophage T7. J Mol Biol 200: 351–365.
40. Cornelissen A, Ceyssens PJ, T'Syen J, Van Praet H, Noben JP, et al. (2011) The T7-related *Pseudomonas putida* phage phi15 displays virion-associated biofilm degradation properties. PLoS One 6: e18597.
41. Casjens SR, Molineux IJ (2012) Short noncontractile tail machines: adsorption and DNA delivery by podoviruses. Adv Exp Med Biol 726: 143–179.
42. Friman VP, Ghoul M, Molin S, Johansen HK, Buckling A (2013) *Pseudomonas aeruginosa* Adaptation to Lungs of Cystic Fibrosis Patients Leads to Lowered Resistance to Phage and Protist Enemies. PLoS One 8: e75380.
43. Uchiyama J, Rashel M, Matsumoto T, Sumiyama Y, Wakiguchi H, et al. (2009) Characteristics of a novel *Pseudomonas aeruginosa* bacteriophage, PAJU2, which is genetically related to bacteriophage D3. Virus Res 139: 131–134.
44. Mooij MJ, Drenkard E, Llamas MA, Vandenbroucke-Grauls CM, Savelkoul PH, et al. (2007) Characterization of the integrated filamentous phage Pf5 and its involvement in small-colony formation. Microbiology 153: 1790–1798.
45. Webb JS, Lau M, Kjelleberg S (2004) Bacteriophage and phenotypic variation in *Pseudomonas aeruginosa* biofilm development. J Bacteriol 186: 8066–8073.
46. Rice SA, Tan CH, Mikkelsen PJ, Kung V, Woo J, et al. (2009) The biofilm life cycle and virulence of *Pseudomonas aeruginosa* are dependent on a filamentous prophage. ISME J 3: 271–282.
47. Wozniak DJ, Ohman DE (1994) Transcriptional analysis of the *Pseudomonas aeruginosa* genes algR, algB, and algD reveals a hierarchy of alginate gene expression which is modulated by algT. J Bacteriol 176: 6007–6014.
48. Rodriguez-Rojas A, Mena A, Martin S, Borrell N, Oliver A, et al. (2009) Inactivation of the hmgA gene of *Pseudomonas aeruginosa* leads to pyomelanin hyperproduction, stress resistance and increased persistence in chronic lung infection. Microbiology 155: 1050–1057.
49. Vallet-Gely I, Sharp JS, Dove SL (2007) Local and global regulators linking anaerobiosis to cupA fimbrial gene expression in *Pseudomonas aeruginosa*. J Bacteriol 189: 8667–8676.
50. Hossain MJ, Rahman Kh S, Terhune JS, Liles MR (2012) An outer membrane porin protein modulates phage susceptibility in *Edwardsiella ictaluri*. Microbiology 158: 474–487.
51. Randall-Hazelbauer L, Schwartz M (1973) Isolation of the bacteriophage lambda receptor from *Escherichia coli*. J Bacteriol 116: 1436–1446.
52. de Vries GE, Raymond CK, Ludwig RA (1984) Extension of bacteriophage lambda host range: selection, cloning, and characterization of a constitutive lambda receptor gene. Proc Natl Acad Sci U S A 81: 6080–6084.
53. Rau MH, Marvig RL, Ehrlich GD, Molin S, Jelsbak L (2012) Deletion and acquisition of genomic content during early stage adaptation of *Pseudomonas aeruginosa* to a human host environment. Environ Microbiol 14: 2200–2211.
54. Krylov SV, Kropinski AM, Pleteneva EA, Shaburova OV, Burkal'tseva MV, et al. (2012) Properties of the new D3-like *Pseudomonas aeruginosa* bacteriophage phiPMG1: genome structure and prospects for the use in phage therapy. Genetika 48: 1057–1067.
55. Brussow H, Hendrix RW (2002) Phage genomics: small is beautiful. Cell 108: 13–16.
56. Casjens SR (2005) Comparative genomics and evolution of the tailed-bacteriophages. Curr Opin Microbiol 8: 451–458.
57. Braid MD, Silhavy JL, Kitts CL, Cano RJ, Howe MM (2004) Complete genomic sequence of bacteriophage B3, a Mu-like phage of *Pseudomonas aeruginosa*. J Bacteriol 186: 6560–6574.
58. Juhala RJ, Ford ME, Duda RL, Youlton A, Hatfull GF, et al. (2000) Genomic sequences of bacteriophages HK97 and HK022: pervasive genetic mosaicism in the lambdoid bacteriophages. J Mol Biol 299: 27–51.

GBA2-Encoded β-Glucosidase Activity Is Involved in the Inflammatory Response to *Pseudomonas aeruginosa*

Nicoletta Loberto[2,❡], Maela Tebon[1,❡], Ilaria Lampronti[3], Nicola Marchetti[4], Massimo Aureli[2], Rosaria Bassi[2], Maria Grazia Giri[5], Valentino Bezzerri[1], Valentina Lovato[1], Cinzia Cantù[1], Silvia Munari[1], Seng H. Cheng[6], Alberto Cavazzini[4], Roberto Gambari[3], Sandro Sonnino[2], Giulio Cabrini[1], Maria Cristina Dechecchi[1*]

1 Laboratory of Molecular Pathology, Department of Pathology and Diagnostics, University Hospital of Verona, Verona, Italy, **2** Department of Medical Biotechnology and Translational Medicine, University of Milano, Milano, Italy, **3** Department of Life Sciences and Biotechnology, Section of Biochemistry and Molecular Biology, University of Ferrara, Ferrara, Italy, **4** Department of Chemistry and Pharmaceutical Sciences, University of Ferrara, Ferrara, Italy, **5** Medical Physics Unit, Department of Pathology and Diagnostics, University Hospital of Verona, Verona, Italy, **6** Genzyme, a Sanofi Company, Framingham, Massachusetts, United States of America

Abstract

Current anti-inflammatory strategies for the treatment of pulmonary disease in cystic fibrosis (CF) are limited; thus, there is continued interest in identifying additional molecular targets for therapeutic intervention. Given the emerging role of sphingolipids (SLs) in various respiratory disorders, including CF, drugs that selectively target the enzymes associated with SL metabolism are under development. Miglustat, a well-characterized iminosugar-based inhibitor of β-glucosidase 2 (GBA2), has shown promise in CF treatment because it reduces the inflammatory response to infection by *P. aeruginosa* and restores F508del-CFTR chloride channel activity. This study aimed to probe the molecular basis for the anti-inflammatory activity of miglustat by examining specifically the role of GBA2 following the infection of CF bronchial epithelial cells by *P. aeruginosa*. We also report the anti-inflammatory activity of another potent inhibitor of GBA2 activity, namely *N*-(5-adamantane-1-yl-methoxy)pentyl)-deoxynojirimycin (Genz-529648). In CF bronchial cells, inhibition of GBA2 by miglustat or Genz-529648 significantly reduced the induction of IL-8 mRNA levels and protein release following infection by *P. aeruginosa*. Hence, the present data demonstrate that the anti-inflammatory effects of miglustat and Genz-529648 are likely exerted through inhibition of GBA2.

Editor: Dominik Hartl, University of Tübingen, Germany

Funding: This research was supported by Italian Cystic Fibrosis Research Foundation (grant FFC # 14/2012) with the contribution of "Picasso. Capolavori dal Museo Nazionale Picasso di Parigi", Festa d'Estate Villa Sigurtà Verona, Delegazione FFC Lago di Garda e Arezzo. The funders had no role in study design, data collection and analysis, decision to publish, or preparation of the manuscript.

Competing Interests: Seng H. Cheng is an employee and shareholder of Genzyme, a Sanofi Company, when the work was performed. This work is also part of a patent application titled "Amorphous and a crystalline form of Genz 112638 hemitartrate as inhibitor of glucosylceramide synthase" (International Application No: PCT/US20130137743A1). However, this does not alter the authors' adherence to all the PLOS ONE policies on sharing data and materials.

* Email: cristina.dechecchi@ospedaleuniverona.it

❡ These authors contributed equally to this work.

Introduction

Cystic fibrosis (CF) lung disease is characterized by progressive chronic infection and inflammation of the airways. The prolonged airway inflammation is an important aspect of the obstructive lung disease noted in CF patients. Resultant progressive remodeling leads to irreversible damage and fibrosis, which is a major cause of mortality in patients [1]. Significant efforts have been invested into developing therapies that address the underlying basis of CF. For example, recent efforts to identify small-molecule drugs that target a mutant CF transmembrane conductance regulator (CFTR) led to the successful development of a potentiator (Kalydeco) for patients who harbor the mutant G551D-CFTR [2]. Moreover, phase 3 clinical trials of Kalydeco in combination with the corrector lumacaftor for people with two copies of the F508del-CFTR mutation showed significant improvements in lung function and other key measures of the disease (http://www.cff.org/about CFFoundation/NewsEvents/2014NEWSArchive/6-24-Vertex Phase-3-Results_Lumacaftor_Ibvacaftor.cfm). However, despite these very encouranging results, adjuvant therapies that abate the decline in pulmonary function in other patients are still needed. Examples include the potential deployment of new antibiotics, anti-mucolytic and anti-inflammatory drugs [3]. To date, the only non-steroidal anti-inflammatory agent that has been shown to be beneficial in CF patients is ibuprofen; however, its use can be associated with severe adverse effects, such as gastrointestinal bleeding [4]. Hence, the identification and development of novel and more potent anti-inflammatory drugs for CF airway disease remains a priority. The chemokine IL-8 is abundantly expressed at sites of chronic inflammation and appears to play a major role in driving the formation of neutrophil (PMN)-rich exudates in the lungs of CF patients [5–8]; thus its reduction is a key therapeutic goal in CF.

Sphingolipids (SLs) are a large group of lipids that are thought to modulate the pathophysiology of several respiratory disorders, including CF [9–11]. Ceramide, the central hub of SL metabolism, is generated by *de novo* synthesis or hydrolysis of complex SLs, such as sphingomyelin (SM) by acid sphingomyelinase (ASM) and glucosylceramide (GlcCer) by glucocerebrosidases [12]. Ceramide plays an important role in the infection by *P. aeruginosa* by reorganizing lipid rafts on cellular membranes into larger signaling platforms, which is a feature conducive to internalizing bacteria, inducing apoptosis and regulating the cytokine response [13]. Controversial findings on the association between abnormalities in SL metabolism and inflammation in CF have been reported. For example, ceramide has been identified as a key regulator of inflammation in CF airways in different CFTR-/- mouse models [14]. In contrast, decreased ceramide levels have been demonstrated in CFTR KO mice [15], and no significant difference has been found in basal ceramide levels in CFTR KO lung homogenates compared to wild type mice [16]. The possible explanation for this discrepancy appears to be the special diet required for the survival of CFTR KO mice, which severely affects the concentration of SLs [14]. Interestingly, an accumulation of ceramide, which has been directly correlated with neutrophilic lung inflammation, has been demonstrated in the lower airway of CF patients [17]. These findings suggest that the CF pathophysiology associated with infection by *P. aeruginosa* can be corrected, in part, by modulating ceramide levels to their normal physiological range, independent of the conflicting results obtained in different CF models. To date, there is some evidence that supports pharmacological interventions in SL metabolism as therapeutic agents for CF lung disease [14–21].

Given the emerging importance of SLs in respiratory disorders, novel drugs that selectively target different enzymes involved in SL metabolism are under development. Recently developed iminosugar-based inhibitors of GBA2 are of particular interest because of their good oral bioavailability and specific immune modulatory and chaperoning activities [22]. A well-characterized inhibitor is miglustat (*N*-butyldeoxynojirimycin, NB-DNJ), which is FDA-approved and EMA-designated for use in Europe and the USA for the treatment of type I Gaucher and other SL storage diseases. We previously demonstrated that miglustat exhibits an anti-inflammatory effect *in vitro* and *in vivo* by reducing *P. aeruginosa* induced immunoreactive ceramide levels [20,23]. Moreover, miglustat can restore F508del-CFTR chloride channel activity in respiratory and pancreatic cells *in vitro* [24,25] and in CF mice [26]. However, a recent clinical trial in CF patients did not provide evidence of efficacy, which may be related to the intra-individual variability of nasal potential difference (NPD) measurements or the short duration of exposure [27]. Nevertheless, a drug that is able to correct both the CF channel defect and reduce the inflammatory response is of interest and warrants further attention. Miglustat inhibits the enzyme ceramide glucosyl-transferase (GlcCerT), which catalyzes the first step in the glycosphingolipid biosynthetic pathway [28] with IC50 values in the low micromolar range. It also inhibits the activities of two different GlcCer degrading enzymes, glucocerebrosidase (GBA1) and the non-lysosomal β-glucosidase 2 (GBA2), with IC50 values in the high micromolar and nanomolar range, respectively [29,30]. In addition, it is also a potent inhibitor of α-glucosidase [31]. Therefore, miglustat could affect the host response to *P. aeruginosa* through one or more of these SL metabolism pathways. The galactose analog of miglustat, *N*-butyldeoxygalactonojirimycin (NB-DGJ), also inhibits GlcCerT and GBA2, whereas its effect on GBA1 is less clear [30,32,33]. Similar to miglustat, NB-DGJ produces an anti-inflammatory effect in bronchial epithelial cells [25], which suggests a potential involvement of GlcCerT and/or GBA2 in the response of bronchial cells to *P. aeruginosa*. The non-lysosomal β-glucosidase GBA2, which is extremely sensitive to deoxynojirimycin-type inhibitors [34], is a membrane-associated enzyme located in the plasma membrane and ER of cells [29,35]. GBA2 has been described as a single pass transmembrane protein with its catalytic domain facing the extracellular environment [29]. Because this enzyme can hydrolyze GlcCer directly at the cell surface, it might be involved in affecting transient local changes in bioactive SL concentrations.

To gain greater insights into the molecular basis of the anti-inflammatory activity of miglustat, we explored the potential involvement of GBA2 in the ceramide-mediated signaling processes following *P. aeruginosa* infection of CF bronchial epithelial cells. The effects of a potent inhibitor of GBA2, *N*-(5-adamantane-1-yl-methoxy)pentyl)- deoxynojirimycin or Genz-529648 as it is referred to in this report [4,36], on the inflammatory response to *P. aeruginosa* were investigated and compared to miglustat and NB-DGJ. We also examined the impact of lowering the expression of GBA2 in human CF bronchial epithelial cells exposed to *P. aeruginosa* using siRNA oligonucleotides. The results obtained here demonstrate that GBA2 is a target of the anti-inflammatory effects of miglustat and Genz-529648. Thus, these compounds provide novel insights into the role of GBA2 in the signaling cascade activated by *P. aeruginosa* in CF bronchial epithelial cells.

Methods

Cell models

IB3-1 (LGC Promochem GmbH, Teddington, Middlesex, United Kingdom)[37] and CuFi-1 (a generous gift of A. Klingelhutz, P. Karp and J. Zabner, University of Iowa, Iowa City)[38] are human bronchial epithelial cells grown as previously described [24]. Primary airway epithelial cells, i.e., mainstem human bronchi, derived from CF individuals were obtained from "Servizio Colture Primarie" of the Italian Cystic Fibrosis Research Foundation and cultured as previously described [39].

Bacterial strains

The reference *P. aeruginosa* strain, PAO1, was kindly provided by A. Prince (Columbia University, New York) and grown in trypticase soy broth (TSB) or agar (TSA) (Difco) as previously described [25]. Some experiments were conducted with organisms killed by heating to 65°C for 30 minutes.

Inhibitors of SL metabolism

Miglustat and NB-DGJ were obtained from Toronto Research Chemicals, North York, ON, Canada. Genz-529648 was obtained from Genzyme, a Sanofi Company; amitriptyline was obtained from Sigma.

Inflammatory response *in vitro*

Cells were treated with different inhibitors or solvent alone and then infected with PAO1 for 4 hours at 37°C as previously described [25]. The inflammatory response to PAO1 infection was studied at the transcriptional level by measuring IL-8 chemokine expression as previously described [20]. An enzyme-linked immunosorbent assay for the quantitative measurement of IL-8 protein release was performed using the Human IL-8 Instant ELISA kit (Bender MedSystems, Vienna, Austria).

Cell toxicity

The effects of Genz-529648 on cell proliferation, viability and apoptosis were studied to evaluate the potential toxicity as detailed in the Supplement S3.

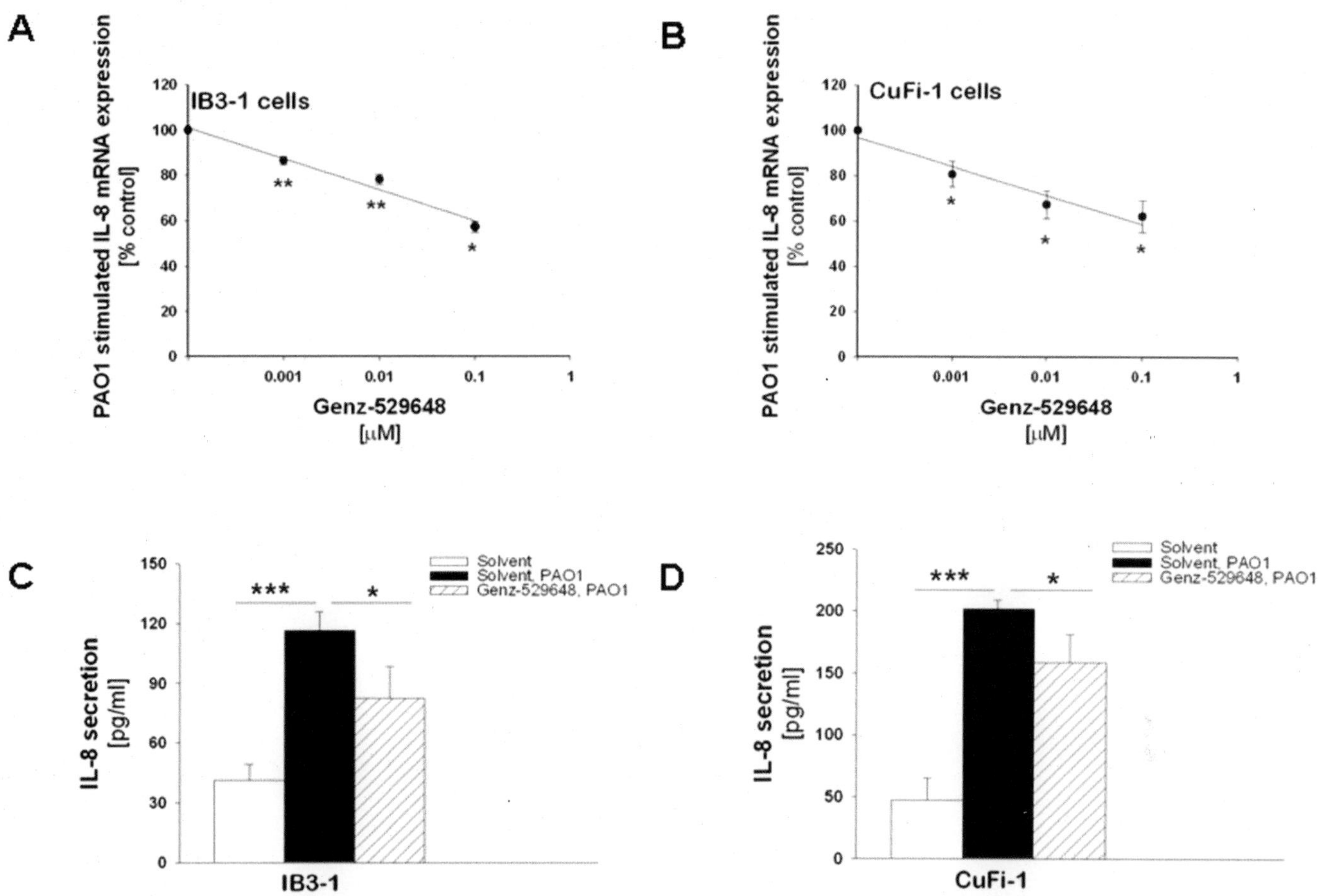

Figure 1. Genz-529648 reduces *P. aeruginosa* stimulated IL-8 mRNA expression and protein release. *Panels A and B. Genz-529648 reduces P. aeruginosa stimulated IL-8 mRNA expression.* IB3-1 (A) and CuFi-1 (B) cells were treated with a range of doses of Genz-529648 (1–100 nM) or solvent alone for 1 hour and then infected with PAO1 for 4 hours at 37°C. The inflammatory response was evaluated by studying the expression of IL-8 mRNA, which was measured by Real-time qPCR and obtained by comparing the ratio IL-8 and the housekeeping gene GAPDH between non-infected and infected cells. The results are expressed as the % of untreated cells and represent the mean ± standard error of the mean of 4 independent experiments in duplicate. Comparisons between groups were made by using Student's *t* tests. *Panels C and D. Genz-529648 reduces the P. aeruginosa induced IL-8 secretion.* IB3-1 (C) and CuFi-1(D) cells were treated with Genz-529648 (100 nM) for 1 hour prior to infection with heat killed PAO1 for 24 hours. Data reported are the mean ± standard error of the mean of 4 independent experiments in duplicate. Comparisons between groups were made by using Student's *t* tests.

GBA2 silencing

To perform silencing experiments of the GBA2 gene, a TriFECTa RNAi Kit (Integrated DNA technologies, Coralville, Iowa, IA) was used. Cells were transiently transfected with specific siRNA for GBA2 (sequence GGAUCAUGUUUGGAGCUA) or scrambled (CGUUAAUCGCGUAUAAUACGCGUAT) duplexes complexed with cationic liposomes Lipofectamine 2000 (Invitrogen, Carlsbad, CA) diluted in 1 ml serum-free cell culture medium. GBA2 siRNA or scrambled duplexes (10 nM) were added and incubated for 10 minutes. Liposome:duplex complexes (500 μL) were added to the cells grown in 2 cm^2 wells and incubated at 37°C for 6 hours. The cells were washed twice with culture medium and maintained at 37°C for an additional 18 or 42 hours.

Analysis of cell ceramide content

The analysis of cell ceramide content was performed via two different approaches: by the LC-MS and LC-MS/MS method [40] and by the metabolic labeling of cell SLs using (^{3}H)sphingosine as a precursor. Both methods are detailed in the Supplement S1 and S2.

Enzymatic activity

IB3-1 or CuFi-1 cells were treated with 2 μM miglustat, 10 nM Genz-529648 or solvent alone for 1 hour and the infected with heat-killed PAO1 for 4 hours. The cells were then scraped and centrifuged; the cellular pellets were resuspended in water containing protease inhibitors and sonicated. After protein determination, the β-glucosidase activities were assayed in the total cell lysates using the fluorigenic substrate 4-methylumbelliferyl-β-D-glucopyranoside (MUB-Glc) as previously described [41]. To discriminate between GBA1 and GBA2 β-glucosidase activity, the enzymatic assays were performed in the presence of 5 nM of Genz-529648 or 500 μM of Conduritol B Epoxide (CBE), respectively.

Statistics

Results are expressed as the mean ± standard error of the mean. Comparisons between groups were made using Student's t

Table 1. Inhibition of *P. aeruginosa* stimulated IL-8 mRNA expression by alkylated iminosugars in IB3-1 and CuFi-1 cells.

	IB3-1 cells				CuFi-1 cells			
Inhibitor	*IC_{50}*	*CI*	*Maximal Inhibition*	*CI*	*IC_{50}*	*CI*	*Maximal Inhibition*	*CI*
	(µM)	*(µM)*	*(%)*	*(%)*	*(µM)*	*(µM)*	*(%)*	*(%)*
Miglustat	2.2	1.4–3.4	51.6	51.1–53.3	1.98	1.4–2.7	51.5	51.0–57.3
NB-DGJ	0.27	0.16–0.44	45.0	39.0-52-0	0.39	0.004–3.8	53.0	41.0–55.0
Genz-529648	0.009	0.004–0.018	51.4	46.0–57.0	0.002	0.002–0.003	46.0	38.0–53.0

IB3-1 and CuFi-1 cells were treated with a range of doses of the alkylated iminosugars miglustat or NB-DGJ (0.5–100 µM) or Genz-529648 (1–100 nM) for 1 hour prior to infection with PAO1 (10–50 CFU/cell) for 4 hrs, and IL-8 mRNA expression was measured. IC_{50} values were calculated by fitting with a non-linear regression experimental data obtained in 4 different independent experiments performed in each cell line treated with each inhibitor.
IC_{50} values (*i.e.*, inhibitor concentration that results in 50% inhibition) were calculated by fitting experimental data with a non-linear regression according to the following formula: -log(*I*) = *pKi* + log (V−v)/v.
I = inhibitor concentration; v = % inhibition; *pKi* = IC_{50}; V = maximal inhibition; CI = confidence interval 95%.

tests. Statistical significance was defined by $p<0.05$. In order to calculate the IC_{50} values, experimental data were fitted by nonlinear regression using the software "R Core Team, 2013, "R: A language and environment for statistical Computing", R Foundation for Statistical Computing, Vienna, Austria, URL http://www.R-project.org.

Results

Genz-529648 reduces the expression of IL-8 in CF bronchial epithelial cells

Several hydrophobic deoxynojirimycin derivatives have been generated that can be used as research tools to probe the physiological relevance of GBA2. Complete inhibition of GBA2 can be realized in cells treated with low nanomolar concentrations of *N*-(5-adamantane-1-yl-methoxy)pentyl)- deoxynojirimycin (Genz-529648). GlcCerT and oligosaccharide chain-trimming glucosidases, which are sensitive to other hydrophobic deoxynojirimycin derivatives, are unaffected by Genz-529648 [34]. To determine a possible involvement of GBA2 in the inflammatory response to *P. aeruginosa* in bronchial epithelial cells, the effect of Genz-529648 was investigated and compared to miglustat and NB-DGJ. IB3-1 and CuFi-1 cells were treated with increasing amounts (1–100 nM) of the inhibitors for 1 hour prior to infection with *P. aeruginosa* (strain PAO1), and the IL-8 expression was then analyzed 4 hours post-infection. As shown in panels A and B in figure 1, Genz-529648 reduced the PAO1 induced increase in IL-8 mRNA levels by approximately 40% in both cell lines. These experiments were extended by measuring IL-8 chemokine secretion in the supernatants of IB3-1 and CuFi-1 cells. Thus, the cells were treated with Genz-529648 (100 nM) for 1 hour prior to infection with heat killed PAO1, and the supernatants were collected 24 hours later. Heat killed organisms were used to prevent bronchial cell death during the 24 hours of bacterial challenge. Figure 1, panels C and D, shows that Genz-529648 significantly decreased the amount of IL-8 released from the CF bronchial cells infected by PAO1 by approximately 30%, which is consistent with the results obtained at the transcriptional level (figure 1, panels A and B).

The effects of Genz-529648 in bronchial cells were then compared to miglustat and NB-DGJ, which also exhibit anti-inflammatory effects [25]. IB3-1 and CuFi-1 cells were treated with different concentrations of miglustat, NB-DGJ or Genz-529648 and infected with PAO1 as previously described; the IL-8 mRNA levels were then measured. As summarized in table 1, a similar maximal inhibition of approximately 50% was observed in both cell lines treated with miglustat, NB-DGJ or Genz-529648. However, the IC_{50} values of Genz-529648 in IB3-1 and CuFi-1 cells were considerably lower compared to miglustat or NB-DGJ, which indicated that it is a more potent inhibitor of the inflammatory response in CF bronchial cells. Moreover, the IC_{50} values of Genz-529648 at inhibiting IL-8 expression were of the same order of magnitude compared to that reported at inhibiting GBA2 [35], which suggests that the reduction in the inflammatory response to *P. aeruginosa* may have been mediated through its action on GBA2.

Although Genz-529648 is active at nanomolar concentrations, its potential toxicity on bronchial epithelial cells was investigated. To determine the impact on cell proliferation, IB3-1 cells were treated with increasing concentrations of Genz-529648 (from 0.001 to 1 µM), and the cell number/ml was analyzed after 4, 24, 48 and 72 hours. The results, which were derived from three independent experiments, indicate that the IC_{50} values calculated at these time points were always greater than 1 µM, which

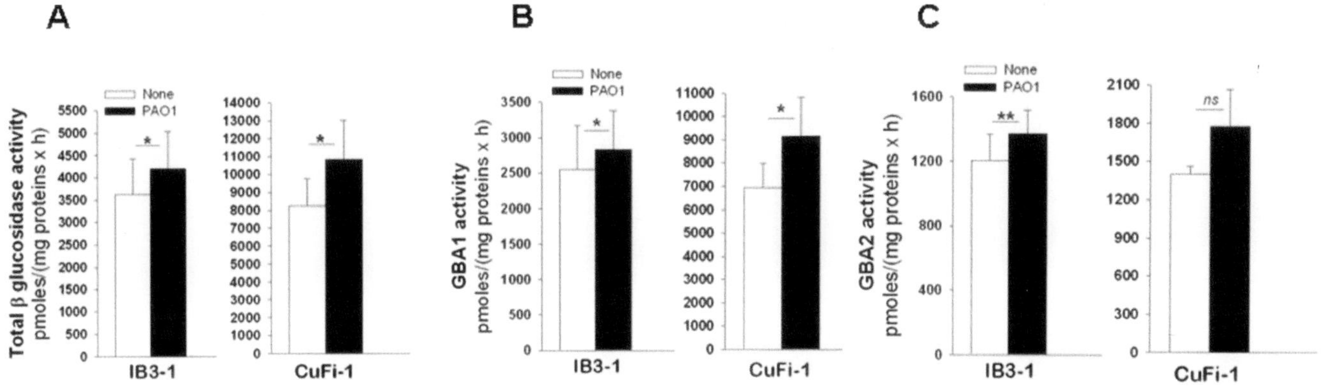

Figure 2. Infection with PAO1 increases β-glucosidase activity in IB3-1 and CuFi-1 cells. IB3-1 and CuFi-1 cells were infected with heat-killed PAO1 for 4 hours. The cells were then scraped and centrifuged; the cellular pellets were resuspended in water containing protease inhibitors and sonicated. Similar amounts of cellular proteins were used to perform the enzymatic assays to detect the activities of total β-glucosidase (A), GBA1 (B) and GBA2 (C), as reported in the Methods section. The data reported are the mean ± standard error of the mean of 4 (IB3-1) or 3 (CuFi-1) independent experiments in triplicate. Comparisons between groups were made by using Student's *t* tests.

supports the concept that this compound is not cytotoxic at nanomolar concentrations and does not display inhibitory activity on CF bronchial cells. Cell viability, which was measured after 4 and 24 hours of treatment (figure S1), was always similar to the untreated cells and between 91.3 and 97.6%. At the same time points, treatment with Genz-529648 did not cause apoptotic effects, even when used at the 1 μM concentration (figures S2 and S3).

Miglustat and Genz-529648 inhibit GBA2 activity in *P. aeruginosa* infected CF bronchial epithelial cells

To ascertain the possible involvement of GBA2 in the signaling processes associated with *P. aeruginosa* infection, total β-glucosidase, GBA1 and GBA2 activities in the lysates of both IB3-1 and CuFi-1 cells infected by heat killed PAO1 were measured. To prevent potential interference because of bacterial glucosidase activities, the infected cells were subjected to washes with PBS that removed most bacteria; moreover, heat killed instead of living organisms were used. In addition, the residual GBA1 and GBA2 activities associated with heat killed bacteria were measured by enzymatic assays on the amounts of heat killed PAO1 from 20 to 30-fold higher compared to those used for the cell infection. The fluorescence associated with the PAO1 samples, which was the result of hydrolysis of the artificial substrate MUB-Glc, was less or the same extent of that identified in the negative controls, which indicates that heat killed PAO1 does not have detectable β-glucosidase activity. As shown in figure 2, a significant increase in total β-glucosidase (figure 2, panel A), GBA1 (figure 2, panel B) and GBA2 (figure 2, panel C) activities were observed in response to infection. The effects of pre-treatment with miglustat or Genz-529648 on β-glucosidase activity were then studied in both IB3-1 and CuFi-1 cells infected with PAO1. Total β-glucosidase was slightly reduced in both cell lines treated with the two inhibitors (figure 3, panel A), whereas GBA1 activity remained unchanged (figure 3, panel B). Importantly, both miglustat and Genz-529648 significantly decreased GBA2 activity in bronchial cells infected with *P. aeruginosa* (figure 3, panel C). These results demonstrate that miglustat and Genz-529648 inhibited the activity of GBA2 and support the hypothesis that GBA2 could be a target of the anti-inflammatory effects of deoxynojirimycin-type inhibitors.

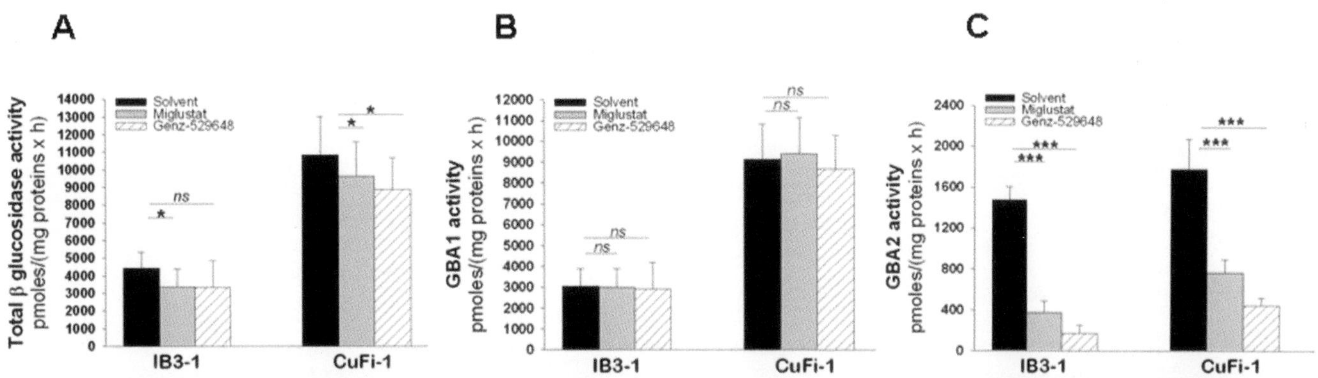

Figure 3. Miglustat and Genz-529648 inhibit GBA2 activity in IB3-1 and CuFi-1 cells infected by *P. aeruginosa*. IB3-1 and CuFi-1 cells were treated with [2 μM] miglustat, [10 nM] Genz-529648 or solvent alone for 1 hour prior to infection with heat-killed PAO1 for 4 hours. Total β-glucosidase (A), GBA1 (B) and GBA2 (C) activities were measured as indicated in figure 2. The data reported are the mean ± standard error of the mean of 3 (IB3-1) or 2 (CuFi-1) independent experiments in triplicate. Comparisons between groups were made by using Student's *t* tests.

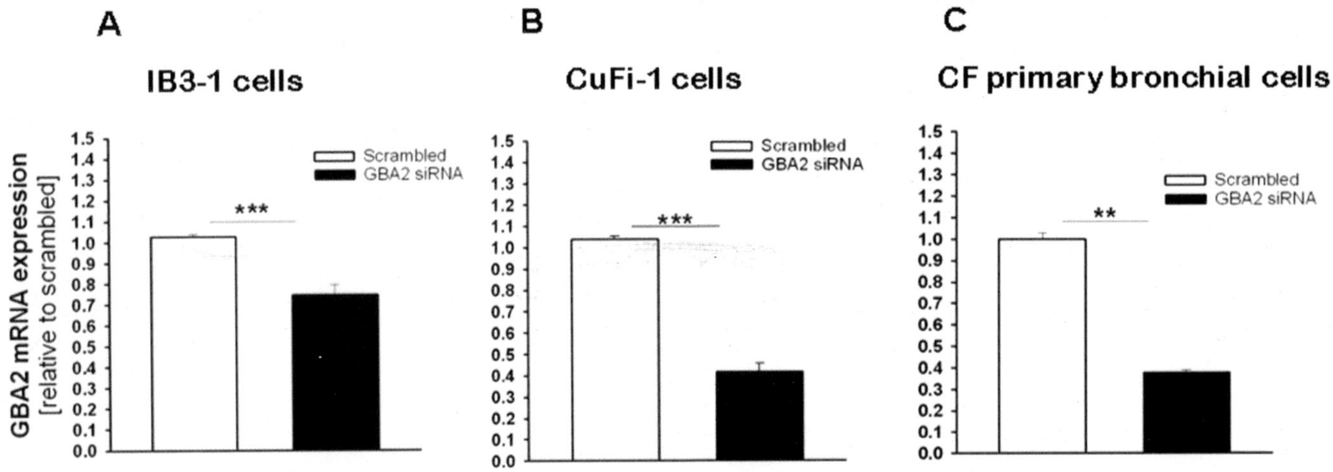

Figure 4. Transfection with GBA2 siRNA reduces the expression of GBA2 in CF bronchial cells. IB3-1 (A), CuFi-1 (B) or CF primary bronchial cells (C) were transfected with GBA2 siRNA or scrambled oligonucleotides for 24 h. GBA2 mRNA expression was measured by Real-time qPCR and obtained by comparing the ratio GBA2 and the housekeeping gene GAPDH between scrambled or siRNA treated cells. The data reported on the y-axis are relative to scrambled-treated cells and represent the mean ± SE of five (IB3-1, panel A), eight (CuFi-1, panel B) and four (CF primary bronchial, panel C) independent experiments performed in duplicate. Comparisons between groups were made by using Student's *t* tests.

siRNA-mediated silencing of GBA2 in CF bronchial cells decreases IL-8 expression

To confirm if GBA2 is involved in the signaling cascade activated by *P. aeruginosa* infection of CF bronchial cells, the levels of IL-8 were measured following GBA2 silencing with siRNA oligonucleotides. The cells were transiently transfected with a siRNA that specifically targeted the degradation of human GBA2 mRNA or a control duplex scrambled siRNA. As shown in figure 4, panel A, transfection of IB3-1 cells with the GBA2-specific siRNA significantly reduced (30%) the level of expression of GBA2 mRNA. Transfection of CuFi-1 cells with the GBA2 siRNA produced a greater decrease (60%) in GBA2 mRNA levels (figure 4, panel B). The experiments were then repeated in primary CF bronchial cells, a cell model that closely resembles the native epithelium, where a decrease of GBA2 expression (~60%) was also identified after transfection with the GBA2 specific siRNA (figure 4, panel C). As shown in figure 5, the silencing of GBA2 expression decreased IL-8 transcription in both uninfected cells (figure 5, panels A, B and C) and cells infected by *P. aeruginosa* (figure 5, panels D, E and F); however, in IB3-1 cells, the IL-8 reduction was not significant (figure 5, panels A and D). These findings were confirmed by measuring IL-8 protein levels in the supernatants of CuFi-1 cells at 4 hours post-infection with PAO1. As expected, the decrease in IL-8 mRNA expression was accompanied by a significant reduction in the secretion of IL-8 into the supernatant (figure 6). To provide evidence that the reduction of IL-8 levels is related to a decrease in GBA2 function, GBA2 activity was measured in GBA2 silenced CuFi-1 cells. Therefore, the cells were transiently transfected as previously described, and the total β-glucosidase and GBA2 activities in cell lysates were measured 18 and 42 hours after transfection. As shown in figure 7, panel A, GBA2 activity was significantly decreased at 18 hours after transfection. A further reduction of GBA2 activity resulted from measurements performed 42 hours after silencing. In these experimental conditions, transfection with siRNA that targeted GBA2 had an impact only on GBA2 activity, as demonstrated by the slight decrease of total β-glucosidase activity identified in GBA2 silenced cells (figure 7, panel B). These data, which demonstrate that lowering the expression and activity of GBA2 leads to a concomitant reduction in IL-8 levels, suggest a role for GBA2 in the inflammatory response induced by *P. aeruginosa* infection of CF bronchial cells.

Increase of cell ceramide content induced by *P. aeruginosa* in CF bronchial cells

Inhibiting the catabolism of GlcCer by GBA2 could also lower ceramide levels and thereby reduce pulmonary inflammation in CF patients. We have previously shown that miglustat reduced the expression of immunoreactive ceramides (measured by immuno-fluorescence) induced by *P. aeruginosa* [20]. To assess the effect of *P. aeruginosa* infection on the total cell ceramide content, LC-MS and LC-MS/MS analyses were performed as detailed in the Supplement S1. In the PAO1 infected IB3-1 and CuFi-1 cells, a significant increase in ceramides was identified (figure 8, panels A and B), which indicated that the infection up-modulated whole cell ceramide levels. Treatment with miglustat or Genz-529648 significantly reduced whole cell ceramide in IB3-1 cells by approximately 50% (figure 8, panel A), whereas in CuFi-1 cells, a small, albeit not significant decrease in ceramide levels was identified (figure 8, panel B).

To better evaluate the contribution of GSL catabolism to the ceramide increase following PAO1 infection, cell SL metabolic labeling was performed with the radioactive precursor sphingosine, which enables labeling of SLs at the steady-state. Thus, the effects of drug treatment on the radioactive ceramide content are only because of the modulation of the SL catabolism, thereby excluding the *de novo* pathway. To discriminate between the ceramide derived from SM catabolism and GSLs, we treated cells with amitriptyline alone, which is an inhibitor of ASM activity, or in combination with Genz-529648. IB3-1 and CuFi-1 cells were also subjected to the SL metabolic labeling with (1-^{3}H) sphingosine and were then differently treated with 10 μM amitriptyline alone or in combination with 10 nM Genz-529648 and infected with PAO1 as detailed in the Supplement S2. The total lipid extracts (ELT) obtained from cells were subjected to HPTLC separation to distinguish ceramide from the other SLs. The radioactive ceramide was quantified by digital autoradiography (figure 9, panel A). In the CuFi-1 cells, the ceramide levels were under the

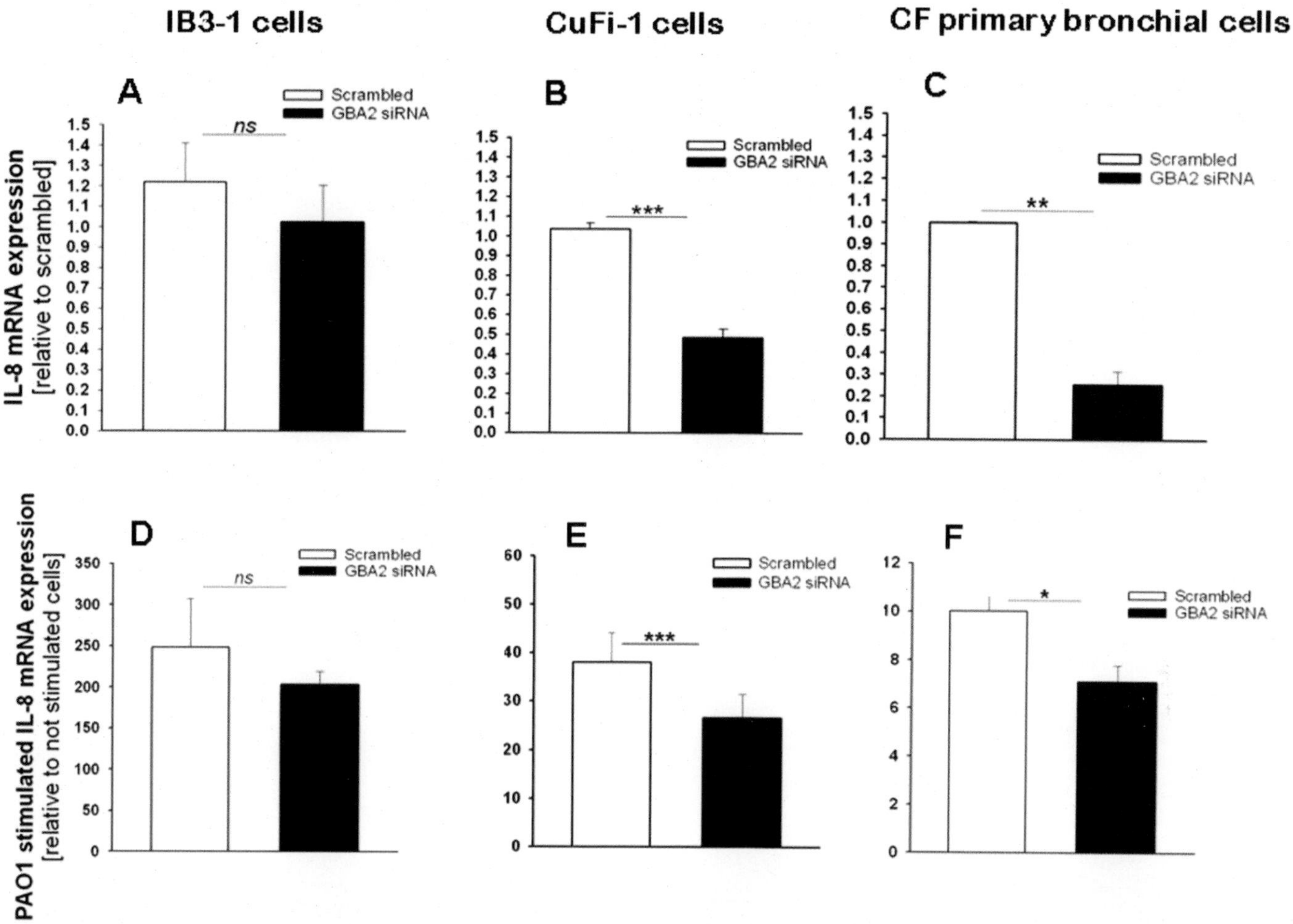

Figure 5. Reduction of IL-8 is associated with a relevant decrease of GBA2 expression in CF bronchial cells. IB3-1 (A), CuFi-1 (B) or CF primary bronchial cells (C) were transfected with GBA2 siRNA or scrambled oligonucleotides for 24 h and then infected with PAO1 (10–50 CFU/cell). IL-8 mRNA expression was measured as indicated in figure 1. The data reported on the y-axis are relative to scrambled-treated cells (A, B and C) or scrambled-treated uninfected cells (D, E and F) and represent the mean ± SE of five (IB3-1, panels A and D), eight (CuFi-1, panels B and E) and four (CF primary bronchial, panels C and F) independent experiments performed in duplicate. Comparisons between groups were made by using Student's *t* tests.

sensitivity threshold of the digital autoradiograph used. By contrast, a significant increase in the ceramide content after PAO1 infection was observed in the IB3-1 cells. The treatment of cells with amitriptyline caused a slight reduction of ceramide, whereas a significant decrease of the ceramide content was observed when infected cells were treated with both amitriptyline and Genz-529648; these findings support a direct involvement of GBA2 in ceramide production (figure 9, panel B).

Discussion

Recent advances in glycobiology have encouraged a search for novel drug molecules that address new biochemical targets. Iminosugars, which are carbohydrate-mimetics with a nitrogen atom replacing oxygen, have many attributes that make them suitable as small-molecule drug candidates. Pharmaceutical interest in these compounds is related to their ability to modulate carbohydrate processing, control cancer cell glycosylation, reduce viral and bacterial infectivity, alter immune responses and bind carbohydrate receptors [22]. The iminosugar miglustat, which was approved to treat type I Gaucher disease and Niemann-Pick type C disease, exerts an anti-inflammatory effect in CF human bronchial epithelial cells infected by *P. aeruginosa* and down modulates the neutrophil chemotaxis in murine lungs *in vivo* [20,23]. Here, we report that the non-lysosomal β-glucosidase 2, is a target of the anti-inflammatory effects of miglustat and other deoxynojirimycin-type inhibitors used in this study. This contention is supported by the findings that: *i*) treatment of *P. aeruginosa* infected CF bronchial cells with Genz-529648, a potent inhibitor of GBA2, reduced the extent of inflammation; *ii*) the IC_{50} value of the anti-inflammatory effect of Genz-529648 was similar compared to the effect reported toward inhibiting GBA2 activity (33); *iii)* treatment of CF bronchial cells with miglustat or Genz-529648 inhibited GBA2; and *iv)* inhibition of GBA2 by siRNA lowered the expression of IL-8.

The alkylated iminosugars miglustat, NB-DGJ and Genz-529648 employed in this study inhibit GlcCerT, GBA1 and GBA2. However, the impact of these compounds on GlcCerT and GBA activities depends greatly on their dosage [30]. Lower concentrations of iminosugars primarily affect GBA2, whereas higher doses inhibit all enzymes. Notably, we obtained a reduction of *P. aeruginosa* stimulated IL-8 mRNA expression in CF bronchial cells treated with Genz-529648 at very low nanomolar

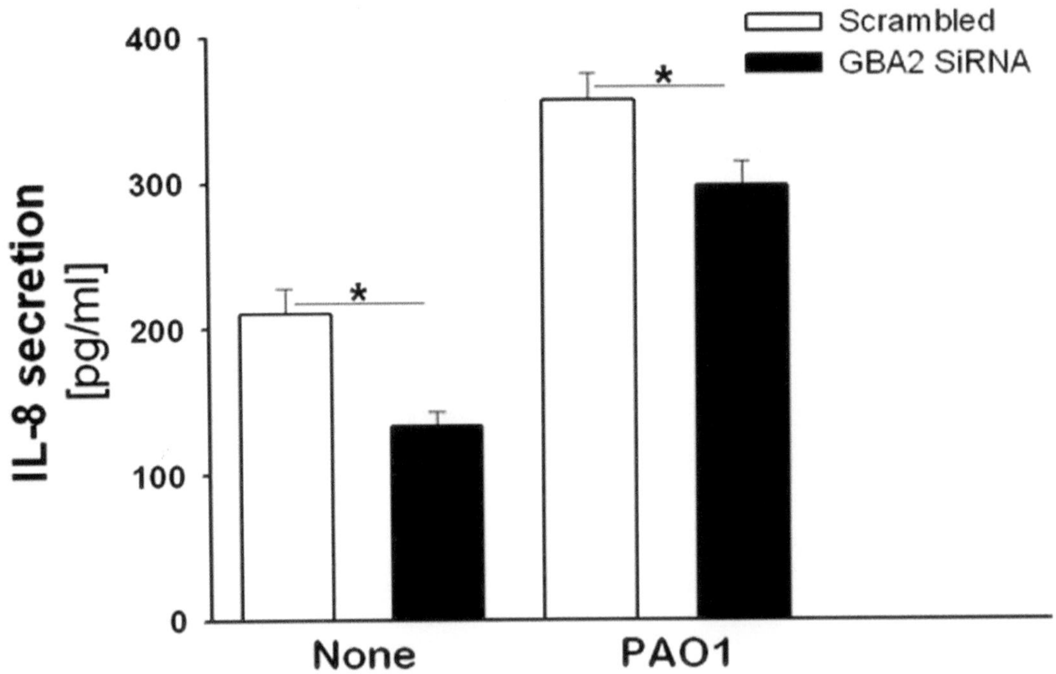

Figure 6. GBA2 silencing reduces the IL-8 protein release in CuFi-1 cells. CuFi-1 cells were transfected with GBA2 siRNA or scrambled oligonucleotides and then infected with PAO1 as indicated in figure 5. The supernatants were collected at the end of infection, and IL-8 protein release was measured as detailed in the "Methods" section. The data reported are the mean ± SE of eight independent experiments performed in duplicate. Comparisons between groups were made by using Student's *t* tests.

concentrations, which completely inhibited GBA2 activity, but not GBA1 or GlcCerT [34]. Measurements of the sensitivity of GlcCerT, GBA1 and GBA2 to the inhibition by miglustat in different mammalian cells/tissues revealed IC_{50} values in the low μM, high μM and nM range, respectively. This finding indicates that GBA2 is more sensitive to miglustat compared to GlcCerT and GBA1 [30]. Although the IC_{50} values of miglustat at inhibiting *P. aeruginosa* stimulated IL-8 mRNA expression in CF bronchial cells (table 1) are higher compared to the IC_{50} values for inhibiting GBA2, they are substantially lower compared to GlcCerT and GBA1. Hence, GlcCerT and GBA1 are unlikely to have been the targets of the anti-inflammatory effects of miglustat. Furthermore, we previously reported that miglustat down modulates neutrophil chemotaxis *in vivo* at doses that are lower (100 mg/Kg) [20] compared to the doses necessary to affect GlcCerT (1800–2400 mg/Kg) [42], which further supports the notion that the primary effect of miglustat is on GBA2 activity.

GBA2 plays a role in extra-lysosomal GlcCer catabolism, producing ceramide that can then be rapidly converted into sphingomyelin [29]. Although the mechanism and function of extra-lysosomal GlcCer degradation are not well understood, GBA2 has recently been implicated in various pathologic conditions, such as neuronal diseases [43] or cancer [44], which supports a role of GlcCer in cell growth, proliferation and immunity. The present novel findings suggest that GBA2 may also be involved in modulating the inflammatory response to *P. aeruginosa* infection in CF bronchial epithelial cells. Indeed, total β-glucosidase, GBA1 and GBA2 activities were elevated in CF bronchial cells infected by *P. aeruginosa* (figure 2). As for the effects of infection on SLs, it should be noted that infection of host epithelial cells with *P. aeruginosa* activates host ASM levels, which leads to the generation of plasma membrane ceramide-enriched platforms that promote the internalization of bacteria, induce apoptosis and regulate the cytokine storm [13]. Based on the observations noted in our studies, it is possible that in addition to ASM, an overall activation of β-glucosidase activity may also be involved in the host cell response to infection. However, additional studies are needed to validate this assumption. Importantly, miglustat or Genz-529648, at the concentrations used in this study, strongly inhibited only GBA2 activity (figure 3); in parallel, we demonstrated a reduction of *P. aeruginosa* stimulated IL-8 mRNA expression and protein release in CF bronchial cells when GBA2 expression (figure 5) and function (figures 1 and 7) were decreased. These findings support the contention that GBA2 is involved in the inflammatory response to *P. aeruginosa*. GBA2 is typically associated with plasma- and/or ER-membranes in close proximity to the sites of GlcCer synthesis and ceramide conversion to SM [45]. Therefore, as GBA2 is in a key position for GlcCer-mediated signaling, it could be activated following interactions between *P. aeruginosa* and the host cell. It has been shown that GBA2 activation causes the phosphorylation of eukaryotic initiation factor 2α (eIF2α), and this event is associated with an increased expression of the ATF4 family of transcription factors [44]. Interestingly, phosphorylation of eIF2α has been observed in models of acute infection with *Clostridium difficile*, as part of the mucosal inflammatory response [46]. It can be speculated that GBA2 activation by *P. aeruginosa* leads to increased expression of the transcription factors that regulate the pro-inflammatory genes in CF bronchial cells.

The airway epithelium is known to play a key role in the initiation and regulation of inflammatory processes in response to pathogens. In addition to the classical cytokines and chemokines that are released by the respiratory epithelium, ceramide is another important factor in pulmonary host defense [11]. Here, we report an increase in whole cell ceramides in response to infection by *P. aeruginosa* (figures 8 and 9) in CF bronchial

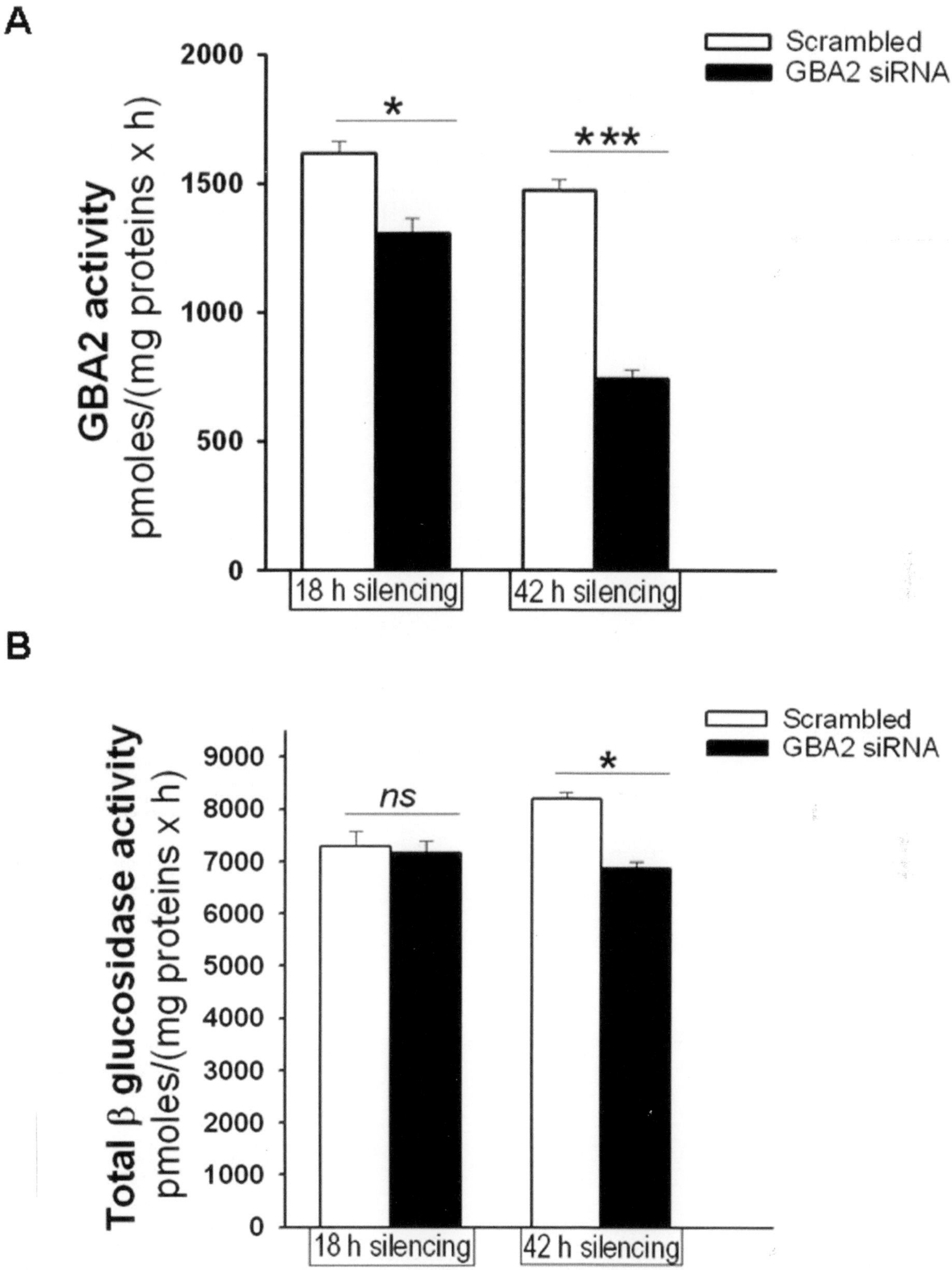

Figure 7. GBA2 silencing reduces GBA2 activity in CuFi-1 cells. CuFi-1 cells were transfected with GBA2 siRNA or scrambled oligonucleotides as indicated in figure 5. Eighteen or 42 hours after transfection, the cells were scraped and treated as indicated in figure 2. Total β-glucosidase (B) and GBA2 (A) activities were measured as reported in the Methods section. The data reported are the mean ± standard error of the mean of 2 independent experiments in triplicate. Comparisons between groups were made by using Student's *t* tests.

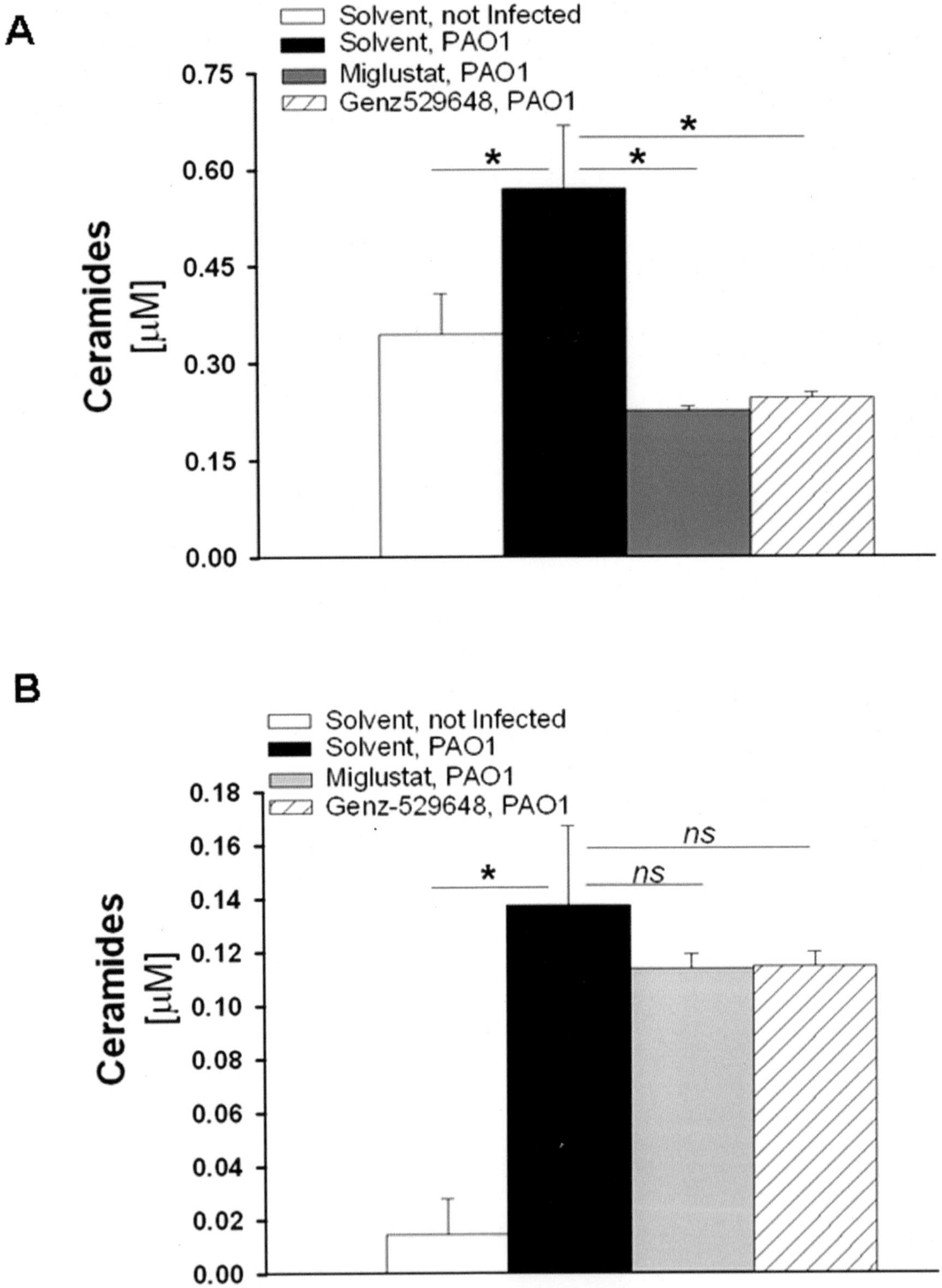

Figure 8. Infection with PAO1 increases whole cell ceramides in CF bronchial epithelial cells. IB3-1 (A) and CuFi-1 (B) cells were treated with [2 μM] miglustat, [10 nM] Genz-529648 or solvent alone and infected with PAO1 as indicated in figure 3. After infection, whole cell ceramides were analyzed by LC-MS and LC-MS/MS methods as described in the online supplement. The data reported are the mean ± SE of three independent experiments performed with both cell lines. Comparisons between groups were made by using Student's *t* tests.

epithelial cells, which is consistent with the rise of ceramide levels at the plasma membrane previously described [20]. In CuFi-1 cells, which have a lower ceramide content compared to IB3-1 cells, we observed a slight decrease in ceramide levels by miglustat or Genz-529648 (figure 8, panel B). By contrast, IB3-1 cells infected with PAO1 and treated with both miglustat and Genz-

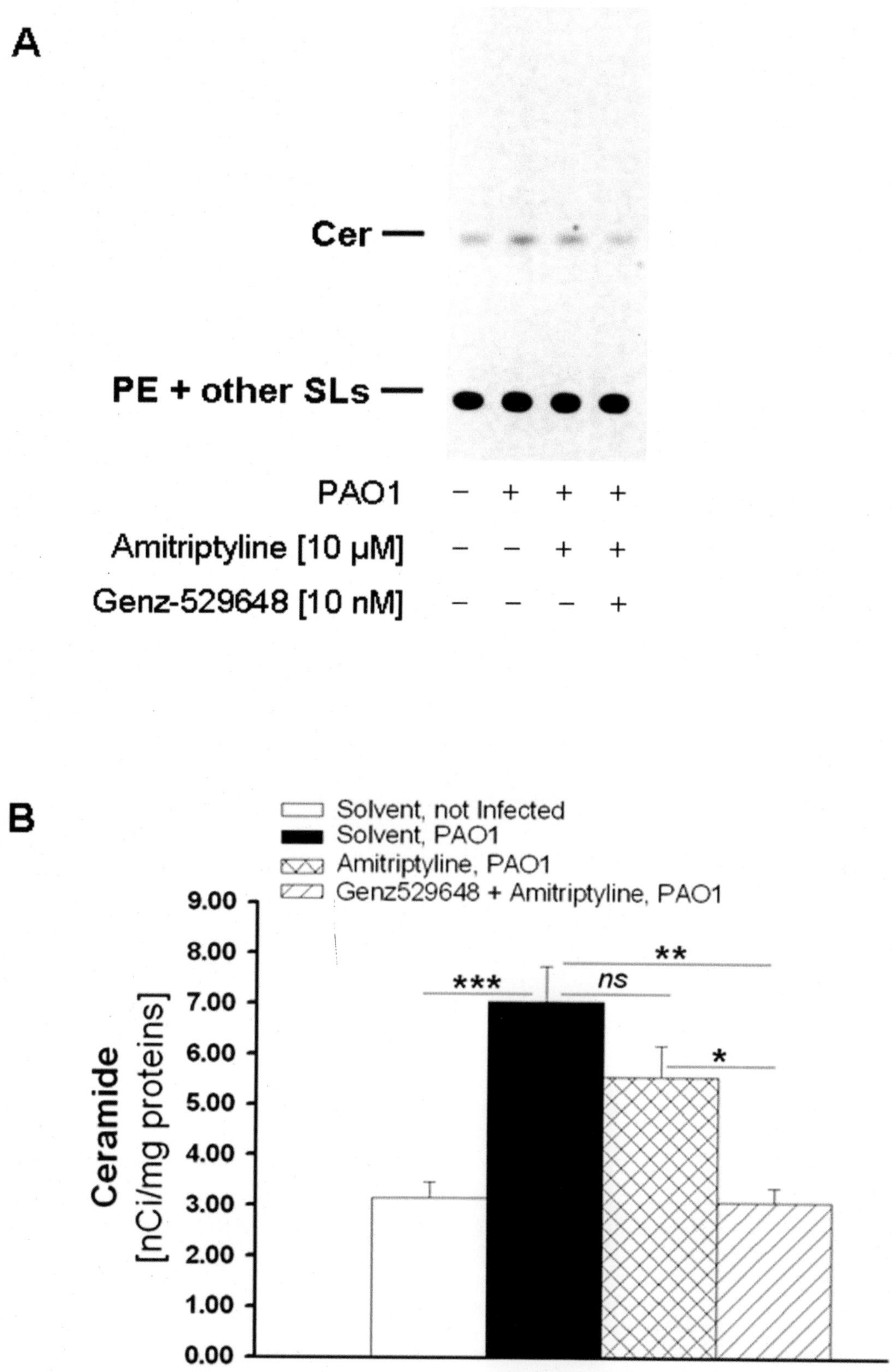

Figure 9. Treatment with Genz-529648 reduces the ceramide content in IB3-1 cells infected with PAO1. IB3-1 cells subjected to the SL metabolic labeling with (1-^{3}H)sphingosine were treated with [10 µM] amitriptyline alone, in combination with [10 nM] Genz-529648, or with solvent alone and infected with PAO1 as indicated in figure 3. After lipid extraction, (^{3}H)ceramide was separated from the other radioactive SLs by HPTLC, as detailed in the online supplement, and detected by digital autoradiography (total lipid extracts amounts corresponding to 4 µg of cellular proteins were applied on a 4-mm line. Time of acquisition: 48 hours). The digital autoradiography represents data obtained in three different experiments (A). The ceramide content was quantified by specific β-Vision software, and the data reported are the mean ± SE of three independent experiments. Comparisons between groups were made by using Student's *t* tests (B).

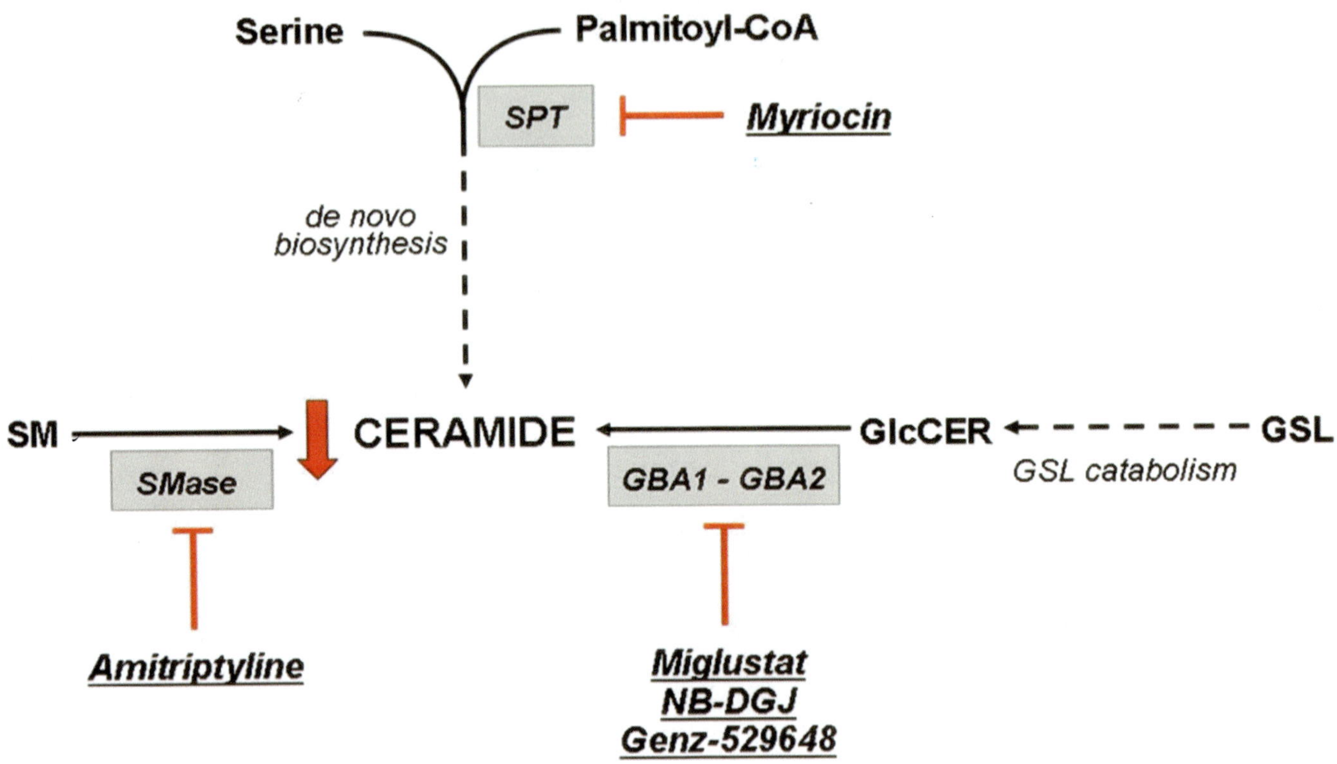

Figure 10. Metabolic pathways involved in ceramide formation. Schematic representation of the primary metabolic pathways involved in ceramide production. Ceramide can be produced by the *de novo* biosynthesis, the hydrolysis of sphingomyelin (SM) by the action of sphingomyelinases and the catabolism of glycosphingolipids (GSL). In particular, it has been observed that in CF bronchial epithelial cells, the use of inhibitors of these pathways resulted in a reduction of ceramide. Myriocin acts on the first step of the *de novo* biosynthesis through the inhibition of the Serine-palmitoyl transferase (SPT); amitriptyline inhibits the acid SMase (ASM) responsible for SM catabolism; and miglustat, NB-DGJ and Genz-529648 are inhibitors of the β-glucosidases GBA1 and GBA2, which are involved in the hydrolysis of the glucosylceramide (GlcCer).

529648 showed a marked decrease of ceramide content (figure 8, panel A). The increase in ceramide content following infection by PAO1 could be a result of different pathways, including the *de novo* biosynthesis [21], SM catabolism [13] and GSL degradation. When we evaluated the effects of drug treatment on the radioactive ceramide content that resulted only because of the modulation of SL catabolism, thus excluding the *de novo* pathway, we identified a marked increase in the cell ceramide content after PAO1 infection (figure 9). After ASM inhibition, we observed a slight decrease and a further, more significant ceramide reduction after the addition of the specific inhibitor of GBA2, Genz-529648 (figure 9), which strongly supports the direct involvement of GBA2 in the ceramide production after PAO1 infection of human bronchial epithelial cells. Thus, the information derived from the literature and the data presented here provide evidence that different inhibitors, such as miglustat and Genz-529648, amitriptyline [14] and myriocin [21], that target GBA2, ASM and ceramide *de novo* synthesis, respectively, could represent therapeutic tools to reduce ceramide levels and limit excessive lung inflammation in CF patients (figure 10). Nevertheless, drugs that target SL metabolism must be carefully titrated to normalize ceramide levels in CF airways, but not reduce ceramide concentrations below a critical level that would impair normal biological functions. Notably, systemic inhibition of ASM could negatively affect the host defense, which has been demonstrated by studies in mice that completely lack ASM and are unable to control infections [13]. Interestingly, no increased susceptibility to bacterial infections has been identified in patients affected by Gaucher disease, treated with miglustat [47] or in a mouse model of Sandhoff disease treated with Genz-529648 [48].

In summary, our study proposes GBA2 as a novel target to reduce the inflammatory response to *P. aeruginosa* in CF bronchial cells. These results further support the use of modulators of SL metabolism for CF lung inflammation. In addition, as GBA2 is sensitive to very low doses of miglustat, other alkylated iminosugars (NB-DGJ) and Genz-529648, our findings provide evidence to develop therapeutic options for CF lung inflammation using iminosugars, which can be effective at even low doses, thus limiting potential adverse effects.

Supporting Information

Figure S1 Viability profile of IB3-1 cells treated for 24 hours with the indicated concentrations of Genz-529648.

Figure S2 Apoptosis profile of IB3-1 cells treated for 24 hours with the indicated concentration of Genz-529648.

Figure S3 Apoptotic IB3-1 cells after 4 and 24 hours of treatment with the indicated concentrations of Genz-529648.

Supplement S1 Analysis of cell ceramide levels using LC-MS and LC-MS/MS.

Supplement S2 Analysis of cell ceramide levels by cell SLs labeling with (^{3}H)sphingosine.

Supplement S3 Cellular toxicity of Genz-529648.

Acknowledgments

We are grateful to: A. Tamanini for helpful discussions, A. Prince for the *P. aeruginosa* laboratory strain PAO1, "In Vitro Model and Cell Culture Care" of the University of Iowa, Iowa, U.S.A. for providing CuFi-1 cells and to "Servizio Colture Primarie" of the Italian Cystic Fibrosis Research Foundation at the Laboratory of Molecular Genetics, G. Gaslini Institute, Genova, Italy, for CF primary cells. This research was supported by the Italian Cystic Fibrosis Research Foundation (grant FFC # 14/2012) with the contribution of *"Picasso. Capolavori dal Museo Nazionale Picasso di Parigi", Festa d'Estate Villa Sigurtà Verona, Delegazione FFC Lago di Garda e Arezzo.*

Author Contributions

Conceived and designed the experiments: MCD MA SS GC. Performed the experiments: NL MT IL NM RB VB VL CC SM. Analyzed the data: MCD MA NL NM MGG AC RG. Contributed reagents/materials/analysis tools: SHC MGG. Wrote the paper: MCD SHC MA RB NL .

References

1. Welsh JM, Ramsey BW, Accurso F, Cutting GR (2001) Cystic Fibrosis in Scriver CR, Beaudet AL, Sly WS, Valle D (Eds). *The Metabolic and Molecular Bases of Inherited Diseases*. McGraw-Hill, New York.
2. Ramsey BW, Davies J, McElvaney NG, Tullis E, Bell SC, et al. (2011) VX08-770-102 Study Group A CFTR Potentiator in Patients with Cystic Fibrosis and the *G551D* Mutation. New England J of Medicine 365: 1663–1672.
3. Hoffman LR, Ramsey BW (2013) Cystic Fibrosis Therapeutics. The road ahead. Chest 143(1): 207–213.
4. Konstan MW, Schluchter MD, Xue W, Davis PB (2007) Clinical use of Ibuprofen is associated with slower Fev1 decline in children with cystic fibrosis. Am J Respir Crit Care Med 176 (11): 1084–1089.
5. Khan TZ, Wagener JS, Bost T, Martinez J, Accurso FJ, et al. (1995) Early pulmonary inflammation in infants with cystic fibrosis. Am J Respir Crit Care Med 151: 1075–1082.
6. Noah TL, Black HR, Cheng PW, Wood RE, Leigh MW (1997) Nasal and bronchoalveolar lavage fluid cytokines in early cystic fibrosis. J Infect Dis 175: 638–647.
7. Tirouvanziam R, de Bentzmann S, Hubeau C, Hinnrasky J, Jacquot J, et al. (2000) Inflammation and infection in naive human cystic fibrosis airway grafts. Am J Respir Cell Mol Biol 23(2): 121–127.
8. Chmiel JF, Berger M, Konstan MW (2002) The role of inflammation in the pathophysiology of CF lung disease. Clin Rev Allergy Immunol 23: 5–27.
9. Lahiri S, Futerman AH (2007) The metabolism and function of shingolipids and glycoshingolipids. Cell Mol Life Sci 64: 2270–2284.
10. Uhlig S, Gulbins E (2008) Sphingolipids in the lungs. Am J Respir Crit Care Med 178(11): 1100–1114.
11. Yang Y, Uhlig S (2001) The role of sphingolipids in respiratory disease. Ther Adv Respir Dis 5: 325–344.
12. Hannun YA, Obeid LM (2008) Principles of bioactive lipid signalling: lessons from sphingolipids. Nat Rew Mol Cell Biol 9: 139–150.
13. Grassme' H, Jendrossek V, Riehle A, von Kürthy G, Berger J, et al. (2003) Host defense against *Pseudomonas aeruginosa* requires ceramide-rich membrane rafts. Nature Medicine 9: 322–330.
14. Teichgraber V, Ulrich M, Endlich N, Riethmüller J, Wilker B, et al. (2008) Ceramide accumulation mediates inflammation, cell death and infection susceptibility in cystic fibrosis. Nature Med 14: 382–391.
15. Guilbault C, De Sanctis JB, Wojewodka G, Saeed Z, Lachance C, et al. (2008) Fenretinide corrects newly found ceramide deficiency in cystic fibrosis. Am J Respir Cell Mol Biol 38(1): 47–56.
16. Yu H, Zeidan YH, Wu BX, Jenkins RW, Flotte TR, et al. (2009) Defective acid sphingomyelinase pathway with *Pseudomonas aeruginosa* infection in cystic fibrosis. American Journal of Respiratory Cell and Molecular Biology 41: 367–375.
17. Brodlie M, McKean MC, Johnson GE, Gray J, Fisher AJ, et al. (2010) Ceramide is Increased in the Lower Airway Epithelium of People with Advanced Cystic Fibrosis Lung Disease. Am J Respir Crit Care Med 182 (3): 369–375.
18. Bodas M, Min T, Mazur S, Vij N (2011) Critical modifier role of membrane-cystic fibrosis transmembrane conductance regulator-dependent ceramide signaling in lung injury and emphysema. J Immunol 186: 602–613.
19. Nährlich L, Mainz JG, Adams C, Engel C, Herrmann G, et al. (2013) Therapy of CF-patients with amitriptyline and placebo-a randomised, double-blind, placebo-controlled phase IIb multicenter, cohort-study. Cell Physiol Biochem 31(4–5): 505–312.
20. Dechecchi MC, Nicolis E, Mazzi P, Cioffi F, Bezzerri V, et al. (2011) Modulators of sphingolipid metabolism reduce lung inflammation. Am J Respir Cell Mol Biol 45(4): 825–833.
21. Caretti A, Bragonzi A, Facchini M, De Fino I, Riva C, et al. (2014) Anti-inflammatory action of lipid nanocarrier-delivered myriocin: therapeutic potential in cystic fibrosis. Biochim Biophys Acta 1840(1): 586–594.
22. Nash RJ, Kato A, Yu C-Y, Fleet GWJ (2011) Iminosugars as therapeuthic agents:recent advances and promising trends. Future Med Chem 3(12): 1–9.
23. Dechecchi MC, Nicolis E, Mazzi P, Paroni M, Cioffi F, et al. (2012) Pharmacological modulators of sphingolipid metabolism for the treatment of cystic fibrosis lung inflammation. In Dinesh D and Sriramulu D editors. Cystic Fibrosis - the Human Agony, ISBN 979-953-307-059-8, Germany.
24. Norez C, Noel S, Wilke M, Bijvelds M, Jorna H, et al. (2006) Rescue of functional delF508-CFTR channels in cystic fibrosis epithelial cells by the α-glucosidase inhibitor miglustat. FEBS Lett 580: 2081–2086.
25. Dechecchi MC, Nicolis E, Norez C, Bezzerri V, Borgatti M, et al. (2008) Anti-inflammatory effect of miglustat in bronchial epithelial cells. J Cyst Fibros 7(6): 555–565.
26. Lubamba B, Lebacq J, Lebecque P, Vanbever R, Leonard A (2009) Airway delivery of low-dose miglustat normalizes nasal potential difference in F508del cystic fibrosis mice. Am J Respir Crit Care Med 179: 1022–1028.
27. Leonard A, Lebecque P, Dingemanse J, Leal T (2012) A randomized placebo-controlled trial of miglustat in cystic fibrosi based on nasal potential difference. J Cystic Fibrosis 11(3): 231–236.
28. Inokuchi J, Mason I, Radin NS (1987) Antitumor activity via inhibition of glycosphingolipid biosynthesis. Cancer Lett 38: 23–30.
29. Boot RG, Verhoek M, Donker-Koopman W, Strijland A, van Marle J, et al. (2007) Identification of the non-lysosomal glucosylceramidase as beta-glucosidase 2. J Biol Chem 282: 1305–1312.
30. Ridley CM, Thur KE, Shanahan J, Thillaiappan NB, Shen A, et al. (2013) β-Glucosidase 2 (GBA2) activity and imino sugar pharmacology. J Biol Chem 288(36): 26052–26066.
31. Dwek RA, Butters TD, Platt FM, Zitzmann N (2002) Targeting glycosylation as a therapeutic approach. Nat Rev Drug Discov 1: 65–75.
32. Platt FM, Neises GR, Karlsson GB, Dwek RA, Butters TD (1994) N-butyldeoxygalactonojirimycin inhibits glycolipid biosynthesis but does not affect N-linked oligosaccharide processing. J Biol Chem 269 (43): 27108–27114.
33. Weenekes T, Meijer AJ, Groen AK, Boot RG, Groener JE, et al. (2010) Large-Scale synthesis of the glucosylceramide synthase inhibitor N-[5-(Adamantan-1-yl-methoxy)-pentyl]-1-deoxynojirimycin. J Med Chem 53: 689–698.
34. Overkleeft HS, Renkema Hg, Neele J, Vianello P, Hung IO, et al. (1998) Generation of specific deoxynojirimycin-type inhibitors of the non-lysosomal glucosylceramidase. J Biol Chem 273 (41): 26522–26527.
35. Yildiz Y, Matern H, Thompson B, Allergood JC, Warren RL, et al. (2006) Mutation of beta-glucosidase 2 causes glycolipid storage disease and impaired male fertility. J Clin Invest 116: 2985–2994.
36. Aerts JM, Ottenhoff R, Powlson AS, Grefhorst A, van Eijk M, et al. (2007) Pharmacological inhibition of glucosylceramide synthase enhances insulin sensitivity. Diabetes 56(5): 1341–1349.
37. Zeitlin PL, Lu L, Rhim J, Cutting G, Stetten G, et al. (1991) A cystic fibrosis bronchial epithelial cell line: immortalization by adeno-12-SV40 infection. Am J Respir Cell Mol Biol 4: 313–319.
38. Zabner J, Karp P, Seiler M, Phillips Sl, Mitchell CJ, et al. (2003) Development of cystic fibrosis and non cystic fibrosis airway cell lines. Am J Physiol Lung Cell Mol Physiol 284: L844–L854.
39. Scudieri P, Caci E, Bruno S, Ferrera L, Schiavon M, et al. (2012) Association of TMEM16A chloride channel overexpression with airway goblet cell metaplasia. J Physiol 590 (23): 6141–6155.
40. Sullards MC, Allegood JC, Kelly S, Wang E, Haynes CA, et al. (2007) Structure-specific, quantitative methods for analysis of sphingolipids by LC-tandem MS: "inside-out" sphingolipids. Methods in Enzymology 432: 83–115.
41. Aureli M, Loberto N, Bassi R, Ferraretto A, Perego S, et al. (2012) Plasma membrane-associated glycohydrolases activation by extracellular acidification due to proton exchangers. Neurochem Res 37(6): 1296–1307.
42. Platt FM, Reinkensmeier G, Dwek RA, Butters TD (1996) Extensive glycosphingolipid depletion in the liver and lymphoid organs of mice treated with *N*- butyldeoxynojirimycin. J Biol Chem 272: 19365–19372.
43. Martin E, Schüle R, Smets K, Rastetter A, Boukhris A, et al. (2013) Loss of function of glucocerebrosidase GBA2 is responsible for motor neuron defects in hereditary spastic paraplegia. Am J Hum Genet 92(2): 238–244.
44. Sorli SC, Colié S, Albinet V, Dubrac A, Touriol C, et al. (2013) The nonlysosomal β-glucosidase GBA2 promotes endoplasmic reticulum stress and impairs tumorigenicity of human melanoma cells. FASEB J 27(2): 489–498.
45. Körschen HG, Yildiz Y, Raju DN, Schonauer S, Bönigk W, et al. (2013) The non-lysosomal β-glucosidase GBA2 is a non-integral membrane-associated protein at the endoplasmic reticulum (ER) and Golgi. J Biol Chem 288(5): 3381–3393.

46. Sadighi Akha AA, Theriot CM, Erb-Downward JR, McDermott AJ, Falkowski NR (2013) Acute infection of mice with Clostridium difficile leads to eIF2α phosphorylation and pro-survival signalling as part of the mucosal inflammatory response. Immunology 140(1): 111–122.
47. Hollak CE, Hughes D, van Schaik IN, Schwierin B, Bembi B (2009) Miglustat (Zavesca) in type 1 Gaucher disease: 5-year results of a post-authorisation safety surveillance programme. Pharmacoepidemiol Drug Saf 18(9): 770–777.
48. Ashe KM, Bangari D, Li L, Cabrera-Salazar MA, Bercury SD, et al. (2011) Iminosugar-based inhibitors of glucosylceramide synthase increase brain glycosphingolipids and survival in a mouse model of Sandhoff disease. PLoS One 6(6): 1–11.

Permissions

All chapters in this book were first published in PLOS ONE, by The Public Library of Science; hereby published with permission under the Creative Commons Attribution License or equivalent. Every chapter published in this book has been scrutinized by our experts. Their significance has been extensively debated. The topics covered herein carry significant findings which will fuel the growth of the discipline. They may even be implemented as practical applications or may be referred to as a beginning point for another development.

The contributors of this book come from diverse backgrounds, making this book a truly international effort. This book will bring forth new frontiers with its revolutionizing research information and detailed analysis of the nascent developments around the world.

We would like to thank all the contributing authors for lending their expertise to make the book truly unique. They have played a crucial role in the development of this book. Without their invaluable contributions this book wouldn't have been possible. They have made vital efforts to compile up to date information on the varied aspects of this subject to make this book a valuable addition to the collection of many professionals and students.

This book was conceptualized with the vision of imparting up-to-date information and advanced data in this field. To ensure the same, a matchless editorial board was set up. Every individual on the board went through rigorous rounds of assessment to prove their worth. After which they invested a large part of their time researching and compiling the most relevant data for our readers.

The editorial board has been involved in producing this book since its inception. They have spent rigorous hours researching and exploring the diverse topics which have resulted in the successful publishing of this book. They have passed on their knowledge of decades through this book. To expedite this challenging task, the publisher supported the team at every step. A small team of assistant editors was also appointed to further simplify the editing procedure and attain best results for the readers.

Apart from the editorial board, the designing team has also invested a significant amount of their time in understanding the subject and creating the most relevant covers. They scrutinized every image to scout for the most suitable representation of the subject and create an appropriate cover for the book.

The publishing team has been an ardent support to the editorial, designing and production team. Their endless efforts to recruit the best for this project, has resulted in the accomplishment of this book. They are a veteran in the field of academics and their pool of knowledge is as vast as their experience in printing. Their expertise and guidance has proved useful at every step. Their uncompromising quality standards have made this book an exceptional effort. Their encouragement from time to time has been an inspiration for everyone.

The publisher and the editorial board hope that this book will prove to be a valuable piece of knowledge for researchers, students, practitioners and scholars across the globe.

List of Contributors

Ben Ryall, Marta Carrara, James E. A. Zlosnik, Volker Behrends, Xiaoyun Lee, Zhen Wong, Kathryn E. Lougheed and Huw D. Williams
Department of Life Sciences, Faculty of Natural Sciences, Imperial College London, Sir Alexander Fleming Building, London, United Kingdom

Gabriella Wojewodka and Danuta Radzioch
Department of Human Genetics, McGill University, Montreal, Quebec, Canada

Juan B. De Sanctis
Institute of Immunology, Central University of Venezuela, Caracas, Venezuela

Joanie Bernier, Jim Gruber, Jennifer Landry and Elias Matouk
Adult Cystic Fibrosis Clinic, Montreal Chest Institute, McGill University Health Center, Montreal, Quebec, Canada

Julie Bérube
McGill University Health Center Research Institute, Montreal, Quebec, Canada

Heather G. Ahlgren, Dao Nguyen, Simon Rousseau, Andrea Benedetti and Danuta Radzioch
Department of Medicine, McGill University, Montreal, Quebec, Canada

Larry C. Lands
Division of Pediatric Respiratory Medicine, Montreal Children's Hospital, McGill University Health Center Research Institute, Montreal, Quebec, Canada

Andrea Benedetti
Department of Epidemiology, Biostatistics and Occupational Health, Montreal Chest Institute, McGill University Health Center, Montreal, Quebec, Canada

Ha Won Lee, Jie Cheng, Mark Donowitz and William B. Guggino
Department of Physiology, Johns Hopkins University, School of Medicine, Baltimore, Maryland, United States of America

Olga Kovbasnjuk
Department of Medicine, Johns Hopkins University, School of Medicine, Baltimore, Maryland, United States of America

Serena Schippa, Valerio Iebba, Floriana Santangelo, Antonella Gagliardi, Riccardo Valerio De and Maria Pia Conte
Public Health and Infectious Diseases Department, Microbiology Unit, 'Sapienza' University of Rome, Rome, Italy

Riccardo Valerio De Biase, Antonella Stamato, Serenella Bertasi and Serena Quattrucci
Regional Cystic Fibrosis Centre, Paediatrics and Infant Neuropsychiatry Department, 'Sapienza' University of Rome, Rome, Italy

Marco Lucarelli
Department of Haematology and Cellular Biotechnologies, Sapienza University of Rome, Rome, Italy

Natalie Jiricny, Kevin Foster, Pauline D. Scanlan, Melanie Ghoul, Lorenzo A. Santorelli and Ashleigh S. Griffin
Department of Zoology, Oxford University, Oxford, United Kingdom

Søren Molin
Department of Systems Biology, Technical University of Denmark, Lyngby, Denmark

Stephen P. Diggle
School of Life Sciences, Centre for Biomolecular Sciences, University Park, University of Nottingham, Nottingham, United Kingdom

Helle Krogh Johansen
Institute for International Health, Immunology and Microbiology, University of Copenhagen, Copenhagen, Denmark

Roman Popat
Centre for Immunity, Infection and Evolution, University of Edinburgh Ashworth Labs, King's Buildings, West Mains Road, Edinburgh, United Kingdom

Valia Verrière, Gerard Higgins, Mazen Al-Alawi, Brian J. Harvey and Valérie Urbach
Department of Molecular Medicine, RCSI Education and Research Centre, Beaumont Hospital, Dublin, Ireland

Raphaël Chiron
CRCM, Montpellier, France

Mazen Al-Alawi and Richard W. Costello
Department of Respiratory Medicine, Beaumont Hospital, Dublin, Ireland

Gerard Higgins, Paul McNally and Valérie Urbach
National Children's Research Centre, Our Lady's Children's Hospital Crumlin, Dublin, Ireland

Matthew T. Cabeen
Department of Molecular and Cellular Biology, Harvard University, Cambridge, Massachusetts, United States of America

Hanna Renk and Dominik Hartl
University Children's Hospital, Eberhard-Karls-University, Tuebingen, Germany

Nicolas Regamey
Department of Paediatrics, Inselspital and University of Bern, Bern, Switzerland

Arianna Pompilio, Domenico Ciavardelli, Valentina Crocetta, Ada Consalvo, Carmine Di Ilio and Giovanni Di Bonaventura
Clinical Microbiology Unit, Center of Excellence on Aging, "G. d'Annunzio" University Foundation, Chieti, Italy

Arianna Pompilio, Valentina Crocetta, Roberta Zappacosta, Carmine Di Ilio and Giovanni Di Bonaventura
Department of Experimental and Clinical Sciences, School of Medicine, "G. d'Annunzio" University, Chieti, Italy

Domenico Ciavardelli
School of Engineering, Architecture and Motor Science, "Kore" University, Enna, Italy

Anil J. Trindade, Douglas A. Medvetz, Nicole A. Neuman, Faina Myachina, Jane Yu, Carmen Priolo and Elizabeth P. Henske
Division of Pulmonary and Critical Care Medicine, Brigham and Women's Hospital and Harvard Medical School, Boston, Massachusetts, United States of America

Anthony Tang and Stuart E. Turvey
Department of Microbiology and Immunology, University of British Columbia, Vancouver, British Columbia, Canada

Ashish Sharma, Roger Jen, Pascal M. Lavoie and Stuart E. Turvey
Department of Experimental Medicine, University of British Columbia, Vancouver, British Columbia, Canada

Aaron F. Hirschfeld, Mark A. Chilvers, Pascal M. Lavoie and Stuart E. Turvey
Department of Pediatrics, British Columbia Children's Hospital and Child and Family Research Institute, Vancouver, British Columbia, Canada

David A. Ngan
Centre for Heart Lung Innovation, St. Paul's Hospital, University of British Columbia, Vancouver, British Columbia, Canada

Bradley S. Quon, Pearce G. Wilcox, S. F. Paul Man and Don D. Sin
Division of Respiratory Medicine, St. Paul's Hospital, University of British Columbia, Vancouver, British Columbia, Canada

Matthew L. Workentine and Michael G. Surette
Farncombe Family Digestive Health Research Institute, McMaster University, Hamilton, Ontario, Canada
Department of Medicine, McMaster University, Hamilton, Ontario, Canada

Michael G. Surette
Department of Biochemistry and Biomedical Sciences, McMaster University, Hamilton, Ontario, Canada

Christopher D. Sibley, Bryan Glezerson, Swathi Purighalla, Jens C. Norgaard-Gron, Michael D. Parkins, Harvey R. Rabin and Michael G. Surette
Department of Microbiology, Immunology and Infectious Diseases, University of Calgary, Calgary, Alberta, Canada

Michael D. Parkins and Harvey R. Rabin
Department of Medicine, University of Calgary, Calgary, Alberta, Canada
Adult Cystic Fibrosis Clinic, University of Calgary, Calgary, Alberta, Canada

Sanhita Roy
Department of Ophthalmology and Visual Sciences, Case Western Reserve University, Cleveland, Ohio, United States of America

Tracey Bonfield
Department of Pediatrics, Case Western Reserve University, Cleveland, Ohio, United States of America

Alan M. Tartakoff
Pathology Department and Cell Biology Program, Case Western Reserve University, leveland, Ohio, United States of America

Mette Kolpen, Thomas Bjarnsholt, Claus Moser, Arsalan Kharazmi and Peter Østrup Jensen
Department of Clinical Microbiology, Rigshospitalet, Copenhagen, Denmark

Mette Kolpen, Thomas Bjarnsholt and Niels Høiby
Department of International Health, Immunology and Microbiology, Faculty of Health Sciences University of Copenhagen, Copenhagen, Denmark

Michael Kühl and Lars Liengaard
Marine Biological Section, Department of Biology, University of Copenhagen, Helsingør, Denmark

Michael Kühl
Plant Functional Biology and Climate Change Cluster, University of Technology Sydney, Sydney, Australia
Singapore Centre on Environmental Life Sciences Engineering, Nanyang Technological University, Singapore, Singapore

Christine Rønne Hansen and Tanja Pressler
Copenhagen CF Centre, Rigshospitalet, Copenhagen, Denmark

Bettina Schaible, Andrew Selfridge and Cormac T. Taylor
UCD School of Medicine and Medical Science and The Conway Institute, University College Dublin, Dublin, Ireland

Bettina Schaible
School of Pharmacy, Queens's University, Belfast, United Kingdom

Siobhán McClean
Institute of Technology Tallaght, Dublin, Ireland

Alexis Broquet and Karim Asehnoune
Laboratoire UPRES EA 3826, Thérapeutiques cliniques et expérimentales des infections, Facultéde médecine, Université de Nantes, Nantes, France

Karim Asehnoune
Centre Hospitalier Universitaire de Nantes, Service anesthé sie réanimation chirurgicale, Hôtel Dieu-HME, Nantes, France

Kirsten Schaffer
Department of Microbiology, St. Vincent's University Hospital, Dublin, Ireland

Rossella Baldan, Francesca Testa and Daniela M. Cirillo
Emerging Bacterial Pathogens Unit, San Raffaele Scientific Institute, Milan, Italy

Cristina Cigana, Irene Bianconi, Maura De Simone and Alessandra Bragonzi
Infection and Cystic Fibrosis Unit, San Raffaele Scientific Institute, Milan, Italy

Danilo Pellin and Clelia Di Serio
University Centre for Statistics in the Biomedical Sciences, Universita` Vita-Salute San Raffaele, Milan, Italy

Rashmi Tripathi, Nathalie Benz, Pascal Trouvé and Claude Férec
INSERM UMR1078, Brest, France

Rashmi Tripathi and Claude Férec
Université de Bretagne Occidentale, Faculté de Medecine et des sciences de la santé, Brest, France

Nathalie Benz
Association Gaétan Saleün, Brest, France

Bridget Culleton and Claude Férec
Hôpital Morvan, Laboratoire de Génétique Moléculaire et d'Histocompatibilité, Brest, France

Claude Férec
Etablissement Français du Sang-Bretagne, Brest, France

Randal C. Fowler and Nancy D. Hanson
Creighton University School of Medicine, Department of Medical Microbiology and Immunology, Center for Research in Anti-Infectives and Biotechnology, Omaha, Nebraska, United States of America

Libera Latino, Christiane Essoh, Yann Blouin and Christine Pourcel
Univ Paris-Sud, Institut de Génétique et Microbiologie, UMR 8621, Orsay, France, CNRS, Orsay, France

Hoang Vu Thien
Hôpital Armand Trousseau, Assistance Publique-Hôpitaux de Paris (APHP), Bactériologie, Paris, France

Maela Tebon, Valentino Bezzerri, Valentina Lovato, Cinzia Cantù, Silvia Munari, Giulio Cabrini and Maria Cristina Dechecch
Laboratory of Molecular Pathology, Department of Pathology and Diagnostics, University Hospital of Verona, Verona, Italy

Nicoletta Loberto, Massimo Aureli, Rosaria Bassi and Sandro Sonnino
Department of Medical Biotechnology and Translational Medicine, University of Milano, Milano, Italy

Ilaria Lampronti and Roberto Gambari
Department of Life Sciences and Biotechnology, Section of Biochemistry and Molecular Biology, University of Ferrara, Ferrara, Italy

Nicola Marchetti and Alberto Cavazzini
Department of Chemistry and Pharmaceutical Sciences, University of Ferrara, Ferrara, Italy

Maria Grazia Giri
Medical Physics Unit, Department of Pathology and Diagnostics, University Hospital of Verona, Verona, Italy

Seng H. Cheng
Genzyme, a Sanofi Company, Framingham, Massachusetts, United States of America

Index